DENTAL LABORATORY PROCEDURES
COMPLETE DENTURES

VOLUME ONE

DENTAL LABORATORY PROCEDURES

COMPLETE DENTURES

ROBERT M. MORROW, D.D.S., F.A.C.D., F.I.C.D.

Associate Dean for Advanced Education,
Professor and Head, Postdoctoral Division, Department of Prosthodontics,
The University of Texas Health Science Center
at San Antonio, Dental School,
San Antonio, Texas

KENNETH D. RUDD, D.D.S., F.A.C.D., F.I.C.D.

Associate Dean for Continuing Education,
Professor of Prosthodontics, Department of Prosthodontics,
The University of Texas Health Science Center
at San Antonio, Dental School,
San Antonio, Texas

HAROLD F. EISSMANN, D.D.S., F.A.C.D.

Clinical Professor, Department of Fixed Prosthodontics,
University of California at San Francisco,
School of Dentistry,
San Francisco, California

with **2141** illustrations

The C. V. Mosby Company

ST. LOUIS • TORONTO • LONDON   1980

Copyright © 1980 by The C. V. Mosby Company

All rights reserved. No part of this book may be reproduced in any manner without written permission of the publisher.

Printed in the United States of America

The C. V. Mosby Company
11830 Westline Industrial Drive, St. Louis, Missouri 63141

Library of Congress Cataloging in Publication Data

Main entry under title:

Dental laboratory procedures.

    Bibliography: v. 1, p.
    Includes index.
    CONTENTS: v. 1. Complete dentures.
    1. Dental technology. I. Morrow, Robert M.,
1931- II. Rudd, Kenneth D. III. Eissmann,
Harold F. [DNLM: 1. Denture, Complete—Laboratory
manuals. 2. Technology, Dental—Laboratory manuals.
WU530 R914d]
RK652.D47   617.6   79-16785
ISBN 0-8016-3513-6 (v. 1)

GW/CB/B 9 8 7 6 5 4 3 2 1   01/D/085

CONTRIBUTORS

WILLIAM B. AKERLY, D.D.S., M.S.

Associate Professor, Restorative Dentistry, The University of Mississippi Medical Center, School of Dentistry, Jackson, Mississippi

JAMES S. BRUDVIK, D.D.S.

Colonel USA DC, Commander Regional Dental Activity, Fort Sam Houston, Texas; Consultant for Laboratory Prosthodontics to the Surgeon General United States Army

A. ANDERSEN CAVALCANTI, D.D.S.

Associate, Professional Research, Dentsply International Inc., York, Pennsylvania

R. NEAL EDWARDS, D.D.S.

Formerly Assistant Professor, Department of Prosthodontics, The University of Texas Health Science Center at San Antonio, Dental School, San Antonio, Texas

AMBROCIO V. ESPINOZA, C.D.T.

The University of Texas Health Science Center at San Antonio, Dental School, San Antonio, Texas

EARL E. FELDMANN, D.D.S., F.A.C.D.

Professor and Chairman, Department of Prosthodontics, The University of Texas Health Science Center at San Antonio, Dental School, San Antonio, Texas

GERALD T. GAUBERT, C.D.T.

Baton Rouge, Louisiana

ALEXANDER R. HALPERIN, D.D.S.

Assistant Professor, Department of Prosthodontics, The University of Texas Health Science Center at San Antonio, Dental School, San Antonio, Texas

FRANK F. KOBLITZ, B.S.

Section Head, Physical Chemistry, Central Research Laboratory, Dentsply International Inc., York, Pennsylvania

CLARENCE L. KOEHNE, C.D.T.

Supervisor, Dental Laboratory, Audie Murphy Veteran's Administration Hospital, San Antonio, Texas

JESSE S. LEACHMAN, C.D.T.

The University of Texas Health Science Center at San Antonio, Dental School, San Antonio, Texas

MICHAEL J. MAGINNIS, D.D.S., M.S.

Baton Rouge, Louisiana

FREDRICK M. MATVIAS, D.M.D., M.S.

Senior Staff, Henry Ford Hospital, Detroit, Michigan

ROBERT M. MORROW, D.D.S., F.A.C.D., F.I.C.D.

Associate Dean for Advanced Education, Professor and Head, Postdoctoral Division, Department of Prosthodontics, The University of Texas Health Science Center at San Antonio, Dental School, San Antonio, Texas

LAURENCE T. OLIVER, C.D.T.

Dental Technician, Dentsply International Inc., York, Pennsylvania

KENNETH D. RUDD, D.D.S., F.A.C.D., F.I.C.D.

Associate Dean for Continuing Education, Professor of Prosthodontics, Department of Prosthodontics, The University of Texas Health Science Center at San Antonio, Dental School, San Antonio, Texas

WALTER L. SHEPARD, D.D.S., F.A.C.D.

Associate Professor of Prosthodontics, Emory University, School of Dentistry, Atlanta, Georgia

RICHARD A. SMITH, D.D.S.

Director of Professional Research, Dentsply International Inc., York, Pennsylvania

HUGH E. WOLFE, C.D.T.

Technical Director, Removable Prosthodontics, Dentsply International Inc., York, Pennsylvania

TO

Mrs. LIDIE DYER

our medical editor and longtime friend

PREFACE

Except for those procedures completed directly in the oral cavity, successful restorations may depend significantly on the quality of the dental laboratory procedures incident to their construction.

As a result of this relationship, we believe there is a need for a comprehensive, yet concise, text that clearly describes and illustrates dental laboratory procedures in a sequential manner. In *Dental Laboratory Procedures: Complete Dentures*, we present a selection of methods and techniques used in constructing complete dentures, immediate overdentures, and maxillofacial prostheses. We hope the descriptions and illustrations will prove useful to students, dentists, dental technicians, and assistants as an aid for improving existing skills and adding new ones. Definitions used throughout the text are from the second edition of Boucher's *Current Clinical Dental Terminology* (1974) and the third edition of The Academy of Prosthodontics' *Glossary of Prosthodontic Terms* (1968).

In such an undertaking we depended on the assistance and support of many individuals. We acknowledge with thanks the excellent work of our contributors, who were selected because of their knowledge and abilities in their respective areas. The outstanding support provided by the Medical Photography Section at The University of Texas Health Science Center at San Antonio should also be acknowledged. We particularly wish to recognize the splendid assistance provided by Mrs. Lidie Dyer, to whom this book is dedicated. We recognize her for what she is, an outstanding medical editor and, more importantly, our good friend.

Robert M. Morrow
Kenneth D. Rudd
Harold F. Eissmann

CONTENTS

DENTAL LABORATORY PROCEDURES
COMPLETE DENTURES

CHAPTER 1

PRELIMINARY IMPRESSIONS: CARE AND POURING

KENNETH D. RUDD and ROBERT M. MORROW

preliminary impression An impression made for the purpose of diagnosis or construction of a tray.

preliminary cast A positive reproduction of the upper or lower jaw tissues that is made in an impression and over which impression trays may be fabricated.

A complete denture depends on an artificial stone cast for its dimensions, contours, and ultimate clinical success. This artificial stone cast is the direct link between clinical procedures completed in the dentist's office and the complete denture constructed in the dental laboratory. Therefore proper care and handling of the impression are essential for a high-quality cast.

REQUIREMENTS

A cast should possess the following qualities:

1. All surfaces to be contacted by the tray and denture should be accurate and free of voids or nodules. (It is essential to remove nodules resulting from voids or inclusion of air in the impression, but handcarving in critical areas is not acceptable.)

2. The surface of a cast should be hard, dense, and free of any grinding sludge left by the cast trimmer.

3. A cast should extend sufficiently to include all of the area available for denture support. For example, a mandibular cast should extend 3 to 4 mm beyond the retromolar pads.

4. The peripheral roll should be complete and no deeper than 3 to 4 mm, and the edge of a cast extending out from this roll should be approximately 3 to 4 mm wide.

5. The side walls of a cast should be vertical or slightly tapered outward, but not undercut.

6. The base of a cast should not be less than 15 to 16 mm at the thinnest point.

7. The tongue space on a mandibular cast should be flat and smooth when trimmed, but the lingual peripheral roll should remain intact (Fig. 1-1).

8. A cast should not show signs of having been wet or washed with tap water.

The two materials used most frequently for complete denture preliminary impressions are alginate irreversible hydrocolloid and modeling plastic, often referred to as *impression compound*. Care of the impression and pouring procedures for these materials are not the same because of differences in physical properties. This chapter describes the care and pouring of preliminary impressions made from alginate and from modeling plastic.

ALGINATE PRELIMINARY IMPRESSIONS

Alginate irreversible hydrocolloid is an impression material that is used extensively (Rudd et al., 1969). Generally, it is used to make impressions for diagnostic casts and removable partial dentures. It also is used frequently in making preliminary impressions for complete dentures (Sharry, 1974). Alginate impression materials were developed during World War II when the halting of agar imports from Japan resulted in a scarcity.

Alginates are the salts of alginic acid, which is obtained from kelp. By an irreversible chemical reaction,

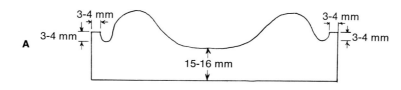

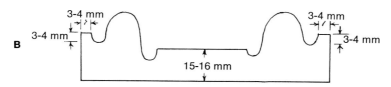

Fig. 1-1. Sides of cast should be vertical and perpendicular to base. They should not incline inward or outward. Tongue space on mandibular casts should be trimmed flat. Note recommended dimensions for maxillary cast, **A,** and mandibular cast, **B.**

alginates change from sol to gel, thereby accounting for the designation irreversible hydrocolloid. The sol form is a soluble salt of alginic acid, and the gel is an insoluble salt. (Guide to Dental Materials and Devices 1976-1978). For the best results, it is necessary to pour impressions made with alginate irreversible hydrocolloid soon after making the impression. Two-stage pouring usually results in better cast surfaces (Young, 1975). It is impossible to store alginate impressions in air or water, since they dehydrate in air and absorb water if stored in it for any significant length of time. If an alginate impression dehydrates, it shrinks; conversely, if it absorbs water, it expands. Both types of changes result in an inaccurate cast. Therefore it is mandatory to pour alginate impressions as soon as possible to minimize distortion. A delay in pouring the stone mix to form the cast is probably the most common error associated with the use of this material.

PROCEDURE

1. Prior to pouring, examine the impression carefully for voids in critical areas and possible pulling away of the alginate from the tray (Fig. 1-2). It is better to reject a poor impression than to attempt to use it, since remaking the impression because of defects costs less than remaking the completed restoration.

2. Run cold tap water over the impression gently to wash it (Fig. 1-3). Sprinkle artificial stone on the impression to disclose films of saliva; then wet the impression and scrub in the stone gently with a soft camel's

hair brush (Fig. 1-4). Flush the impression with water to make certain that no stone remains on the impression.

3. Remove excess moisture from the impression with a gentle stream of air (Fig. 1-5). Do not use a strong blast of air because it can dislodge the impression material from the tray. Once loosened from the tray, it cannot be returned to position accurately. The surface of the alginate impression should not be thoroughly dry; it should glisten or shine. However, no droplets or liquid film should be discernible. To prevent dehydration of the impression, mix the stone immediately. Usually it is best to avoid filling in the tongue space with wax, since it is difficult to make wax stick to the alginate, and the procedure requires more time.

4. With a sharp knife trim excess alginate that extends beyond the back of the tray (Fig. 1-6). This step prevents any alginate from touching the laboratory bench when the impression rests on it (Fig. 1-7). If excess material comes in contact with the bench top, distortion of the impression could result. If use of excess material is vital to the impression, making trimming impossible, support the impression by the tray handle. An excellent tray holder can be made by cutting a horizontal slot wide enough to accept the handle in a length of wood 1 × 2 inches (2.5 × 5 cm), or nail two boards together with a suitable spacer between them (Fig. 1-8). When fastened to a wall or case pan, this block may be used to hold a tray so that it avoids contact with the bench top (Fig. 1-9).

5. Weigh the artificial stone, and mix it with the rec-

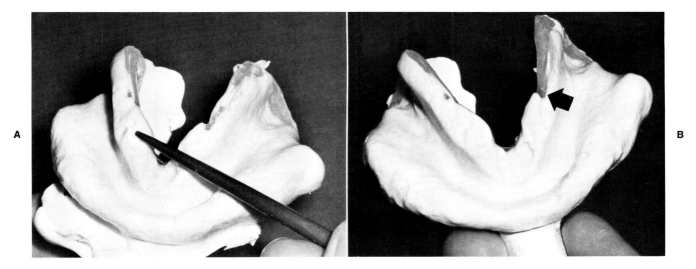

Fig. 1-2. A, Alginate impression is examined carefully under good light. **B,** Impression is examined for voids in critical areas and for evidence of alginate impression material pulling away from tray (arrow).

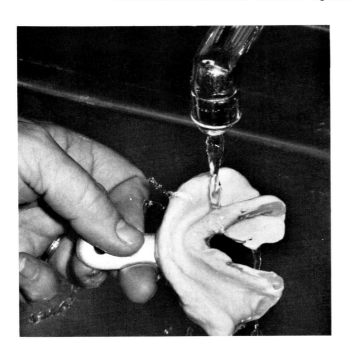

Fig. 1-3. Cold tap water is run over impression gently to remove all traces of saliva.

ommended volume of water (Phillips, 1973). Since the proper powder-water ratio is essential for a good cast surface, weigh the stone on a balance scale (Fig. 1-10). Preweighing stone in the required amounts for individual impressions also results in economy of material by reducing the amount of waste when handling too large a mix. The majority of impressions require 200 gm of stone. A 4-ounce (112-gm) ointment jar is a convenient container for 100 gm portions of preweighed stone (Fig. 1-11). Use a larger container for larger mixes of stone (Fig. 1-12). When stored in open containers or bins, stone is subject to hydration and is not usable in pour-

ing impressions for high-quality casts (Fig. 1-13). However, stone stored in bins is satisfactory for mounting casts in articulators, flasking, and pouring indexes. Stone stored in open containers is subject to contamination from water droplets and other types of stone or plaster when using the same scoop for several containers (Fig. 1-14).

6. Mix the preweighed stone in a mechanical spatulator* under reduced atmospheric pressure (Fig. 1-15).

Text continued on p. 9.

*Combination Vac-U-Vestor/Power Mixer, Whip-Mix Corp., Louisville, Ky.

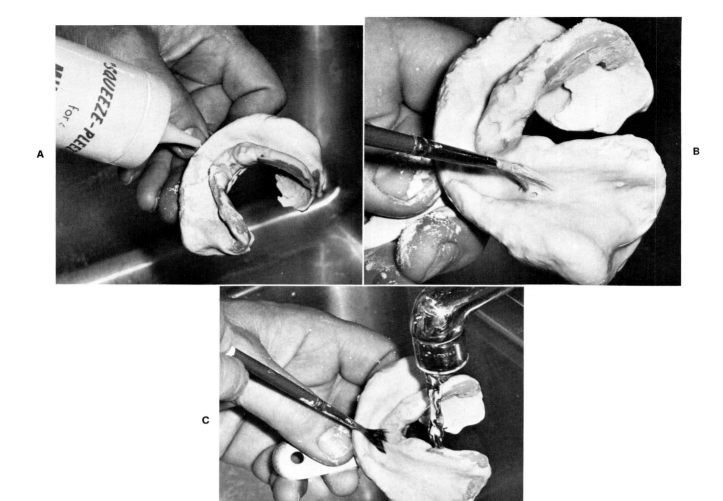

Fig. 1-4. **A,** Plastic mustard or catsup dispenser can be used to sprinkle stone into impression. **B,** Soft camel's hair brush is used to scrub stone into impression gently. **C,** Impression is placed under running cold tap water, and camel's hair brush is used to remove all traces of stone.

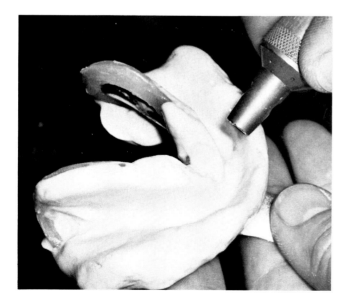

Fig. 1-5. Excess moisture is removed from impression with gentle stream of air. Strong blast of air can cause separation of impression from tray.

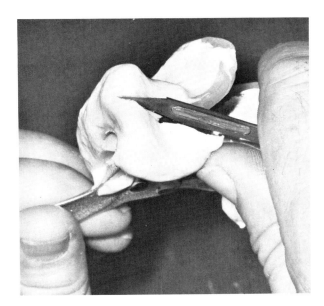

Fig. 1-6. Excess alginate protruding beyond posterior extension of tray is removed with sharp knife. Sharp Bard-Parker blade in knife is excellent for this purpose.

Fig. 1-7. Tray is trimmed of excess alginate to keep remaining alginate from making contact with surface of laboratory bench (arrow). If alginate is not trimmed and is allowed to contact surface of bench by being placed on it, impression can be distorted.

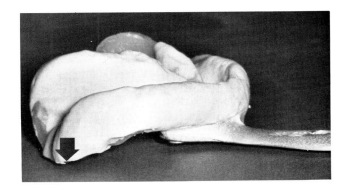

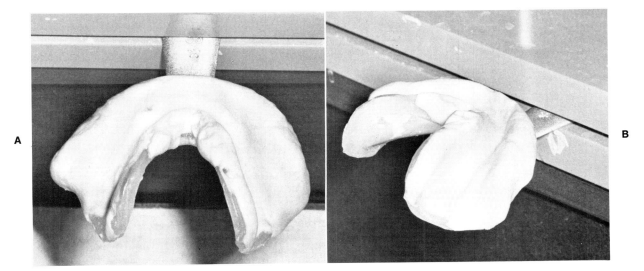

Fig. 1-8. A, Two boards nailed together, with spacer between them that is wide enough to permit placement of tray handle, make excellent device for suspending impression. **B,** Boards attached to wall or workbench are readily available for use. Impression is suspended by handle to eliminate any possibility of distortion, resulting from resting on heel portion.

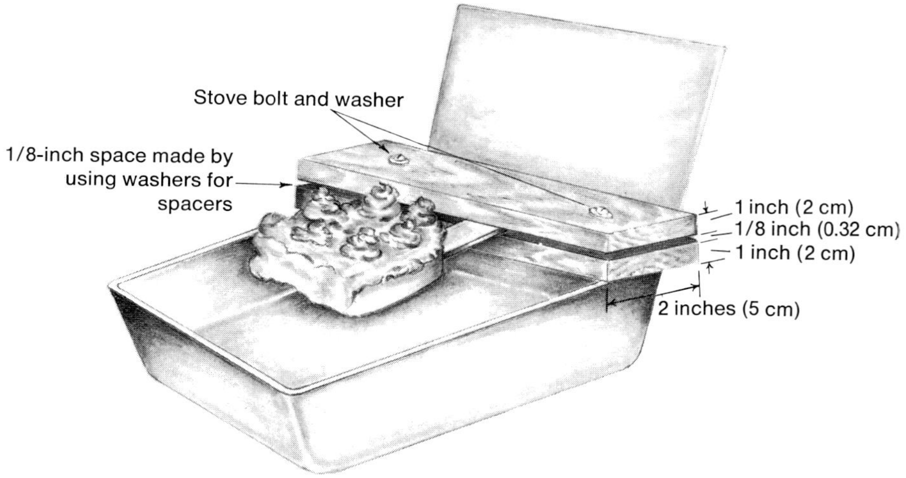

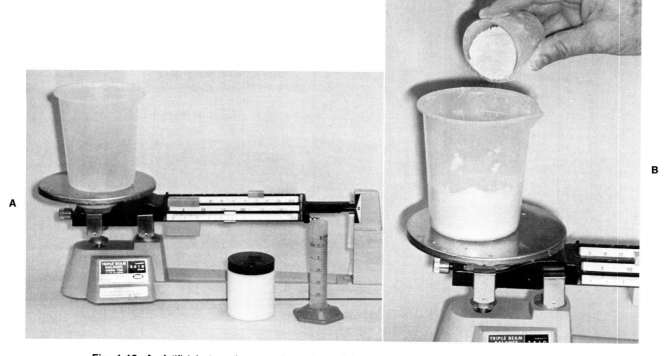

Stove bolt and washer

1/8-inch space made by using washers for spacers

1 inch (2 cm)
1/8 inch (0.32 cm)
1 inch (2 cm)
2 inches (5 cm)

Fig. 1-9. Two pieces of wood 1 × 2 inches (2.5 × 5 cm) have been fastened together with spacer between them and attached to case pan to support impression tray.

A

B

Fig. 1-10. A, Artificial stone is proportioned by weight, using small balance scale. After stone is weighed, it can be stored in suitable jar with tight-fitting lid. Then weighed stone is mixed with manufacturer's recommended amount of water. **B,** Usually 200 gm of stone are sufficient for majority of impressions.

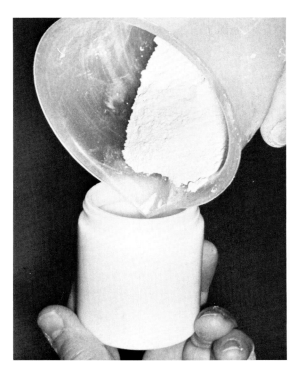

Fig. 1-11. Four-ounce (112-gm) ointment jar can be used for storing smaller mixes, such as 100 gm of stone or less. This quantity generally is used to pour very small impressions or impressions for removable dies. Lid is placed on jar securely, and jar is labeled to indicate type of stone, amount, and required volume of water to make mix.

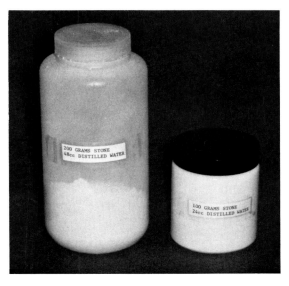

Fig. 1-12. Larger container, such as plastic bottle, *left,* can be used to store larger mixes of stone. Four-ounce (112-gm) ointment jar, *right,* is used for smaller mixes, such as 100 gm or less. Both are excellent containers for storing stone.

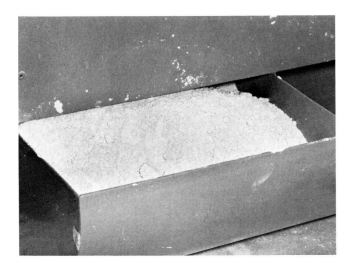

Fig. 1-13. Storage in bins is satisfactory for stone used to mount casts in articulators or to flask, but it is poor storage method for stone used to make casts.

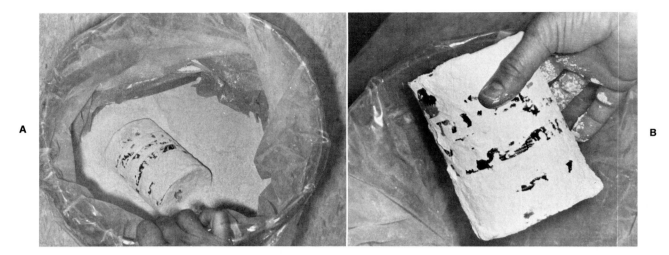

Fig. 1-14. A, Stone stored in open containers is subject to contamination from use of same scoop in various types of stone and from water droplets. Contamination should be avoided to obtain best results. **B,** Stone adhering to scoop can contaminate future mixes.

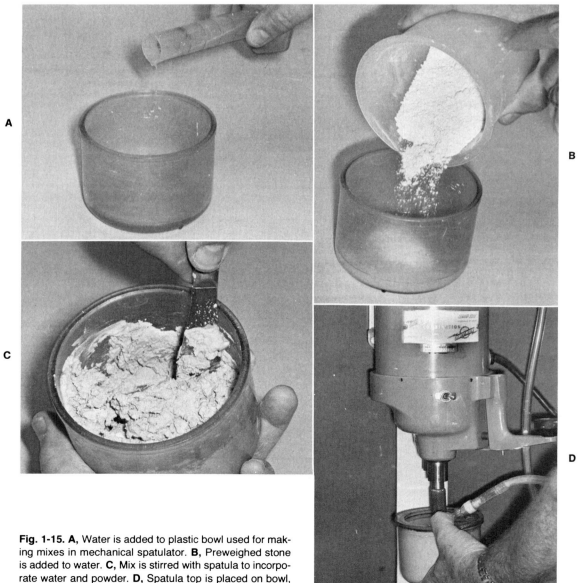

Fig. 1-15. A, Water is added to plastic bowl used for making mixes in mechanical spatulator. **B,** Preweighed stone is added to water. **C,** Mix is stirred with spatula to incorporate water and powder. **D,** Spatula top is placed on bowl, and stone is mixed in mechanical mixer for approximately 20 seconds.

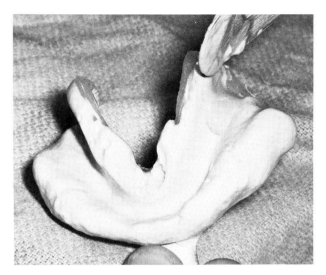

Fig. 1-16. Stone is vibrated into impression gently by adding stone in small increments to posterior portion of impression.

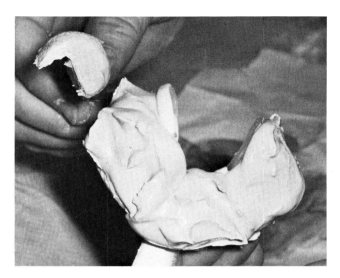

Fig. 1-17. Stone is added until impression is filled.

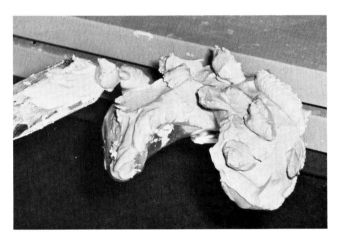

Fig. 1-18. Small droplets of stone are added to poured impression to create mechanical undercuts, which form firm attachment between first and second pours of casts.

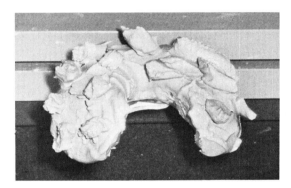

Fig. 1-19. Poured impression is placed in slot of tray holder and allowed to set.

Stone mixed in this manner contains less air and results in a dense cast.

7. Gently vibrate the stone into the impression (Fig. 1-16). Avoid harsh or prolonged vibration, and exercise care in handling the alginate in the tray to keep it from touching the vibrator, which may result in separation and distortion.

8. Continue to add stone in only one distal corner of the impression (Fig. 1-17). This procedure will help prevent voids, which result from the entrapment of air. Observe the flowing stone carefully during this stage, and add stone slowly until the impression is full. Cover the entire anatomic portion of the impression during the first pour.

9. Apply the remaining stone in droplets on the pre-

viously poured stone to make irregular undercuts (Fig. 1-18). In the final, or base, pour, stone will engage the undercuts and produce a strong cast that will not separate during the usual dental laboratory procedures.

10. Insert the handle in a tray holder, and suspend the poured impression while it sets (Fig. 1-19).

11. After the stone has set initially, and while it is still warm from the heat of crystallization, place the impression containing the stone in clear slurry water* for 3 to 5 minutes (Fig. 1-20).

12. Remove the impression and blow off excess slurry

---

*Slurry water is made by placing stone debris or particles in a container of water and allowing them to soak for 48 hours; the resultant supernatant solution is used for rinsing or soaking casts.

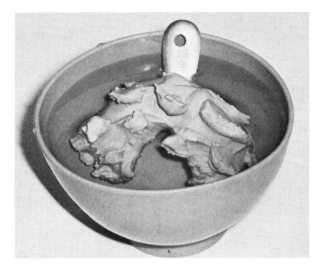

Fig. 1-20. Poured impression is placed in clear slurry water for 3 to 5 minutes to wet surface of first-pour stone and assure good bond between first and second pours.

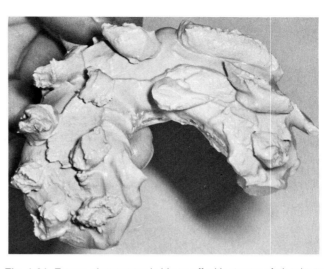

Fig. 1-21. Excess slurry water is blown off with stream of air prior to pouring base. Avoid overdrying; surface of stone should glisten.

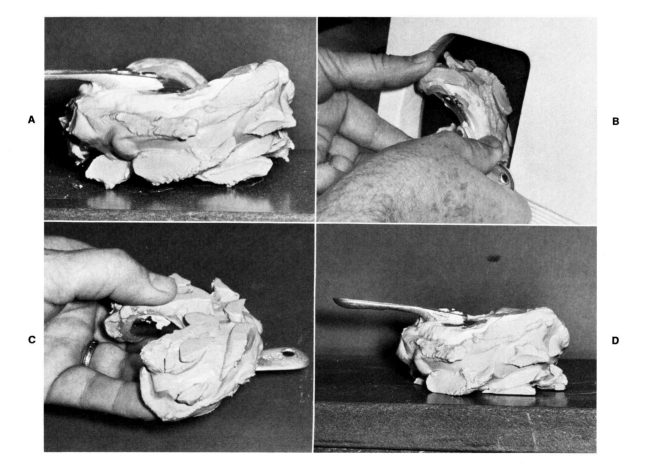

Fig. 1-22. A, First pour is inverted on bench top to determine whether or not stone droplets are too high. **B,** If too high, first pour is reduced easily on cast trimmer. **C,** Portions of stone droplets added to first pour to serve as mechanical undercuts have been reduced in height to make cast thinner. **D,** Trimmed first pour is placed on bench top to determine its thickness after correction.

water with a stream of air prior to pouring the base in the same kind of stone as used for the first portion. Do not overdry; the surface of the stone should glisten (Fig. 1-21). Invert the first pour, and check the height prior to pouring the base (Fig. 1-22). If it is too high, reduce the height by grinding on a model trimmer; then recheck the height.

13. Make a mix of stone in the power-mixer using the same powder-water ratio, and place a patty on a glass or plastic slab (Fig. 1-23). Shape the patty to the approximate size and thickness needed for the base.

14. With a spatula add a small amount of stone to the undercuts of the first pour (Fig. 1-24).

15. Invert the poured cast into the stone patty, and draw the stone up onto the sides of the first-pour stone (Fig. 1-25).

16. Remove the excess carefully, particularly in the area lingual to the mandibular ridge, and shape it until the surface is flat (Fig. 1-26).

17. Separate the cast from the impression approximately 45 minutes to 1 hour after the first pour (Fig. 1-27). If the alginate remains in contact with the stone longer, it can make the surface of the stone cast rough or soft. Do not remove the cast too soon, because the second-pour stone may not have set.

18. Examine the cast carefully to determine its acceptability. Remove small nodules of stone and alginate particles (Fig. 1-28). Do not rinse or soak the cast in tap

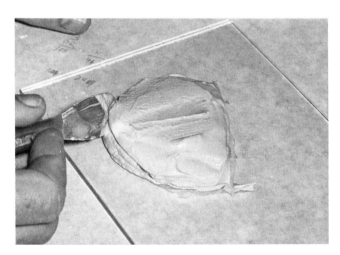

Fig. 1-23. Second mix of stone using correct powder-water ratio is made, and patty is placed on glass slab. Patty should approximate contours of base of cast.

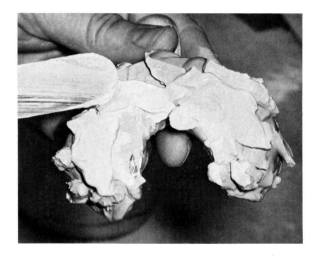

Fig. 1-24. Small amount of mix is wiped into undercuts of first pour with spatula to minimize voids.

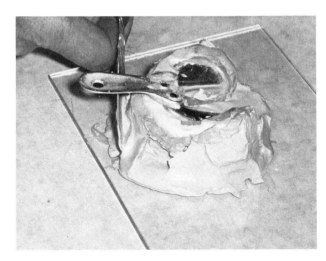

Fig. 1-25. Impression with first pour is settled into stone patty carefully, and stone is drawn up around borders of first pour.

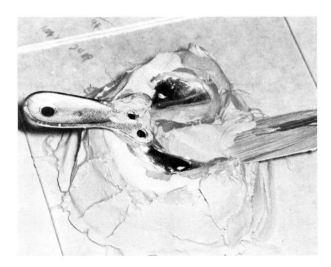

Fig. 1-26. Excess stone, particularly in area lingual to mandibular ridge, removed and surface shaped. Unless area is flat, it will require trimming later. It is exceedingly difficult to trim at that time.

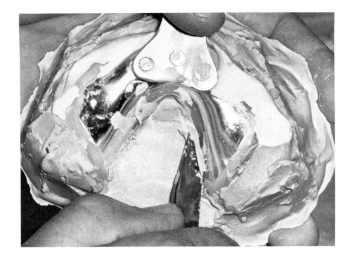

Fig. 1-27. Prior to attempt at removing impression from poured cast, excess stone is cleared away carefully from sides of tray to free it.

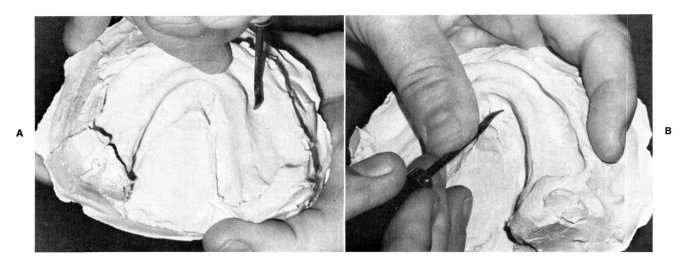

Fig. 1-28. A, Cast is examined carefully, and small nodules or projections are removed. Small scraper is ideal for this procedure. **B,** Small nodules of stone on cast are smoothed before cast is trimmed on cast trimmer.

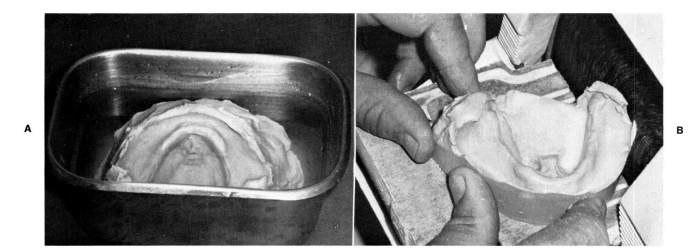

Fig. 1-29. A, Stone cast is soaked in clear slurry water prior to trimming it on cast trimmer. **B,** This procedure keeps sludge created during trimming from adhering to cast.

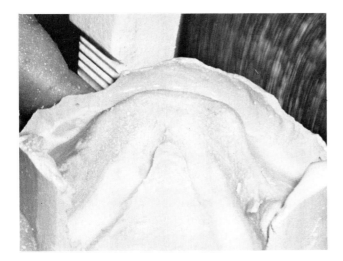

Fig. 1-30. Dry sludge is difficult to remove without damaging cast.

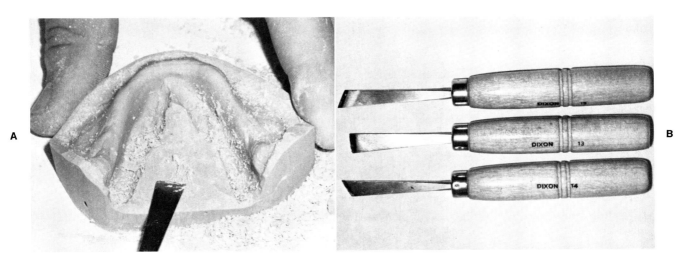

Fig. 1-31. A, Chisels can be used to smooth lingual area of mandibular casts. **B,** Right-, straight-, and left-bevel chisels (Dixon) are available.

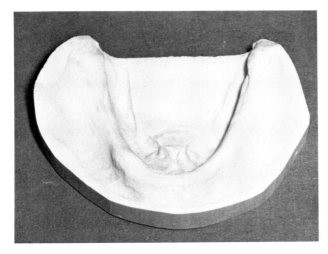

Fig. 1-32. Examine trimmed cast carefully to make certain that essential areas have not been trimmed away.

water because it can dissolve the surface of the cast (Rudd et al., 1969). Perhaps this problem is not too critical in a preliminary cast used to make a tray; however, it is exceedingly important in a master cast.

19. Soak the cast in slurry water for a few minutes and then trim it on a cast trimmer (Fig. 1-29). The soaking will keep sludge created during trimming from sticking to the cast. Rinse the cast in slurry water as needed to remove the sludge. Do not allow sludge to dry on the cast, since it is exceedingly difficult to remove (Fig. 1-30). Be careful in trimming to avoid removing essential areas of the cast; otherwise, it may be necessary to make a new impression. Smooth the lingual space of mandibular casts to improve access later (Fig. 1-31).

20. Permit the trimmed cast to dry, and then examine it critically (Fig. 1-32).

21. Identify the cast by labeling it with a pencil (Fig. 1-33).

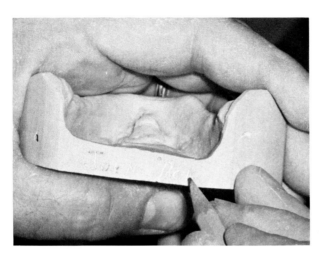

Fig. 1-33. Each cast is identified by marking patient's name or case number on it in pencil.

PROBLEM AREAS

Problems associated with pouring alginate irreversible hydrocolloid impressions are (1) failure to identify a faulty impression, (2) too long a delay in pouring the impression, (3) poor pouring technique, and (4) incorrect trimming on the cast trimmer (Table 1-1). Examine impressions carefully before pouring, and obtain another impression instead of using a defective one. To proceed with an inadequate impression is poor economy for everyone involved. Pour the alginate impression as soon as possible after making it. Do not wrap the impression in a wet towel for transporting to the laboratory. Follow the recommended procedures for pouring the cast, use a two-stage technique, and avoid so-called shortcuts that can compromise quality. Trim the cast, so that it is no thinner than 15 to 16 mm at the thinnest point. Trim the sides perpendicular to the base, but do not remove anatomic portions of the cast. On mandibular casts, smooth the area lingual to the mandibular ridge

Table 1-1. Alginate preliminary impressions

Problem	Probable cause	Solution
Voids in impression	Voids in impression material during making of impression	Obtain another impression if first defective
Impression separated from tray	Too much time between impression and pouring	Pour alginate impression as soon as possible
Alginate pulled away from tray and dry	Too much time between making of impression and pouring	Pour alginate impressions soon after making them
Cast surface chalky and soft	Impression not separated from cast within 1 hour after pouring	Separate cast from impression within 1 hour after pouring
	Incorrect powder-water ratio, making mix too thin	Weigh stone and mix with recommended amount of water
Voids on surface of cast	Mechanical spatulator not used	Mix stone in mechanical spatulator under reduced atmospheric pressure
	Stone poured into impression too quickly	Pour slowly into only one distal corner of impression to minimize voids
Cast too thin or too thick	Cast trimmed improperly on cast trimmer	Exercise care when trimming cast on cast trimmer; check thickness of base frequently to prevent overtrimming
	First-pour stone not checked for thickness and not reduced prior to pouring of base	Check first-pour stone to determine that it is not too thick; if needed, thin cast on cast trimmer prior to pouring base
Critical areas of cast trimmed away	Trimmed improperly on cast trimmer	Check cast frequently when trimming to prevent overtrimming
Cast broken easily	Improper powder-water ratio in mix	Use recommended powder-water ratio; mix in mechanical spatulator under reduced atmospheric pressure
	Cast trimmed too thin	Do not overtrim
Slurry sludge stuck on cast, making surface rough	Cast not dipped in clear slurry water prior to trimming on cast trimmer	Soak or wet cast in clear slurry water when trimming on cast trimmer to prevent sludge from sticking to cast

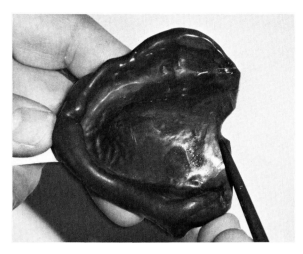

Fig. 1-34. Modeling plastic impression is examined carefully prior to pouring in artificial stone. It is checked for chips and voids, which could make cast unusable.

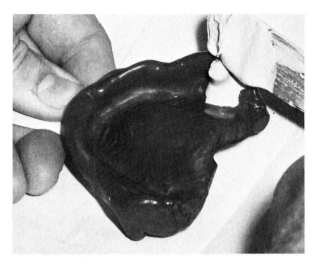

Fig. 1-35. Modeling plastic impression is poured on vibrator, and stone is added in small amounts at only one corner of impression.

to permit access to the lingual area during fabrication of the tray. Do not allow sludge from the cast trimmer to dry on the cast, and do not dissolve the cast by repeated rinsing in tap water.

MODELING PLASTIC IMPRESSIONS

Modeling plastic, or impression compound, is a thermoplastic material usually composed of gum dammar, prepared chalk, and other materials (Boucher, 1974). It is used especially for making complete denture impressions. The material is available in a variety of consistencies, often identified by color. For example, black modeling plastic may soften at a higher temperature than red, and green, gray, and white may soften at progressively lower temperatures. Black and red modeling plastics are probably the ones used most frequently for complete denture preliminary impressions. Some dentists use modeling plastic impressions as trays for the final impression, whereas others use modeling plastic to make preliminary impressions and then pour them in stone. They construct a tray on the cast as when using alginate preliminary impressions. The care and pouring procedure for modeling plastic impressions differ from those for alginate impressions. Modeling plastic is not a hydrocolloid and, being rigid, it is less subject to distortion. However, modeling plastic changes as a result of flow or memory and, although the changes are not as critical as for alginates, it is recommended that it be poured as soon as practicable.

PROCEDURE

1. Examine the impression to make certain that it has not been broken or chipped while in transit between the dental office and the laboratory (Fig. 1-34).

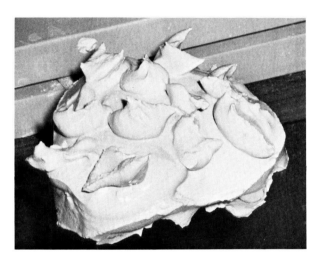

Fig. 1-36. Modeling plastic impression with first pour of stone is placed in tray holder again and allowed to set. Two-pour method gives good base thickness control.

2. Place the impression in a holder, and make a mix of stone, as described earlier.

3. Pour the stone mix into the modeling plastic impression, taking care to avoid entrapping air and the resultant voids (Fig. 1-35).

4. Fill the impression, and make certain to cover the anatomic portion, as described previously.

5. Replace the poured impression in the tray holder (Fig. 1-36).

6. After the initial set, make another mix of stone, and pour the base, as described earlier.

7. Approximately 45 minutes to 1 hour after the first pour, place the poured impression in warm slurry water to soften the modeling plastic (Fig. 1-37). Lift the soft-

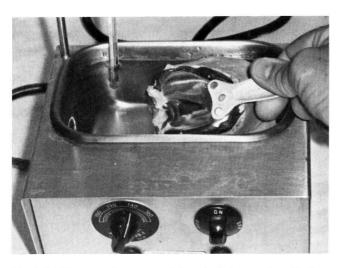

Fig. 1-37. After stone has set, modeling plastic impression with stone is placed in low temperature–water bath to soften modeling plastic before separation is attempted.

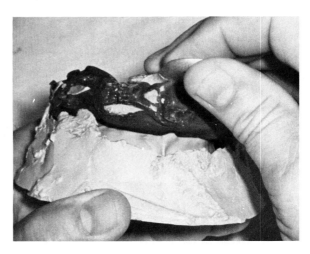

Fig. 1-38. Softened modeling plastic impression is lifted away from stone cast carefully. If modeling plastic is not soft enough, placing it back in water bath will allow it to soften longer, thereby avoiding breaking cast.

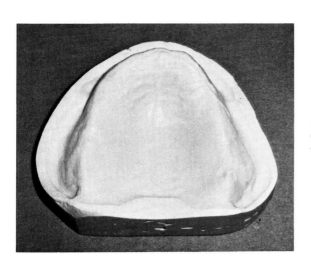

Fig. 1-39. On separation, stone cast is examined carefully to make certain that there are no voids. Then cast can be trimmed on trimmer, as described previously.

Table 1-2. Modeling plastic impressions

Problem	Probable cause	Solution
Cast broken during separation from impression	Modeling plastic not softened adequately before removal attempted	Immerse poured impression in warm water to soften modeling plastic before separating from cast
Modeling plastic stuck to cast at time of separation	Modeling plastic overheated when placed in water that is too warm	Do not oversoften modeling plastic; place in warm water only long enough to soften and remove; do not overheat or use dry heat
Cast too thin or too thick	Cast poured or trimmed too thin Thick base as a result of first pour being too thick	Pour cast to proper thickness; do not trim too thin Check thickness of first pour before pouring base; trim on cast trimmer if needed

ened modeling plastic impression off the cast carefully (Fig. 1-38).

8. Examine the cast and, if it is acceptable, trim it on the cast trimmer, as described earlier.

9. The preliminary cast is ready for fabrication of the tray (Fig. 1-39).

PROBLEM AREAS

Problems associated with pouring modeling plastic impressions arise with failure to soften the material adequately before separating the cast from the impression (Table 1-2). Frequently, the cast breaks during the separation. Conversely, overheating the modeling plastic makes it stick to the cast tenaciously, and removal may be impossible. As with the use of alginate, proper pouring and trimming procedures are essential to the successful use of modeling plastic.

SUMMARY

This chapter presents methods for the care and pouring of preliminary complete denture impressions made of alginate irreversible hydrocolloid and of modeling plastic. Making accurate casts demands systematic attention to a multitude of minor details that, singly, may be of little consequence. It is the cumulative effect of many errors in technique that assures poor results. Use of the procedures described will make it possible to pour accurate, hard, dense casts in alginate or in modeling plastic impressions. An accurate, properly extended, preliminary cast is a significant step toward a successful complete denture.

REFERENCES

Boucher, C. O., editor: Current clinical dental terminology, ed. 2, St. Louis, 1974, The C. V. Mosby Co.

Martinelli, N.: Dental laboratory technology, St. Louis, 1975, The C. V. Mosby Co., pp. 100-115.

Phillips, R. W.: Skinner's science of dental materials, ed. 7, Philadelphia, 1973, W. B. Saunders Co., p. 130.

Rudd, K. D., Morrow, R. M., and Bange, A. A.: Accurate casts, J. Prosthet. Dent. **21:**545-554, 1969.

Sharry, J. J.: Complete denture prosthodontics, ed. 3, New York, 1974, McGraw-Hill Book Co., pp. 209-210.

Sowter, J. B.: Dental laboratory technology, prosthodontic techniques, Chapel Hill, N.C., 1968, University of North Carolina Press, pp. 11-14.

Young, J. M.: Surface characteristics of dental stone: impression orientation, J. Prosthet. Dent. **33:**336-341, 1975.

CHAPTER 2

IMPRESSION TRAYS

KENNETH D. RUDD and ROBERT M. MORROW

impression tray A receptacle or device used to carry the impression material to the mouth, confine the material in apposition to the surfaces to be recorded, and control the impression material while it sets to form the impression.

LaVere and Freda (1976) classified impression trays as stock trays of various sizes made by manufacturers and individualized trays made specifically for one patient and discarded later. Jamieson (1954) stated that individual, or custom-made, trays should adapt to the cast readily; be rigid, but not bulky; retain their shape; and be easy to trim. Ellinger (1973) further added that the impression tray should simulate the finished denture in size and shape, be able to carry the impression material to the mouth, and control and confine the material to enable it to record accurately minute details of the denture-bearing area.

REQUIREMENTS FOR IMPRESSION TRAYS

The requirements for individualized impression trays are as follows:

1. The tray should be rigid but not overly thick.
2. It should retain its shape throughout the construction and pouring of the impression.
3. The method of construction should be simple enough so that an acceptable impression tray can be made in a minimal amount of time at a reasonable cost.
4. It should be possible to trim or thin the tray readily with a bur, mounted stone, scissors, or an arbor band.
5. The tray should be smooth because sharp edges may injure oral tissues.

IMPRESSION TRAY MATERIALS

Materials used to make impression trays are special autopolymerizing acrylic resin impression tray materials,* conventional autopolymerizing acrylic resins,† thermoplastic resin sheets used in vacuum- or pressure-adapting devices,‡ and thermoplastic shellac baseplate materials. Probably the most commonly used impression tray materials are the special autopolymerizing resin tray materials that are modified to improve their adaptability to a cast. If finger adapted to a cast, these tray resins satisfy many of the requirements for impression trays; they are available in a variety of colors, and are excellent for the purpose. Thermoplastic vacuum-adapted resins also are popular. Their principal advantages are the ease and rapidity with which it is possible to make an impression tray, but they require special equipment. Thermoplastic shellac baseplate material, generally in a double thickness, is usable for impression trays, although its dimensional instability can be a distinct disadvantage.

Impression trays usually are fabricated on preliminary stone casts made from alginate irreversible hydrocolloid or impression compound impressions. Since it is customary to overextend preliminary impressions, a dentist should indicate the extension of the impression tray, as well as the outline and type of relief desired when drawing the tray outline on the cast (Fig. 2-1).

---

*Formatray, Kerr Manufacturing Co., Romulus, Mich., or equivalent.
†Repair Resin, The L. D. Caulk Co., Milford, Del., or equivalent.
‡Vacu-Press, Dentsply International, Inc., York, Pa., or Sta-Vac Vacuum Adapter, Buffalo Dental Manufacturing Co., Inc., Brooklyn, N.Y., or equivalent.

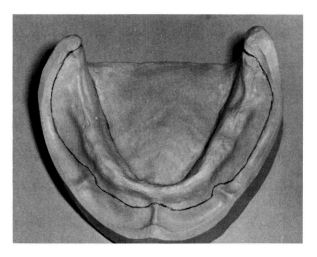

Fig. 2-1. Preliminary impressions usually are overextended; consequently, outline of tray border is short of cast border.

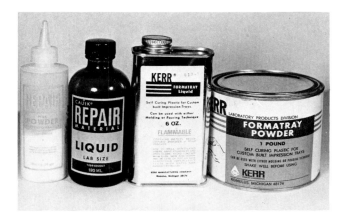

Fig. 2-2. Specially modified autopolymerizing resin is used for impression trays. Conventional autopolymerizing repair resin also is used for impression trays.

Autopolymerizing resin impression trays

Autopolymerizing acrylic resin specially modified for trays and conventional autopolymerizing resin used for repairs and baseplates are the materials frequently used for impression trays (Fig. 2-2). Resin materials are easy to use, require no special equipment, and when manipulated properly make excellent impression trays. Resin impression trays can be made thin but reasonably rigid, modified easily by grinding with an arbor band or an acrylic bur, and smoothed or polished readily. Properly constructed resin impression trays have sufficient dimensional stability to make an accurate impression.

The two methods of using these materials are the sprinkle-on method and the finger-adapted dough method.

Sprinkle-on method

Although the sprinkle-on method is commonly used for constructing acrylic resin baseplates (McCracken, 1964), it is not the most frequently used method for constructing resin impression trays. Some tray resin powders do not wet well with liquid monomer dispensed from an eyedropper in the sprinkle-on method (Fig. 2-2). Factory modifications in the autopolymerizing tray resin formula have made it possible to finger adapt this material easily and rapidly when it is in the dough stage. However, if tray resin is unavailable, the sprinkle-on method with conventional autopolymerizing resin* can certainly be used (Fig. 2-2).

Martone (1963) identified the two methods of achieving relief as grinding out the material from the interior surface of the tray and providing required relief during

*Caulk Repair Resin, The L. D. Caulk Co., Milford, Del.

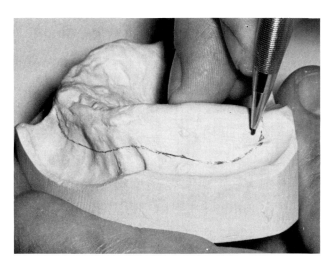

Fig. 2-3. Pencil is used to outline tray border on cast. Tray outline can be beaded to facilitate trimming if desired.

construction of the tray. In the work-order request, the dentist should specify the preferred method, as well as areas that require additional relief such as sharp bony ridges and soft displaceable hyperplastic tissues. The usual method is to warm a sheet of baseplate wax 1 mm thick and adapt it over those portions of the cast in need of relief.

PROCEDURE

1. Make an outline of the impression tray on the cast with a pencil (Fig. 2-3). Although the dentist may have specific requirements for this outline, the borders usually are short of the vestibular reflections of the cast. Often the posterior border is determined by a line extend-

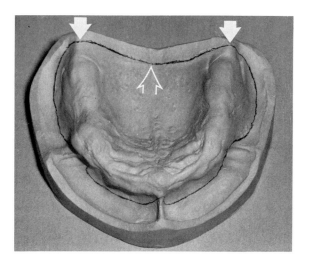

Fig. 2-4. Posterior border is determined by hamular notches on each side (arrows) and midpoint approximately 2 mm distal to fovea palatina (center arrow).

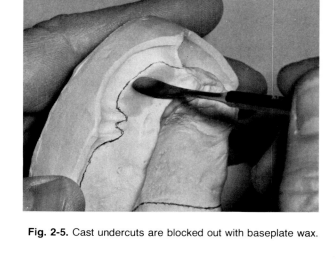

Fig. 2-5. Cast undercuts are blocked out with baseplate wax.

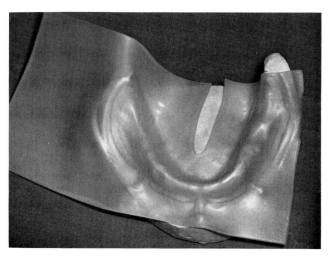

Fig. 2-6. Sheet of baseplate wax is adapted to cast. Slit in wax facilitates adaptation without wrinkles.

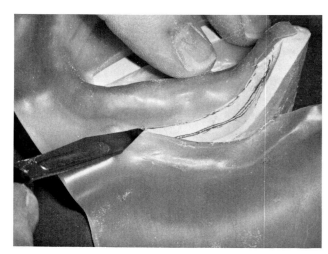

Fig. 2-7. Baseplate wax is trimmed to desired outline.

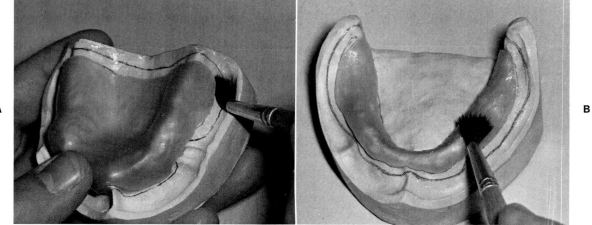

Fig. 2-8. A, Tinfoil substitute is painted on cast. **B,** Tinfoil substitute is painted on relief wax to aid in removing it from tray later.

ing between the hamular notches, with the midpoint approximately 2 mm distal to the fovea palatina (Fig. 2-4).

2. Block out the severe undercuts with wax, and adapt a layer of baseplate wax to the cast for relief (Figs. 2-5 and 2-6). Trim the relief wax to the desired outline (Fig. 2-7).

3. Paint tinfoil substitute on the stone cast and over the relief wax (Fig. 2-8). The tinfoil substitute facilitates later removal of wax from the impression tray. If the tinfoil substitute does not wet the baseplate wax relief, often 1 or 2 drops of surface tension–reducing agent* added to the tinfoil substitute will increase the wettability and result in easier separation later.

---

*Ti-Sol, Ticonium, Albany, N.Y.

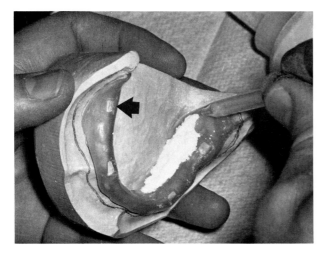

Fig. 2-9. Polymer powder is sifted onto cast and relief wax and wet with liquid monomer from eyedropper. Note rectangular sections of wax removed to create tissue stops (arrow).

4. Sift powdered polymer onto the cast and relief wax, and saturate it with liquid monomer from an eyedropper (Fig. 2-9). Apply more powder and liquid until there is a uniform layer approximately 2 mm thick. The same considerations apply when sifting resin onto the cast for impression trays as when sifting resin for baseplates (Chapter 4). The cast should be tilted during sifting to prevent unnecessary buildup of resin in the palatal region of maxillary casts or in the mucobuccal fold areas of mandibular casts.

5. Cure the impression tray under an inverted plaster bowl to reduce the porosity.

6. Mix more resin in a paper cup and, when it is in the dough stage, form handles and adapt them to the impression tray. Some dentists prefer only one handle in the anterior portion of the tray (Dresen, 1958), whereas others have suggested three handles or finger rests for mandibular impression trays (Merkeley, 1959; Martone, 1963) (Fig. 2-10). Position the handles in the first molar region and the anterior region of mandibular impression trays. Make the handles approximately 3 to 4 mm thick, 8 mm long, and approximately 8 mm high. Place horizontal grooves across the facial and lingual surfaces of the handles to improve the grip. If necessary, the dentist can adjust the handles easily. Usually anterior handles do not protrude horizontally unless requested (Fig. 2-11). When handles protrude, they can interfere with lip movements of patients and make an impression faulty. Handles on the impression tray should approximate the position of the teeth on the finished denture (Fig. 2-12).

7. Adapt the resin dough to the approximate size of the handle, and wet the resin tray at the point of attachment with liquid acrylic monomer in an eyedropper or a cotton pledget saturated with it to facilitate chemical bonding (Fig. 2-13).

8. After setting, remove the impression tray from the

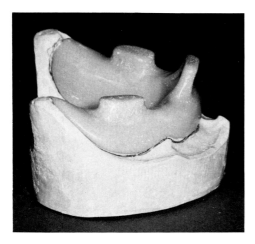

Fig. 2-10. Some dentists prefer mandibular impression tray with three handles or finger rests.

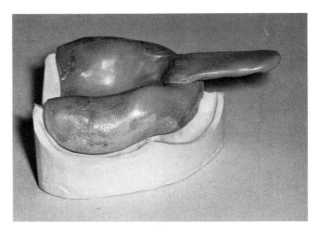

Fig. 2-11. Anterior handles protruding horizontally can interfere with lip movements while making impression. This design should be avoided unless specifically requested.

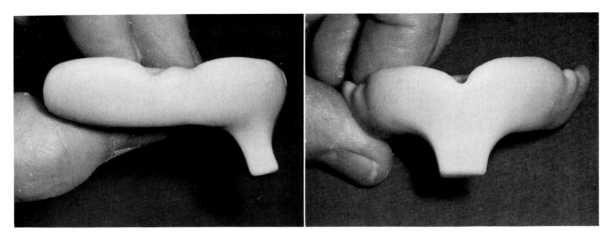

Fig. 2-12. Handle on impression tray should approximate position of anterior teeth.

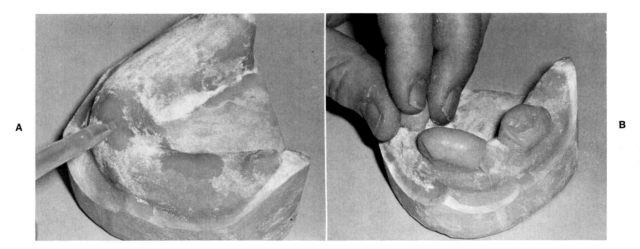

Fig. 2-13. A, Eyedropper bottle is used to place liquid monomer on tray in area where handle is to be attached. **B,** Resin dough is shaped and positioned on tray.

cast, and trim it with an arbor band or bur (Fig. 2-14).

9. Examine the completed tray, and adjust and polish rough areas that can cause discomfort to the patient. Pumice the borders of the tray lightly to make the surface smooth (Fig. 2-15).

10. Store the impression tray on the cast until needed (Fig. 2-16).

PROBLEM AREAS

The principal problem with the sprinkle-on method is the difficulty in controlling the thickness of the impression tray (Table 2-1). During sifting and wetting, the resin tends to flow into the deeper recesses of the cast and make the impression tray too thick in the palate and too thin over the convex or ridge portions of the cast. Tilting the cast while applying the resin powder and liquid can compensate for the flow characteristics. If severe undercuts are not blocked out, the impression tray or cast can be broken during separation. The sprinkle-on method is better for conventional autopolymerizing acrylic resin, such as repair resins, and the finger-adapted dough method is better for the modified acrylic tray resins.

Finger-adapted dough method

The finger-adapted dough method is used extensively for making resin impression trays. Specially modified resin tray materials can be formed into a dough that can be thinned readily or rolled to the desired thickness and adapted to the cast with finger pressure. The method is quick, and the resultant impression trays fit well and have acceptable dimensional stability.

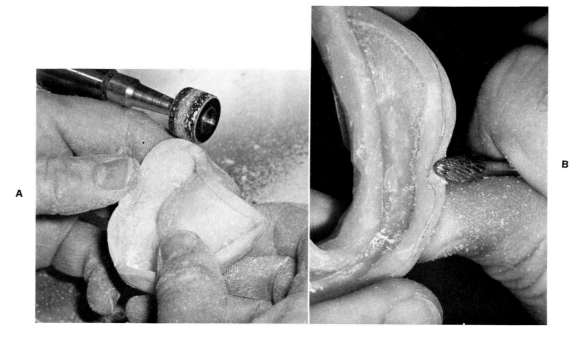

Fig. 2-14. A, Mounted arbor band is used to trim tray borders. **B,** Bur in handpiece also is used for trimming. Cast beading simplifies border trimming of tray.

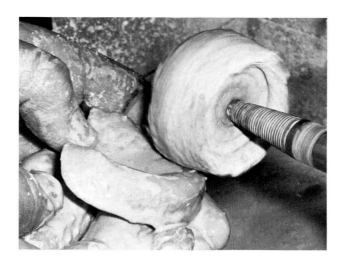

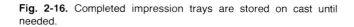

Fig. 2-15. Tray can be pumiced lightly to smooth surface.

Fig. 2-16. Completed impression trays are stored on cast until needed.

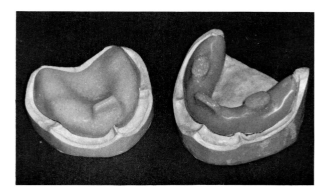

Table 2-1. Sprinkle-on method

Problem	Probable cause	Solution
Entire impression tray too thick	Too much resin buildup on cast from too generous application of powder and liquid	Control applications of powder and liquid to create uniform layer approximately 2 mm thick; check thickness of resin with periodontal probe
Impression tray too thin over ridges and too thick in palate	Resin flow not controlled by tilting cast during sprinkle on and resultant pooling of resin in palate region	Tilt cast while sifting resin to minimize pooling Thin palate with bur on arbor band
Impression tray or cast broken during separation	Undercuts not blocked out	Identify undercuts and block them out with wax before sifting resin on cast
	Tinfoil substitute contaminated or not used	Paint tinfoil substitute on cast; avoid using contaminated tinfoil substitute
Impression tray too flexible	Impression tray too thin or anterior ridge on lower cast flat	Make impression tray approximately 2 mm thick; use wire reinforcement for added strength and rigidity

PROCEDURE

1. Place the outline for the resin impression tray on the cast, and bead the outline with a sharp instrument if desired (Fig. 2-17). The resultant beading on the cured resin tray serves as a guide when trimming (Fig. 2-18).

2. Place the outline for areas of relief on the cast (Fig. 2-19).

3. Block out undercut areas with wax, and adapt the relief wax to the cast (Fig. 2-20). Removal of 4-mm squares of relief wax will expose the cast, thereby providing tissue stops (Fig. 2-21).

4. Paint tinfoil substitute on the cast and relief wax (Fig. 2-22).

5. Proportion the impression tray material according to the manufacturer's recommendations, and mix in a paper cup or other suitable container.

6. Check the consistency of the resin periodically, and remove it from the paper cup when it reaches the dough stage. Roll the resin to the desired thickness with a roller* or use a special form† to make the impression tray uniformly thick (Figs. 2-23 and 2-24).

7. Hand adapt the material to the cast carefully to avoid overthinning the resin on the convex portions of the cast (Fig. 2-25). It is easy to overthin the impression tray by applying too much finger pressure. Light-colored impression tray resins offer an advantage, since it is frequently possible to see the relief wax through them and avoid overthinning.

8. Remove excess tray material from the cast borders.

9. Form the excess material into handles, and adapt them to the tray as described previously. Put more acrylic monomer on the impression tray with a cotton pledget or an eyedropper at the point of attachment to improve bonding of the handles to the tray (Fig. 2-26).

10. Make the handles small, so that they require only a minimal amount of time for finishing to the proper size (Fig. 2-27).

11. Continue finger adaptation until the impression tray material remains adapted to the cast and does not rebound.

12. Cure the impression tray on the bench or under an inverted plaster bowl.

13. After setting, remove the impression tray from the cast, and trim the borders (Fig. 2-28).

14. Smooth all rough areas and store the tray on the cast (Figs. 2-29 and 2-30).

PROBLEM AREAS

Problems with the finger-adapted dough method usually are related to the finger adaptation (Table 2-2). There is a tendency to overthin the impression tray material by finger pressure over the convex or ridge portions of the cast. Adaptation should begin when the resin is in the dough stage. If allowed to progress beyond that stage, the resin becomes rubbery and impossible to adapt to the cast accurately. Failure to roll out impression tray material to a uniform thickness before adapting it to the cast can make the tray too thick, require too much time to finish, and increase the cost. Unless finger adaptation continues until the resin begins to set, it may rebound and lift off the cast, making the tray fit poorly. However, it is easy to master this technique and make excellent impression trays.

*Rollette Unit, Kerr Manufacturing Co., Romulus, Mich.
†Stone mold.

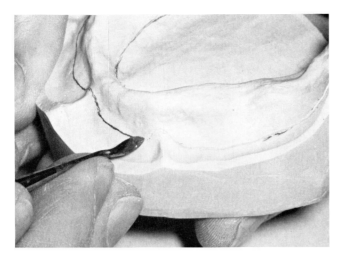

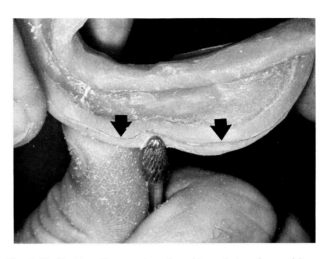

Fig. 2-17. Tray outline can be beaded on cast to facilitate border trimming.

Fig. 2-18. Cast beading now transferred to resin tray (arrows) is excellent guide during trimming.

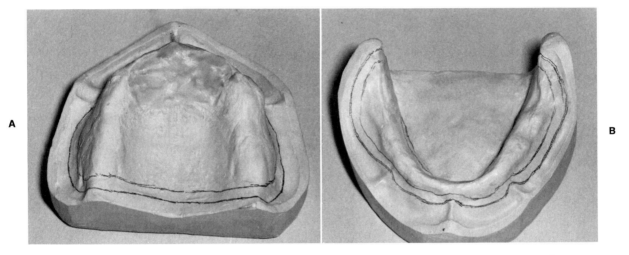

Fig. 2-19. A, Outline for relief wax is drawn on cast. **B,** Edge of relief wax is usually 2 to 3 mm short of tray border.

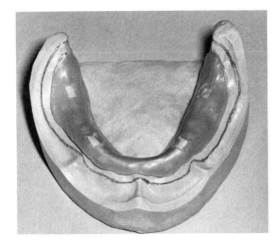

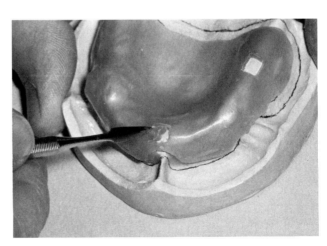

Fig. 2-20. One layer of baseplate wax is adapted to cast and trimmed to previously drawn outline.

Fig. 2-21. Tissue stops are made by removing 4 mm squares of wax to expose cast. Exact location of tissue stops can vary.

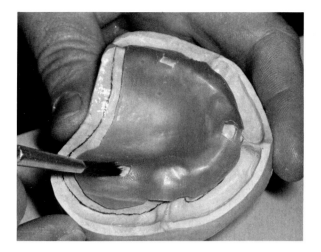

Fig. 2-22. Tinfoil substitute is painted on cast and relief wax. Note cutout tissue stops. Tissue stops may or may not be requested. Their size and position may also vary according to the dentist's requirements.

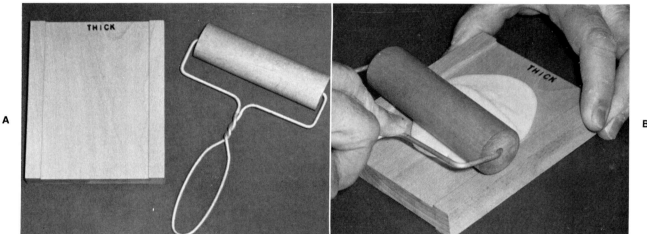

Fig. 2-23. A, Rollette unit is convenient for rolling resin into sheets of uniform thickness. **B,** Resin dough is rolled into sheets before adapting it to cast. Roller and wood block should be lightly lubricated to minimize sticking.

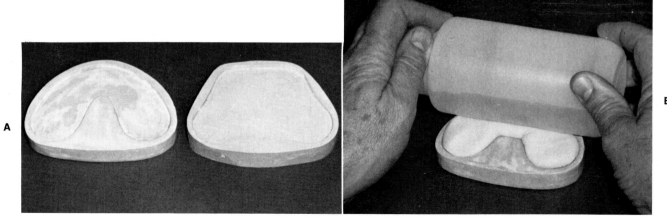

Fig. 2-24. A, Stone mold made by impressing double-thickness shellac baseplate material also is used to make tray resin sheets of uniform thickness. **B,** Plastic bottle serves as roller when making resin sheets in stone mold. Both should be lubricated to prevent sticking.

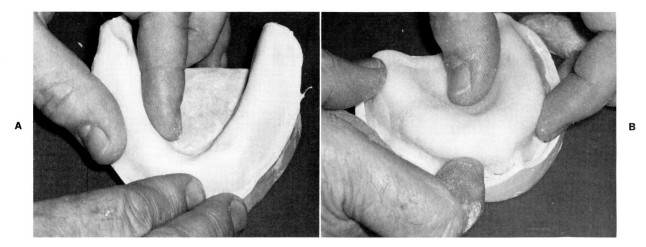

Fig. 2-25. **A,** Resin dough is adapted to cast carefully. **B,** Do not overthin resin over ridge portion of cast.

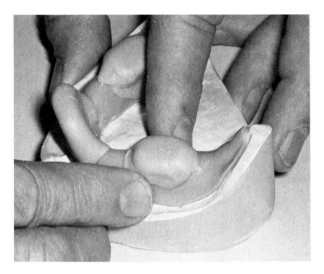

Fig. 2-26. Excess resin is shaped into handles or finger rests and adapted to tray that has been moistened with monomer.

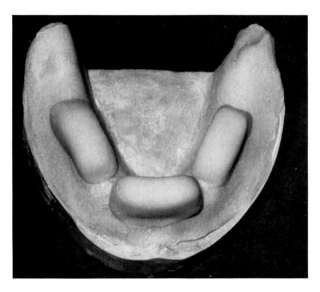

Fig. 2-27. Handles are too large and require too much time for finishing.

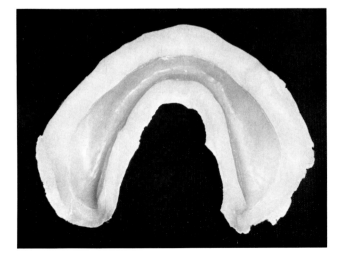

Fig. 2-28. Tray is removed from cast prior to trimming borders. Note that relief wax remains in tray.

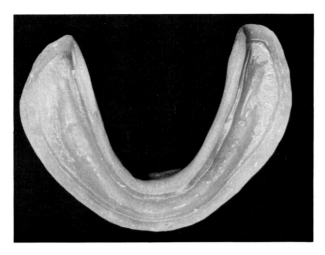

Fig. 2-29. Tray borders have been trimmed and smoothed. Borders can be pumiced lightly.

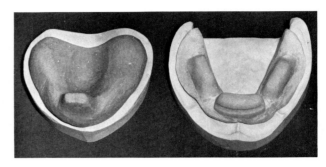

Fig. 2-30. Completed impression trays are stored on casts until needed. Note groove in anterior handle of mandibular tray for ease in holding while making impression.

Table 2-2. Finger-adapted dough method

Problem	Probable cause	Solution
Impression tray too thin in some areas and too thick in others	Impression tray material overthinned by finger pressure over residual ridges and allowed to become too thick in concave areas	Exercise care during adaptation to avoid exerting too much pressure on resin over convex portions of cast
	Resin not rolled to uniform thickness prior to adaptation	Use roller to make sheet of resin of proper thickness
Failure of tray to fit cast	Resin past dough stage before start of finger adaptation and adaptation inaccurate	Start adaptation when resin is in dough stage; do not wait until resin is rubbery
	Finger adaptation discontinued too soon	Continue adaptation until resin begins to set to prevent rebound
Impression tray or cast broken on separation	Undercuts not blocked out or tinfoil substitute not used	Block out undercuts; paint cast with tinfoil substitute

Vacuum-adapted method

Vacuum- or pressure-formed thermoplastic resin sheets can make good impression trays; the method is quick and easy, but it requires special equipment* for adapting the resin sheet to the cast (Fig. 2-31). The materials are available in a variety of colors and thicknesses as well as different degrees of flexibility. Although manufacturers issue specific instructions for their equipment, the vacuum-adapted methods for making impression trays are similar.

*Omnivac, Sta-Vac, Mini-lab Vacuum Adapter, Buffalo Dental Manufacturing Co., Inc. Brooklyn, N.Y.; Dentsply Vacu-Press, Dentsply International, Inc., York, Pa.

PROCEDURE

1. Place the outline of the impression tray on the cast with a pencil, or bead the outline with a sharp instrument if desired (Fig. 2-32).

2. Block out the undercuts and place the relief on the cast with a material, such as a wet sheet of nonasbestos casting ring lining material (Fig. 2-33), that will not melt during heating of the resin sheet.

3. Center the cast on the vacuum-adapter plate (Fig. 2-34).

4. Place a resin sheet of the appropriate color and thickness in the heating frame, and rotate the heating unit into position (Fig. 2-35).

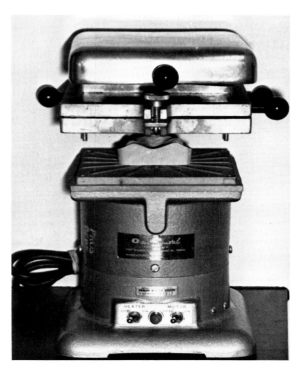

Fig. 2-31. Omnivac vacuum adapter can be used to make impression trays quickly and easily. Vacuum-adapting equipment is available from several manufacturers.

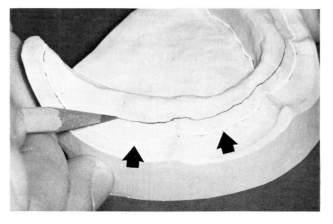

Fig. 2-32. After outline of tray has been beaded on cast (arrows), outline of relief is drawn on cast.

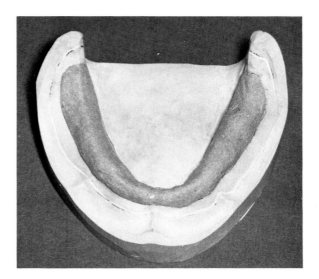

Fig. 2-33. Wet sheet of nonasbestos casting ring lining material has been adapted to cast for required relief. Wetting material thoroughly with water improves adaptability.

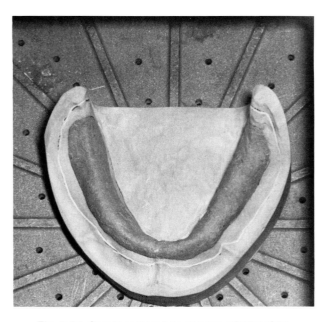

Fig. 2-34. Cast is centered on vacuum-adapter plate.

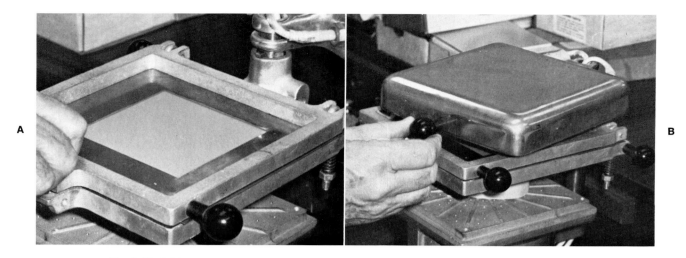

Fig. 2-35. A, Tray-weight resin sheet is placed in adapter frame. **B,** Heating unit is rotated into position before activating switch.

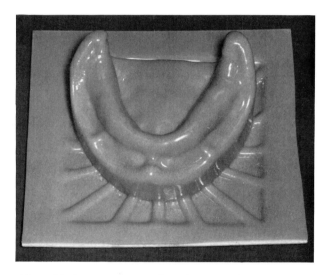

Fig. 2-36. Adapted resin is allowed to cool prior to trimming.

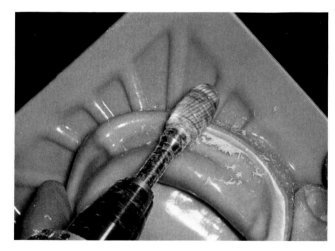

Fig. 2-37. Lathe-mounted large carbide bur is used to trim excess tray material.

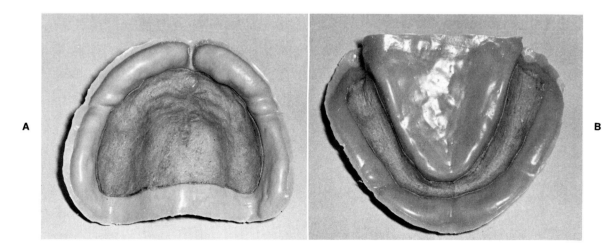

Fig. 2-38. Vacuum-adapted trays are removed from cast prior to trimming. **A,** Maxillary tray. **B,** Mandibular tray.

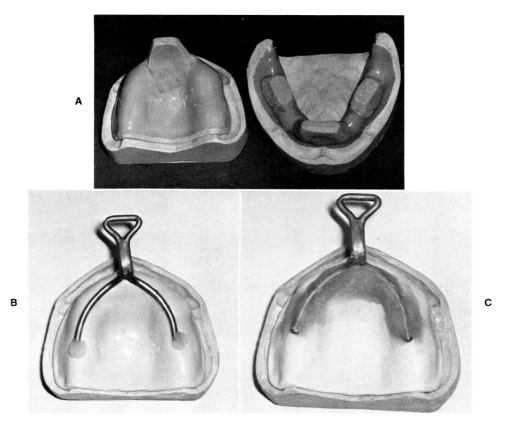

Fig. 2-39. A, Resin handles can be adapted to tray. **B,** Preformed metal handle can be used. **C,** Metal handle can be bonded to tray with autopolymerizing resin.

5. Activate the heating switch, and continue heating until the specified sag in the material occurs.

6. Lower the frame and resin sheet onto the cast, and start vacuum adaptation. After adaptation is complete, allow the resin sheet to cool, and then remove it from the vacuum-adapting unit (Fig. 2-36).

7. Trim the excess material with a large bur and lathe (Fig. 2-37).

8. Remove the tray from the cast, and trim the borders (Fig. 2-38).

9. Add handles made of autopolymerizing acrylic resin or use preformed metal handles (Fig. 2-39).

10. Store the tray on the cast until ready to use (Fig. 2-40).

PROBLEM AREAS

The principal limitation of the vacuum-adapted method is the need for special equipment and materials to vacuum-adapt impression trays. In addition, some tray-weight materials are not rigid enough after being formed into a tray (Table 2-3). Providing relief in the impression tray is difficult, particularly if it is necessary to retain the relief in the impression tray during part of

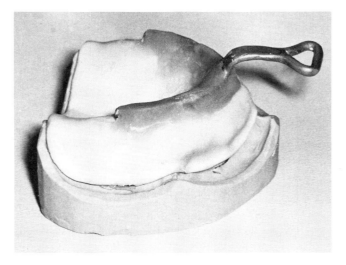

Fig. 2-40. Completed tray with metal handle is stored on cast until needed. Metal handle should not interfere with lip movements. The bend in this handle should prevent such interference.

Table 2-3. Vacuum-adapted method

Problem	Probable cause	Solution
Impression tray too flexible	Impression tray material too thin	Use thicker stock material for tray; reinforce it with wire to improve rigidity
Cast or tray broken during separation	Undercuts not blocked out	Identify and block out undercuts before vacuum adaptation

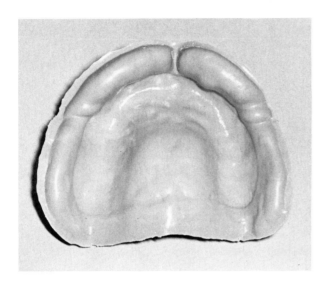

Fig. 2-41. Nonasbestos relief material must be removed from tray prior to use. Here it was removed prior to trimming the borders.

the impression-making procedure. Wax relief is unsatisfactory because it melts during vacuum adapting. Use of wet nonasbestos casting ring lining material as a heat-resistant relief on the cast during vacuum adaptation is satisfactory; however, it must be removed from the tray prior to use (Fig. 2-41).

The advantages of this method are the ease and rapidity with which it is possible to fabricate an impression tray from resin sheets of a variety of thicknesses and colors.

Shellac method

The dental profession has used shellac baseplate material for many years, primarily for baseplates. Although it is possible to make an adequate impression tray from shellac, autopolymerizing resins specially modified for constructing impression trays seem to have displaced shellac to a large extent.

Double-thickness shellac baseplate material is essential for fabricating an impression tray. An advantage of this method is the rapidity with which the shellac baseplate material can be adapted to the cast and the tray fabricated. The serious disadvantage is the lack of di-

mensional stability of the material, especially during the application of heat when border molding the tray with impression compound.

PROCEDURE

1. Place an outline of the impression tray on the cast, and bead if desired, as described previously.

2. Block out undercuts on the cast with a plaster and pumice mix or with wet nonasbestos casting ring lining material.

3. Provide relief as required with a layer of wet nonasbestos casting ring lining material (Fig. 2-42). Baseplate wax used for relief will melt during adaptation of the shellac baseplate material.

4. Center a sheet of double-thickness shellac baseplate material over the cast, and wilt it onto the cast with flame (Fig. 2-43).

5. Fold the excess shellac material at the borders back onto itself to make them of the proper thickness (Fig. 2-44).

6. Continue adaptation until the shellac material makes intimate contact with the cast and relief material (Fig. 2-45).

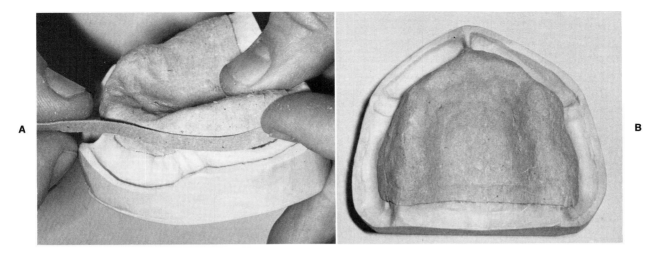

Fig. 2-42. A, Wet nonasbestos casting ring lining material strip is adapted to cast to provide relief. **B,** Completed relief is seen on cast.

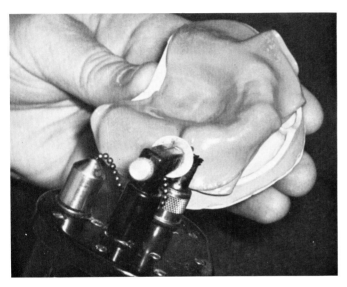

Fig. 2-43. Sheet of double-thickness shellac baseplate material is heated with alcohol torch or Bunsen burner and wilted onto cast. Exercise care to avoid overheating and charring shellac material.

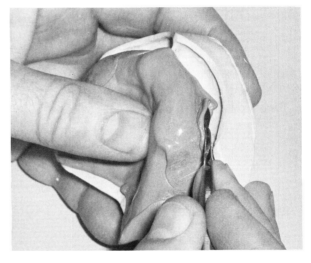

Fig. 2-44. Excess shellac is folded back onto itself to make borders of proper thickness.

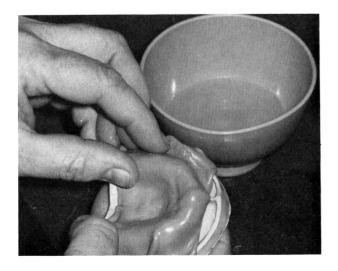

Fig. 2-45. Shellac material is adapted until it makes intimate contact with cast and relief material. Dip fingers in cool water when adapting.

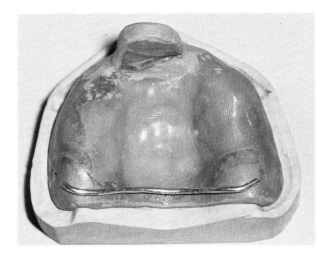

Fig. 2-46. Handle is made by warming and shaping shellac baseplate material into handle. Embedding paper clip wire across posterior border improves tray rigidity.

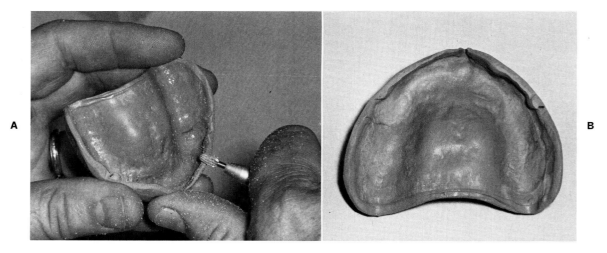

Fig. 2-47. A, Large bur can be used to trim shellac tray if rotated slowly and used with light pressure to avoid clogging and loss of effectiveness. **B,** Tray borders are trimmed to desired outline.

Fig. 2-48. All relief material is removed from tray.

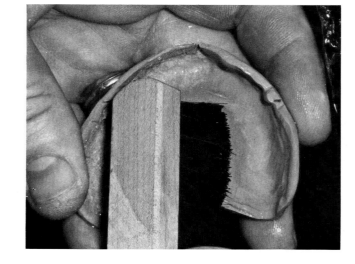

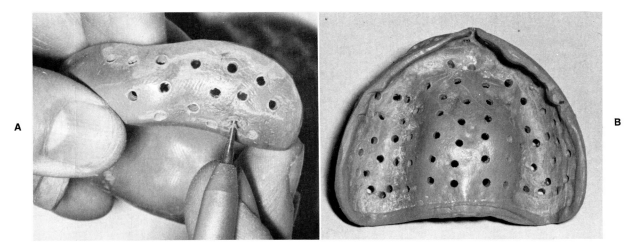

Fig. 2-49. A, Tray is perforated to aid in retaining alginate impression material. **B,** Completed tray has multiple perforations.

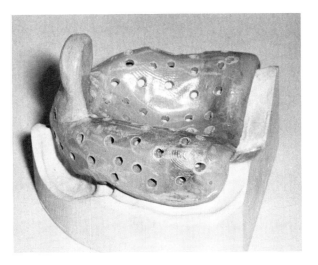

Fig. 2-50. Completed tray is stored on cast to minimize dimensional change.

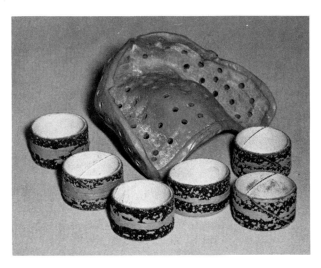

Fig. 2-51. Arbor band can be used to trim shellac tray if shellac is not overheated.

7. Form a handle from scrap shellac baseplate material, warm it, and adapt it to the impression tray (Fig. 2-46).

8. Allow the impression tray to cool, then remove it from the cast, and trim it to the border outline (Fig. 2-47). If the cast has been beaded, use the beading on the tray as a guide when trimming. Remove the relief from the tray (Fig. 2-48).

9. Perforate the shellac tray with a No. 8 round bur if using alginate impression material (Fig. 2-49).

10. Store the impression tray on the cast until ready for use (Fig. 2-50).

PROBLEM AREAS

The primary problem in using shellac baseplate material for an impression tray is the inherent lack of di-

mensional stability and rigidity associated with its thermoplastic nature (Table 2-4). The incorporation of relief in the impression tray is more difficult because baseplate wax relief can melt during adaptation of the shellac material, and it is difficult to remove the relief after the tray has cooled. Since many dentists prefer to have the relief remain in the tray during part of the impression procedures, it is more difficult to satisfy this requirement when using shellac baseplate material. In addition, adjusting or trimming shellac impression trays is particularly difficult because the material tends to ruin or clog arbor bands and burs (Fig. 2-51). The use of wire reinforcement, as discussed in Chapter 4 for shellac baseplates, improves the rigidity and dimensional stability of shellac impression trays. Shellac baseplate materials are not as satisfactory for making impression trays

Table 2-4. Shellac method

Problem	Probable cause	Solution
Warping of impression tray and failure to fit cast	Shellac baseplate material warped during cooling	Readapting shellac baseplate material
Impression tray too flexible	Shellac baseplate material not rigid enough, and anterior ridge on mandibular cast flat	Using double-thickness shellac baseplate material and reinforcing anterior ridge region with wire
Tray stuck to cast	Shellac baseplate material overheated during adaptation	Wetting cast before heating shellac baseplate material and not overheating and charring shellac baseplate material

as modified autopolymerizing acrylic resin or thermoplastic vacuum-adapted resin materials.

IMPRESSION TRAYS FOR IMMEDIATE DENTURES

Appleby and Kerchoff (1955); Lutes, Ellinger, and Terry (1967); Campagna (1968); Lambrecht (1968); Cupero (1972); and Javid, Tanaka, and Porter (1974) have described impression trays for immediate dentures.

When making trays for immediate dentures the considerations are different from making trays for conventional complete dentures because of the presence of teeth on the cast. The immediate denture treatment sequence used by many dentists consists of removing the posterior teeth; after a healing period, making an impression of the relatively well-healed posterior ridges; completing the denture; and then removing the anterior teeth and inserting the denture. Therefore two areas of impression trays for immediate dentures that require consideration are (1) the impression of the edentulous ridges and (2) the impression of the remaining natural teeth.

Each of the three impression methods for immediate dentures requires a different type of tray (Fig. 2-52). In one method, a one-piece full-arch impression tray covers the edentulous ridges and natural teeth. The disadvantage of this type of tray is its tendency to be bulky because it is necessary to have the relief over the natural teeth to block out undercuts. A second method of making an immediate denture impression is to use a custom-made impression tray for the posterior edentulous portion of the impression, and then make an overall impression over the posterior tray and natural teeth. The third method is to use a two-piece tray. The first impression tray is made over the edentulous portion of the arch, and the second over the anterior portion of the arch and the anterior teeth joining the first tray. Several meth-

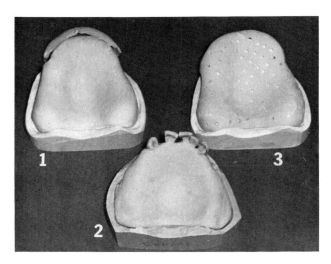

Fig. 2-52. Impression trays for immediate dentures are of three types: two-piece tray *(1)*, custom posterior tray *(2)*, and one-piece full-arch tray *(3)*.

ods of keying the two impression trays are available, and the principal advantage is that these trays are less bulky than the stock trays or one-piece custom trays. The disadvantage is the increased time required to construct the keyed two-piece trays.

Full-arch impression trays

Appleby and Kerchoff (1955) have described a method of making an overall acrylic resin impression tray for an immediate maxillary denture impression. Their method requires placing the tray outline on the cast, blocking out the natural teeth on the cast with wax, and adapting a layer of baseplate wax over the cast that extends to the border outline. The purpose of this relief is to provide space for the impression material. Autopolymerizing resin is used to make the overall impression tray. The procedure for making the full-arch

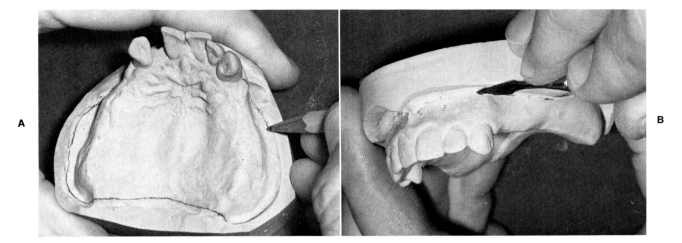

Fig. 2-53. **A,** Outline for impression tray and relief is drawn on cast with pencil. **B,** Outline can be beaded for use as guide in trimming.

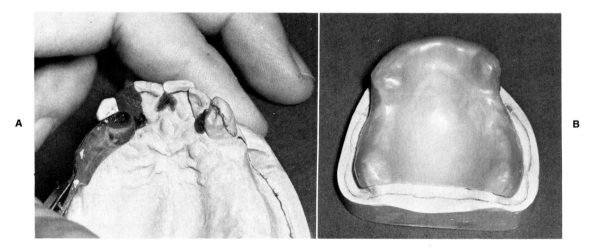

Fig. 2-54. **A,** Teeth on cast are blocked out with wax. **B,** A sheet of baseplate wax is adapted over the cast and trimmed to relief outline.

impression trays involves the finger-adapted vacuum-adapted, or the sprinkle-on method.

Finger-adapted dough method
PROCEDURE

1. Outline the border of the impression tray on the cast with a pencil, and bead it if desired (Fig. 2-53).

2. Block out the teeth on the cast with baseplate wax, so that the tray can be removed without breaking the teeth, adapt a layer of baseplate wax over the cast, and trim to the relief outline (Fig. 2-54).

3. Paint tinfoil substitute on the stone cast and baseplate relief wax, as described earlier in this chapter.

4. Proportion the autopolymerizing tray resin according to the recommendation of the manufacturer, and

mix it in a paper cup. Immediately prior to reaching the dough stage, remove some material from the cup with a spatula, and place it in the border areas of the cast (Fig. 2-55).

5. When the material reaches the desired dough stage, remove it from the cup, and roll it into a sheet of the proper thickness (2 mm).*

6. Adapt the resin sheet over the relieved cast (Fig. 2-56). Fold or trim the excess resin extending over the borders of the cast (Fig. 2-57).

7. Continue finger adaptation until the resin begins to set.

---

*Rollette Unit, Kerr Manufacturing Co., Romulus, Mich.

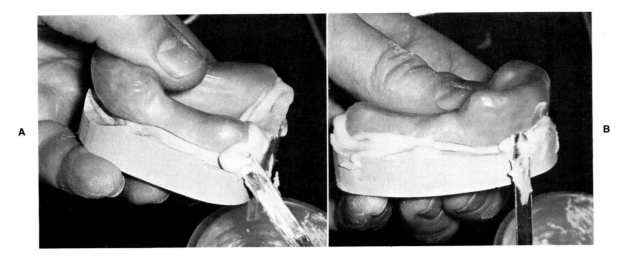

Fig. 2-55. Resin dough is placed in border reflections of cast with spatula to minimize voids.

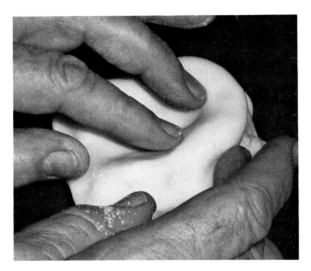

Fig. 2-56. Resin sheet is adapted to cast and relief wax.

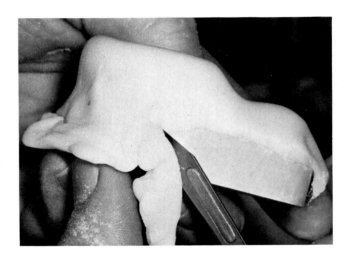

Fig. 2-57. Excess resin is trimmed with knife.

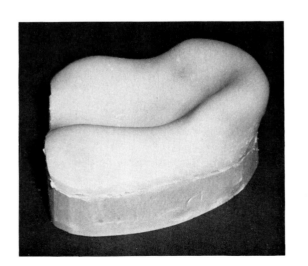

Fig. 2-58. Resin tray is left on cast to cure.

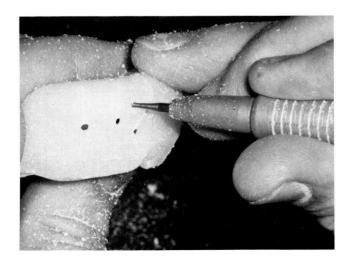

Fig. 2-59. Resin tray can be perforated with bur to improve retention of impression material.

8. Permit the resin to cure on the cast, and then carefully remove the tray from the cast (Fig. 2-58).

9. Finish and polish the borders, and smooth rough areas to avoid discomfort for the patient. Perforate the tray with a No. 8 bur to aid in retaining elastic impression materials if desired (Fig. 2-59).

The finger-adapted dough method is preferable to the sprinkle-on method for full-arch impression trays, but either is usable.

PROBLEM AREAS

A potential problem with the finger-adapted dough method is the difficulty in maintaining tray thickness when applying pressure (Table 2-5). There is a distinct tendency to overthin the material over the convex areas of the cast and teeth, thereby making the impression tray too thin in these areas (Fig. 2-60). Another prob-

lem is the overall bulk of the tray required over the blocked-out teeth and edentulous portions of the cast (Fig. 2-61).

Vacuum-adapted method

It is possible to make a one-piece full-arch immediate denture impression tray by vacuum adaptation. The procedure is similar to that described previously for conventional complete dentures with a modification in the blockout. The principal advantage of this method is the minimal amount of time used in constructing a tray, and the principal disadvantage is the investment required for specialized equipment.

PROCEDURE

1. Place the outline of the tray on the cast with a pencil or bead it with a sharp instrument (Fig. 2-53).

Table 2-5. Full-arch impression tray: finger-adapted dough method

Problem	Probable cause	Solution
Tray thick in some areas; thin in other areas	Resin overthinned over convex areas of cast by too much finger pressure	Exercise care when adapting resin to cast, particularly over ridges and teeth; use only enough pressure to achieve adaptation
Tray or cast broken during removal of tray from cast	Teeth on cast not blocked out adequately; and undercuts elsewhere on cast not blocked out	Block out teeth on cast with baseplate wax to eliminate undercuts; identify and block out other undercuts on cast
	Tinfoil substitute contaminated or not used	Coat cast with uncontaminated tinfoil substitute
	Too much force used in prying tray from cast	Use minimal force when removing tray; pry gently around borders of tray to lift it from cast without breaking it

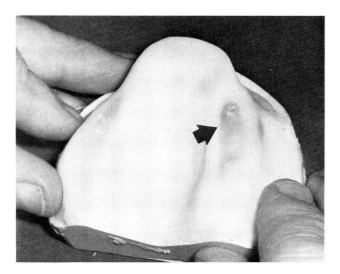

Fig. 2-60. Care should be exercised to avoid overthinning resin over convex portions of cast. Note relief wax showing through (arrow).

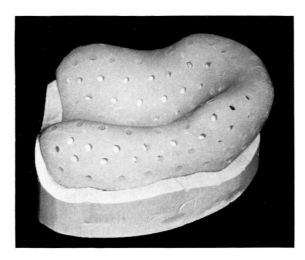

Fig. 2-61. One-piece full-arch impression trays often are bulky because of presence of teeth and relief wax.

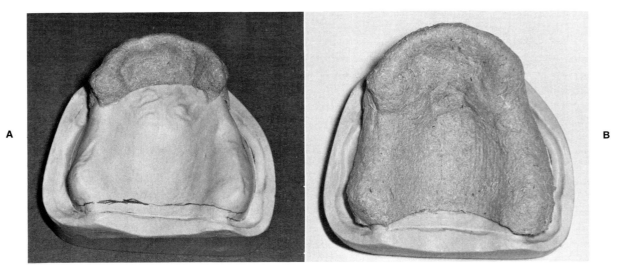

Fig. 2-62. A, Wet nonasbestos casting ring lining material strips are adapted to teeth on cast to block out undercuts. **B,** Additional layer of relief is adapted to desired outline before vacuum adapting resin tray.

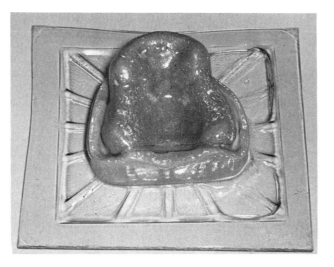

Fig. 2-63. Resin is permitted to cool before trimming.

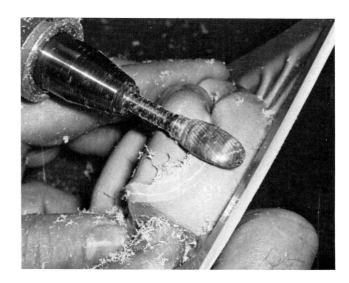

Fig. 2-64. Large lathe-mounted bur is convenient for trimming excess resin.

2. Block out undercuts and relief areas with a heat-stable relief material (Fig. 2-62).

3. Position a sheet of resin of the proper thickness in the heating frame of the vacuum adapter as described previously.

4. Center the blocked out cast in the vacuum former (Fig. 2-34).

5. Start the heater and, when the recommended amount of sag occurs, lower the heating frame and activate the vacuum.

6. After completing the adaptation, allow the resin to cool and trim the borders with a large bur in a lathe (Figs. 2-63 and 2-64).

7. Remove the tray, and trim it to the previously established outline.

8. Smooth and finish all borders.

9. Use the resin that projects over the anterior teeth as a handle for this type of tray (Fig. 2-65).

10. Remove all traces of blockout and relief material from the interior of the impression tray (Fig. 2-66).

11. If specified, perforate the tray with a bur to improve retention of the impression material in the tray (Fig. 2-66).

12. Store the completed tray on the cast until needed (Fig. 2-66).

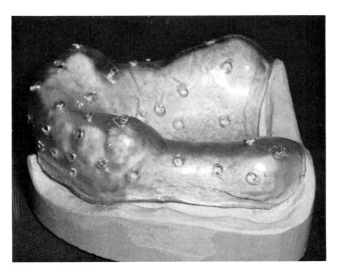

Fig. 2-65. Usually, resin projecting over anterior teeth serves as handle on this type of tray. Perforations in tray aid in retaining impression material.

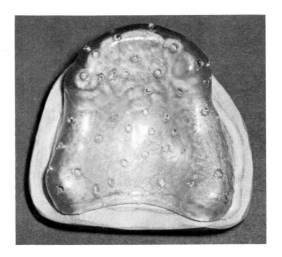

Fig. 2-66. Perforations made in tray with No. 8 or 10 bur. Note all of relief material has been removed from interior of tray. Tray is stored on cast until needed.

Table 2-6. Full-arch impression tray: vacuum-adapted method

Problem	Probable cause	Solution
Cast or tray broken on separation	Undercuts or teeth on cast not blocked out	Examine cast carefully to identify undercuts; block them out
Tray not adapted to cast in some areas	Tray material not heated sufficiently before vacuum adaptation started	Make certain that recommended amount of sag occurs in tray resin before activating vacuum
Tray too flexible	Stock material used for tray too thin	Use tray-weight resin sheet to assure adequate rigidity

PROBLEM AREAS

Problems with the vacuum-adapted method are minimal (Table 2-6). Occasionally, tray-weight resin sheets do not adapt to all areas of the cast, particularly in the border reflections. It is possible to minimize this problem by making certain that the recommended amount of sag has occurred before starting adaptation. Occasionally the tray is too flexible, probably as a result of using a sheet of resin that is too thin. The principal disadvantage to this method is the requirement for specialized equipment.

Custom posterior trays

A simple form of the sectional impression tray for an immediate denture is a tray made over only the edentulous portion of the cast. A second overall impression is made of the teeth and anterior vestibule with a stock tray. Making a custom posterior tray is quick and easy with tray resin and the finger-adapted dough method. It also can be made by the sprinkle-on or vacuum-adapted method by using the procedures discussed previously.

Finger-adapted dough method
PROCEDURE

1. Place an outline of the tray on the cast with a pencil (Fig. 2-67).
2. Extend the impression tray outline to contact lingual surfaces of the anterior teeth. This extension aids in positioning the tray in the patient's mouth and increases the accuracy of the impression (Fig. 2-68). An alternate method is to use a wax ledge approximately 2 mm wide anterior to the incisive edges of the teeth (Ellinger and Terry, 1967). It allows the tray to extend in front of the teeth and aids in positioning the tray (Fig. 2-69).
3. Block out spaces between the teeth with wax to keep resin from entering the undercut areas and to prevent the teeth from breaking when removing the tray from the cast (Fig. 2-70). After blocking out the spaces

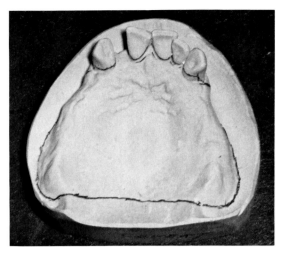

Fig. 2-67. Outline of posterior impression tray is placed on cast.

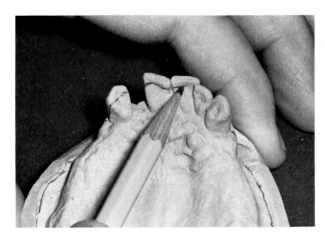

Fig. 2-68. Impression tray can be extended onto lingual surfaces of teeth to aid in positioning tray when making impressions.

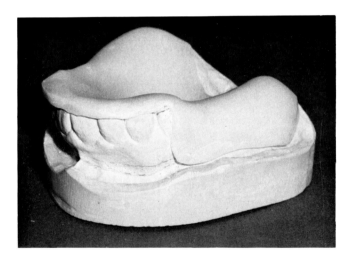

Fig. 2-69. Alternate method to extend this type of tray over incisal edges of teeth to aid in positioning tray while making impression.

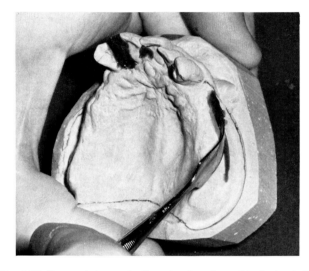

Fig. 2-70. Spaces between teeth and undercuts are blocked out with baseplate wax to prevent extrusion of resin into spaces during making of tray and resultant breakage of teeth on cast on separation.

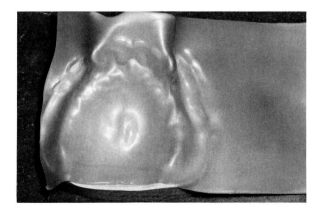

Fig. 2-71. Single thickness of baseplate wax is adapted over blocked out teeth and trimmed to desired relief outline.

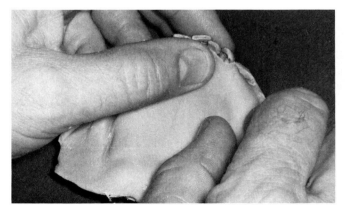

Fig. 2-72. Adaptation of resin to cast is continued until it begins to set.

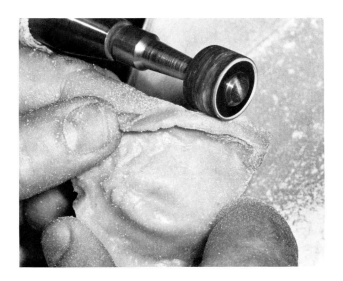

Fig. 2-73. Tray borders are trimmed to previously established outline with lathe-mounted arbor band.

Table 2-7. Custom posterior impression tray: finger-adapted dough method

Problem	Probable cause	Solution
Teeth on cast broken on removal of tray	Spaces between anterior teeth on cast not blocked out with wax	Examine cast to find spaces between teeth and other undercut areas; block them out with wax
Tray too thick	Resin not rolled to uniform thickness prior to adaptation	Roll resin into sheet approximately 2 mm thick before adapting to cast
Tray stuck to cast	Tinfoil substitute contaminated or not used	Paint cast with uncontaminated tinfoil substitute

and undercuts, adapt one layer of baseplate wax for relief (Fig. 2-71).

4. Paint tinfoil substitute on the cast and relief wax.

5. Using a paper cup, mix the resin according to the manufacturer's recommendations.

6. When the resin reaches the desired state, remove it from the paper cup and roll it into a sheet 2 to 3 mm thick, using a template mold or special roller. Adapt the resin to the cast, but do not overthin it on the cast prominences. Trim excess resin from the cast with a knife.

7. Continue adaptation of the resin until it begins to set (Fig. 2-72). After setting, remove the impression tray from the cast and trim it to the previously established outline with an arbor band or an acrylic bur (Fig. 2-73).

PROBLEM AREAS

A problem arises with this method when the anterior teeth have spaces between them (Table 2-7). If the acrylic resin extrudes between the teeth during construction of the tray, usually the teeth break from the cast on removal of the tray. Blocking out the spaces between the teeth with baseplate wax will solve this problem.

Two-piece trays

It is possible to construct two-piece impression trays for immediate dentures with autopolymerizing resin tray materials (Javid et al., 1974). The first-stage impression tray is fabricated over the posterior edentulous portion of the cast. The second-stage tray, which is constructed for placing over the first-stage tray, covers the anterior teeth and labial flange portion of the cast. The two sections of the tray assemble and allow removal as a unit or in sections after completion of the impression.

The advantage of the two-piece tray method is that it permits the dentist to make the impression for an immediate denture in a two-stage procedure. The principal disadvantage is the additional time required to make the two-piece tray.

Finger-adapted dough method

The finger-adapted dough method should be used for this tray.

PROCEDURE

1. Draw the outline for the posterior section of the tray on the cast with a pencil.

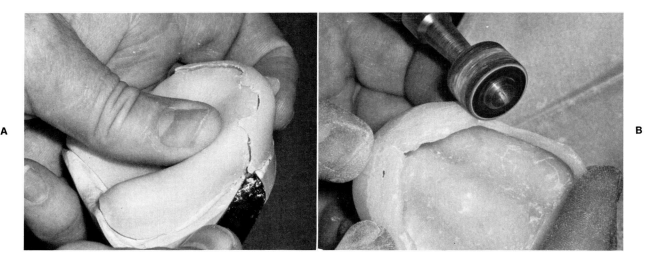

Fig. 2-81. **A,** After curing, anterior tray section is removed. **B,** Sections are reassembled and then trimmed to proper thickness.

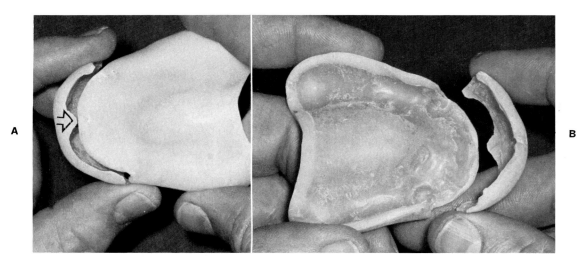

Fig. 2-82. **A,** Sections of tray should interlock positively. Note projection in midline to aid in assembly (arrow). **B,** Interior view of two-piece tray.

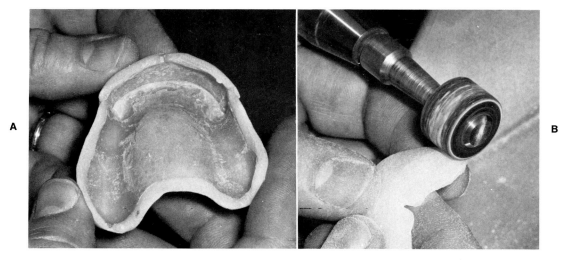

Fig. 2-83. **A,** Completed impression tray is examined for sharp edges. **B,** Edges are smoothed wherever necessary.

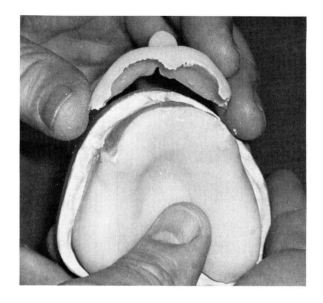

Fig. 2-84. Completed impression tray is assembled and stored on cast until needed.

Table 2-8. Two-piece impression trays: finger-adapted dough method

Problem	Probable cause	Solution
Tray sections stuck together and unable to be separated	First-stage tray not coated with separating medium, such as silicone lubricant or tinfoil	Coat part of first-stage tray that contacts second section to prevent chemical bonding and resultant inability to separate tray sections

PROBLEM AREAS

In addition to many of the previously discussed problems, the two-piece impression tray method can present another problem associated with failure to apply a separating medium to the first tray before making the second, or anterior, tray. In this instance, the two trays become bonded together (Table 2-8). Making two-piece trays also requires considerable time and effort.

SUMMARY

Methods of constructing impression trays for conventional complete dentures and immediate dentures have been described. Conventional and tray autopolymerizing resins, shellac baseplate material, and thermoplastic resins make satisfactory impression trays. Tray resins are easy to use, require minimal equipment, make excellent impression trays when manipulated properly and, consequently, enjoy widespread usage. Vacuum-forming equipment also can produce good impression trays, particularly when minimal construction time is a requirement. Although used extensively in the past for baseplates and impression trays, shellac is less satisfactory for impression trays because of its lack of dimensional stability.

REFERENCES

Appleby, R. C., and Kerchoff, W. F.: Immediate maxillary denture impression, J. Prosthet. Dent. **5:**443-451, 1955.

Barone, J. V.: Physiologic complete denture impression, J. Prosthet. Dent. **13:**800-809, 1963.

Boos, R. H.: Physiologic denture technique, J. Prosthet. Dent. **6:**726-740, 1956.

Campagna, S. J.: An impression technique for immediate dentures, J. Prosthet. Dent. **20:**196-203, 1968.

Carlton, J. R.: Complete denture prosthesis, J. Prosthet. Dent. **5:**342-349, 1955.

Chase, W. W.: Adaptation of rubber base impression materials to remove denture prosthetics, J. Prosthet. Dent. **10:**1043-1050, 1960.

Choudhary, S. C.: Modified pressure impression techniques for edentulous patients, J. Prosthet. Dent. **23:**199-204, 1970.

Cupero, H. M.: Technique for making complete maxillary immediate denture impression, J. Prosthet. Dent. **28:**546-548, 1972.

Dresen, O. M.: The rubber base impression materials, J. Prosthet. Dent. **8:**14-18, 1958.

Ellinger, C. W.: Minimizing problems in making a complete lower impression, J. Prosthet. Dent. **30:**553-558, 1973.

Filler, W. H.: Modified impression techniques for hyperplastic alveolar ridges, J. Prosthet. Dent. **25:**609-612, 1971.

Fusayama, T., and Nakazato, M.: The designs of stock trays and the retention of irreversible hydrocolloid impressions, J. Prosthet. Dent. 21:136-142, 1969.

Harris, L. W.: Facial templates and stabilized baseplates with the new chemical set resins, J. Prosthet. Dent. 1:156-160, 1951.

Jamieson, C. H.: A complete denture impression technique, J. Prosthet. Dent. 4:17-29, 1954.

Javid, N., Tanaka, H., and Porter, M.: Split tray impression technique for immediate upper dentures, J. Prosthet. Dent. 32:348-351, 1974.

Klein, I. E.: Complete denture impression technique, J. Prosthet. Dent. 5:739-755, 1955.

Lambrecht, J. R.: Immediate denture construction: The impression phase, J. Prosthet. Dent. 19:237-245, 1968.

LaVere, A., and Freda, A. L.: An individualized impression tray utilizing the patient's existing denture, J. Prosthet. Dent. 36:334-346, 1976.

Leathers, L. L.: Overcoming obstacles and objections to immediate dentures, J. Prosthet. Dent. 10:5-13, 1960.

Lutes, M. R., Ellinger, C. W., and Terry, J. M.: An impression procedure for construction of maxillary immediate dentures, J. Prosthet. Dent. 18:202-210, 1967.

Martone, A. L.: Clinical applications of concepts of functional anatomy and speech science to complete denture prosthodontics, part VII, Recording Phases, J. Prosthet. Dent. 12:4-33, 1963.

McCracken, W. L.: Externally stabilized mandibular impression, J. Prosthet. Dent. 14:5-11, 1964.

Merkeley, H. J.: Mandibular rearmament, part II, denture construction, J. Prosthet. Dent. 9:567-577, 1959.

Munz, F. R.: Impressions in transparent trays, J. Prosthet. Dent. 4:596-605, 1954.

Parker, H. C.: Biomechanical procedures based on anatomic considerations in full denture prosthesis, J. Prosthet. Dent. 2:477-490, 1952.

Rosenthal, L. E., Boyer, R., Lane, J. V., and Lane, S. L.: Rehabilitation after partial glossectomy, J. Prosthet. Dent. 10:270-277, 1960.

Schieffer, F. J., Jr.: The neutral zone and polished surfaces in complete dentures, J. Prosthet. Dent. 14:854-865, 1964.

Sowter, J. B.: Custom impression trays from complete dentures, dental laboratory technology, Prosthodontic technique, Chapel Hill, N.C., 1968, University of North Carolina Press.

Tilton, G. E.: A minimum pressure complete denture impression technique, J. Prosthet. Dent. 6:6-23, 1956.

Wagner, A. G.: Making duplicate dentures for use as final impression trays, J. Prosthet. Dent. 24:111-113, 1970.

Woelfel, J. B.: Contour variations in impressions of one edentulous patient, J. Prosthet. Dent. 12:229-254, 1962.

CHAPTER 3

FINAL IMPRESSIONS, BOXING AND POURING

KENNETH D. RUDD, ROBERT M. MORROW, and EARL E. FELDMANN

boxing an impression Building up vertical walls around an impression, usually in wax, to produce the desired size and form of the base of the cast and to preserve certain landmarks of the impression.

BOXING IMPRESSIONS

Boxing final impressions before pouring preserves the extension, as well as the thickness, of the border; controls the form and thickness of the base of the cast; facilitates placing remounting plates* in the cast; and conserves artificial stone (Sowter, 1968; Air Force Manual 160-29, 1959; Bolouri, Hilger, and Gowrylock, 1975). Several methods and a variety of materials are available for boxing impressions (Air Force Manual 160-29, 1959; Boucher, 1964; Sowter, 1968). The materials are wax, metal strips, plaster of Paris alone or modified by adding pumice, and caulking compound.

Boxing with wax is especially suitable for impressions made in zinc-oxide impression paste, since wax beading adheres to this material readily. However, boxing a rubber base or silicone impression with wax is more difficult because it is almost impossible to make the wax stick to these materials. Another method of boxing makes it necessary to settle the impression into a mix of plaster and, after setting, to trim the plaster to the desired border outline, box the impression, and pour it in artifi-

*Split Remounting Plate Assembly Complete, Teledyne Dental Products Co., Hanau Division, Buffalo, N.Y.

cial stone. In a modification of this procedure, the addition of pumice to the plaster mix weakens it, thereby facilitating retrieval of the cast from the boxed impression (Harris, 1960; Sowter, 1968; Heartwell and Rahn, 1974; Bolouri, Hilger, and Gowrylock, 1975). This method, which is excellent for boxing impressions made in elastomeric materials, serves equally well for zinc-oxide paste impressions.

It is also possible to use caulking compound for boxing impressions. Beading the border of the impression with strips of caulking compound makes the border of the cast the desired width. The beaded impression is then boxed with metal or wax boxing strips. Blank (1961) describes the use of a "paddle grip" wax technique for boxing impressions. The impression is sealed to wax on a paddle, which is used as a handle for holding the boxed impression while pouring it on the vibrator.

This chapter presents three methods of boxing impressions and the technique for pouring and indexing casts.

Wax boxing method

Wax boxing is effective for zinc-oxide paste impressions and is usable also for rubber base or silicone impressions, but only after thoroughly drying them before adapting the beading wax. This wax is available in round or square strips* (Fig. 3-1). Orthodontic wax† or utility wax‡ also is usable for beading an impression. Some orthodontic tray waxes, which are especially flexible,

---

*Beading Grip Wax, The L. D. Caulk Co., Milford, Del.
†Orthodontic Tray Wax, Hygienic Dental Manufacturing Co., Akron, Ohio.
‡Utility Wax Strips, Hygienic Dental Manufacturing Co., Akron, Ohio, or equivalent.

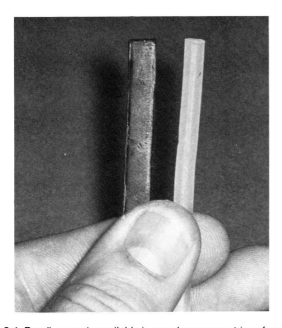

Fig. 3-1. Beading wax is available in round or square strips of various sizes.

adapt to the impression easily. After the beading wax is adapted and sealed, the impression is boxed with a wax strip, and the cast is poured.

PROCEDURE

1. Place the impression on the bench with impression surface up, and use soft wax or modeling clay to align the impression so that the ridge portion is approximately parallel to the bench top (Fig. 3-2). Adjust the height until a boxing wax strip extends approximately 13 mm above the highest point on the impression (Fig. 3-3).

2. Fill in the tongue space of a mandibular impression by adapting and sealing a sheet of baseplate wax cut to the proper form. Use a wax spatula to seal the wax to the impression (Fig. 3-4). Seal it to the impression on both sides (Fig. 3-5). Make the waxed-in tongue area smooth and seal it approximately 3 to 4 mm below the border of the impression (Fig. 3-6). Lower placement will compromise access to parts of the cast, such as when making baseplates.

3. Adapt orthodontic tray wax or beading wax around the periphery of the impression (Fig. 3-7). This wax should be approximately 4 mm wide and 3 to 4 mm below the border of the impression (Fig. 3-8).

4. Adapt another short length of beading wax to the heel region of the mandibular impression and across the posterior edge of the waxed-in tongue area to make the border wider in these areas (Fig. 3-9).

5. Seal the beading wax to the impression with a wax spatula (Fig. 3-10). Handle the hot spatula carefully to avoid damaging the impression or allowing the wax to flow onto the border of the impression.

6. Check the width of the beading by looking down

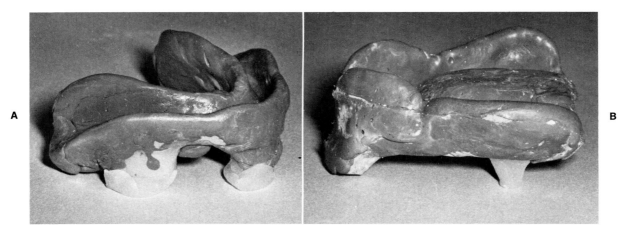

Fig. 3-2. A, Soft wax or modeling clay is used to support impression so that ridges are approximately parallel to bench top. Height of impression should be controlled. **B,** Maxillary impression is oriented to make residual ridges parallel to bench top.

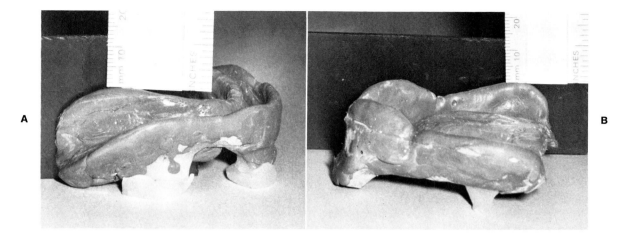

Fig. 3-3. A, Soft wax is used to adjust height of impression. Boxing wax should extend approximately 13 mm above highest point on impression to produce cast of desired thickness. **B,** Maxillary impression is adjusted for height. Note that measurement is made from highest point on border of impression.

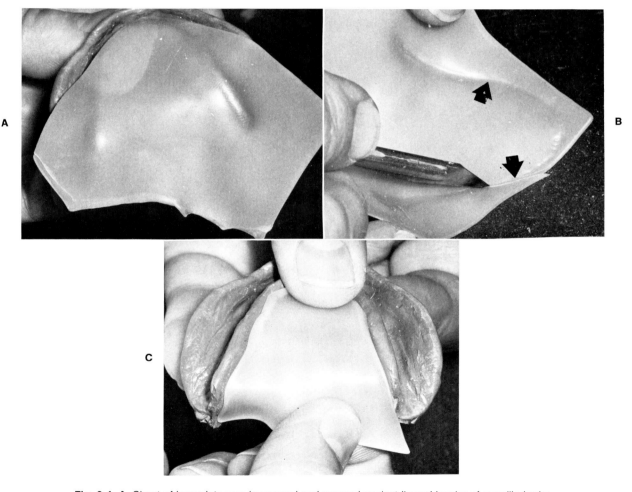

Fig. 3-4. A, Sheet of baseplate wax is warmed and pressed against lingual border of mandibular impression. **B,** Baseplate wax is removed, and indentations (arrows) produced by border of impression are used as guides in trimming wax. **C,** Trimmed wax is adapted to lingual area of mandibular impression.

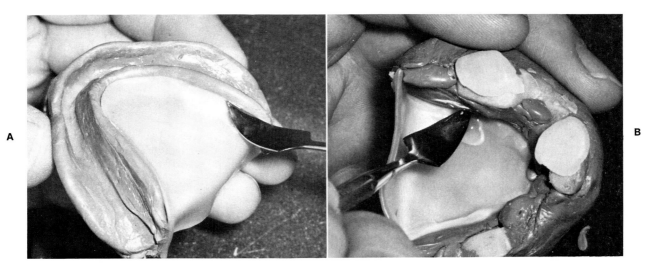

Fig. 3-5. A, Baseplate wax blocking out tongue area of mandibular impression is sealed carefully to impression approximately 3 to 4 mm below border of impression. **B,** Wax is sealed also on underside of impression to make strong junction that will not separate during pouring.

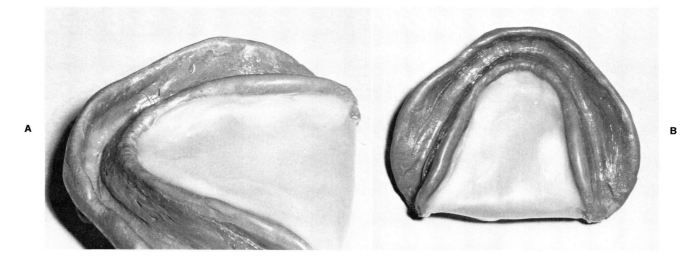

Fig. 3-6. A, Blockout of tongue area has been completed and wax sealed to lingual border of impression. **B,** Wax is sealed approximately 3 to 4 mm below border of impression to preserve thickness of border during fabrication of denture.

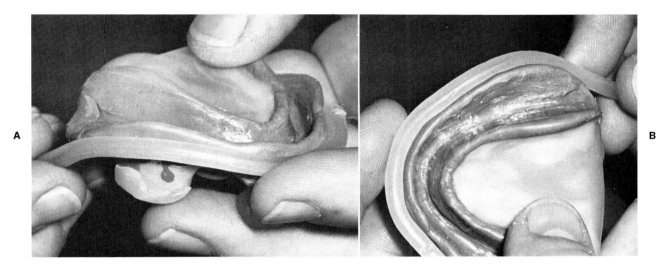

Fig. 3-7. A, Orthodontic tray wax or beading wax is adapted around periphery of impression. **B,** Beading wax is placed approximately 3 to 4 mm below border of impression.

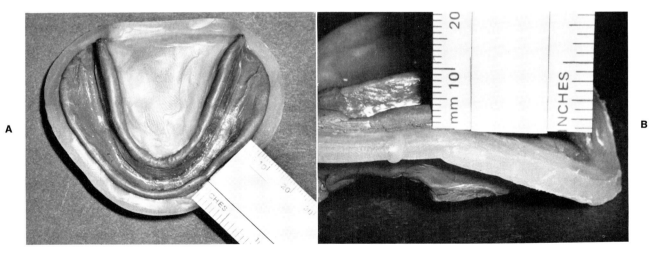

Fig. 3-8. A, Wax beading should be approximately 4 mm wide to make border of cast proper width. **B,** Position of beading wax 3 to 4 mm below border of impression is verified.

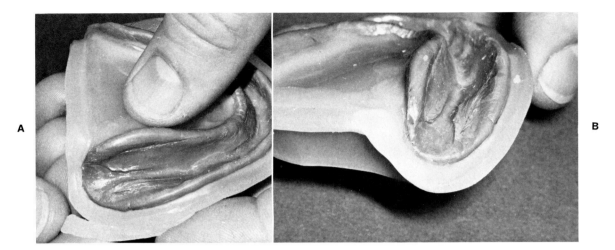

Fig. 3-9. A, Heel area of mandibular impression is widened by applying another short length of beading wax. Beading wax is placed below mandibular impression to permit land area of cast to be above impression surface of cast. **B,** Note position of beading wax in heel area of mandibular impression.

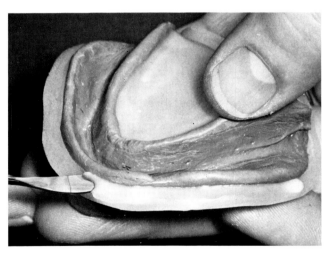

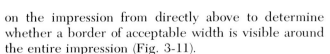

Fig. 3-10. Beading wax is sealed to impression carefully.

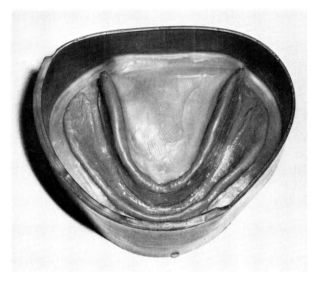

Fig. 3-11. Impression with tongue area blocked out with wax and beading wax in position. Note that uniform width of beading around border of entire impression must be preserved when boxing strip is adapted.

on the impression from directly above to determine whether a border of acceptable width is visible around the entire impression (Fig. 3-11).

7. Set the impression on the bench top, warm a strip of boxing wax* over a Bunsen burner until flexible, and carefully fold it around the impression wax (Fig. 3-12). Take care to avoid distorting and thinning the beading wax while adapting the boxing strip.

*Boxing Grip Wax, The L. D. Caulk Co., Milford, Del.

8. Seal the ends of the boxing strip to the underlying layer of wax (Fig. 3-13).

9. Seal the beading wax to the boxing strip on both the impression side and the underside to make it watertight (Fig. 3-14). Handle the hot spatula carefully to avoid perforating the boxing wax or dripping wax into the impression.

10. Check the boxed impression for adequate width of the border, sealing, and height before pouring it in stone (Fig. 3-15). Fill the impression with cool water to check

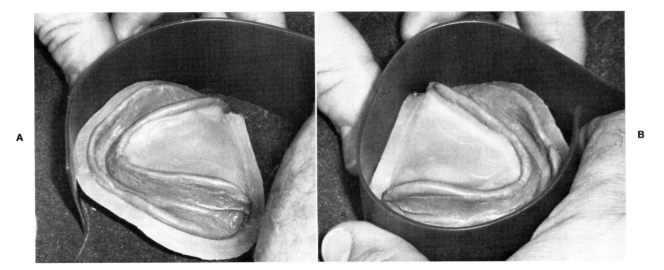

Fig. 3-12. **A,** With beaded impression in position on bench, strip of boxing wax is warmed and adapted around wax beading. **B,** Boxing wax strip is folded around beaded impression to form base of cast.

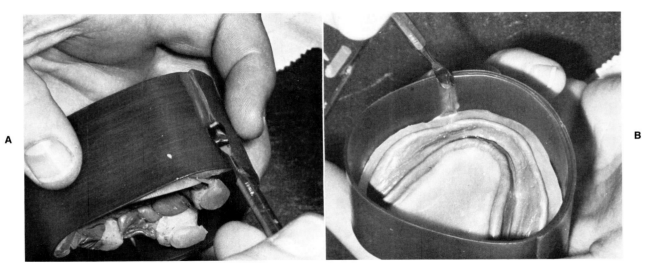

Fig. 3-13. **A,** Boxing wax strip is sealed with hot spatula. **B,** Interior joint of boxing wax is sealed with hot spatula.

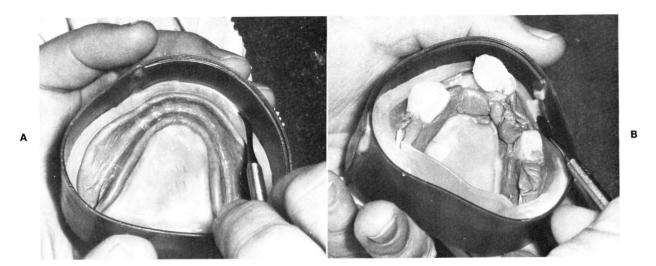

Fig. 3-14. **A,** Beading wax is sealed to boxing wax with hot spatula. **B,** Boxing wax is sealed on underside also to make it watertight and to prevent separation of boxing wax from beading wax when pouring stone cast.

for leaks. Pour the impression in vacuum-spatulated* artificial stone (Fig. 3-16).

_____

*Vac-U-Vestor Combination Power Mixer, Whip-Mix Corp., Louisville, Ky.

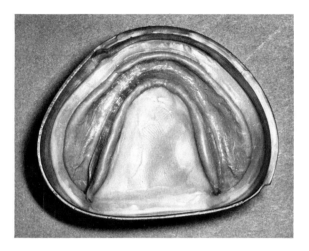

Fig. 3-15. Boxed impression is examined carefully to determine whether border is of correct width and beading wax is sealed to boxing wax properly.

PROBLEM AREAS

Problems arise with the wax boxing method when the beading wax is of the wrong width and, consequently, the border is too narrow or too wide (Table 3-1). It is easy to correct a border that is too wide by trimming it on the cast, but it is difficult to correct a land area that is too narrow (Fig. 3-17). Thinning the beading wax border may occur during adaptation of the boxing strip; if the strip is too stiff, it may distort and thin the borders. Placing beading wax too near the border of the impression results in inadequate preservation of the border contour (Fig. 3-18).

Beading wax placed too low makes the border of the cast too high and necessitates its trimming. A common error when boxing impressions is placing the beading wax too high in the heel area of mandibular impressions (Fig. 3-19) and across the posterior border of maxillary impressions (Fig. 3-20). This error makes the casts too low in these areas (Fig. 3-21). When boxing an impression it is necessary to think in reverse to determine the effect on the cast; for example, when a section of beading wax on the impression is too high, it will be too low on the cast.

Control the thickness of the base of the cast by making the impression the proper height within the boxing

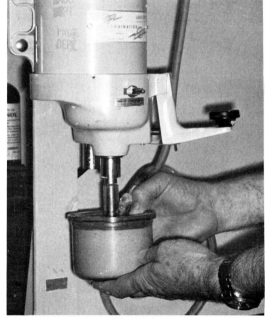
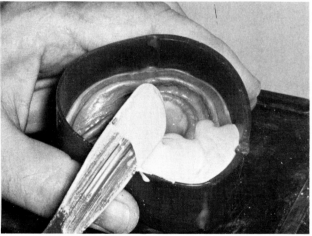

Fig. 3-16. A, Artificial stone is proportioned by weight and mixed with recommended volume of water in vacuum spatulator. Stone mixed under reduced atmospheric pressure results in cast that is dense and free of bubbles and voids. **B,** Boxed impression is placed on vibrator, and vacuum-mixed stone is added slowly at one corner of impression and permitted to flow over entire surface of impression. Initial pouring should be done slowly to minimize entrapment of air and resultant voids in master cast.

Table 3-1. Wax boxing method

Problem	Probable cause	Solution
Borders of cast too narrow or too wide	Beading wax too narrow or too wide	Make beading wax approximately 4 mm wide
	Cast overtrimmed on cast trimmer	Exercise care in adapting boxing wax to avoid reducing width of beading wax Be careful when trimming cast on cast trimmer
Border of cast not high enough to preserve thickness of impression flanges	Beading wax placed too high on impression	Adapt beading wax; seal it 3 to 4 mm below border of impression
Border of cast too high	Beading wax placed too low on impression	Place beading wax 3 to 4 mm below border of impression Trim cast to reduce border height
Base of master cast too thin (less than 13 mm in thinnest area)	Boxing strip is not extended high enough above impression	Extend boxing strip approximately 13 mm above highest area on impression
Base of master cast too thick (more than 13 mm in thickest area)	Boxing strip extended too high above impression	Keep boxing strip approximately 13 mm above impression and no higher.
Cast lopsided (high on one side and low on other side)	Impression not oriented properly prior to boxing	Position impression to make ridges approximately parallel to bench top; use soft wax or modeling clay to maintain position when boxing
Boxing wax separated from beading wax during pouring of cast	Beading wax not properly luted to boxing strip	Exercise care to see that boxing strip is luted to beading wax securely; use hot spatula to make watertight seal

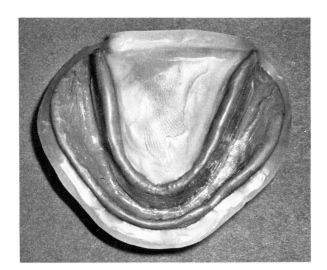

Fig. 3-17. Beading wax in posterior areas of impression is to narrow, and border of resultant cast will be too narrow. This error is difficult to correct.

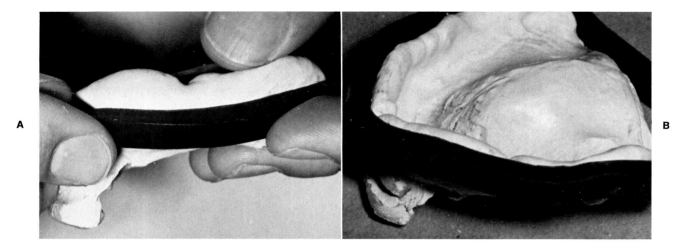

Fig. 3-18. **A,** Beading wax has been placed too low on impression. Border of cast will be too high and is likely to fracture on separation of impression from cast. **B,** Beading wax has been placed too high on impression. Border of cast will be too low and may not preserve thickness of impression.

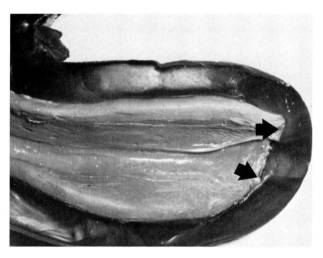

Fig. 3-19. Beading wax has been placed too high in heel area of mandibular impression (arrows). In this area, border of cast will be below surface of impression. Beading wax in heel areas of mandibular impressions always should be below impression. When beading and boxing impressions, it is always necessary to think in reverse, that is, if high on impression, it will be low on poured cast.

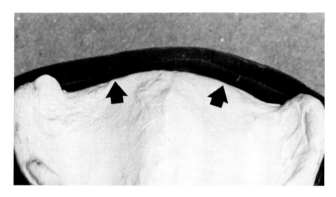

Fig. 3-20. Beading wax has been placed too high across posterior border of maxillary impression (arrows). In some instances, posterior border may be below surface of impression.

wax; otherwise, the resultant cast may be too thick or too thin. Although it is possible to reduce a thick cast by trimming, the presence of a split mounting plate complicates the trimming. It is more difficult to correct the error when a cast is too thin than when it is too thick, but it is best to avoid both situations. Occasionally, rough handling or excessive vibration during the pouring procedure may cause separation of the boxing wax from the beaded impression and make it necessary to reaccomplish the procedure. In this case, rinse the stone from the impression immediately.

Plaster of Paris and pumice boxing method

The plaster of Paris and pumice boxing method is excellent for boxing impressions of rubber base or silicone materials because maintaining contact between the boxing material and the impression material presents no problem.

PROCEDURE

1. Make a 1:1 mixture by volume of plaster of Paris* and flour of pumice, and stir thoroughly while dry to assure uniformity (Fig. 3-22). The pumice weakens the set plaster and facilitates separation of the cast after pouring. Approximately 200 gm of plaster usually is adequate for the majority of impressions.

---

*Laboratory Plaster, Whip-Mix Corp., Louisville, Ky., or equivalent.

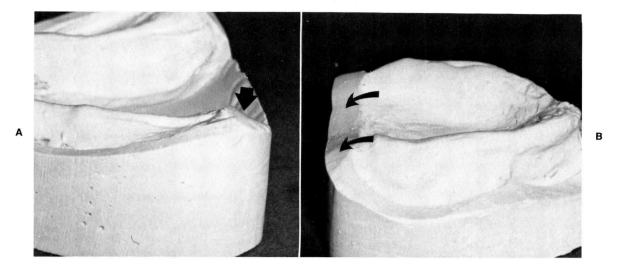

Fig. 3-21. A, Cast was poured in impression with beading wax placed incorrectly. Note that land area (arrow) is below surface of impression. B, Posterior border of maxillary impression was beaded incorrectly, and border of resultant cast is below surface of impression (arrows). It is necessary to think in reverse to determine effect on cast; placing beading wax too high on impression results in border that is too low on cast.

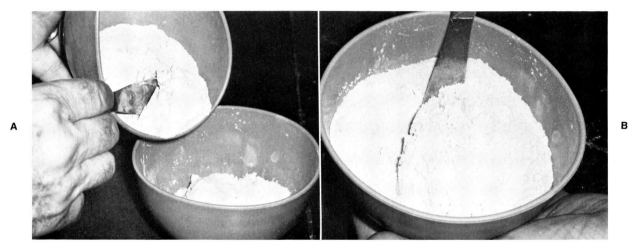

Fig. 3-22. A, Plaster of Paris and flour of pumice are mixed in approximately 1:1 ratio while dry. B, Plaster and pumice are mixed thoroughly with spatula before water is added.

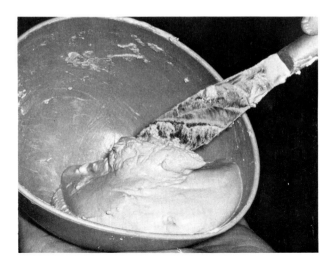

Fig. 3-23. Water is added to make stiff mix. It is spatulated thoroughly to reduce setting time.

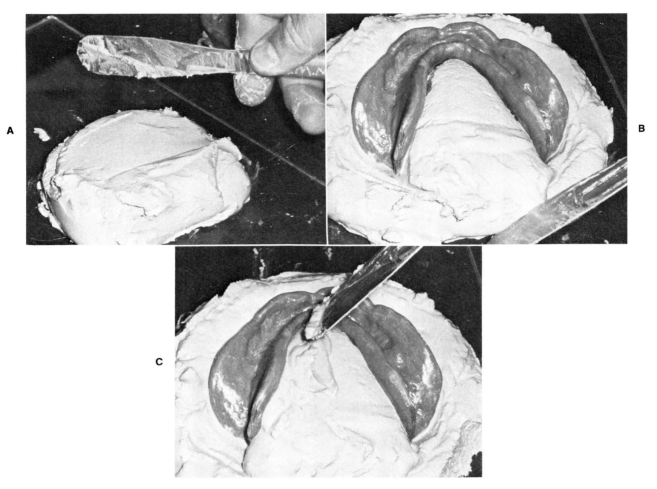

Fig. 3-24. A, Patty of plaster and pumice mix is placed on glass slab. **B,** Impression is settled into plaster and pumice patty gently, and ridge portion of impression is kept parallel to bench top. **C,** Spatula is used to draw the plaster and pumice mix to height of approximately 3 to 4 mm below border of impression.

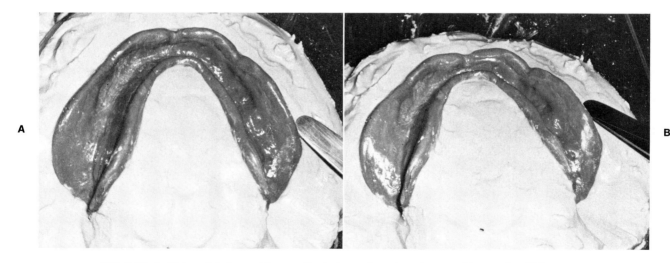

Fig. 3-25. A, Wet spatula is used to smooth plaster and pumice mix around impression. This procedure will result in cast with smooth surfaces in border area. **B,** Wet spatula should be handled carefully when smoothing plaster and pumice mix to keep plaster 3 to 4 mm high below border.

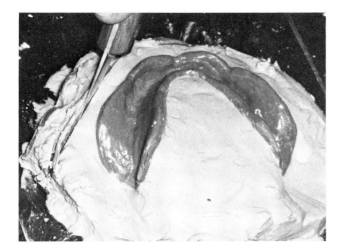

Fig. 3-26. As plaster and pumice mix begins to set, excess material can be cut away carefully with sharp knife. It should be done cautiously to prevent breakage of plaster and pumice mix.

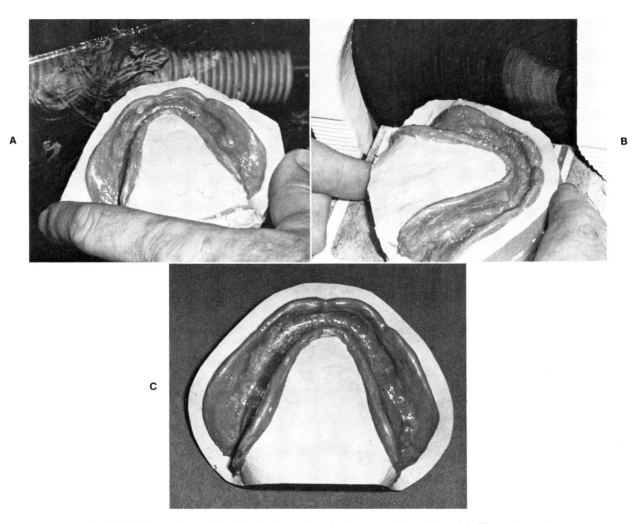

Fig. 3-27. A, Impression enclosed in plaster and pumice is removed from glass slab. Flowing tap water on glass slab and gently sliding impression off slab makes removal easy. **B,** Plaster and pumice boxing material is trimmed on cast trimmer until border is desired width. Care is required to keep from overthinning border. **C,** Impression boxed in plaster and pumice and with border trimmed to correct height and width.

2. Add enough water to make a stiff mix and spatulate thoroughly (Fig. 3-23).

3. Place a patty of the mix on a glass slab (Fig. 3-24, *A*).

4. Keeping the ridge portion of the impression parallel to the bench top, settle the impression into the patty (Fig. 3-24, *B* and *C*). Use a spatula to draw the plaster mix around the impression until it is 3 to 4 mm below the border.

5. Smooth the plaster mix around the impression with a wet spatula to make the border of the cast smooth (Fig. 3-25).

6. As the plaster and pumice mix begins to set, trim it to remove excess material. Do not trim closer than 5 to 6 mm (Fig. 3-26).

7. After the plaster has set, remove it from the glass slab, and trim it on a cast trimmer until the border is 4 mm wide (Fig. 3-27). Set the cast trimmer table to produce sides on the cast that are perpendicular to the base.

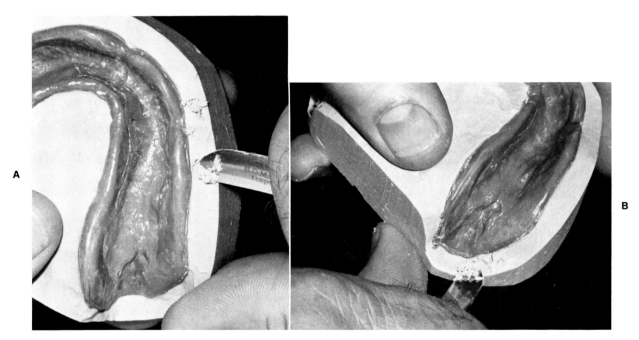

Fig. 3-28. A, Height of plaster and pumice boxing can be adjusted with sharp plaster knife. **B,** It is of primary importance to see that boxing in heel area of mandibular impression is below surface of impression.

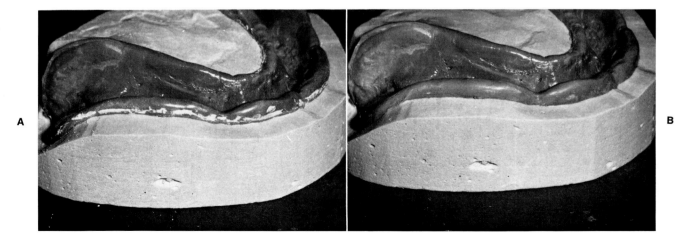

Fig. 3-29. A, After trimming with knife, some plaster still adheres to surface of impression. **B,** Plaster has been removed with soft-bristle toothbrush.

8. Trim the plaster with a sharp knife until it is 3 to 4 mm below the border of the impression. This is especially necessary in the heel region of mandibular impressions and across the posterior border of maxillary impressions (Fig. 3-28). In these regions the plaster may be 2 mm below the border.

9. Remove the plaster that adheres to the border of the impression by brushing gently with a soft-bristle toothbrush (Fig. 3-29).

10. Adapt the boxing wax to the invested impression so that the wax extends at least 13 mm above the highest point on the impression (Fig. 3-30).

11. Seal the boxing strip to the plaster with a hot spatula and wax (Fig. 3-31).

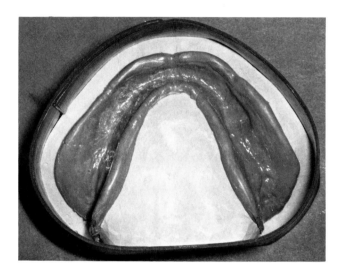

Fig. 3-30. Boxing wax adapted to invested impression should stand at least 13 mm above highest point on impression.

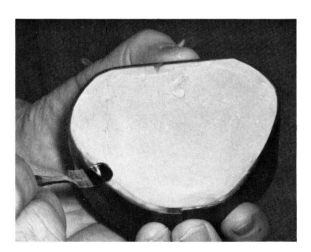

Fig. 3-31. Boxing wax strip is sealed to plaster and pumice investment with hot spatula.

12. Paint the plaster surfaces with a separating medium* (Fig. 3-32).

13. Fill the boxed impression with cool water to check for leaks. The water also wets the plaster, thereby minimizing voids in the stone cast that can occur when pouring stone onto dry plaster.

14. Proportion the stone by weight, according to the manufacturer's recommendation, mix it in a vacuum spatulator under reduced atmospheric pressure, and pour the cast (Fig. 3-33). Generally 200 gm of artificial stone is enough to pour most impressions, but large ones may require more.

15. After setting, cut away the plaster and pumice boxing, and remove the impression and cast.

16. Place the impression and cast in a plaster bowl containing warm water to soften the impression material, permitting separation without breaking the cast (Fig. 3-34). Do not overheat, or the compound may stick to the cast.

17. Using a sharp knife, reduce the height of the border on the cast where necessary (Fig. 3-35).

18. Adjust the width of the border of the cast on a cast trimmer until it is approximately 4 mm. Soak the cast in clear slurry water for 3 to 4 minutes before trimming it to prevent slurry splatter from the cast trimmer from sticking to the cast (Fig. 3-36). Trim the sides of the cast perpendicular to the base (Fig. 3-37).

19. The trimmed cast is ready for fabrication of the baseplate (Fig. 3-38).

---

*Super-Sep Separating Fluid, Kerr Manufacturing Co., Romulus, Mich.

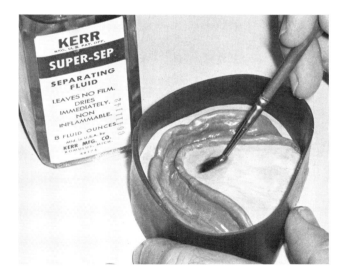

Fig. 3-32. Separating medium is painted on plaster and pumice investment. Failure to do this will allow cast to adhere to plaster and pumice investment and may result in breakage of cast on separation.

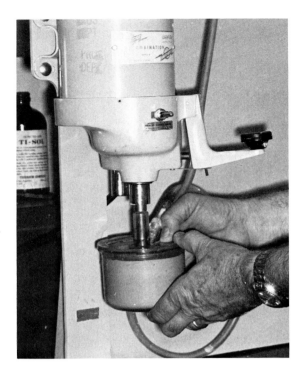

Fig. 3-33. Boxed impression is poured with artificial stone that has been mixed in vacuum spatulator under reduced atmospheric pressure. Usually 200 gm of artificial stone is adequate for boxed impression.

A 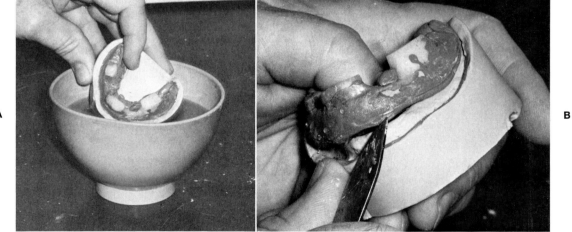 B

Fig. 3-34. A, Cast with impression is placed in plaster bowl containing warm water. This procedure will soften impression material and facilitate removal of impression from cast without breaking. **B,** After cast with impression is removed from warm water, impression is pried from cast gently. This procedure should be done slowly and carefully to prevent fracture of cast.

Fig. 3-35. Height of border on cast can be reduced where necessary with sharp knife.

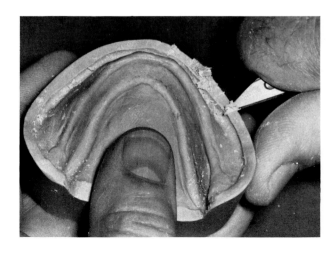

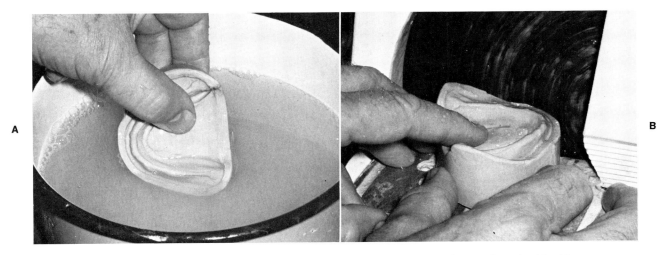

Fig. 3-36. A, Cast is soaked in clear slurry water prior to trimming on cast trimmer. Cast should not be dry when trimming on cast trimmer because splatter from cast trimmer will stick to cast, and removal will be difficult. **B,** Wet cast is trimmed on cast trimmer. Care should be exercised to see that border is not overtrimmed.

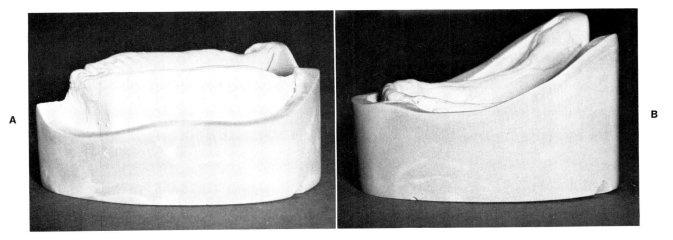

Fig. 3-37. A, Sides of casts are trimmed so that they are perpendicular to base. **B,** Mandibular cast has been trimmed so that sides are perpendicular to base.

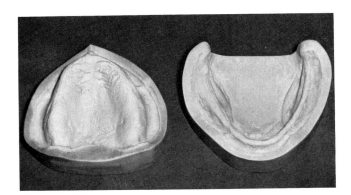

Fig. 3-38. Trimmed casts are ready for fabrication of baseplate.

PROBLEM AREAS

As in the wax boxing method, failure to make the plaster and pumice border the proper height or width results in a poor master cast (Table 3-2). The border of the cast should be 4 mm wide and 3 to 4 mm below the border of the impression. The boxing wax should be high enough above the impression (13 mm) so that the cast will be thick enough. The impression should be parallel to the bench top when settling into the plaster and pumice mixture to ensure that the base of the cast is of uniform thickness. The plaster should have a coat of separating medium before pouring the impression to avoid breaking the cast during separation. The boxing wax strip should not be overly soft prior to its adaptation to the trimmed plaster and pumice–encased impression. It is easy to distort an oversoft wax strip and thereby make the border of the cast too thin (Fig. 3-39). The impression and encasing plaster and pumice should soak in cool water for 3 to 4 minutes prior to pouring. This soaking will reduce the frequency of voids associated with pouring stone against a dry plaster and pumice surface. A good quality artificial stone,* proportioned by weight according to specification and preferably mixed in a vacuum spatulator under reduced atmospheric pressure, will prevent soft casts and voids.

Caulking compound and paddle boxing method

A paddle method for boxing impressions has been described by Blank (1961). The impression is boxed on a paddle, and wax or caulking compound* is used for beading. Then the paddle is used as a convenient holder while vibrating stone into the impression.

PROCEDURE

A table-tennis paddle can be adapted for boxing impressions by attaching metal stripping to the borders of the paddle (Fig. 3-40). Scrap wax is melted into the metal enclosure to serve as a wax base for boxing impressions (Fig. 3-41).

1. Use strips of caulking compound rope to bead impressions, particularly for those made in zinc-oxide impression paste (Fig. 3-42). Carefully adapt a strip of caulking compound rope 3 to 4 mm below the border of the impression (Fig. 3-43).

2. Adapt the caulking compound rope 2 to 4 mm be-

---

*Quickstone, Whip-Mix Corp., Louisville, Ky., or equivalent.

*DAP Rope Caulk, 3/16 inch (0.47 cm) round, Dap, Inc., Dayton, Ohio.

Table 3-2. Plaster of Paris and pumice boxing method

Problem	Probable cause	Solution
Border of cast too high or too low	Plaster of Paris and pumice on border of cast not trimmed to proper level or properly mixed	Trim plaster of Paris and pumice until 3 to 4 mm below border of impression
	Mix of plaster of Paris and pumice too thin, causing it to slump and make border too low on impression	Use thick mix of plaster of Paris and pumice to prevent slumping
Borders of cast too narrow or too wide	Plaster of Paris and pumice border of wrong width	Make plaster of Paris and pumice border approximately 4 mm wide; use thick mix so that plaster and pumice will not slump
Cast unable to be separated from plaster of Paris and pumice boxing	Separating medium not painted on plaster of Paris and pumice investment	Paint separating medium on plaster of Paris and pumice before pouring stone cast
Base of cast too high on one side and too low on other side	Impression not oriented properly prior to boxing	Position impression to make ridges approximately parallel to bench top before boxing
Base of cast too thick or too thin	Height of boxing strip wrong	Place boxing strip 13 mm above highest point on impression; cast too thin if boxing strip is less than 13 mm above; cast too thick if boxing strip is more than 13 mm above impression

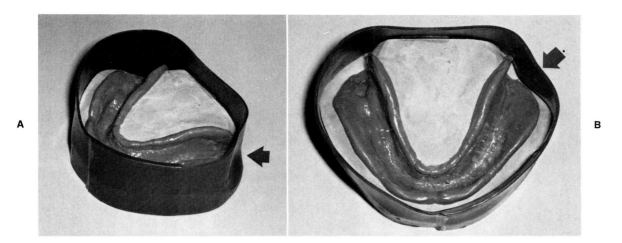

Fig. 3-39. A, Boxing wax was too soft when adapted to impression. Note concavity of boxing wax in heel area (arrow). **B,** Concavity, produced by adapting boxing wax that was too soft, will make cast too thin in heel area (arrow).

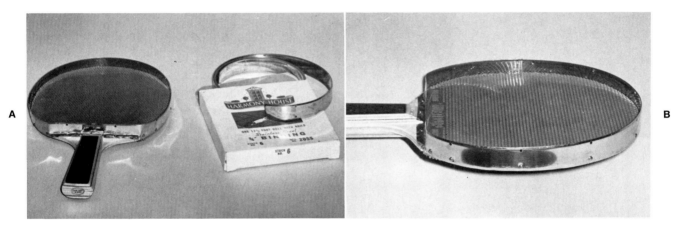

Fig. 3-40. A, Table tennis paddle can be adapted for holding boxed impressions by adding metal stripping. **B,** Table tennis paddle after attachment of metal stripping to borders.

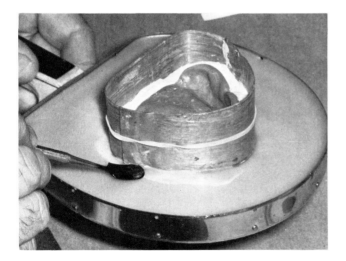

Fig. 3-41. Scrap wax melted into enclosure makes wax base for attaching boxed impression.

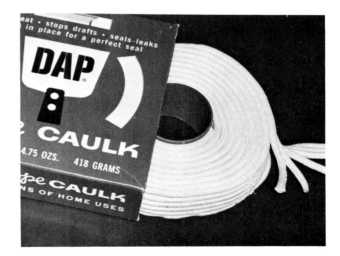

Fig. 3-42. Caulking compound rope is suitable for beading impressions, particularly for those made in zinc-oxide impression pastes.

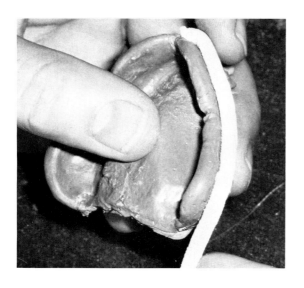

Fig. 3-43. Caulking compound rope is aligned carefully 3 to 4 mm below border of impression.

A

B

Fig. 3-44. A, Strip of caulking compound rope is adapted below level of impression, as in wax beading method. B, Note position of caulking compound rope below level of impression.

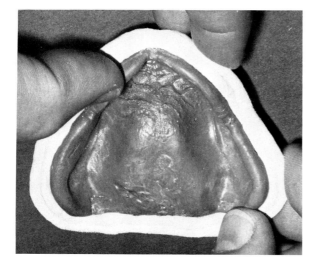

Fig. 3-45. If necessary, another strip of caulking compound rope can be placed over first strip to increase width of border.

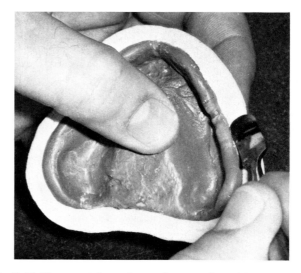

Fig. 3-46. Warm spatula can be used to smooth caulking compound and to seal it to impression.

low the posterior border of maxillary impressions and the heel region of mandibular impressions (Fig. 3-44).

3. If the single caulking strip is too narrow, place another strip over the first one to make the border of the cast 4 to 5 mm wide (Fig. 3-45).

4. Burnish the caulking compound with a warm wax spatula to make the border smooth and to seal it to the impression (Fig. 3-46).

5. Check the width of the caulking compound border before boxing with a wax or metal strip (Fig. 3-47).

6. Fold a metal boxing strip carefully around the impression and caulking cord, and secure it with a rubber band. Make certain that the boxing strip extends approximately 13 mm above the highest point on the impression (Fig. 3-48). Have the ridges of the impression approximately parallel to the top edge of the boxing strip and the bench top.

7. Seal the caulking compound to the metal or wax boxing strip on the impression side and the underside. A warm spatula aids in sealing (Fig. 3-49).

8. Check the boxed impression for the width and height of the border before sealing it to the paddle (Fig. 3-50).

9. Seal the boxed impression securely to the wax on

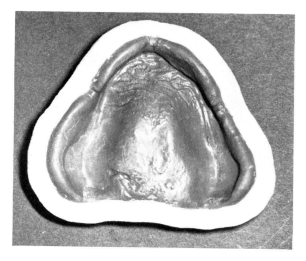

Fig. 3-47. Width and height of caulking compound beading is evaluated before applying boxing strip.

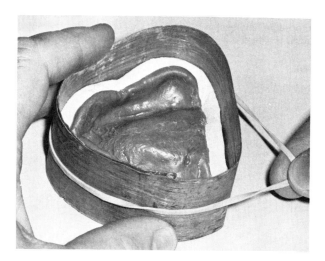

Fig. 3-48. Metal boxing strip is adapted gently to caulking compound beading and secured with rubber bands. It is essential that boxing extend at least 13 mm above highest point on impression.

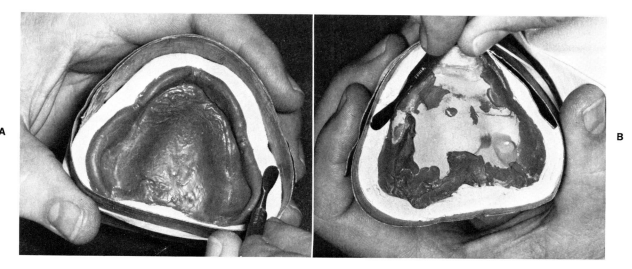

Fig. 3-49. A, Warm spatula is used to seal caulking compound to metal boxing strip. **B,** Caulking compound is adapted closely to metal strip on underside also.

Table 3-3. Caulking compound and paddle boxing method

Problem	Probable cause	Solution
Borders of cast too high or low	Beading placed at wrong level	Place beading material approximately 3 to 4 mm below border of impression
Borders of cast too narrow or wide	Beading too narrow or wide	Keep beading approximately 4 mm wide; exercise care in adapting boxing strip to avoid compressing or narrowing beading
	Cast overtrimmed on cast trimmer	Exercise care when trimming on cast trimmer
Base of cast too thick or thin	Boxing wax at wrong height border of impression	Place boxing strip approximately 13 mm above border of impression
Cast lopsided	Alignment of impression wrong when boxed	Position impression to make ridges nearly parallel to bench top

cial stone,* some dentists may prefer an improved stone.† To achieve the best possible physical properties of a particular stone, it is necessary to proportion it by weight and mix it with the specified amount of water. Mixing the stone in a vacuum spatulator under reduced atmospheric pressure makes the stone mix and cast superior. The resultant stone mix is smooth and free of air bubbles, and the cast is strong and dense.

PROCEDURE

1. Proportion the stone by weight, and add it to the recommended amount of water (Fig. 3-57). Usually, 200 gm of stone is ample for pouring the majority of boxed impressions.
2. Spatulate the stone under reduced atmospheric pressure for 10 to 25 seconds (Fig. 3-58). Usually spatulation for 20 to 25 seconds is sufficient, but it is necessary to follow the manufacturer's recommendations for individual stones.
3. Vibrate the mix into the boxed impression. Add stone in only one area of the impression, and tilt the impression on the vibrator to allow stone to flow over the entire impression, thereby minimizing voids (Fig. 3-59).
4. Continue adding stone until the boxed impression is full (Fig. 3-60)
5. Allow the poured impression to set before separating the cast. Many dental stones set hard enough to separate between 45 minutes and 1 hour after mixing.
6. Trim the border of the cast, as described previously (Fig. 3-61).

PROBLEM AREAS

The principal problems when pouring casts relate to improper powder-water ratios, which can result in a markedly inferior, soft cast of inadequate strength (Table 3-4). Incorporating voids or air bubbles during pouring and incorrect trimming of the poured cast also can be problems. Omission of the separating medium can result in broken casts when using the plaster and pumice boxing method. Adherence to the powder-water ratios recommended by the manufacturer (weighing the artificial stone and mixing it with the recommended amount of water), mixing in a vacuum spatulator under reduced atmospheric pressure, and careful pouring technique contribute to producing strong, dense casts with superior surfaces.

Careful attention when trimming the cast on the cast trimmer will result in fewer overtrimmed borders. Wetting the cast in clear slurry water prior to trimming will reduce the incidence of slurry splatter sticking to the cast, which is difficult to remove. A separating medium always should be painted on the plaster and pumice boxing prior to pouring the stone cast.

INDEXING THE CAST

Indexing casts prior to mounting them in an articulator permits removal of the casts and accurate replacement in the articulator. Indexing is particularly helpful during remounting procedures, such as when correcting processing errors after curing a denture. Indexed casts also are useful during the split-cast method for verifying jaw relation records. Grooves, notches, or special metal* or plastic remounting plates are placed in the cast for indexing (Fig. 3-62).

*Quickstone, Whip-Mix Corp., Louisville, Ky., or equivalent.
†Vel Mix, Kerr Manufacturing Co., Romulus, Mich.

*Split Remounting Plate Assembly Complete, Teledyne Dental Products Co., Hanau Division, Buffalo, N.Y.

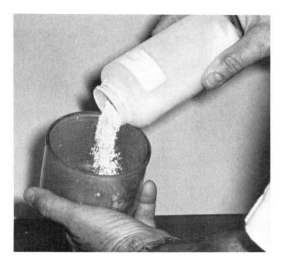

Fig. 3-57. Artificial stone is proportioned by weight and mixed with recommended amount of water. Usually 200 gm of stone is ample for impression.

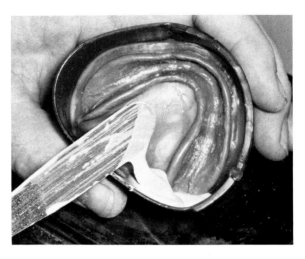

Fig. 3-58. Artificial stone mixed in vacuum spatulator under reduced atmospheric pressure is used to pour cast.

A 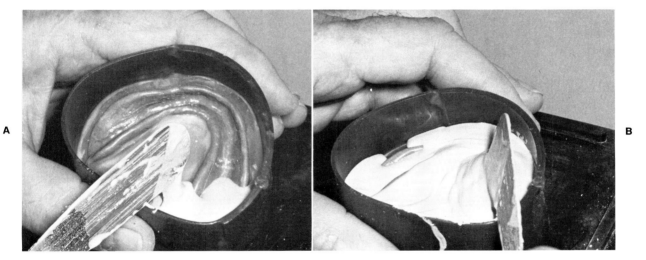 B

Fig. 3-59. A, Boxed impression is tilted on vibrator when stone is added initially. **B,** Stone is always added in same area and allowed to flow over entire surface of impression to preclude formation of voids.

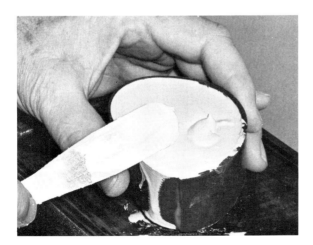

Fig. 3-60. Stone is added until boxed impression is full.

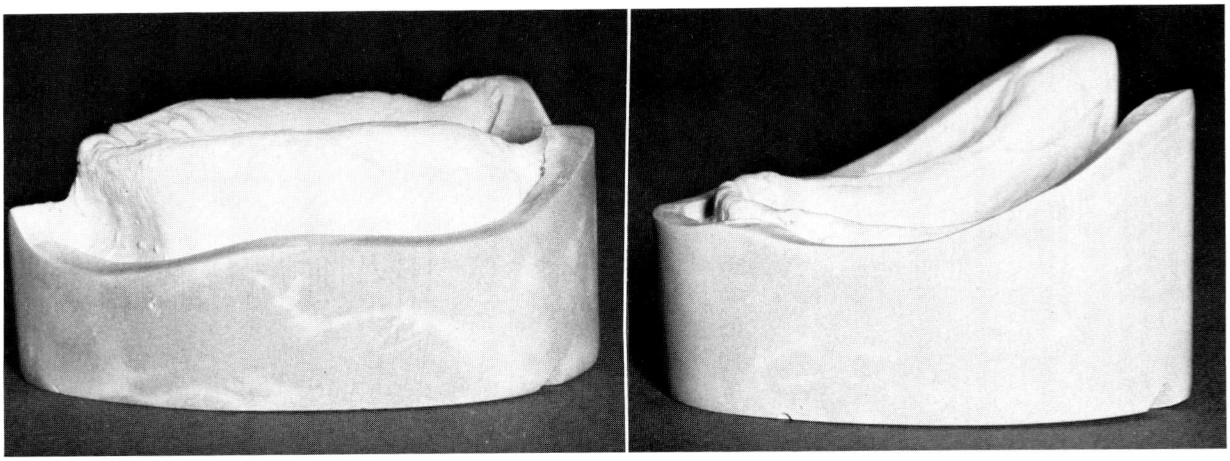

Fig. 3-61. A, Maxillary cast with sides trimmed perpendicular to base. **B,** Mandibular cast with sides trimmed perpendicular to base.

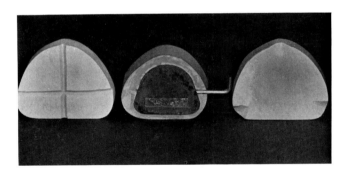

Fig. 3-62. Indexing can be accomplished by placing grooves in cast *(left),* by using metal remounting plates *(center),* or by notching cast *(right).*

Table 3-4. Pouring the cast

Problem	Probable cause	Solution
Surface of cast too soft and not strong enough	Powder-water ratio wrong	Adhere to powder-water ratio recommended by manufacturer; weigh stone and mix with recommended amount of water; mix in vacuum spatulator under reduced atmospheric pressure
Numerous voids in cast	Vacuum spatulator not used	Mix stone in vacuum spatulator under reduced atmospheric pressure
Cast rough from slurry splatter	Cast not wet in clear slurry water before and during trimming on cast trimmer	Dip cast in clear slurry water before trimming on cast trimmer and repeat frequently during trimming procedure to prevent slurry splatter from sticking to cast

Requirements for indexing

It is axiomatic that the indexing should not weaken the cast so that it breaks during routine laboratory procedures. Neither grooves nor notches used for indexing should be undercut to form a mechanical lock with the mounting stone. The indexing should remain functional in the event that the size of the cast must be reduced to fit the flask at the time of processing (Fig. 3-63). The index should provide a positive three-dimensional fit between the cast and mounting stone, permitting easy

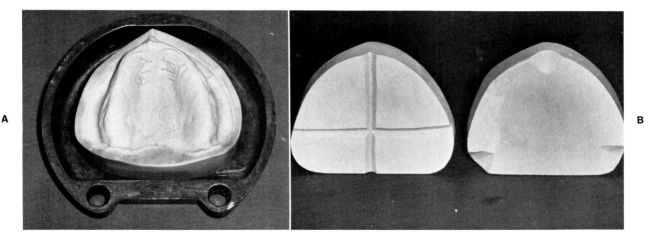

Fig. 3-63. A, Occasionally, cast must be reduced in size to fit within confines of denture flask. **B,** When it is necessary to reduce size of cast to fit within flask, groove indexing *(left)* is preferable to notch indexing *(right)*. Although cast on left can be reduced significantly, enough of groove will be left to allow remounting on original articulator mount. Cast on right (with notch indexing) can be reduced to point at which notches are eliminated, making it impossible to remount on original articulator mount.

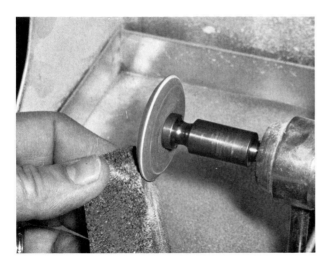

Fig. 3-64. Lathe-mounted wheel should be shaped with trueing stone to create V-shape edge.

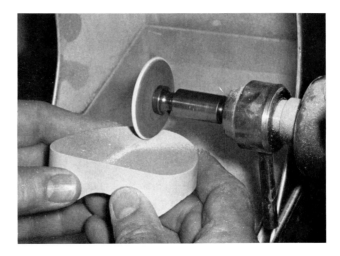

Fig. 3-65. One groove is placed in center of base of cast from front to back with lathe-mounted wheel.

removal and accurate replacement without damage to the cast or mounting. It should be possible to do the indexing easily and rapidly with the equipment and materials generally available.

Groove indexing method

Indexing a cast by grooving the base of the cast with a lathe-mounted wheel offers several advantages. Contouring the lathe wheel will produce a smooth V cut without undercuts. Groove indexing allows reduction of the cast border if necessary while retaining a positive index. It is possible to modify the position of the index groove as needed to avoid thin areas in the cast.

PROCEDURE

1. Shape the lathe-mounted wheel* with a trueing stone to make a V-shape edge (Fig. 3-64).
2. Groove the center of the base of the cast from front to back with the wheel (Fig. 3-65).
3. Groove the rest of the cast perpendicular to the first groove, intersecting approximately in the center of the cast (Fig. 3-66).
4. Where lingual flanges result in thin areas on man-

---

*No. 21 Green Line lathe wheels 3 inches × ⅜ inch (7.6 × 0.97 cm) Buffalo Dental Manufacturing Co., Brooklyn, N.Y.

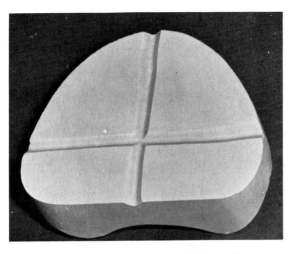

Fig. 3-66. Another groove is placed perpendicular to first groove and intersecting approximately in center of cast.

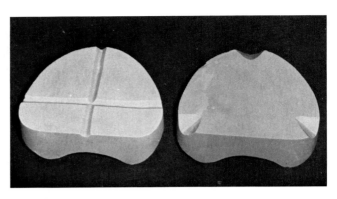

Fig. 3-69. Groove indexing, *left,* is preferable to notch indexing, *right.*

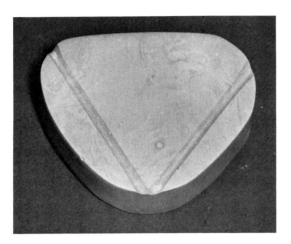

Fig. 3-67. Deep lingual flanges in mandibular impressions occasionally produce thin areas in cast. Breakage of thin areas can be avoided by placing groove directly opposite thickest areas of cast and parallel to ridges.

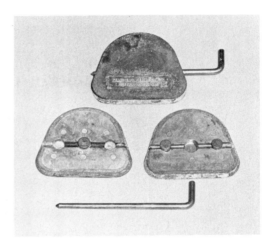

Fig. 3-70. Split remounting plates within master cast offer advantages. They permit rapid removal of cast from articulator and replacement on it. Contact between cast and mounting stone is made through precisely fitting metal plates.

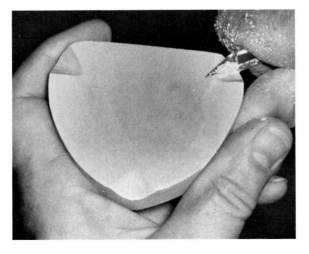

Fig. 3-68. Notches can be placed at widely separated points on cast with lathe-mounted wheel or sharp knife.

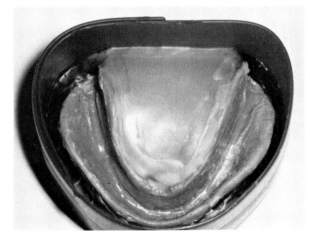

Fig. 3-71. Impression is boxed by method of choice.

dibular casts, place the grooves opposite the ridges in thicker portions of the cast (Fig. 3-67).

Notch indexing method

Notches cut in the base of the cast at three or more points provide a positive index. The notch method is especially suitable for split-cast jaw relation record verification techniques. This method has a potential disadvantage in the event that it is necessary to reduce the cast significantly to fit in a flask. In this instance, the removal of peripheral notches can result in the loss of the index.

PROCEDURE

Notch the base of the cast in the anterior midline and in the right and left distobuccal regions. Use a lathe-mounted wheel or sharp knife to make smooth non-undercut notches (Fig. 3-68).

PROBLEM AREAS

The principal problems in the groove or the notch method of indexing casts are making the grooves or notches too deep, thereby weakening the cast, and undercutting the notches or grooves, resulting in mechanical locks between the cast and mounting stone (Table 3-5). As discussed earlier, it is necessary to reduce the size of a cast occasionally to fit a flask. Cutting away notch indexing in these instances will eliminate the index; as a result, the groove method is preferable (Fig. 3-69).

SPLIT REMOUNTING PLATES

Split remounting plates offer several advantages compared to groove or notch indexing methods (Fig. 3-70). Contact between the cast and mounting stone is through precisely fitting metal plates, which also permit rapid removal and replacement of the cast in the articulator. The dentist or technician can remove the cast from the mounting, set teeth, adjust the position of the teeth or wax the denture, and replace it on the articulator quickly to check the occlusion.

The principal disadvantages are the cost of remounting plates and the time required both to place them in the cast and retrieve them from the cast and mounting stone after completing the denture.

PROCEDURE

1. Box the impression by the method of choice (Fig. 3-71).
2. Make a split-plate positioning aid by embedding one section of a split remounting plate in a 6 × 6 inch (15.2 × 15.2 cm) sheet of Plexiglas ½ inch (1.2 cm) thick. Embed this section of the plate flush with the surface of the Plexiglas, with the indexing surface up (Fig. 3-72).
3. Cut a groove in the plastic plate to accommodate the pin that secures both sections (Fig. 3-73).
4. Attach the opposing section of the split remounting plate to the embedded half, and use a pin to secure it (Fig. 3-74).
5. Position the sheet of Plexiglas with the remounting plate attached over the boxed impression to center the plate over the impression (Fig. 3-75). A small notch cut in the boxing wax will hold the metal pin.
6. Pour the boxed impression in stone (Fig. 3-76).
7. Place more stone in the undercuts of the remounting plate attached to the sheet of Plexiglas (Fig. 3-77).
8. Center the sheet of Plexiglas and the remounting plate over the poured impression (Fig. 3-78).
9. Gently settle the sheet of Plexiglas onto the boxed impression. Since the edges of the boxing wax are visible through the sheet of Plexiglas, it is easy to center the remounting plate in the cast (Fig. 3-79).
10. After setting, remove the pin and lift the Plexiglas

Table 3-5. Indexing the cast

Problem	Probable cause	Solution
Cast broken by improperly cut index	Indexing grooves too deep	Place indexing grooves with trued lathe mounted wheel; make them approximately 3/16 inch (0.47 cm) deep
Cast unable to be separated from mounting stone	Indexing notches or grooves undercut or separating medium not applied prior to mounting	Do not incorporate undercuts in grooves or notches; paint separating medium on cast base prior to mounting
Lingual flange area of cast perforated by indexing groove	Indexing groove too deep	Do not make groove too deep; in mandibular cast with deep lingual extensions, place grooves opposite ridges, not in thinner portions of cast

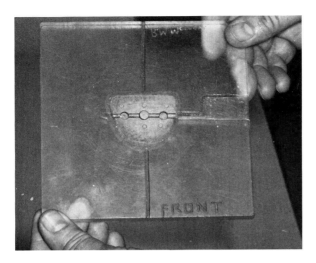

Fig. 3-72. A 6 × 6 inch (15.2 × 15.2 cm) sheet of Plexiglas ½ inch (1.25 cm) thick with one section of split remounting plate embedded in it aids considerably in placing split remounting plates in cast.

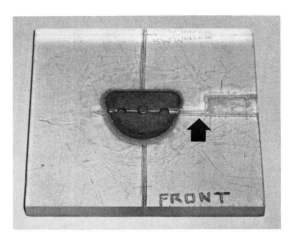

Fig. 3-73. Sheet of Plexiglas with embedded section of remounting plate. Note groove cut in remounting plate for pin (arrow).

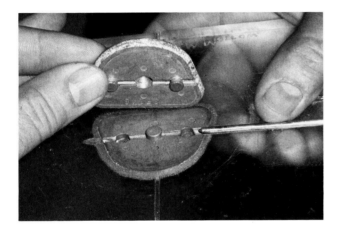

Fig. 3-74. Opposing section of split remounting plate is attached to embedded half and secured in position with pin.

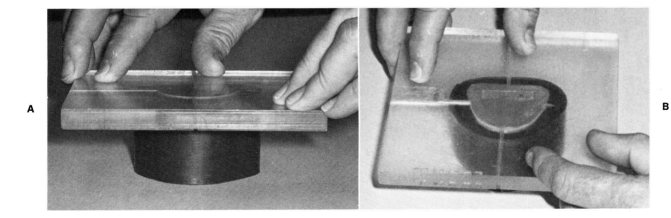

Fig. 3-75. A, Sheet of Plexiglas with remounting plate attached is placed over boxed impression to center remounting plate in boxed impression. **B,** Sheet of Plexiglas facilitates centering of metal remounting plate.

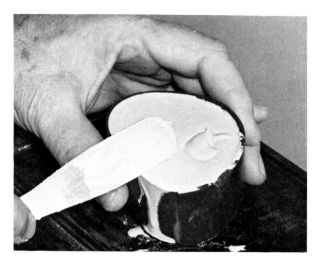

Fig. 3-76. Boxed impression is poured in stone, as described in Fig. 3-59.

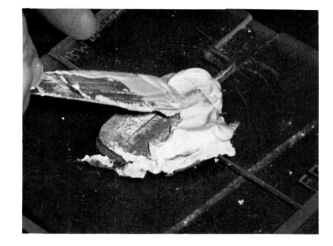

Fig. 3-77. More stone is wiped into undercuts of split remounting plate attached to sheet of Plexiglas.

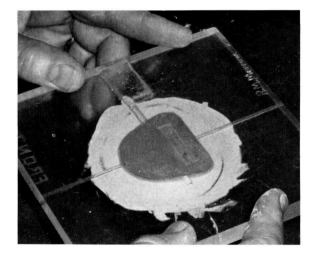

Fig. 3-78. Sheet of Plexiglas with remounting plate attached is centered over boxed impression and settled into place.

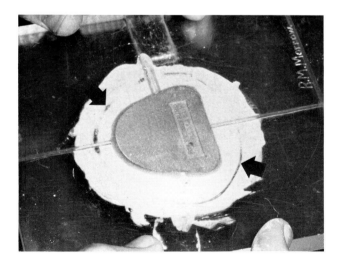

Fig. 3-79. Note edges of boxing wax visible through sheet of Plexiglas. Transparency of Plexiglas facilitates centering of remounting plate in cast.

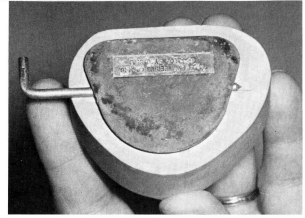

Fig. 3-80. A, After setting of stone, pin is removed, and Plexiglas is separated from cast. **B,** Other section of remounting plate is attached to section of remounting plate embedded in cast, and pin is inserted. **C,** Split remounting plate is mounted in maxillary cast. Removal of pin permits rapid separation and replacement of cast in articulator mounting.

Table 3-6. Split remounting plates

Problem	Probable cause	Solution
Remounting plate sinking into stone while being placed in cast	Sheet of Plexiglas not used to suspend remounting plate	Use 6 × 6 inch (15.2 × 15.2 cm) sheet of Plexiglas ½ inch (1.25 cm) thick during setting of stone
Remounting plate too far off-center	Sheet of Plexiglas not used to suspend and align remounting plate	Use 6 × 6 inch (15.2 × 15.2 cm) sheet of Plexiglas ½ inch (1.25 cm) thick to aid in centering remounting plate
Remounting plate loose in cast	Stone not in intimate contact with remounting plate	Use spatula to wipe stone into all border areas of remounting plate; once in position, do not disturb it until stone sets
Cast too thick or thin	Height of boxing wax wrong	Exercise care in making boxing wax approximately 13 mm above highest point on impression

positioner from the cast. Attach the other section of the remounting plate to the section in the cast in preparation for mounting (Fig. 3-80).

PROBLEM AREAS

In the split remounting plate method, it is difficult to keep the metal remounting plates from sinking into the stone without using a plexiglass split-plate positioner (Table 3-6). Another problem is failure to center the remounting plate. Failure to place stone in the undercut of the remounting plate during the pouring procedures can allow voids, which may cause the plate to move slightly within the cast. If the boxing wax is more than 13 mm above the highest point on the impression, the cast can be too thick. The only solution is to remove the remounting plates and thin the cast. Removal of the remounting plates to correct cast thickness can weaken the cast. For the best results, it is essential to use the Plexiglas positioner, place stone around the borders of the split remounting plates to minimize voids, and center the remounting plates when pouring.

SUMMARY

This chapter describes three methods of boxing impressions, techniques for pouring and trimming casts, and methods of indexing casts with grooves, notches, and remounting plates. Since casts are the direct link between laboratory and clinical procedures, it is axiomatic that a properly boxed, poured, and trimmed cast is essential for a successful restoration.

REFERENCES

Air Force Manual 160-29 Dental Laboratory Technicians Manual, Washington, D.C. 1959, U.S. Government Printing Office.

Blank, H. H.: Impression materials for maxillary immediate dentures, J. Prosthet Dent. 11:414-419, 1961.

Bolouri, A., Hilger, T. C., and Gowrylok, M. D.: Boxing impressions, J. Prosthet. Dent. 33:692-695, 1975.

Boucher, C. O.: Swenson's complete dentures, ed. 5, St. Louis, 1964, The C. V. Mosby Co.

Harris, L. W.: Boxing and cast pouring, J. Prosthet. Dent. 10:390, 1960.

Heartwell, C. M., Jr., and Rahn, A. O.: Syllabus of complete dentures, ed. 2, Philadelphia, 1974, Lea & Febiger.

Sowter, J. B.: Dental laboratory technology, prosthodontic technique, Chapel Hill, N.C., 1968, The University of North Carolina Press.

CHAPTER 4

BASEPLATES AND OCCLUSION RIMS

KENNETH D. RUDD and ROBERT M. MORROW

baseplate *(record base, temporary base, trial base)* A temporary form representing the base of a denture. The baseplate is used for making maxillomandibular (jaw) relation records, arranging artificial teeth, or trial placement in the mouth.

stabilized baseplate A baseplate lined with a plastic, or other material, to improve its adaptation and stability.

occlusion rim An occluding surface built on temporary or permanent denture bases for the purpose of making maxillomandibular records and arranging teeth.

Keyworth (1929) states that the purposes of baseplates are (1) to act as carriers for occlusal rims on which jaw relations are recorded, (2) to hold the teeth in the wax setup for the try-in stage, and (3) to check the accuracy of the previously recorded records.

Dentists use the baseplates and attached occlusion rims to transmit important information to the dental laboratory technician. Jaw relationships, the midline, occlusal plane, high and low lip line, cuspid line, amount of horizontal and vertical overlap, and desired support for lips and cheeks can be indicated on the baseplate and occlusion rim (Fig. 4-1). The success of a dentist's treatment depends on the accurate communication of this information. Therefore it is essential that baseplates meet specific requirements for the liaison between dentist and dental technician to be effective.

REQUIREMENTS FOR BASEPLATES

Elder (1955) gave the following requirements for baseplates:

1. The baseplate should adapt to the basal seat area as the finished denture base.
2. The baseplate should have the same border form as the finished denture base.

3. The baseplate should be sufficiently rigid to resist biting forces.
4. The baseplate should be dimensionally stable.
5. The baseplate as constructed should permit its use as a base for setting up teeth.
6. It should be possible to construct baseplates quickly, easily, and inexpensively.
7. Baseplates should have no undesirable color.

Tucker (1966) added that the baseplate should not abrade the cast during removal and replacement; it should take advantage of desirable undercuts and be of a material that bonds with that used to block out undercuts on the cast so that it becomes part of the baseplate.

Baseplates should fit the cast accurately, be sufficiently rigid to resist closing forces, and have sufficient dimensional stability to maintain fit and ridigity throughout the clinical and laboratory procedures used in denture construction. Although they should satisfy these requirements, unduly thick baseplates might encroach on the space available for setting teeth. They should be of an acceptable color, and the borders should be smooth, rounded, and similar to those of the prospective denture. Removal of the baseplate from the cast or replacement should cause no damage to either.

BASEPLATE MATERIALS

Materials used, singly or in combination, for constructing baseplates are autopolymerizing resins, shellac baseplate material, thermoplastic resins, heat-curing resins, baseplate wax, and metal. Zinc-oxide impression paste, elastomeric impression materials, and hard- or soft-curing resins are other types of material used in combination to stabilize baseplates by improving their

82

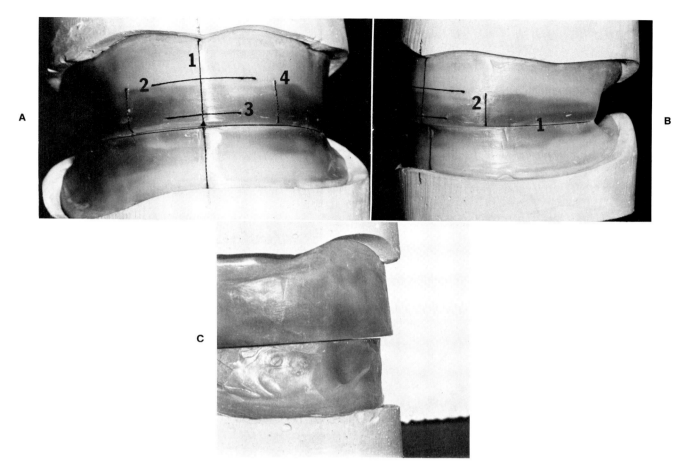

Fig. 4-1. A, Baseplates and attached occlusion rims indicate midline *(1),* high and low lip line *(2* and *3),* cuspid line *(4),* and support desired for lips and cheeks in addition to jaw relation records. **B,** Side view of baseplates and occlusion rims indicates occlusal plane *(1)* and cuspid line *(2).* **C,** Alignment and position of anterior teeth are determined by contour of wax occlusion rim. Note horizontal overlap in anterior region.

adaptation and rigidity. Lining the baseplate with soft-curing resins* and elastomeric impression materials† permits extension of the baseplate into moderate undercuts and removal or replacement of the baseplate on the cast without damage to either.

AUTOPOLYMERIZING RESIN BASEPLATES

Autopolymerizing resins (cold-curing or self-curing resins‡ require an activator and a catalyst for polymerization and no external heat. They are readily available at a reasonable cost, set hard and rigid or soft and flexible according to the formulation, and take color satisfactorily. Generally, their handling characteristics are suit-

able for constructing baseplates that are both serviceable and economical. Therefore autopolymerizing resins, singly or in combination, probably are the materials used most frequently for baseplates. Four methods of construction from these materials will be described.

Sprinkle-on method

The sprinkle-on method is excellent; it consists of coating the cast with tinfoil substitute, sifting polymer powder on it, and saturating it with liquid monomer. Alternate applications of powder and liquid continue until the baseplate is of the desired thickness. It is essential that this method be performed in a hood or a well-ventilated area to minimize exposure to resin fumes. Placing the baseplate in a pressure pot* or under an inverted

---

*Coe-soft, Coe Laboratories, Inc., Chicago, Ill., or equivalent.
†Kerr Permlastic, Kerr Manufacturing Co., Romulus, Mich., or equivalent.
‡Acralite 88, Kerr Manufacturing Co., Romulus, Mich.: Caulk Repair Material, L. D. Caulk Co., Milford, Del., or equivalent.

---

*Acri-Dense Pneumatic Curing Unit, Coe Laboratories, Inc., Chicago, Ill., or equivalent.

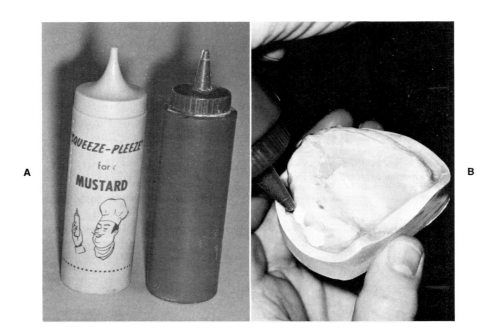

Fig. 4-9. A, Plastic mustard or catsup dispensers make excellent sifters for acrylic resin powder. **B,** Autopolymerizing resin powder is sifted onto cast before it is saturated with monomer. Use nonfibered powder, which sifts readily without clogging.

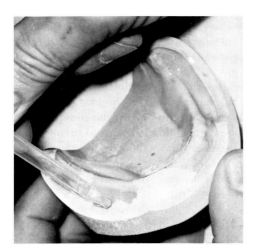

Fig. 4-10. Eyedropper is used to control amount of monomer applied.

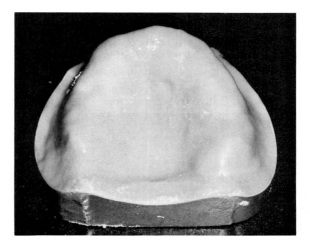

Fig. 4-11. Autopolymerizing resin has been built up to thickness of approximately 2 mm and is ready to be cured.

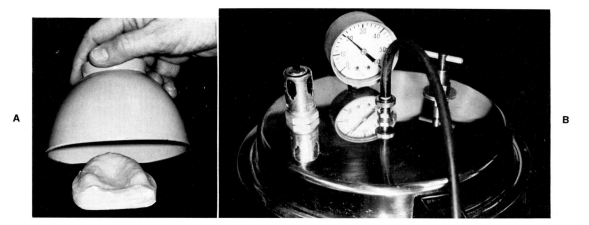

Fig. 4-12. A, Curing baseplate under plaster bowl significantly reduces porosity and makes it fit well. **B,** Curing baseplate under increased pressure reduces porosity, but does not seem to fit cast as well as baseplate cured at atmospheric pressure.

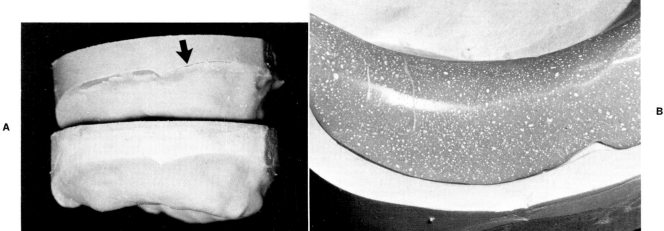

Fig. 4-13. Baseplates constructed from autopolymerizing resin. **A,** Upper baseplate cured in pressure pot does not fit cast (arrow) as well as lower baseplate cured under plaster bowl at atmospheric pressure. **B,** Baseplates cured in open air may demonstrate considerable surface porosity.

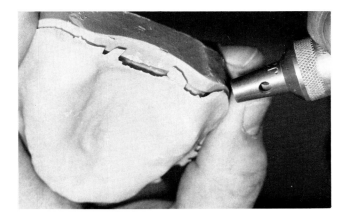

Fig. 4-14. When undercuts are minimal or are blocked out properly, cured baseplate often can be removed from cast by directing stream of air at border.

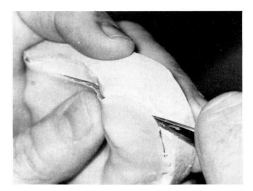

Fig. 4-15. If necessary to pry baseplate from cast, do it gently and on side opposite undercuts to prevent breakage of cast.

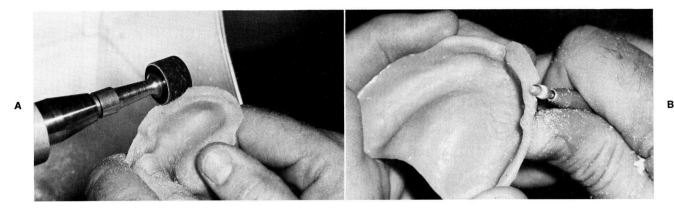

Fig. 4-16. A, Arbor band on lathe can be used to reduce resin flash. Protective goggles should be worn. **B,** Excess resin can be trimmed with suitable bur in handpiece.

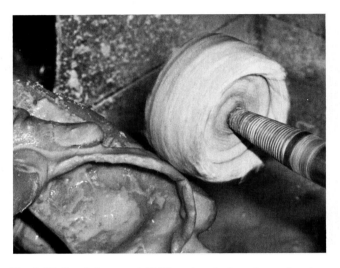

Fig. 4-17. Slow lathe speed (1740 rpm) and adequate pumice slurry reduce buildup of heat in baseplate, minimize warpage, and expedite polishing. Protective goggles should be worn.

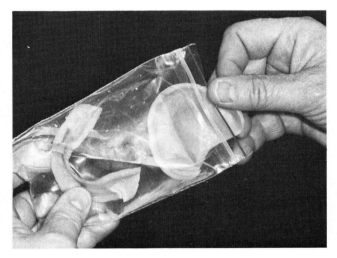

Fig. 4-18. Self-sealing plastic bag containing water or diluted mouthwash is excellent for storing completed baseplate.

10. Smooth the borders and any rough spots on the baseplates with a wet rag wheel and a slurry of water and flour of pumice. A slow speed (1740 rpm) on the lathe with plenty of pumice slurry reduces the buildup of heat in the baseplate during polishing and speeds the procedure (Fig. 4-17). Heat built up as a result of polishing can warp the baseplate and ruin its adaptation. Usually a "high shine" on the baseplate is not essential, since the surface is smooth enough after pumicing. Additional polishing can warp an otherwise satisfactory baseplate.

11. Store the finished baseplate in water until ready for use (Fig. 4-18).

PROBLEM AREAS

Several problems can arise with the sprinkle-on method. The problems, their probable causes, and solutions are presented in Table 4-1.

1. It is impossible to remove the baseplate from the cast without breaking one or both during separation. A common cause of this problem is failure to identify and block out undercuts on the cast adequately. Blockout of extensive undercuts is essential because soft-curing resin can compensate for only moderate undercuts. Examine the cast carefully for undercuts, and note their depth and extent. Use a surveyor to locate the undercuts. Block out extensive undercuts with wax and confirm the blockout. When applying soft-curing resin to moderate undercuts, make certain that it is thick enough, remains in place, and does not flow out of the undercut before applying the conventional resin. Soft-curing resin must be thick enough and in the proper position to protect the cast. Failure to coat the cast or coating it with contaminated tinfoil substitute makes the baseplates stick to the cast tenaciously, usually resulting in damage to the cast on

Table 4-1. Sprinkle-on method

Problem	Probable cause	Solution
Baseplate unable to be removed from cast	Undercuts not properly blocked out	Use soft-curing resin on baseplate for only moderate undercuts; block out extensive undercuts with wax
Baseplate broken during removal	Cast not coated with uncontaminated tinfoil substitute	Coat cast with uncontaminated tinfoil substitute before adding resin
Cast chipped or broken during removal	See above	Make soft-curing resin thick enough; prevent displacement by hard-setting resin
Both cast and baseplate broken during removal	See above	See above
Baseplate too thick in some areas and too thin in others	Resin flow not controlled by tilting cast during application	Control resin flow by tilting cast while sprinkling on powder; exercise care in sifting powder on prominent cast areas; use enough powder to prevent flow of mixture
Completed baseplate too flexible	Ratio of soft-cure resin in undercut areas to hard-setting resin too high	Use only enough soft-curing resin to fill undercut; apply adequate layer of hard-setting resin over it
	Wrong liquid or powder used for hard-setting resin	Use correct powder and liquid for both hard-setting and soft-curing acrylic resins
	Baseplate removed from cast too soon; polymerization not completed	Allow adequate time for baseplates to set before removing from cast
	Baseplate to thin or ridge flat	Reinforce baseplates for flat ridges by wire embedded in resin
Baseplate porous	Some areas allowed to dry when resin is applied to cast	Keep all areas moist with monomer to prevent drying when applying resin
		Cure baseplate in pressure pot or under inverted plaster bowl
Failure of baseplate to fit cast	Baseplate removed from cast before polymerization completed	Adequately cure resin before attempting to remove baseplate from cast
	Baseplate heated by grinding or polishing	Do not overpolish; use slow speeds and ample flour of pumice and water while polishing
	Baseplate stored in dry environment	Store completed baseplate in water
	Baseplate warped from prying when removed from cast	Block out undercuts on cast to avoid need for prying baseplate from cast with resultant warping

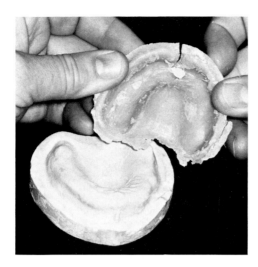

Fig. 4-19. Cast coated improperly with tinfoil substitute; both baseplate and cast broke.

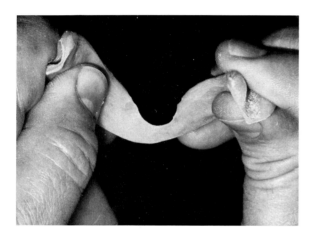

Fig. 4-20. This cured baseplate is too flexible, probably as result of using too much soft-curing autopolymerizing resin or making baseplate too thin.

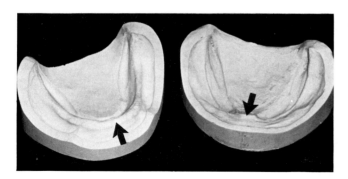

Fig. 4-21. Mandibular cast, *left,* has a well-formed anterior ridge (arrow). Cast on right has especially flat anterior ridge (arrow). Inverted U shape of left cast facilitates construction of rigid baseplate. Flat ridge on right cast will require reinforcement.

separation (Fig. 4-19). Coating the cast with uncontaminated tinfoil substitute before adding the resin will prevent this problem. Pour the tinfoil substitute from the bottle into a container before using, and discard any unused portion. Do not dip the brush into the main storage bottle or return the unused portion into the storage bottle; this will avoid contaminating and ruining its effectiveness.

2. The baseplate is too thick in some areas and too thin in others. This variation is a common defect, particularly in maxillary baseplates in which the palate is too thick and the ridge areas are too thin. Failure to tilt the cast allows the saturated resin to flow from the ridge areas into the palate or vestibules of the cast. Tilting the cast during the sprinkle-on procedure minimizes this problem. Care in sifting polymer on the cast can prevent thin areas. Avoid fumes from the acrylic resin monomer by constructing the baseplate in a hood or some other well-ventilated area.

3. The completed baseplate is too flexible. This condition can occur when the ratio of soft-curing resin in the undercut areas to overlying hard-setting resin is too high (Fig. 4-20). The overlying layer of conventional resin is too thin to give the necessary strength and rigidity. Using the wrong liquid or powder for the overlying hard-setting resin occasionally makes the baseplate flexible. Inadvertent use of soft-curing resin liquid with the conventional powder will keep the resultant baseplate from setting properly and make it entirely too flexible. For adequate rigidity, place sufficient hard-setting resin over the soft-curing resin, and clearly identify the liquid and powders for each resin system. After applying the soft-curing resin to the cast, set the containers aside to pre-

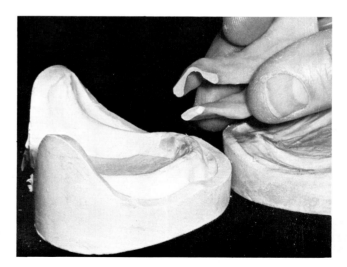

Fig. 4-22. Cross section of top baseplate made on left cast results in greater rigidity than cross section of bottom baseplate made on right cast.

vent their accidental use when applying the conventional resin. If a mandibular cast has an extremely flat ridge in the anterior region, the baseplate constructed on this cast will not be rigid, even after correct application of the resin (Fig. 4-21). A cross section of the baseplate does not have the usual inverted U form in the anterior region with its inherent rigidity (Fig. 4-22). Reinforcing the baseplate with a stiff wire embedded in the resin and extending from premolar to premolar materially improves its strength and increases its rigidity (Fig. 4-23).

4. The completed baseplate is unsightly and too porous. A slight amount of surface porosity in the completed baseplate usually is not a critical defect. Extensive porosity that penetrates to the tissue surface of the baseplate can be a problem because it reduces the rigidity and makes the baseplate unhygienic. Using high-quality autopolymerizing resins and keeping the surface of the resin moistened with monomer during the sprinkle-on procedure minimize porosity. Once started, the sprinkle-on procedure should continue to completion. Do not allow the resin to dry out in one area while adding some in another. Placing the baseplate under an inverted plaster bowl or in a humidor during polymerization also reduces the surface porosity. Pressure-pot curing usually eliminates porosity problems.

5. The completed baseplate does not fit the cast. Adaptation to the cast is critical for acceptability of the baseplate. If the baseplate does not fit the cast, it must be remade. This situation can occur when the baseplate is too flexible as discussed previously, when removal from the cast takes place before adequate polymerization, when the baseplate warps as a result of grinding

and polishing, and when the environment used for storing is too dry. Warping of the baseplate also can occur if the cast is not wet when placed in the curing pot, or if considerable prying is needed to separate the cured baseplate from it. To minimize warpage and construction of an unacceptable baseplate, avoid the previously discussed causes of flexibility. Allow the baseplate to polymerize before removing it from the cast, and do not overpolish it. If prying is necessary to remove it from the cast, do it gently opposite the undercuts.

Finger-adapted dough method

An alternate method of making resin baseplates is the finger-adapted dough method. Instead of sprinkling on powder and saturating it with monomer, mix the powder and liquid together until the mixture is the consistency of dough, form it into a roll or sheet, and adapt it to the cast with finger pressure. A modification of this method is to roll the dough in a sheet of the desired thickness before adapting it to the cast (Fig. 4-24). Although some prefer finger adaptation, which may be quicker than the sprinkle-on method of constructing baseplates, it has several disadvantages. First, unless using gloves, needless repeated contact with resin during adaptation may lead to contamination of the resin or, more importantly, result in contact dermatitis. Second, it is exceedingly difficult to achieve uniform thickness of the baseplate by hand adaptation. Invariably, the resin is too thin over the convex ridge portions and too thick in the less accessible areas. Third, usually it is necessary to continue finger adaptation throughout polymerization to prevent rebound or lift-off of the resin, but this manipu-

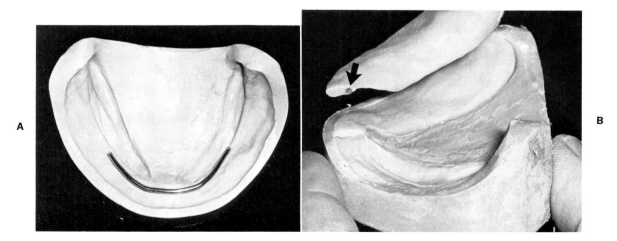

Fig. 4-23. A, Reinforcing wire is adapted to cast lingual to crest of ridge. Note that lingual position prevents interference when setting teeth. **B,** Cross section of baseplate reinforced with wire (arrow). Note position of wire toward lingual border of baseplate.

lation can cause distortion. Finger adaptation also can displace soft-curing resin used to fill in undercuts.

PROCEDURE

1. Identify the undercuts, and decide whether to use wax or soft-curing resin for blockout. Blockout considerations are the same for the finger-adapted dough method as for the sprinkle-on method.

2. Apply tinfoil substitute to the cast.

3. Put baseplate wax in severe undercuts and soft-curing resin in moderate undercuts.

4. Proportion and mix the resin powder and liquid according to the manufacturer's recommendations. When the mixture is in the dough stage, form the resin

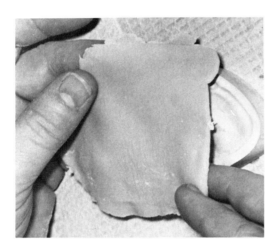

Fig. 4-24. Baseplate resin has been rolled into sheet approximately 2 mm thick before being adapted to cast.

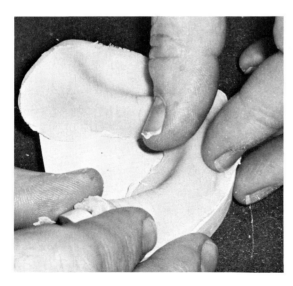

Fig. 4-25. Once resin has reached dough stage, it is formed into roll and adapted to cast.

into a roll, and adapt it to the cast (Fig. 4-25). The resin baseplate should be approximately 2 mm thick. It is possible to make a convenient mold by impressing a double thickness shellac baseplate into a mix of artificial stone (Swenson, 1970) (Fig. 4-26). After the stone has set, remove the baseplate and use the resultant mold to shape a resin sheet of uniform thickness into a baseplate (Fig. 4-27). An alternate, and excellent, procedure is to roll the dough into a sheet of the desired thickness,* trim it to the shape of a baseplate, and adapt it to the cast (Fig. 4-28).

5. Regardless of which method is used, continue finger adaptation until the resin, being well adapted to the cast, does not spring away or rebound (Fig. 4-29).

6. Place the baseplate on the cast under a plaster bowl or in a pressure pot for polymerization, as described previously.

7. After curing, remove the baseplate from the cast, trim it, and smooth it.

8. Replace the baseplate on the cast, and evaluate the adaptation and border thickness (Fig. 4-30). Store the completed baseplate in water until needed.

---

*Rollette Unit, Kerr Manufacturing Co., Romulus, Mich.

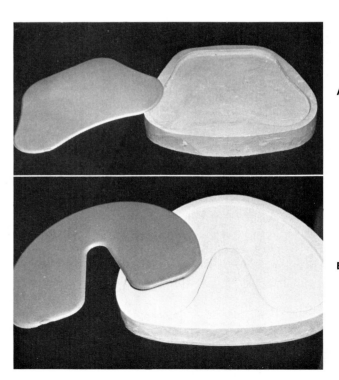

Fig. 4-26. A, Convenient mold can be made by impressing double-thickness shellac baseplate into mix of artificial stone. **B,** Resultant mold is used to make acrylic resin baseplate form for adaptation to cast.

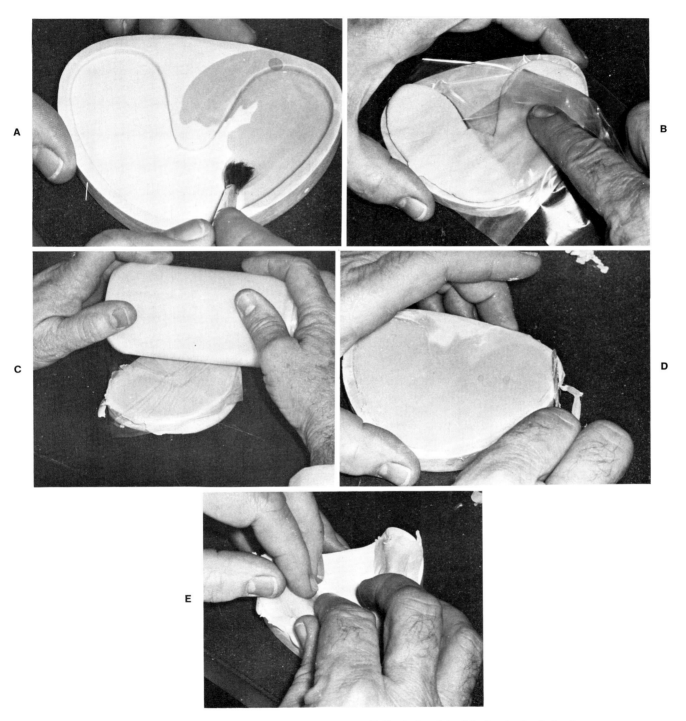

Fig. 4-27. A, Stone mold is coated with tinfoil substitute. **B,** Resin dough is picked up in sheet of cellophane and placed into stone mold. **C,** Resin dough is rolled out to desired thickness. In this instance, plastic bottle is used as roller. **D,** Excess resin is trimmed with spatula. **E,** Resin baseplate is removed from mold and adapted to cast. Continue finger adaptation until resin loses rebound and retains adaptation.

A

B

C

D

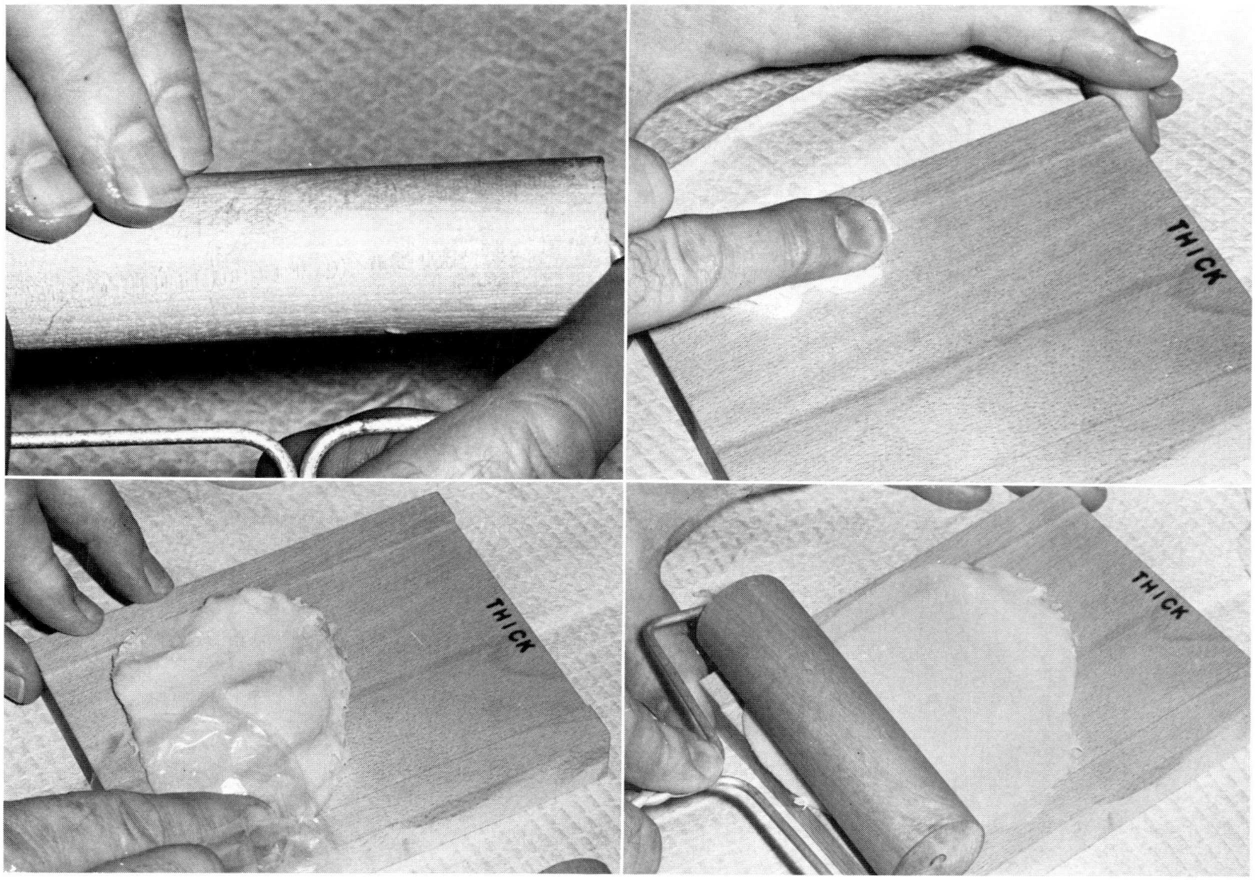

Fig. 4-28. A, Wooden roller is coated with silicone lubricant to keep resin from sticking. **B,** Wooden tray also is coated with silicone lubricant to keep resin from sticking as sheet is rolled to desired thickness. **C,** Use sheet of cellophane to prevent finger contact with resin dough. **D,** Resin dough is rolled to uniform thickness.

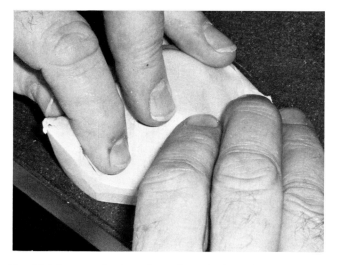

Fig. 4-29. In any method used to make resin sheet, finger adaptation must be continued until resin is well adapted to cast; resin should not spring away or rebound.

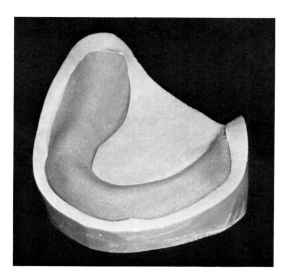

Fig. 4-30. Baseplate fit and adaptation are checked on cast. This baseplate is well adapted.

Table 4-2. Finger-adapted dough method

Problem	Probable cause	Solution
Failure of baseplate to fit cast	Resin beyond dough stage before finger adaptation started	Adapt resin when in dough stage
	Finger adaptation of resin discontinued too early	Continue finger adaptation of resin until it no longer springs away from cast
Baseplate too thin in some areas and too thick in others	Convex areas too thin as result of finger pressure	Do not place too much pressure over convex ridge areas when adapting resin
	Resin not rolled to desired thickness before applying to cast	Roll resin into sheets of proper thickness before adapting to cast

PROBLEM AREAS

The principal problems associated with this method are achieving and maintaining the accurate adaptation to the cast and the uniform thickness of the baseplate (Table 4-2).

1. The completed baseplate does not fit the cast. If the resin progresses beyond the dough stage before starting finger adaptation, it is difficult to obtain intimate contact between the cast and baseplate. The resin becomes rubbery and has a pronounced rebound that defies permanent adaptation. Finger molding the resin at the proper stage is essential because once it reaches the rubbery stage, accurate adaptation by finger pressure is impossible (Fig. 4-31). Finger adaptation must continue until the resin no longer springs away from the cast.

2. The baseplate is too thin in some areas and too thick in others because of inherent difficulties associated with finger molding. Convex areas are excessively thin as a result of finger pressure, and depressions or inaccessible areas are too thick. Care should be taken in molding to avoid placing too much pressure over convex ridge areas. Roll the resin to the desired thickness before adapting it to minimize the thick and thin spots.

Confined dough methods

Investigators have suggested various methods for confining or applying pressure to the autopolymerizing resin during baseplate construction. Elder (1955) has applied pressure with modeling plastic, LaVere and Freda (1974) have confined the resin with wax, and Assadzadik and Yarmond (1975) have made a stone index to mold the baseplate. Their method offers excellent control of thickness, reduced finishing time, and minimal porosity. The disadvantages of this method are an increase in the time required to make the mold and a tendency to form voids in the baseplate.

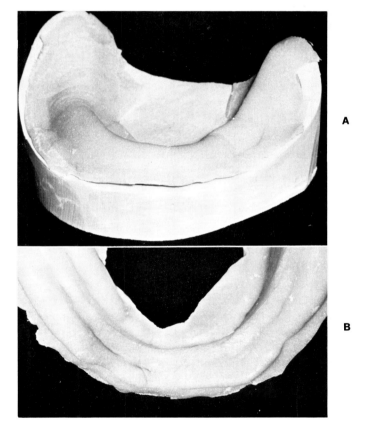

A

B

Fig. 4-31. A, Baseplate did not fit cast, because resin was beyond dough stage before finger adaptation was started. **B,** Interior view of poorly adapted baseplate. Wrinkles, folds, and lack of adaptation make baseplate unacceptable.

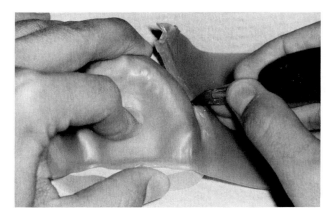

Fig. 4-32. One layer of baseplate wax is adapted to cast and trimmed to size.

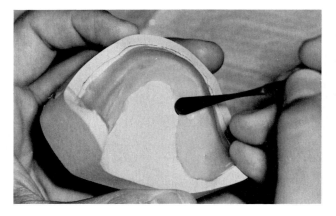

Fig. 4-33. Additional wax is added to fill in borders, and wax pattern is sealed to cast. Borders of cast are marked with pencil to serve as guide when waxing.

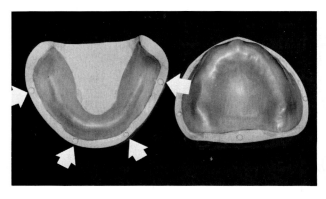

Fig. 4-34. Index indentations are placed at four widely separated points (arrows) on land area of cast. They can be made with large round bur.

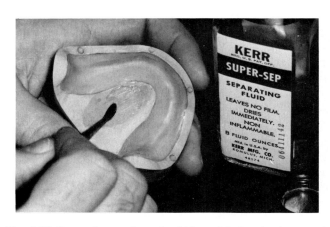

Fig. 4-35. Separating medium should be painted on land areas of stone cast.

Stone-mold method
PROCEDURE

1. Adapt one layer of baseplate wax over the cast, and seal it around the borders to form a wax pattern for the proposed baseplate (Fig. 4-32). Fill in the borders of the baseplate with additional wax to make them of the proper thickness (Fig. 4-33). This pattern should duplicate the finished baseplate in thickness and contour; placing additional wax in undercut areas or over the midline on maxillary casts can increase the thickness.

2. Place index indentations on the land area of the cast at four widely separated points with a large round bur (Fig. 4-34).

3. Paint separating medium on the stone land areas (Fig. 4-35).

4. Box the cast and pattern with boxing wax (Fig. 4-36). This wax should extend above the cast to make the stone at least 15 mm thick (Fig. 4-37).

5. Mix artificial stone with slurry concentrate* to accelerate the set, and vibrate it onto the boxed cast and pattern (Fig. 4-38).

6. Allow the boxed stone to set.

7. After setting, remove the stone index (Fig. 4-39), and lift the wax pattern from the cast (Fig. 4-40).

8. Paint tinfoil substitute on the cast and stone index (Fig. 4-41).

9. Reassemble the index and cast to check the fit (Fig. 4-42).

10. Block out undercuts on the cast with wax or soft-curing resin, as previously described (Fig. 4-43).

11. Proportion the autopolymerizing resin, and mix

---

*Slurry concentrate is a thick mixture of water and stone grindings obtained from a cast trimmer. The collected slurry is allowed to settle overnight, and the clear solution is poured off, leaving a clear layer approximately 1 inch (2.54 cm) thick. The resultant slurry concentrate accelerates the set when mixed with artificial stone.

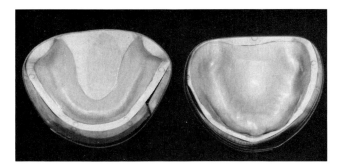

Fig. 4-36. Cast and wax pattern are boxed with boxing wax before pouring stone.

A 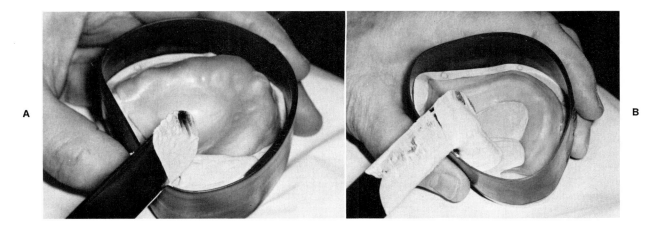 B

Fig. 4-37. A, Boxing wax should extend approximately 15 mm above wax pattern to allow stone to be thick enough to prevent breakage. **B,** Artificial stone is mixed with slurry water to accelerate set and poured onto boxed cast and pattern.

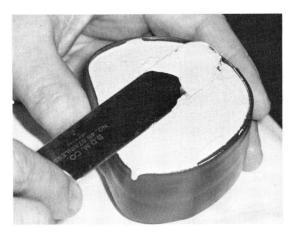

Fig. 4-38. Surface of poured index is smoothed with spatula.

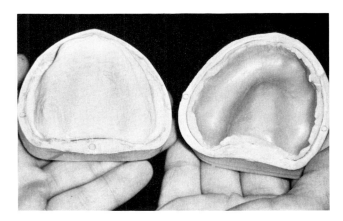

Fig. 4-39. After setting, stone index is separated from cast.

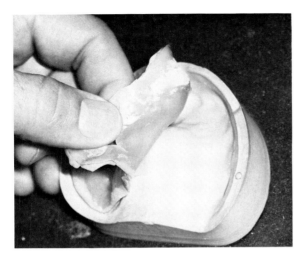

Fig. 4-40. Wax pattern is removed, and care is taken to remove all traces of wax from cast and index.

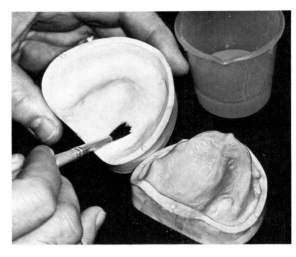

Fig. 4-41. Tinfoil substitute is painted onto cast and stone index. Soak cast and index in clear slurry water before painting.

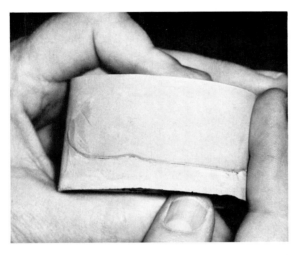

Fig. 4-42. Cast and index are assembled and examined critically to determine fit.

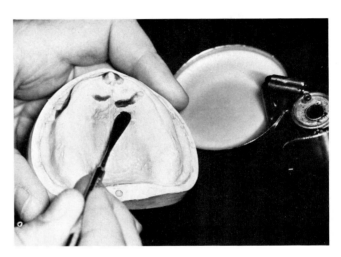

Fig. 4-43. Cast undercuts are blocked out with wax or soft-curing autopolymerizing resin. Adequate blockout assures removal of baseplate from cast without fracturing baseplate or damaging cast.

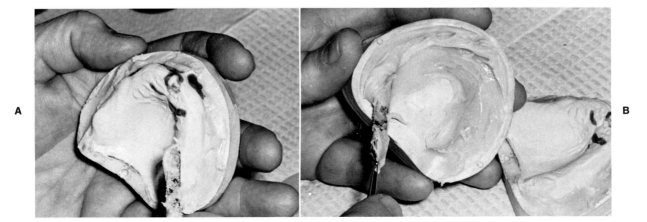

Fig. 4-44. A, Autopolymerizing resin is mixed and applied to cast with spatula. Care should be taken to place resin into peripheral roll to prevent voids. **B,** Additional resin is applied to interior of index with spatula. Careful application of resin to index and cast will reduce voids in completed baseplate.

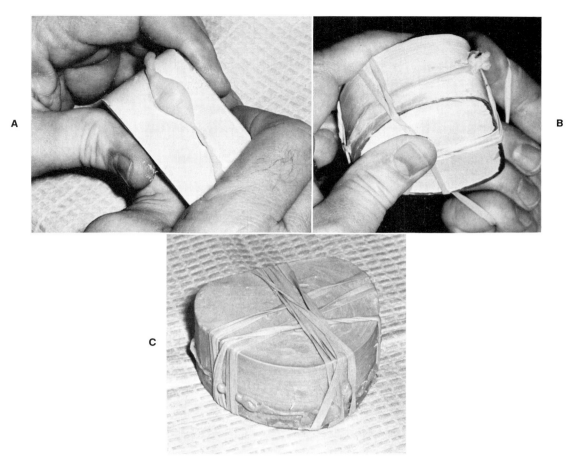

Fig. 4-45. **A,** Cast and index are assembled, and finger pressure is used to express excess resin. Adequate force should be used to achieve stone-to-stone contact because failure to do so would make baseplate too thick. **B,** Heavy rubber bands placed around assembled index and cast assure maintenance of pressure while curing. **C,** Heavy rubber bands in place.

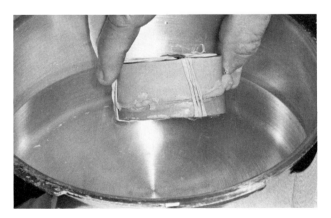

Fig. 4-46. Curing can be accomplished in pressure pot at 20 psi for 20 minutes, or enclosed resin can be bench cured.

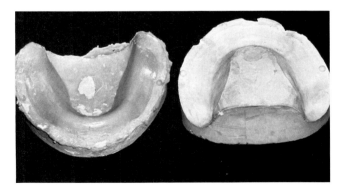

Fig. 4-47. After curing, index and cast are separated, and baseplate is removed, finished, and polished. Note smooth surface on baseplate produced by stone index.

according to the manufacturer's recommendations. When the mix reaches the dough stage, mold it onto the cast (Fig. 4-44). Usually, 8 to 10 ml of monomer and 24 to 30 ml of polymer are enough; use excess resin to minimize voids.

12. Assemble the index and cast, and maintain closure with heavy rubber bands (Fig. 4-45).

13. Cure the mold in a pressure pot in warm water at 20 psi for 20 minutes or bench cure it (Fig. 4-46). Confinement and pressure from the stone index greatly reduce porosity.

14. After the resin has hardened, open the mold, remove the baseplate, and finish it (Fig. 4-47). Generally, only minimal finishing is necessary.

PROBLEM AREAS

Problems are usually improper thickness of the stone index, failure to include adequate resin in the mold, and failure to close the mold completely (Table 4-3).

1. The stone index breaks under pressure when closing the mold. The probable causes are too thin a stone index; failure of the stone to set before pressure is applied; use of too much water in the stone mix making it soft; or use of resin beyond the dough stage when attempting to close the mold. The stone index should be at least 13 to 15 mm thick. Make certain that the stone has set before packing the resin, and pack it only at the dough stage.

2. The baseplate has voids (Fig. 4-48). The prob-

Table 4-3. Confined dough methods: stone mold method

Problem	Probable cause	Solution
Breaking of stone index when pressure applied to close mold	Stone index too thin	Make stone index at least 13 to 15 mm thick
	Stone not completely set before pressure applied	Let stone set before packing resin
	Improper powder-water ratio used when mixing stone for index	Use proper powder-water ratio
	Resin too stiff before attempting to close mold	Pack resin at dough stage
Voids in completed baseplate	Insufficient resin for filling mold	Mix sufficient resin to overfill mold slightly
Baseplate too thick	Mold not completely closed, resulting in thicker baseplate	Pack mold with resin at proper stage to assure closing of mold

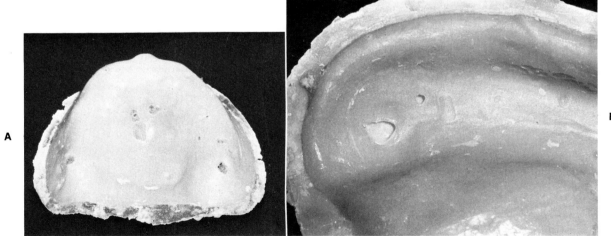

Fig. 4-48. A, Resin baseplate with voids, probably caused by use of insufficient resin in mold during packing or by entrapment of air. Smaller voids can be easily repaired. **B,** Small nonperforating voids on tissue surface of baseplate can be repaired with autopolymerizing resin.

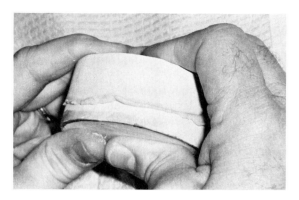

Fig. 4-49. Baseplate will be too thick because cast and index were not closed completely.

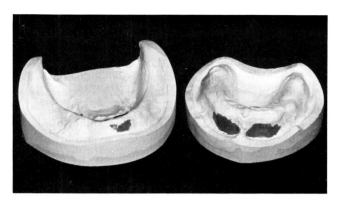

Fig. 4-50. Undercuts should be blocked out with wax prior to adaptation of wax tray.

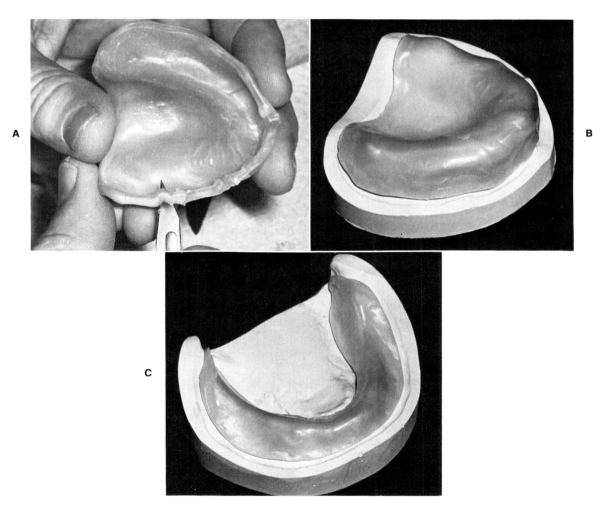

Fig. 4-51. A, Wax tray is trimmed 2 mm short of borders of cast. **B,** Maxillary wax tray on cast is approximately 2 mm short of border reflections. **C,** Mandibular wax tray on cast is trimmed approximately 2 mm short of border reflections.

Table 4-4. Confined dough methods: wax-confined method

Problem	Probable cause	Solution
Resultant baseplate too thin	Wax tray with resin seated too firmly on cast	Seat wax tray with resin so as to form layer of resin approximately 1 to 2 mm thick
Resultant baseplate too thick	Wax tray improperly seated on cast	Same as above
Resin on exterior wax surface of baseplate	Resin inadvertently placed on exterior wax when adapting borders	Carefully adapt and smooth resin borders to keep exterior wax free of resin

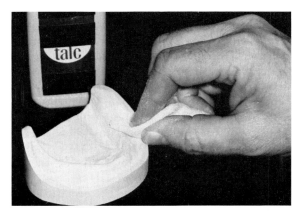

Fig. 4-58. Talc is applied to cast to act as separator for shellac baseplate material.

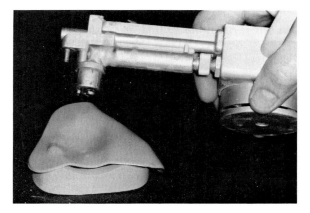

Fig. 4-59. Shellac baseplate is positioned over cast and softened with Bunsen burner. Baseplate should be centered over cast carefully to assure that there is adequate baseplate material for borders.

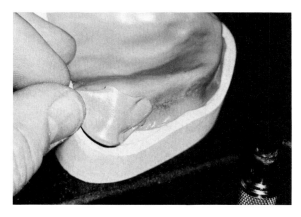

Fig. 4-60. Piece of scrap shellac baseplate material can be added to baseplate where needed to cover more of cast.

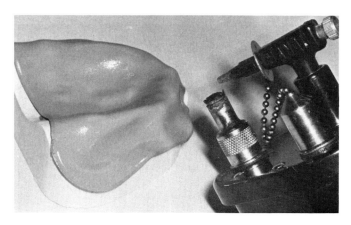

Fig. 4-61. Alcohol torch can be used to soften baseplate material in localized areas for adaptation.

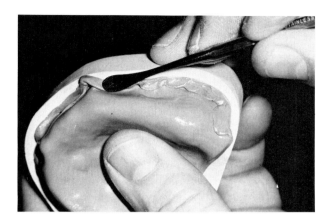

Fig. 4-62. Rounded baseplate borders are formed by folding over shellac baseplate material with spatula.

baseplate on the cast and flame it with a Bunsen burner (Fig. 4-59). When one shellac blank is not large enough to cover a cast, it is simple to add a piece of scrap shellac by flame-softening both pieces and readapting them (Fig. 4-60).

3. Soften the baseplate more with an alcohol torch, as needed (Fig. 4-61). Continue finger molding or use a spatula to adapt the baseplate around the entire border (Fig. 4-62).

4. Cool the baseplate and remove it from the cast. If necessary, trim the borders with an arbor band, fast-cut stone, or bur. If the lathe turns too fast and/too much pressure is exerted, it will gum up the trimmer (Fig. 4-63). Nonclogging rubber abrasive wheels also are available for trimming baseplates.

5. Examine the tissue side for glossy areas that indicate lack of adaptation (Fig. 4-64). Flame these areas, and replace the baseplate on the cast for more adaptation.

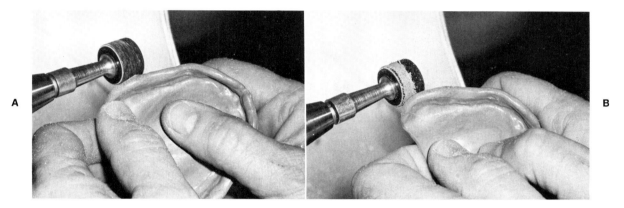

Fig. 4-63. A, Shellac baseplates can be smoothed lightly with arbor band. **B,** Using too much pressure during finishing results in clogged arbor band.

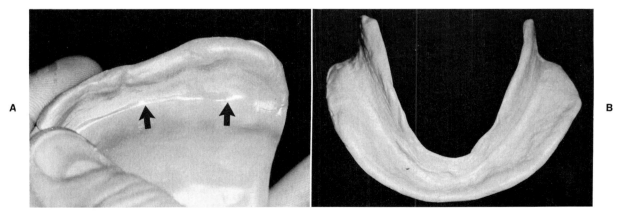

Fig. 4-64. A, Glossy surfaces (arrows) on interior of baseplate indicate lack of adaptation to cast. These surfaces should be flamed and readapted to cast. **B,** Well-adapted shellac baseplate shows excellent surface detail.

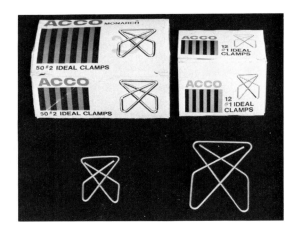

Fig. 4-65. Length of heavy-duty wire paper clip is excellent for reinforcing shellac baseplates.

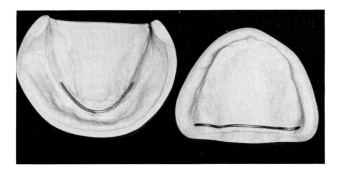

Fig. 4-66. Paper-clip wire is adapted to cast. Note position of mandibular reinforcing wire lingual to crest of alveolar ridge *(left);* it keeps reinforcing wire from interfering with positioning of teeth. Maxillary reinforcing wire is adapted to cast anterior to posterior border *(right).*

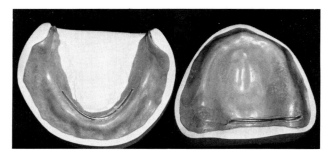

Fig. 4-67. Reinforcing wires are embedded in shellac baseplates.

6. Shellac baseplates should be reinforced. Heavy-duty paper clips are a good source of wire for reinforcement (Fig. 4-65). Adapt the wire to the casts (Fig. 4-66). Embed a piece of wire across the posterior border of the maxillary baseplate (Fig. 4-67). In the mandibular baseplate, embed it lingually to the crest of the ridge from premolar area to premolar area (Fig. 4-67). The reinforcement significantly improves both the strength and rigidity of the baseplate.

7. After cooling, store shellac baseplates on the cast to minimize warpage before use (Fig. 4-68). Readapt them later if necessary. To prevent breakage of a shellac baseplate and/or cast, block out undercuts on the cast, or warm the baseplate prior to separation if it extends into the undercut (Fig. 4-69). Do not overheat or adapt it to a dry cast because it can stick to the cast (Fig. 4-70).

STABILIZED SHELLAC BASEPLATES

Since shellac baseplates tend to warp, investigators such as Fletcher (1951), Boos (1956), Freese (1956), Jamieson (1956), Kapur and Yurkstas (1957), Hall (1958), Bodine (1964), and Malson (1964) have used methods and materials for stabilizing them. The majority of these methods rely on the use of a second material, such as zinc oxide–eugenol impression paste, elastomeric impression material, or autopolymerizing resin, as a liner to produce and maintain the desired adaptation and rigidity.

Baseplates stabilized with zinc oxide–eugenol impression paste

Shellac baseplates reinforced with zinc oxide–eugenol impression paste exhibit better adaptation and dimensional stability and have been in use for some time (Fletcher, 1951; Jamieson, 1956; Kapur and Yurkstas, 1957). Zinc-oxide impression materials adapt well to the cast and can improve the dimensional stability of shellac baseplates. Their disadvantages are that the baseplates are thicker because of the thickness of the impression paste liner, their construction requires additional time, and blockout of undercuts on the cast is essential because the relatively rigid stabilized baseplates cannot extend into the undercuts.

PROCEDURE

1. Identify and block out the undercuts on the cast with wax or a mix of one part plaster to one part flour of pumice (Fig. 4-71).

2. Coat the cast with 0.001-inch (0.0025-cm) thick tinfoil (Fig. 4-72). A toothbrush handle and pencil eraser may be modified to aid in adapting the tinfoil (Fig. 4-73).

3. Adapt a shellac baseplate over the tinfoiled cast as described previously. Cool the baseplate and remove it from the cast.

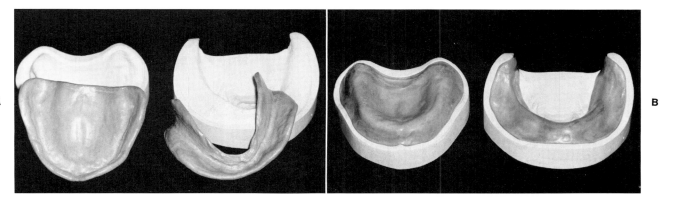

Fig. 4-68. **A,** Completed shellac baseplates, illustrating excellent surface detail. **B,** Completed shellac baseplates should be stored on cast until needed to minimize possibility of distortion.

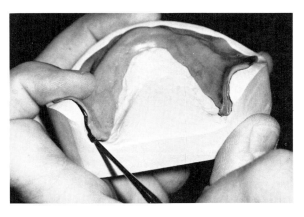

Fig. 4-69. If shellac baseplate is adapted into undercut areas, it should be softened and pried out of undercuts gently to prevent damage to cast or baseplate on separation.

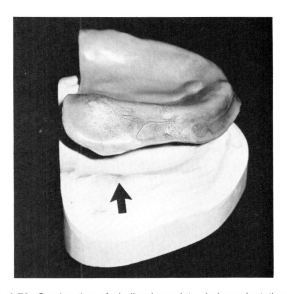

Fig. 4-70. Overheating of shellac baseplate during adaptation resulted in its sticking to cast (arrow).

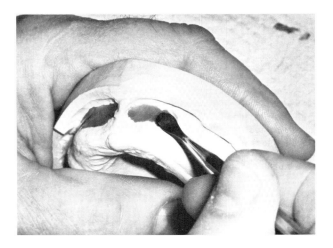

Fig. 4-71. Undercuts on cast are blocked out with wax or with plaster and pumice mixture before adapting tinfoil.

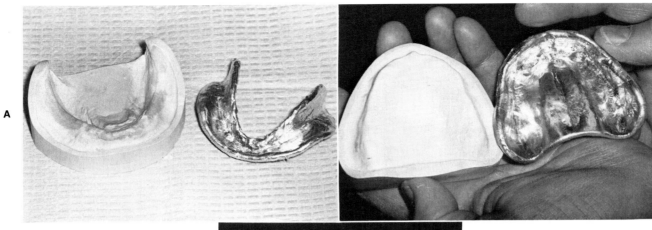

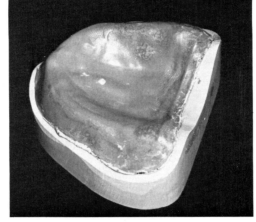

Fig. 4-76. **A,** Mandibular stabilized baseplate removed from cast. It should be stored on cast until ready for use. **B,** Stabilized maxillary baseplate removed from cast shows outstanding adaptation to cast. **C,** Completed maxillary baseplate on cast. Baseplates should be stored on cast until ready for use to prevent distortion.

Table 4-5. Shellac baseplate methods

Problem	Probable cause	Solution
Baseplate unable to be removed from cast	Cast not wet or treated with talc before baseplate adapted	Wet cast in slurry water or coat with talc before adapting baseplate
	Shellac baseplate stuck to cast	Do not overheat shellac baseplate
	Undercuts not blocked out adequately on cast before adapting baseplate	Do not adapt baseplate into undercuts or soften baseplate before removing it from undercuts
Completed baseplate too flexible	Wire reinforcement for stabilization not used	Reinforce shellac baseplate with wire or stabilize it with more material
Completed baseplate too thick	Layer of stabilizing material too thick	Apply finger pressure when adapting baseplate and stabilize material to achieve correct thickness of stabilizer
Void in stabilizing material	Insufficient impression material or inadequate pressure when forming stabilizing liner	Use enough impression material to preclude formation of voids
Completed baseplate unable to fit cast	Baseplate warped by heat	Readapt shellac baseplate by warming
	Baseplate warped by stabilizing material	Remake baseplate if warped by stabilizing material

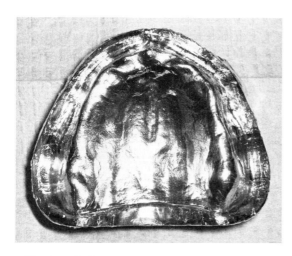

Fig. 4-77. Tinfoil 0.001 inch thick is adapted to cast.

The flexibility of this type of material permits baseplate extensions into moderate undercuts and minimizes the need for blockout of the cast. However, severe undercuts require blockout, since the rubber base impression material liner will not be thick enough to compensate for deep undercuts. The principal disadvantage of this procedure is the added thickness of the baseplate that results from using the elastomeric impression material liner. This type of baseplate costs more because of materials and the increase in construction time.

PROCEDURE

The procedures for constructing a baseplate stabilized with elastomeric impression material are similar to those using zinc-oxide impression material, as described earlier.

1. Apply tinfoil to the cast as previously described (Fig. 4-77).
2. Make additional holes in the adapted shellac baseplate with a No. 8 round bur to increase retention of the liner, and apply adhesive (Fig. 4-78).
3. Proportion and mix the impression material according to the manufacturer's recommendations.
4. Apply the impression material to the interior of the baseplate, and seat it on the tinfoiled cast.
5. After it has set, remove the baseplate, and trim the excess. Peel the tinfoil out of the baseplate.
6. The completed baseplate fits the cast accurately and affords the patient considerable comfort during the jaw relation recording procedures (Fig. 4-79).

Baseplates stabilized with autopolymerizing resin

Boos (1956), Jamieson (1956), and Hall (1958) have stabilized baseplates with autopolymerizing resin. Similar

to zinc oxide–eugenol impression paste and elastomeric impression material, autopolymerizing resin used as a liner improves both the adaptation and rigidity of the baseplate. The disadvantages of this method are the possibility of warping the baseplate as a result of internal stresses being released in the resin liner and the additional time required for fabrication.

PROCEDURE

The technique for stabilizing a baseplate with autopolymerizing resin is similar to those described for zinc oxide–eugenol impression paste.

1. Identify undercuts on the cast, and block them out with wax. Since the resin liner is rigid, the baseplate cannot extend into undercut areas without risk of fracturing the baseplate or damaging the cast on separation.
2. Apply tinfoil to the cast, or coat it with tinfoil substitute.
3. Adapt the shellac baseplate to the cast, and trim it 2 mm short of the borders if using autopolymerizing resin borders.
4. If the cast is not tinfoiled, recoat it with a tinfoil substitute.
5. Place two holes in the canine area and two in the first molar regions of the baseplate with a No. 8 round bur. Place another hole in the palate when constructing a maxillary baseplate.
6. Mix autopolymerizing resin, and place it into the baseplate with a spatula (Fig. 4-80).
7. Seat the baseplate on the cast (Fig. 4-81). Exercise care in seating the baseplate on the cast to assure a thin uniform layer of autopolymerizing resin.
8. After it has hardened, remove the baseplate from the cast, examine it, and polish the borders (Fig. 4-82).

PROBLEM AREAS

The problem areas for resin-stabilized baseplates are essentially the same as those for baseplates stabilized with the materials described in Table 4-5. However, another problem can result after the autopolymerizing resin lining is received. The release of internal stresses in the resin may produce a concomitant warping of the baseplate. Therefore baseplates fabricated in this manner have few advantages over those constructed entirely of autopolymerizing resin.

THERMOPLASTIC RESIN BASEPLATES AND VACUUM-ADAPTED RESIN BASEPLATES

A quick and easy method of making a usable baseplate is to vacuum mold a sheet of thermoplastic resin to a cast. The preformed resin sheet affords excellent thickness control and reasonably good adaptation to the cast, particularly when using thinner sheets. Terry and Wahlberg (1966) have reported obtaining

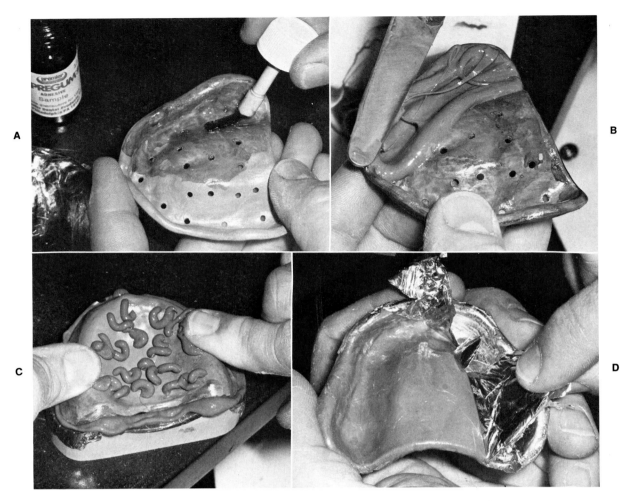

Fig. 4-78. **A,** Holes are placed in shellac baseplate, and adhesive is painted on baseplate to assure adhesion of elastomeric impression material. **B,** Elastomeric impression material is proportioned according to manufacturer's recommendation, mixed, and placed into shellac baseplate. **C,** Baseplate with impression material is seated carefully on cast with finger pressure. Note extrusion of impression material through perforations. **D,** Tinfoil can be peeled from impression material if desired.

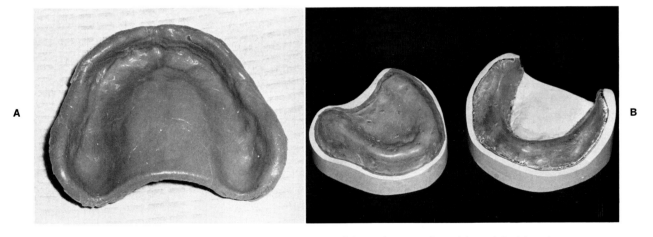

Fig. 4-79. **A,** Liner of elastomeric impression material permits extension of baseplate into minor undercuts. **B,** Baseplates lined with elastomeric impression materials fit cast accurately. These baseplates with soft liners are especially comfortable for patient during jaw relation recording procedures.

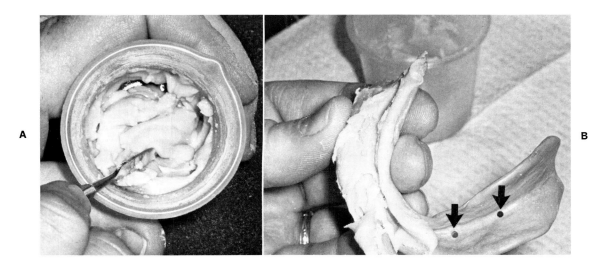

Fig. 4-80. A, Autopolymerizing resin is proportioned according to manufacturer's recommendation and mixed with spatula. **B,** Autopolymerizing resin is placed in baseplate with spatula. Note holes (arrows) placed in cuspid and premolar regions on each side to aid in minimizing voids.

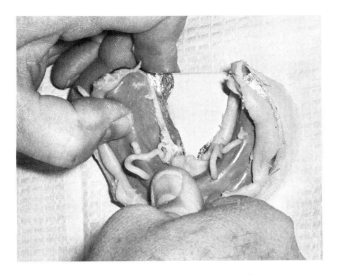

Fig. 4-81. Resin-filled baseplate is seated carefully on cast to develop layer approximately 1 to 2 mm thick. Failure to seat baseplate adequately can result in too thick baseplate.

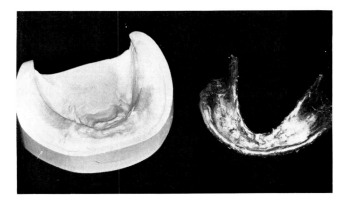

Fig. 4-82. Baseplate stabilized with layer of autopolymerizing resin is removed from cast and should be stored on cast until ready for use.

a more intimate adaptation of baseplate material by vacuum adaptation than by manual adaptation. Allred et al. (1968) have described a method of vacuum molding resin baseplates. The advantages of this method are simple technique; minimal amount of time required; excellent control of thickness; choice of a variety of materials for baseplates, splints, trays, copings, and mouthguards; satisfactory rigidity, particularly when using thicker materials; and, in some instances, excellent adaptation to the cast. The disadvantages are expense of the equipment, difficulty in achieving an intimate adaptation to the cast in deep re-

cesses and border reflections, and the problem of forming smoothly rounded borders from only one layer of a resin sheet.

PROCEDURE

1. Examine the cast and identify the undercuts that require blockout: deep undercuts and delicate creases or folds in the cast. Use a heat-stable blockout compound* to preclude breaking the cast on separation.

---

*Omnidental blockout compound, Buffalo Dental Manufacturing Co., Brooklyn, N.Y.

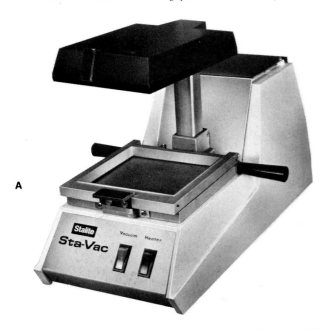

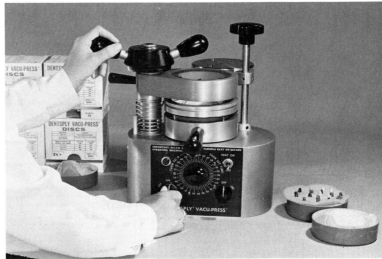

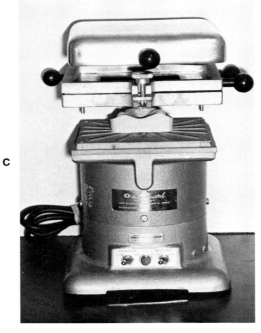

Fig. 4-83. A, Sta-Vac vacuum-adapting equipment. (Courtesy Buffalo Dental Manufacturing Co., Brooklyn, N.Y.) **B,** Dentsply Vacu-Press. (Courtesy Dentsply International, Inc., York, Pa.) **C,** Omnivac vacuum-adapting device.

Do not use wax because it will melt at the temperatures required for adaptation.

2. Select a resin sheet of the proper thickness, usually 0.060 inch (0.15 cm), and rigidity. Thicker material is better for mandibular baseplates, in which achieving adequate rigidity may be a problem.

3. Although the specific directions for molding vary with each manufacturer's equipment and materials, the principles are similar (Fig. 4-83). Place the blocked out cast on the vacuum plate. Make certain that the cast bases are flat, and the sides are not undercut (Fig. 4-84).

4. Position a resin sheet of the desired thickness in the holding frame, and align and activate the heating unit (Fig. 4-85).

5. Watch the resin sheet while heating it and when it

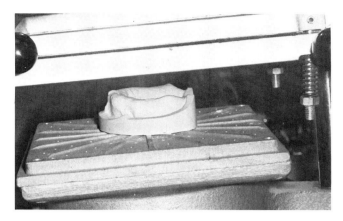

Fig. 4-84. Cast is positioned on vacuum plate (Omnivac) before baseplate is vacuum adapted.

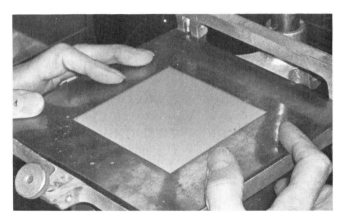

Fig. 4-85. Sheet of resin baseplate material (Omnivac) is placed in frame.

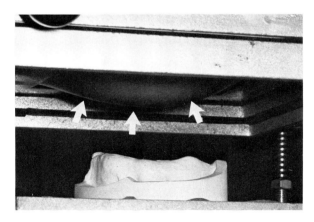

Fig. 4-86. Baseplate resin sheet sags (arrows) as it is heated.

sags approximately ½ inch* (1.3 cm) below the lower edge of the hinged frame,† lower the frame over the vacuum plate (Fig. 4-86).

6. Drape the material over the cast and activate the vacuum to complete the adaptation. Keep the heating unit over the cast until the adaptation is adequate (i.e., 10 to 15 seconds).

7. Move the heating unit away, and continue the vacuum adaptation for 30 seconds more while the baseplate cools. Finger adaptation during this phase can often improve the fit (Fig. 4-87).

8. Remove the adapted baseplate and cast, and permit them to cool before trimming. It is easy to cut the material with a bur or arbor band (Fig. 4-88). Use a small flame to heat areas in need of more adaptation for intimate contact, and adapt them manually with a moistened thumb or finger. If necessary, reinforce the baseplate with a wire and autopolymerizing resin.

PROBLEM AREAS

This method presents few problems. It is sometimes difficult to achieve complete adaptation of the baseplate material into the vestibular reflections of the cast (Table 4-6). The material has a tendency to bridge these areas, particularly when using thick resin sheets. Examination of the tissue side of adapted baseplates often fails to indicate the minute tissue detail typical of intimately adapted baseplates. Often it is necessary to increase the thickness of the border areas with wax or autopolymerizing resin to produce smooth borders of the proper thickness (Fig. 4-89). Primary advantages of this method are the ease and rapidity with which it is possible to fabricate a baseplate (Fig. 4-90). The devices are also useful for constructing mouthguards, impression trays, and coping patterns.

WAX BASEPLATES

Baseplates constructed of hard baseplate wax are satisfactory (Boucher, Hickey, and Zarb, 1975). The principal advantages of this method are that construction of a wax baseplate is easy and rapid, and thinning to gain more space to set teeth is relatively simple. The disadvantage of this type of baseplate is primarily its lack of dimensional stability. Although reinforced with wire, baseplates of wax, a thermoplastic material, are subject to warpage when warmed or cooled. They are more suitable for positioning teeth than for use as bases in recording maxillomandibular relationships.

Text continued on p. 122.

---

*Omnivac baseplate material, 0.060 inch, Buffalo Dental Manufacturing Co., Brooklyn, N.Y.

†Omnivac Precision Vacuum Adapter, Buffalo Dental Manufacturing Co., Brooklyn, N.Y.

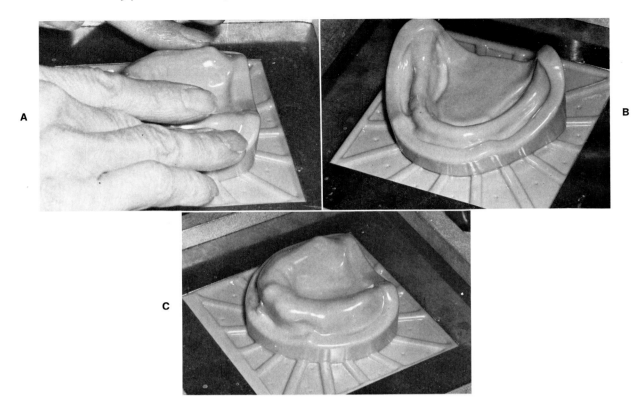

Fig. 4-87. A, Finger adaptation often can improve fit of baseplate; however, care must be taken because baseplate can be quite hot. **B,** Baseplate material is allowed to cool with vacuum-adapting device still in operation. **C,** Maxillary baseplate cooling after vacuum adaptation.

Table 4-6. Thermoplastic resin baseplate and vacuum-adapted resin baseplate methods

Problem	Probable cause	Solution
Baseplate unable to be removed from cast	Deep undercuts not blocked out	Block out deep undercuts with heat stable or nonwax blockout material
Cast chipped on removal of baseplate	Delicate cast undercuts not blocked out	Block out small folds and creases in cast to preclude bridging
Baseplate borders not adapted into vestibular reflections of cast	Vestibular reflections of cast bridged by baseplate material	Fill in borders with wax or autopolymerizing resin for correct thickness and adaptation
Baseplate not intimately adapted to cast	Resin not hot enough when adaptation begun Vacuum molding period too short	Allow resin to develop adequate sag before starting adaptation Continue vacuum adaptation for 30 seconds after discontinuing heating Readapt by manual adaptation

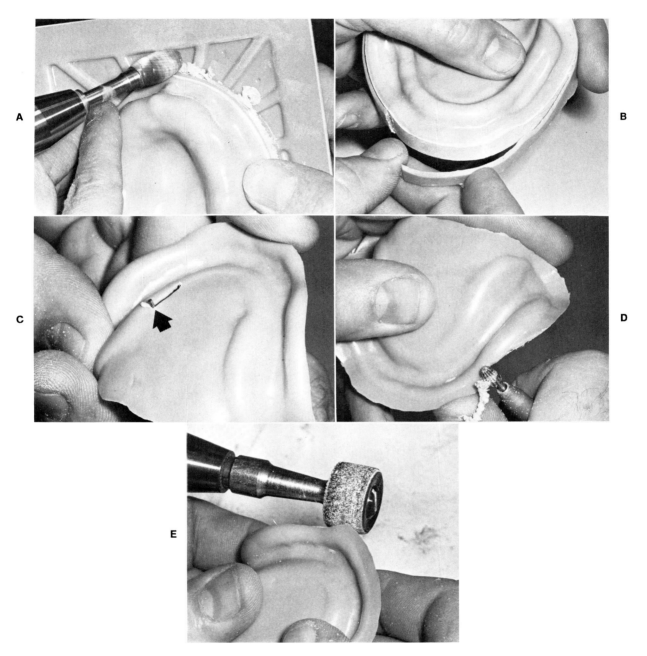

Fig. 4-88. A, Removal of adapted baseplate from cast is accomplished by cutting around periphery with large bur. **B,** After baseplate material has been cut away from cast, borders can be stripped away. **C,** Tongue area (arrow) of mandibular baseplate is removed by using fissure bur and standard handpiece. **D,** Additional finishing can be accomplished easily with large bur in handpiece. **E,** Arbor band also is effective for smoothing borders.

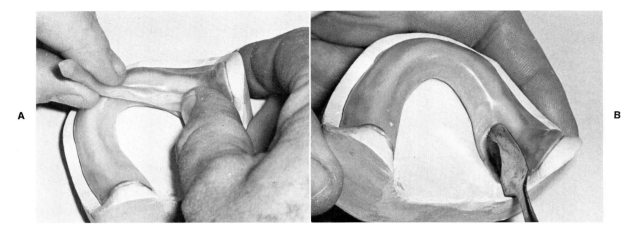

Fig. 4-89. A, Border contours can be thickened and rounded by adding baseplate wax. Baseplate wax should be smoothed to prevent roughness. **B,** Baseplate wax can be flowed into border areas to develop desired thickness and contour.

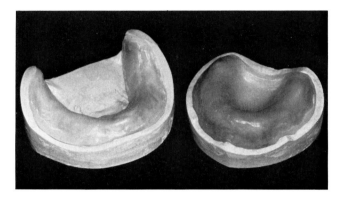

Fig. 4-90. Completed vacuum-adapted baseplates. Principal advantage of this technique is that baseplate can be made in minimal amount of time.

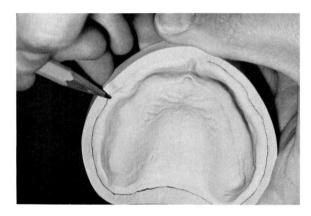

Fig. 4-91. Borders of cast are outlined with pencil to facilitate trimming wax after adaptation.

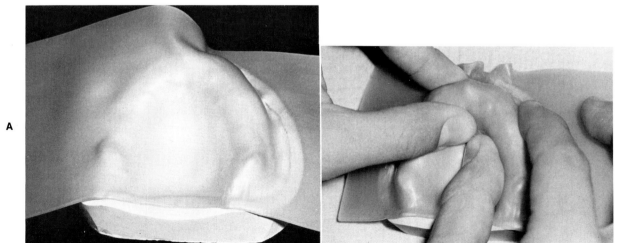

Fig. 4-92. A, Hard baseplate wax is softened and finger adapted to cast. Note pencil-marked border shows through translucent wax. **B,** Care should be taken to assure that baseplate wax is adapted to cast intimately, particularly in palate and peripheral regions.

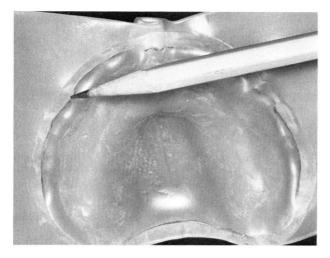

Fig. 4-93. Adapted baseplate wax is removed from cast and trimmed with scissors. Wax should be trimmed approximately 3 to 4 mm beyond pencil line, which readily transfers to wax. Additional wax is folded back onto baseplate to form rounded borders.

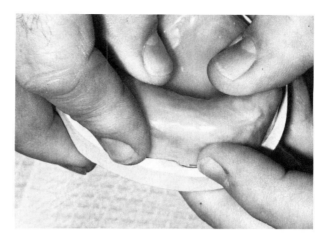

Fig. 4-94. Thickness of baseplate borders is examined, and more wax is added if needed to fill out borders to proper contour.

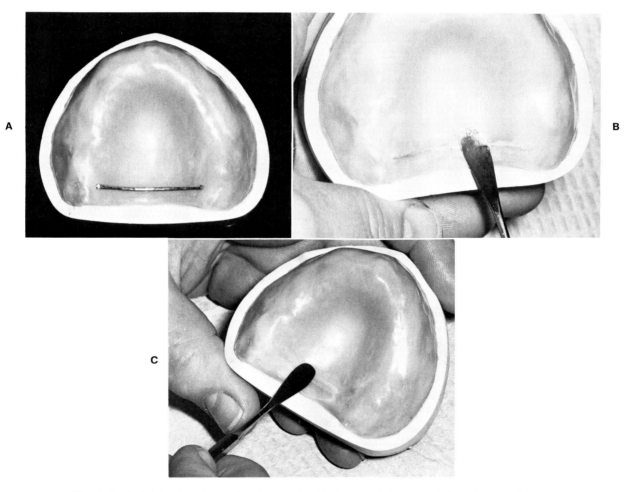

Fig. 4-95. A, Reinforcing wire is placed approximately 3 mm anterior to posterior extension of baseplate. It is embedded in wax baseplate to provide additional rigidity. B, More wax is flowed over wire. C, Wax is flowed over embedded wire and finished to smooth surface.

PROCEDURE

1. Dust powdered talc on the cast surfaces to act as a separator.

2. Adapt a reinforcing wire across the posterior border of the maxillary cast and approximately 2 mm anterior to the posterior border. Position the wire reinforcement for the mandibular baseplate lingual to the ridge crest and extend it from premolar region to premolar region. This wire reinforcement will not interfere with later positioning of the teeth. Remove the wires for the time being.

3. Outline the peripheral border on the cast with a pencil to facilitate trimming the wax (Fig. 4-91).

4. Soften a sheet of hard baseplate wax, and adapt it carefully to the cast to assure its intimate contact with the cast surface (Fig. 4-92).

5. Remove the wax, and trim it with scissors to the approximate contour of the denture border (Fig. 4-93).

6. Fold the wax back on itself at the borders to make a double thickness. Fill out the thickness of the border and extend it with more wax if needed (Fig. 4-94).

7. Embed the previously adapted wire reinforcement in the wax baseplate, and flow additional wax over it to make the surface smooth (Fig. 4-95).

8. Do not adapt the baseplate into deep undercuts because there is no blockout of undercuts on the cast. Warm the wax over the undercuts, and free the baseplate by several removals and insertions (Fig. 4-96). The wax should be smooth and duplicate the border width of the impression (Fig. 4-97). Store the completed wax baseplates on the cast (Fig. 4-98), and readapt them later if necessary.

PROBLEM AREAS

The principal problem with this method results from warpage of the wax baseplate after construction (Table 4-7).

HEAT-CURED COMPRESSION-MOLDED RESIN BASEPLATES

Generally, heat-cured resin baseplates constructed by conventional compression-molding methods serve as record bases and subsequently become denture bases (Brewer, 1962). Wax a pattern on the cast, flask the cast, eliminate the wax, and pack the heat-curing denture resin into the mold. After the recommended curing cycle, deflask the baseplate, remove it from the cast, and polish it. The advantages of this method are (1) the baseplate is strong and rigid, (2) it is possible to control the thickness of the baseplate during the waxing up, (3) it requires only minimal finishing and polishing, and (4) bases constructed in this manner can serve as baseplates for maxillomandibular relationship recording procedures and setting teeth, and subsequently they become part of the denture. The disadvantages of this method are (1) it is much more time consuming and expensive to wax, flask, process, and finish the baseplate; (2) it is necessary to construct mounting casts because flasking and curing usually ruin the master casts; and (3) in the event of a broken or damaged baseplate, no cast is immediately available for constructing another one.

PROCEDURE

1. Do *not* block out cast undercuts.

2. Wax the pattern for the baseplate on the master cast. One layer of baseplate wax is thick enough for the ridge, or convex, portions of the cast. Wax the borders to the full extension and thickness of the cast, as determined from the impression (Fig. 4-99).

3. Place a finish line on the wax pattern to conform to the contours of the baseplate border, and have it approximately 2 to 4 mm from the border. This finish line facilitates waxing of the denture setup prior to flasking and completion of the denture (Fig. 4-100).

4. Flask the cast and wax pattern in a denture flask (Fig. 4-101). Boil out the wax and, after cooling the mold, paint tinfoil substitute on the stone surfaces (Fig. 4-102).

5. Proportion and mix the denture resin, and place it into the mold. Trial pack the resin until eliminating all flash (Fig. 4-103).

6. Use an appropriate curing cycle and, after curing, bench cool and deflask the baseplates (Fig. 4-104).

7. Smooth the borders and polish to complete the

Table 4-7. Wax baseplate method

Problem	Probable cause	Solution
Failure of wax baseplate to fix cast	Wax not adapted properly	Adapt wax to achieve intimate contact
	Wire reinforcement not used	Use wire reinforcement to improve dimensional stability and rigidity
	Baseplate warped after completion	Readapt warped baseplate manually

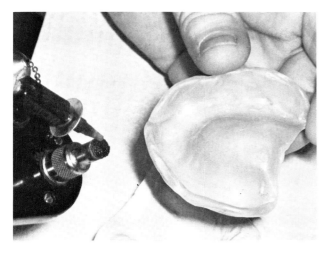

Fig. 4-96. Portions of baseplate extending into undercuts can be softened with alcohol torch. Baseplate is placed on cast and removed several times to prevent adaptation of baseplate into undercuts.

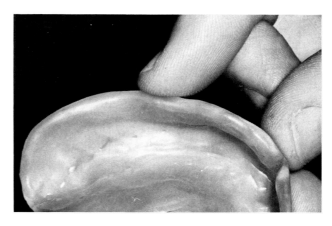

Fig. 4-97. Borders of wax baseplate should be smooth and duplicate borders of impression.

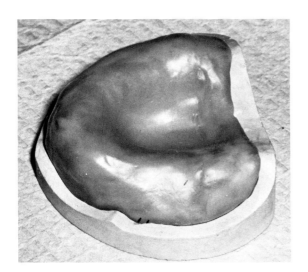

Fig. 4-98. Completed wax baseplates should fit cast accurately and be stored on cast until needed.

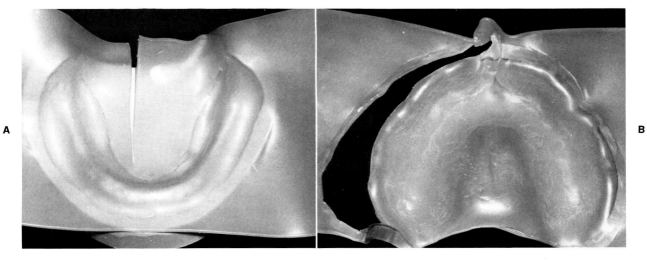

Fig. 4-99. A, One layer of baseplate wax is adapted to cast. Cutting wax through lingual area facilitates smooth adaptation without wrinkles. **B,** Wax pattern for maxillary baseplate is removed from cast and trimmed to border extensions. Borders of wax pattern should duplicate desired border thickness and contour of completed denture.

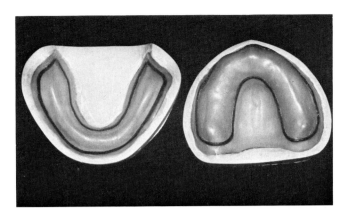

Fig. 4-100. Maxillary and mandibular wax patterns. Note particularly position of finish line on these patterns when used as processed bases.

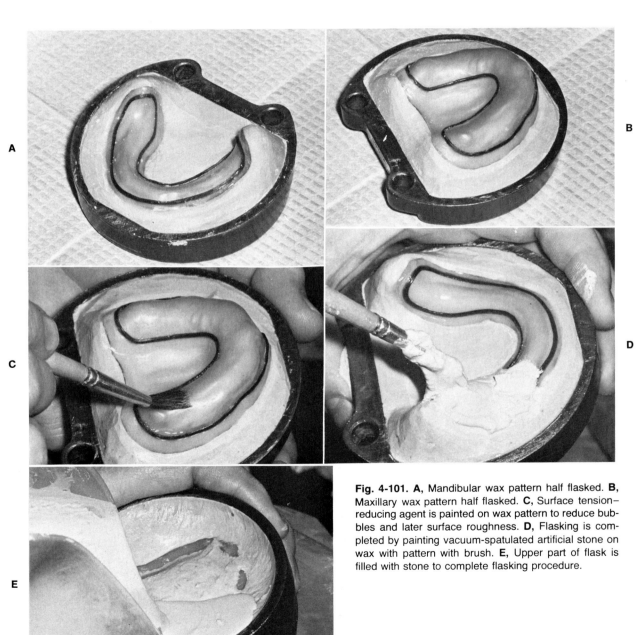

Fig. 4-101. A, Mandibular wax pattern half flasked. **B,** Maxillary wax pattern half flasked. **C,** Surface tension–reducing agent is painted on wax pattern to reduce bubbles and later surface roughness. **D,** Flasking is completed by painting vacuum-spatulated artificial stone on wax with pattern with brush. **E,** Upper part of flask is filled with stone to complete flasking procedure.

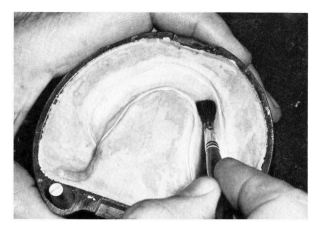

Fig. 4-102. Wax should be eliminated with clean boiling water. After cooling, stone is coated with tinfoil substitute.

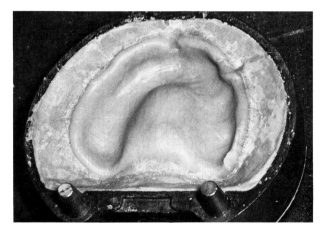

Fig. 4-103. Packing is continued until all flash is eliminated.

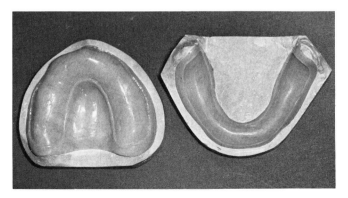

Fig. 4-104. Cured resin baseplate is deflasked carefully.

baseplate (Fig. 4-105). It is preferable to store resin baseplates in water until ready to use them.

PROBLEM AREAS

A potential problem is fracturing the baseplate during deflasking (Table 4-8). Since processing usually ruins the cast, a broken baseplate that is not reparable necessitates making a new impression unless a previously made duplicate master cast is available.

CONSTRUCTING MOUNTING CASTS

Constructing baseplates by the conventional compression-molding techniques or by the fluid resin method usually damages the master casts. Therefore it is necessary to make mounting casts for transferring maxillomandibular relationship records to the articulator and for setting teeth.

PROCEDURE

1. Block out the interior of the processed base with modeling clay to eliminate all interior undercuts (Fig. 4-106). Avoid covering borders to make a firm index on the cast.

2. Make an artificial stone cast for the blocked out baseplate (Fig. 4-107). After the stone has set, separate the baseplate from the mounting cast.

3. Remove the modeling clay from the interior of the processed base, and replace the base on the cast to check its adaptation (Fig. 4-108).

4. Index these casts for use during the maxillomandibular relationship recording procedure (Fig. 4-109).

FLUID RESIN BASEPLATES

Browning (1973) has described a method of using a fluid resin system to make processed bases in a reversible hydrocolloid mold. This method offers the advantage of rapid retrieval of the processed baseplate from the hydrocolloid mold after curing. The disadvantages are the additional time and materials required for waxing, flasking, and processing the processed base or baseplate.

PROCEDURE

1. Block out undercuts with baseplate wax when constructing a baseplate. This step is unnecessary when constructing a processed base.

2. Wax the pattern on the master cast. The waxup determines the thickness of the baseplate, border contours, and extensions. Place a finish line parallel to and 3 to 4 mm away from the border extension when making a permanent base instead of a baseplate (Fig. 4-110). For maxillary bases place a palatal finish line lingual to

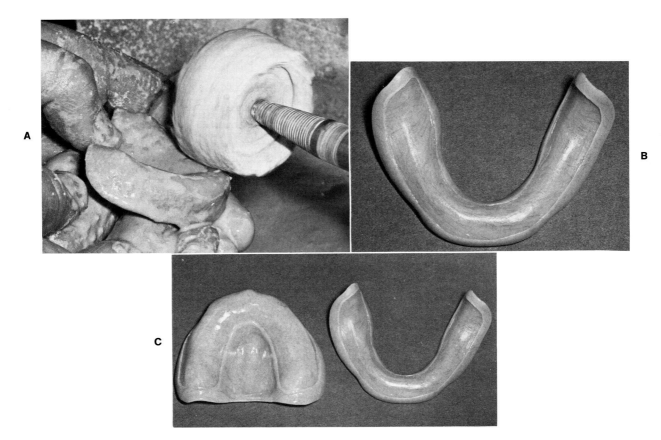

Fig. 4-105. **A,** Borders of resin baseplate are smoothed and polished with flour of pumice and rag wheel. **B,** Completed mandibular processed baseplate. Note sharp finish lines. **C,** Completed maxillary and mandibular processed resin baseplates.

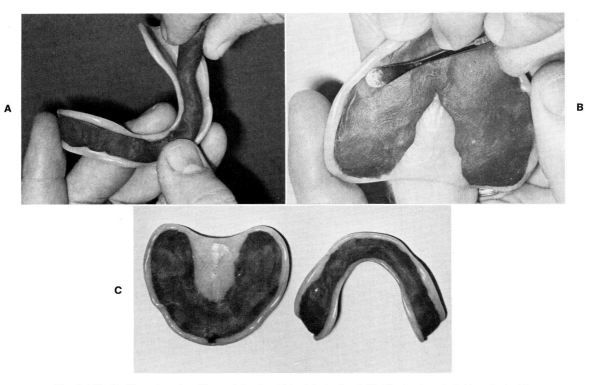

Fig. 4-106. **A,** All undercuts of baseplate should be blocked out. **B,** Blockout material is adapted to borders of baseplate with spatula. **C,** Baseplates blocked out and ready for construction of mounting casts.

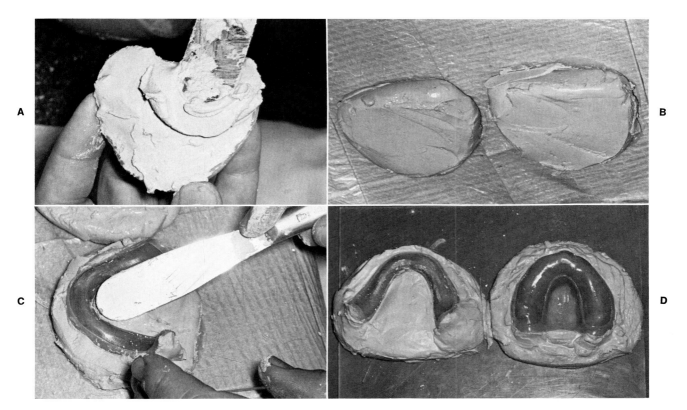

Fig. 4-107. A, Artificial stone is mixed and placed in interior of blocked out baseplate with spatula. **B,** Rest of mix is formed into patties on glass slab. **C,** Baseplate is settled into patty. Care should be taken to avoid submerging baseplate and allowing stone to cover sides of baseplate because it would be impossible to remove baseplates from mounting cast. Tongue area of mandibular casts should be smoothed with spatula. **D,** Maxillary and mandibular baseplates and mounting casts are allowed to set before trimming.

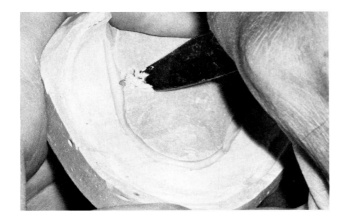

Fig. 4-108. If baseplate cannot be seated readily on mounting cast without interference, some adjustment of mounting cast may be required. Usually, this condition exists when baseplate has been seated too far into stone.

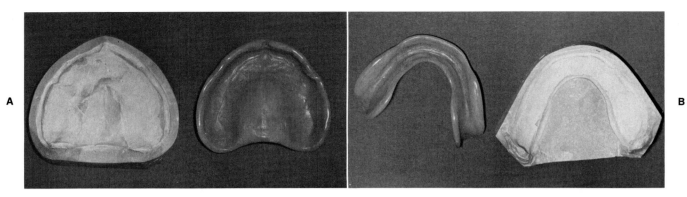

Fig. 4-109. A, Maxillary baseplate and mounting casts. **B,** Mandibular baseplate and mounting casts.

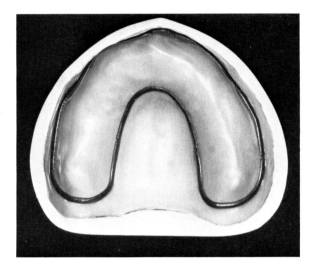

Fig. 4-110. If permanent base is being constructed rather than baseplate, finish line should be placed on wax pattern. Note finish line placed on palate of maxillary wax pattern lingual to crest of ridge.

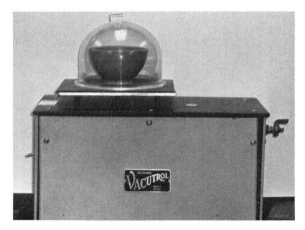

Fig. 4-111. Soaking cast in slurry water under reduced atmospheric pressure expedites wetting of cast and helps to reduce voids in completed baseplate.

Table 4-8. Heat-cured compression-molded resin baseplate method

Problem	Probable cause	Solution
Baseplate broken on removal from cast	Improper prying to remove baseplate from cast	Section cast with saw to remove baseplate
	Cast not painted with tinfoil substitute or tinfoil substitute contaminated	Paint cast with uncontaminated tinfoil substitute before packing
Baseplate too flexible	Wax pattern too thin	Make wax pattern thick enough to provide adequate rigidity

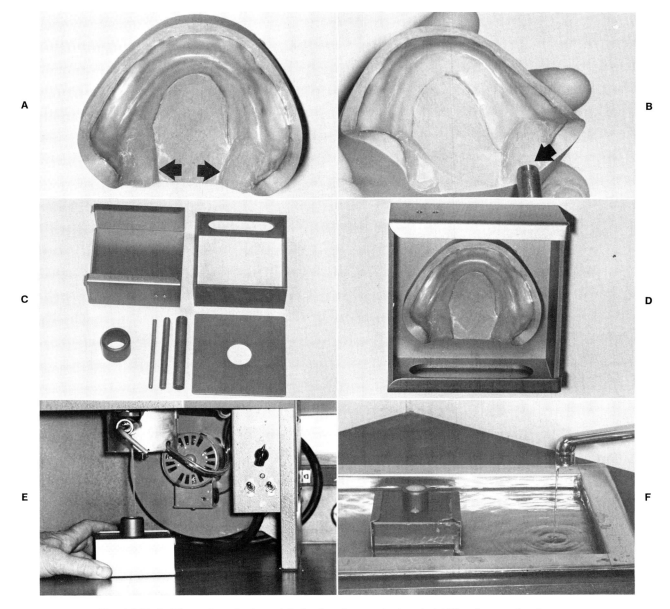

Fig. 4-112. A, Wax pattern for baseplate is placed on soaked cast. Additional wax extensions are placed lingual to heel area of mandibular baseplate or tuberosity of maxillary baseplate (arrows). Sprue feeds will be attached to lingual or palatal wax additions. **B,** Sprue hole cutter is used to cut sprue through hydrocolloid investing material to lingual wax extension (arrow). **C,** Special flask for flasking casts in reversible hydrocolloid. **D,** Cast and wax pattern are placed in assembled flask ready for pouring reversible hydrocolloid. **E,** Flask is filled with reversible hydrocolloid. **F,** Flask containing cast and reversible hydrocolloid is placed in cooling tray, and hydrocolloid is allowed to gel.

the crest of the ridge. Place more wax lingual to the heel region of mandibular baseplates and palatal to the tuberosity region of maxillary baseplates for the sprue attachment.

3. Soak the waxed master cast in clear slurry water for 5 minutes prior to flasking in reversible hydrocolloid. Soaking the cast under reduced atmospheric pressure expedites this step (Fig. 4-111). Invest the cast in a reversible hydrocolloid in a special flask* (Fig. 4-112).

4. Remove the master cast from the set hydrocolloid mold, and remove the wax from the cast with clean boiling water (Fig. 4-113).

---

*Pour N Cure flask, Coe Laboratories, Inc., Chicago, Ill., or equivalent.

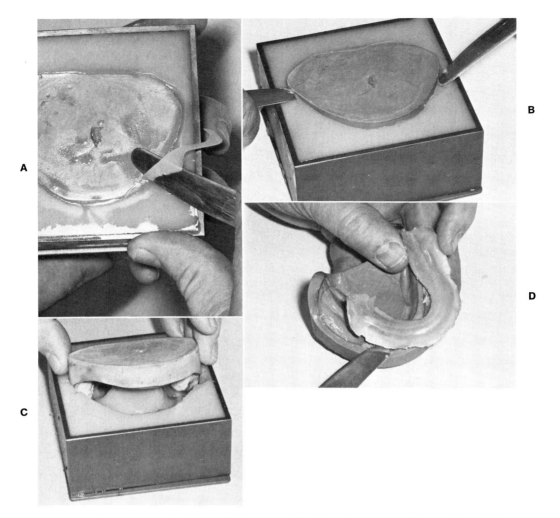

Fig. 4-113. **A,** When reversible hydrocolloid is poured into flask, it sometimes flows underneath base of cast. It can be removed easily with knife prior to removing cast from flask. **B,** Frequently, it is helpful to use two knives, one on each side of cast, to pry upward and separate it from hydrocolloid mold. Care should be taken to avoid damaging hydrocolloid mold. **C,** After cast has been lifted upward from hydrocolloid mold, it can be grasped with fingers and removed. **D,** Wax pattern can be lifted from cast, and residual wax removed with clean boiling water.

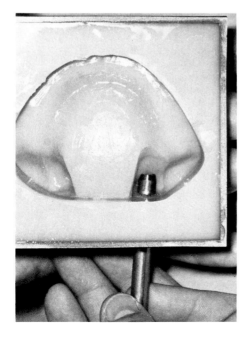

Fig. 4-114. Sprue hole cutter is used to cut sprue hole through reversible hydrocolloid. Diameter of sprue cutter should be as large as possible to facilitate easy pouring of fluid resin.

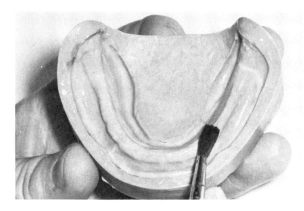

Fig. 4-115. Cast should be coated with tinfoil substitute, allowed to dry, and replaced in hydrocolloid mold.

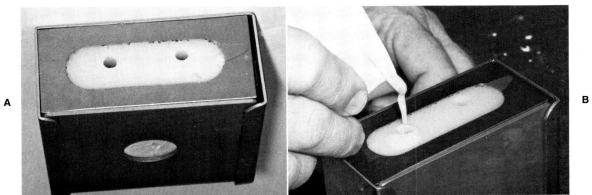

A

B

Fig. 4-116. A, Cast is assembled in hydrocolloid mold ready for pouring fluid resin. B, Autopolymerizing pour-type resin is mixed according to manufacturer's recommendation and poured into one sprue hole. Pouring is continued until resin appears in other sprue hole. Voids can be minimized by rocking flask gently during pouring procedure. Failure to do so can lead to formation of voids and unusable baseplate.

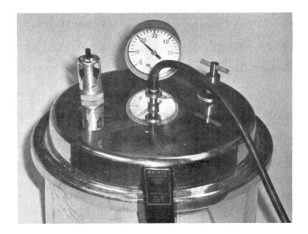

Fig. 4-117. Flask with hydrocolloid mold filled with pour-type autopolymerizing resin is placed upright in pressure pot. Then it is cured at 20 psi in warm water for 20 minutes.

5. Cut sprue holes with a diameter as large as possible in the hydrocolloid mold to facilitate pouring the resin and to serve as a shrinkage compensating reservoir (Fig. 4-114).

6. Paint the cast with tinfoil substitute, allow it to dry, and replace the master cast in the hydrocolloid mold (Fig. 4-115).

7. Mix fluid resin* according to the manufacturer's recommendations, and pour it into only one sprue hole of the hydrocolloid mold (Fig. 4-116). Rock the mold gently to minimize entrapment of air. Continue pouring until the resin becomes visible and fills the other sprue hole.

8. Cure the resin and mold in warm water under 20 psi air pressure (Fig. 4-117).

9. Remove the processed base from the mold (Fig. 4-118) and master cast. Cut off the sprues and slightly polish the borders, thereby completing the fluid resin baseplate (Fig. 4-119). Making a processed base probably will ruin the cast, since there is no need to block out undercuts. In this instance, a mounting cast is essential; tech-

---

*Pour N Cure resin, Coe Laboratories, Inc., Chicago, Ill., or equivalent.

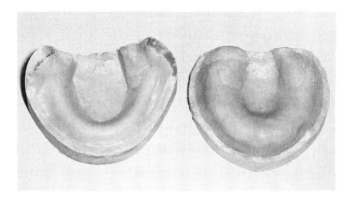

Fig. 4-118. Cured baseplate and cast are removed from hydrocolloid mold. Use of reversible hydrocolloid mold greatly facilitates recovery of baseplates from mold.

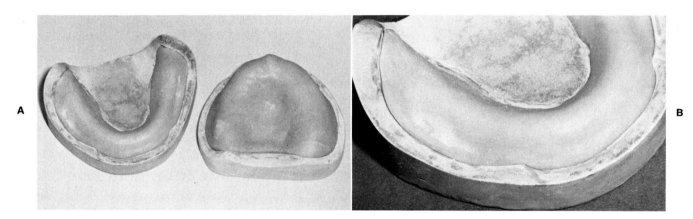

Fig. 4-119. A, Resin baseplates are polished in usual manner and stored in water until ready for use. **B,** Adaptation of baseplate to cast is excellent. Baseplates fabricated by this technique show minimal porosity and require little finishing.

nique for constructing them is described earlier in this chapter.

PROBLEM AREAS

The chief problem in making fluid resin baseplates is the failure to obtain a usable baseplate because of incomplete filling of the mold (Table 4-9). Voids appear or the mold does not fill completely as a result of entrapping air during pouring, making sprues too small or placing them improperly, using insufficient resin, resin curing before completing the pour, pouring resin into both sprues, or not rocking the flask during pouring to express air.

Using sprues of larger diameters and pouring the resin into only one sprue minimize the entrapment of air. Rock the flask slowly while pouring to facilitate the flow of resin into all mold recesses. Introducing sprue feeds below the highest portion of the pattern makes the entrapment of air almost a certainty. Flute the sprue attachment to assure rapid unimpeded flow of resin into the mold. Mix an adequate amount of resin (i.e., one

denture unit), and pour it without unnecessary delay to prevent it from becoming too viscous to pour. Larger sprues also serve as a shrinkage reservoir to feed more resin into the mold as the curing progresses. In spite of the potential problems, baseplates fabricated by this method are excellent.

METAL BASEPLATES

For a detailed description of construction methods for metal bases see Chapter 18.

WAX OCCLUSION RIMS

The majority of occlusion rims are of baseplate wax. The purpose of a wax occlusion rim is to transmit important information to the dental laboratory technician. It includes the maxillomandibular relationships, midline, occlusal plane, high and low lip line, cuspid line, amount of horizontal and vertical overlap, and support for the lips and cheeks. Usually, occlusion rims are furnished to the dentist at average predetermined dimensions; however, the dentist may specify dimensions

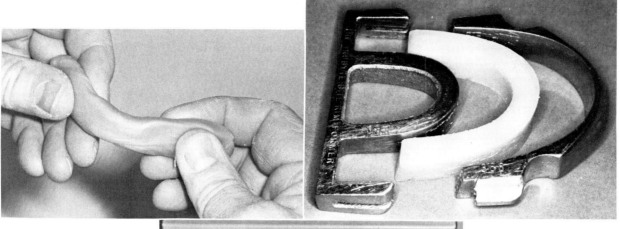

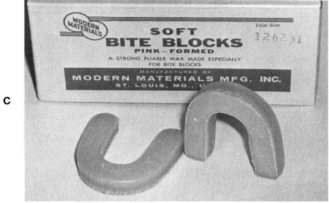

Fig. 4-120. **A,** Occlusion rims can be made from softened roll of baseplate wax. Care should be taken to ensure that wax is homogeneous. Folds and entrapment of air should be avoided. **B,** Metal occlusion rim former can be used to make occlusion rims from baseplate wax or scrap wax; they can be made up in advance to be ready for use when needed. (Courtesy Dentsply International, Inc., York, Pa.) **C,** Occlusion rim forms also can be purchased from different manufacturers. Consistency of wax can be varied from soft to hard as needed.

Table 4-9. Fluid resin baseplate method

Problem	Probable cause	Solution
Baseplate incomplete or voids present	Insufficient resin mixed	Mix enough resin to fill mold, usually one denture unit
	Sprues too small	Use larger diameter sprues
	Sprues improperly placed	Place sprues to prevent entrapment of air in upper recesses of mold
	Resin poured into both sprues	Pour resin into one sprue only
	Pouring delayed and resin set	Pour resin immediately according to manufacturer's directions
	Flask not rocked during pouring	Rock flask gently during pouring to express air

when requesting their construction. Often they are larger than they will be ultimately because the dentist finds it easier to remove wax from an occlusion rim with a warm spatula or knife than to add wax to it. Occlusion rims may be formed with a roll of warmed baseplate wax, shaped with a metal occlusion rim former,* or preformed blanks can be purchased ready to be adapted to the baseplate (Fig. 4-120).

MAXILLARY OCCLUSION RIMS

Jamieson (1956) has indicated that the average distance from the upper sulcus to the incisal edge of the upper central incisor is 22 mm, and the average distance from the lower sulcus to the incisal edge of the lower

---

*Bite Rim Former, Dentsply International, Inc., York, Pa.

central incisor is 18 mm, or a total of 40 mm. Therefore maxillary occlusion rims are usually constructed to measure 22 mm from the highest point on the labial flange to the occlusal surface in the central incisor region (Fig. 4-121). Mandibular occlusion rims should be approximately 18 mm from the lowest part of the lower labial flange to the occlusal surface in the central incisor region. The posterior vertical height of the maxillary occlusion rim should be approximately 6 to 8 mm, i.e., 6 mm when measured above from the baseplate to the top of the occlusion rim, or 8 mm when measured from the tissue surface of the baseplate, to allow for a 2 mm thick baseplate (Fig. 4-122). The facial incisal edge of the maxillary occlusion rim in the central incisor area should be approximately 8 mm anterior to the center of the depression formed by the incisive papilla (Fig. 4-123). The curvature of the maxillary occlusion rim should corres-

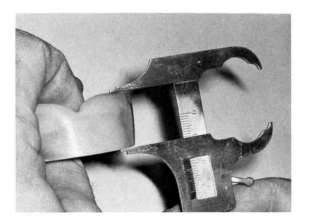

Fig. 4-121. Maxillary occlusion rim should be approximately 22 mm long when measured from highest part of vestibular extension to incisal edge of occlusion rim.

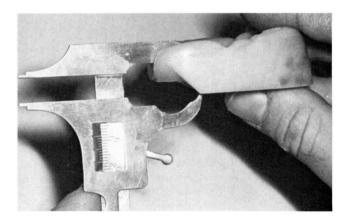

Fig. 4-122. Posterior height of maxillary occlusion rim should be approximately 8 mm when measured from tissue surface of maxillary baseplate to occlusal surface of occlusion rim.

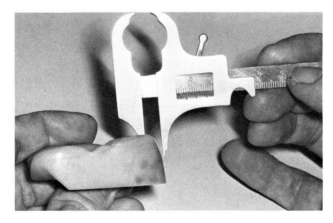

Fig. 4-123. Facial incisal edge of maxillary wax occlusion rim should be approximately 7 to 8 mm anterior to center of depression formed by incisive papilla.

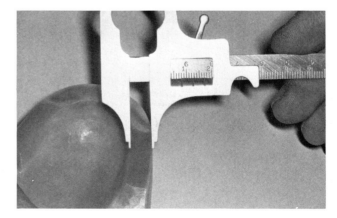

Fig. 4-124. Maxillary occlusion rim should be approximately 8 mm wide.

pond to the overall curvature of the maxillary arch. The occlusion rim should be approximately 8 mm wide (Fig. 4-124), and the maxillary occlusion rim should extend posteriorly to a point approximately 1 cm anterior to the hamular notch.

MANDIBULAR OCCLUSION RIMS

The mandibular occlusion rim should be approximately 18 mm from the incisal edge of the occlusion rim in the central incisor area to the deepest part of the labial vestibule. The occlusion rim should be approximately 8 mm wide, conform to the overall curvature of the mandibular residual ridge, and extend posteriorly to the point on the residual ridge where the ramus of the mandible begins its vertical ascent (Fig. 4-125).

PROCEDURE

1. Warm a sheet of baseplate wax over a Bunsen burner, and form it into a roll approximately 4 inches (10 cm) long (Fig. 4-120, *A*).

2. Adapt the wax roll to the baseplate, and seal it with a spatula (Fig. 4-126).

3. Contour the wax rim to desired shape and dimensions. A large wax melting plate is useful in establishing the occlusal surface (Fig. 4-127).

4. Smooth the wax to eliminate roughness, and check dimensions.

MODELING PLASTIC OCCLUSION RIMS

Occasionally a dentist makes occlusion rims of impression compound to record jaw movement, as in function-

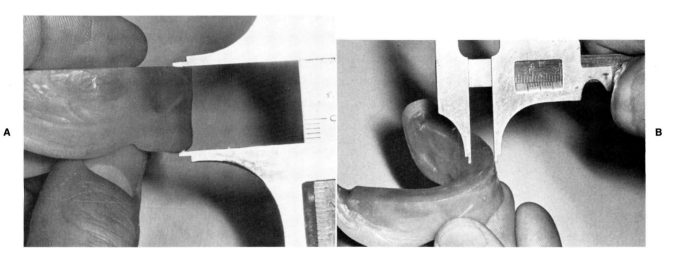

Fig. 4-125. A, Mandibular occlusion rim should be approximately 18 mm from incisal edge of occlusion rim to deepest part of labial vestibule. **B,** Occlusion rim should be approximately 8 mm wide and conform to overall curvature of mandibular residual ridge.

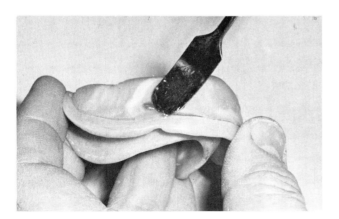

Fig. 4-126. Roll of baseplate wax is sealed to baseplate with hot spatula.

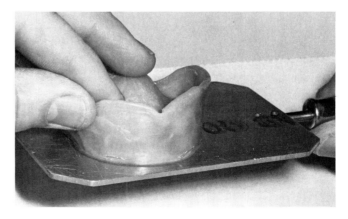

Fig. 4-127. Large flat metal spatula is convenient for developing occlusal surface of occlusion rims.

ally generated path procedures. These occlusion rims are formed from softened modeling plastic and are adapted to the baseplate in a manner similar to those made from softened baseplate wax.

SUMMARY

This chapter describes several methods of constructing baseplates. Some methods use only one material, whereas others require combinations of materials to meet specific requirements. Each combination of methods and materials has advantages and disadvantages. Undoubtedly, it is possible to construct adequate baseplates from all of the materials and according to the various methods described, although some seem to enjoy more widespread use. Resin baseplates made by the sprinkle-on or finger-adapted method satisfy many of the requirements and probably are in more use than others. It is essential to know how to construct baseplates from various materials, using several methods to have a comprehensive knowledge of dental technology.

REFERENCES

Academy of Denture Prosthetics: Principles, concepts and practices in prosthodontics, J. Prosthet. Dent. 19:182-183, 1968.

Air Force Manual 162-6: Dental laboratory technology, Washington, D.C., 1975, Government Printing Office, pp. 3, 6, 17.

Allred, H., Grear, V. D. A., Inglis, A. T., and Jenkins, M. A.: Thermoforming: a new aid in dentistry, Dent. Practit. 18:419-422, 1968; 19:2-7, 39-44, Sept., 1968.

Allred, H., Grear, V. D. A., Inglis, A. T., and Jenkins, M. A.: Application of thermoforming techniques in dentistry, Dent. Practit. 19:2-7, Sept., 1968.

Assadzadek, A., and Yarmond, M. A.: A technique for making temporary bases for complete dentures, J. Prosthet. Dent. 33:333-335, 1975.

Bodine, R. L.: Essentials of a sound complete denture technique, J. Prosthet. Dent. 14:409-431, 1964.

Boos, R. H.: Physiologic denture technique, J. Prosthet. Dent. 6:726-740, 1956.

Boucher, C. O., editor: Current clinical dental terminology, ed. 2. St. Louis, 1974, The C. V. Mosby Co.

Boucher, C. O., Hickey, J. C., and Zarb, G. A.: Prosthodontic treatment of edentulous patients, ed. 7, St. Louis, 1975, The C. V. Mosby Co.

Brewer, A. A., Szmyd, L., and McCall, C. M.: A method for recording information in double processing of denture bases, SAM-TDR 62-102, Aug., 1962, p. 7.

Browning, J. D.: A permanent-base denture technique using fluid resin, J. Prosthet. Dent. 30:468-471, 1973.

Burnett, J. V.: Accurate trial denture bases, J. Prosthet. Dent. 19:338-341, 1968.

Chick, A. O.: Use of cold curing acrylic for baseplates, Dent. Practit. and Dent. Rec. 12:91, Nov., 1961.

Cooperman, M.: Adapting shellac baseplate, Dent. Digest 65:369, Aug., 1959.

Earnshaw, R., and Klineberg, I.: Physical properties of synthetic resin baseplate materials, II, Cold-curing acrylic resins, Aust. Dent. J. 14:255-263, 1969.

Elder, S. T.: Stabilized baseplates, J. Prosthet. Dent. 5:162-168, 1955.

Fletcher, L. S.: Fundamental principles of full denture construction, J. Prosthet. Dent. 1:204-209, 1951.

Freese, A. S.: Stable occlusion rims with rubber impression material, J. Prosthet. Dent. 6:756-757, 1956.

Greener, E. H., Harcourt, J. K., and Lautenschlager, E. P.: Materials science in dentistry, ed. 1, Baltimore, 1972, The Williams & Wilkins Co.

Hall, W. A., Jr.: Important factors in adequate denture occlusion, J. Prosthet. Dent. 8:764-775, 1958.

Harris, L. W.: Facial templates and stabilized baseplates with the new chemical set resins, J. Prosthet. Dent. 1:156-160, 1951.

Harris, L. W.: An advanced use for impression trays, J. Prosthet. Dent. 3:150-154, 1953.

Jamieson, C. A.: A modern concept of complete dentures, J. Prosthet. Dent. 6:582-592, 1956.

Kapur, K. K., and Yurkstas, A. A.: An evaluation of centric relation records obtained by various techniques, J. Prosthet. Dent. 7:770-786, 1957.

Keyworth, R. G.: Monson technic for full denture construction, J. Am. Dent. Assoc. 16:130-162, Jan., 1929.

LaVere, A. M., and Freda, A. L.: Accurate fitting record bases, J. Prosthet. Dent. 32:335-338, 1974.

Malson, T. S.: Equilibrating edentulous mandibles, J. Prosthet. Dent. 14:879-891, 1964.

Martinelli, N.: Dental laboratory technology, ed. 2, St. Louis, 1975, The C. V. Mosby Co.

McCracken, W. L.: Auxillary uses of cold curing acrylic resins in prosthetic dentistry, J. Am. Dent. Assoc. 47:298-304, Sept., 1953.

McKevitt, F. H.: Finding lost prosthodontic terms, J. Prosthet. Dent. 7:738-749, 1957.

Price, R. F.: Molding baseplates, Dent. Digest 64:355, Aug., 1958.

Ringsdorf, W. M.: Ideal baseplate, J. Am. Dent. Assoc. 50:66-68, Jan., 1955.

Schoen, P. E., and Stewart, J. L.: The effect of temporary bases on the accuracy of centric jaw relationships, J. Prosthet. Dent. 18:211-216, 1968.

Sears, V. H.: Essential factors in the trial base and trial denture, J. Am. Dent. Assoc. 21:876-879, 1934.

Shooshan, E. E.: Nonwarping baseplates, J. Prosthet. Dent. 3:331, 1953.

Silverman, S. I.: The management of the trial denture base, Dent. Clin. North Am. 1:231-243, 1957.

Sowter, J. B.: Dental laboratory technology, prosthodontic techniques, Chapel Hill, N.C., 1968, The University of North Carolina Press.

Swenson, M. G., and Boucher, C. O., editors: Swenson's complete dentures, ed. 6, St. Louis, 1970, The C. V. Mosby Co.

Terry, J. M., and Wahlberg, R.: Vacuum adaptation of baseplate materials, J. Prosthet. Dent. 16:26-33, 1966.

Tucker, K. M.: Accurate record bases for jaw relation procedures, J. Prosthet. Dent. 16:224-226, 1966.

Wienski, J. C.: Stability of lower occlusion rims, Dent. Digest 65:31, Jan., 1959.

Woelfel, J. B., and Paffenbarger, G. E.: Stability of plastic impression trays, J. Am. Dent. Assoc. 63:705-706, 1961.

Zuckerman, A.: Baseplate stability, Dent. Surv. 37:594-595, 1961.

CHAPTER 5

ARTICULATORS AND MOUNTING CASTS

KENNETH D. RUDD and ROBERT M. MORROW

articulator A mechanical device that represents the temporomandibular joints and jaw members to which maxillary and mandibular casts can be attached.

mounting The laboratory procedure of attaching maxillary and/or mandibular casts to an articulator or similar instrument

face-bow A caliper-like device that is used to record the relationship of the maxillae to the temporomandibular joint (or opening axis of the mandible) and to orient the cast in this same relationship to the opening axis of the articulator.

A representative variety of articulators available to the dentist is depicted in Figs. 5-1 to 5-4. Jaw relation records obtained by the dentist are used to orient casts for mounting in these articulators. In some instances, a face-bow record may have been made for mounting the maxillary cast in the articulator. After the maxillary cast has been mounted, the mandibular cast is oriented to the maxillary cast according to the jaw relation record and mounted in the articulator. Casts can also be mounted without a face-bow record; then they are positioned in the articulator arbitrarily and attached to the upper and lower members with artificial stone. Although casts can be mounted with plaster of Paris, artificial stone is preferable because it has less setting expansion. Slurry concentrate* is used frequently when mixing the mounting stone to accelerate the set. This chapter presents methods for mounting casts in several articulators.

REQUIREMENTS FOR MOUNTING STONE

To a large extent, the ultimate success of a complete denture restoration depends on an accurate jaw relation record. However, it is equally important that the accurate jaw relation record be transferred to an articulator accurately. The material used to mount casts should set quickly and hard, with only minimal dimensional change; be strong; separate cleanly from the cast after use of a separating medium; and permit reattachment after processing of the denture. It is essential that the mounting material does not damage the cast or the articulator.

Mounting casts
Denar Mark II articulator and ear-bow record

The Denar Mark II articulator is particularly suitable for complete dentures. The instrument is practical, rigid, and easy to use; it also allows casts to be mounted quickly and easily.

PROCEDURE

1. Prepare the articulator to accept the ear-bow.
2. Set the immediate side-shift adjustments at 0 degrees (Fig. 5-5).
3. Set the progressive side-shift at 5 degrees (Fig. 5-6).
4. Set the protrusive condylar paths at 30 degrees (Fig. 5-7).
5. Set the vertical dimension of the incisal pin at 0 (Fig. 5-8).
6. Attach a mounting plate to the upper bow of the articulator and a maxillary cast support to the lower bow (Fig. 5-9).
7. Set the incisal guide table at 0 degrees (Fig. 5-10).

Text continued on p. 143.

---

*Slurry concentrate is a thick liquid made by grinding stone casts on a cast trimmer.

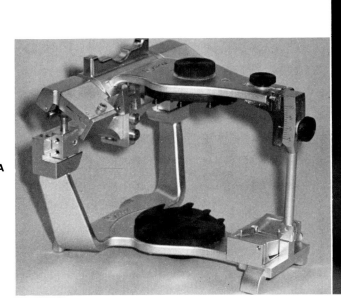
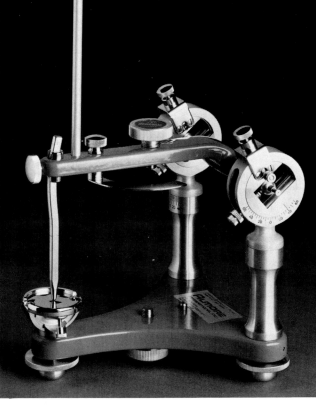

Fig. 5-1. A, Denar Mark II articulator, Denar Corp., Anaheim, Calif. **B,** Dentatus ARH articulator. (**B** courtesy Almore International, Inc., Portland, Ore.)

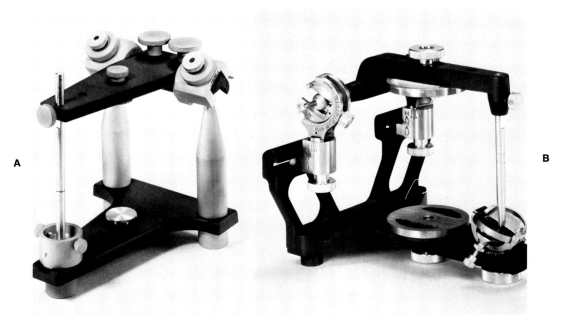

Fig. 5-2. A, Hanau 154-1 articulator. **B,** Hanau 130-1 articulator.

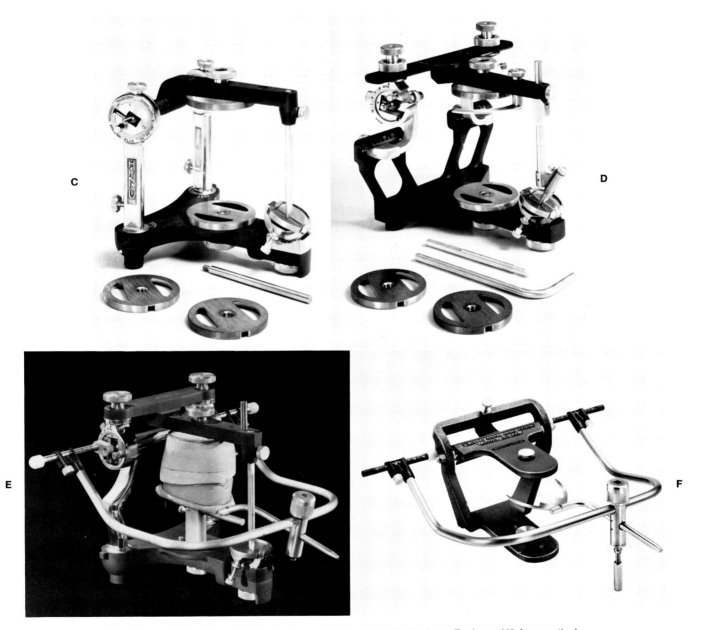

Fig. 5-2, cont'd. C, Hanau 96H2 articulator. **D,** Hanau 130-28 articulator. **E,** Hanau H2 Arcon articulator. **F,** Hanau laboratory technical device. (Courtesy Teledyne Dental Products Co., Hanau Division, Buffalo, N.Y.)

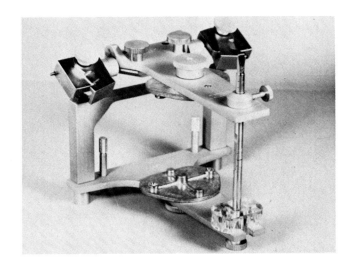

Fig. 5-3. Whip-Mix articulator. (Courtesy Whip-Mix Corp., Louisville, Ky.)

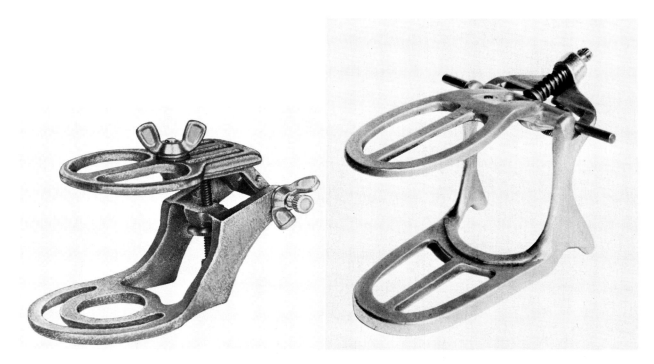

Fig. 5-4. Plainline articulator and Buffalo Dental No. 9 articulator. (Courtesy Buffalo Dental Manufacturing Co., Inc., Brooklyn, N.Y.)

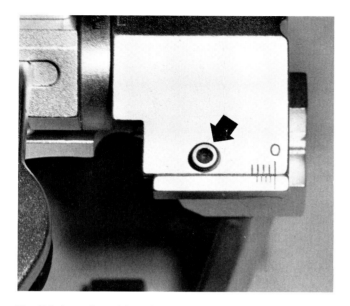

Fig. 5-5. Immediate side-shift adjustment is set at 0 degrees. Lock-screw is medial to scale (arrow).

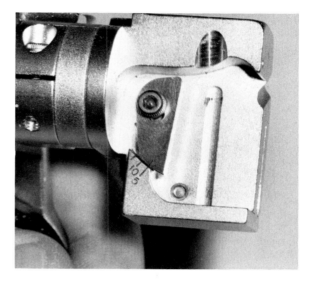

Fig. 5-6. Progressive side-shift is set at 5 degrees.

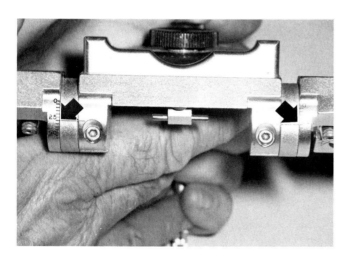

Fig. 5-7. Protrusive condylar paths are set at 30 degrees (arrows).

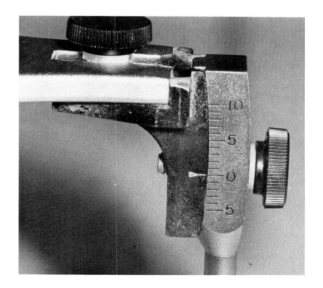

Fig. 5-8. Incisal pin is set at 0.

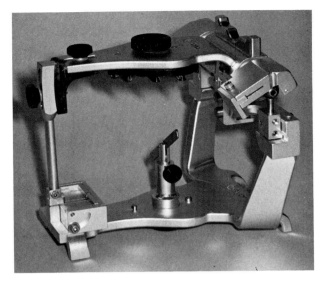

Fig. 5-9. Mounting plate is attached to upper bow, and maxillary cast support to lower bow.

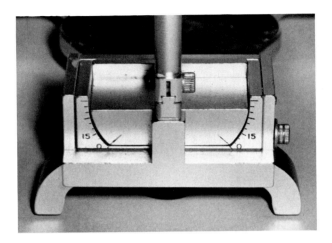

Fig. 5-10. Incisal guide table is set at 0 degrees.

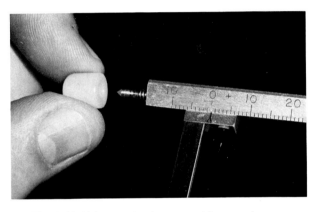

Fig. 5-11. Nylon earplug is removed from ear-bow.

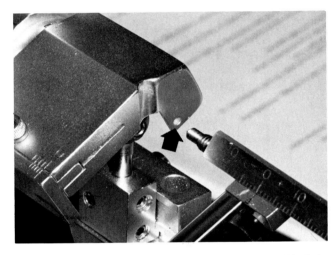

Fig. 5-12. Posterior reference pin of face-bow is placed in index holes (arrow) on lateral aspect of articulator.

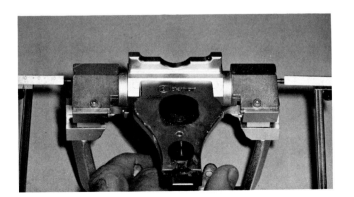

Fig. 5-13. Posterior reference slides are adjusted until they are equal.

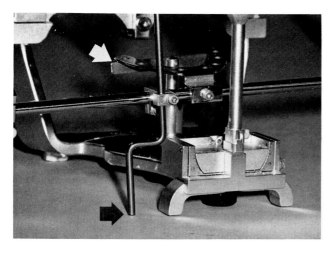

Fig. 5-14. Maxillary cast support crossbar contacts undersurface of fork (white arrow) without lifting reference rod from reference surface (black arrow). Record has been removed to facilitate viewing.

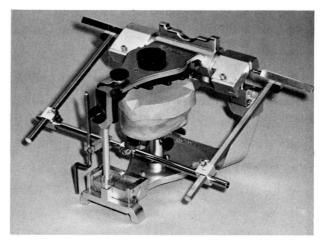

Fig. 5-15. Maxillary cast is seated in face-bow record.

8. Remove the nylon earplugs from the ear-bow to permit its attachment to the articulator (Fig. 5-11).

9. Place the posterior reference pin of the face-bow in the index holes on the lateral aspect of the articulator fossae (Fig. 5-12).

10. Place the face-bow on the articulator, and adjust the posterior reference slides to make both scales equal (Fig. 5-13).

11. Adjust the maxillary cast support until the support crossbar contacts the undersurface of the fork without lifting the reference rod from the bearing surface (Fig. 5-14).

12. Place the maxillary cast in the face-bow record on the bite fork (Fig. 5-15).

13. Paint the upper surface of the cast with a separating medium* (Fig. 5-16).

14. Mix artificial stone with slurry concentrate to accelerate its set and place stone onto the top of the cast and into the upper mounting plate. The artificial stone should completely fill all recesses of the upper mounting plate (Fig. 5-17).

15. Move the upper bow down onto the top of the cast in such a manner that it joins the two layers of stone. Make certain that the condyles maintain centric relation and the incisal pin touches the incisal platform. Smooth the surface of the stone that attaches the maxillary cast to the articulator (Fig. 5-18). After the stone has set, remove the cast support from the articulator and replace it with the lower mounting plate.

16. Allow the stone to set, remove the upper bow from

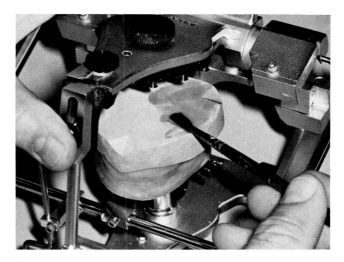

Fig. 5-16. Base of maxillary cast is painted with separating medium.

the articulator, and place it upside down. Orient the mandibular cast to the maxillary cast by using the centric relation record provided (Fig. 5-19). Replace the lower bow of the articulator, and check to see that the space between the articulator and cast is adequate (Fig. 5-20). Lute the two casts together with tongue blades and sticky wax.

17. Paint the base of the lower cast and index grooves with a separating medium (Fig. 5-21). Do not drop the incisal pin to compensate for the thickness of the jaw relation record if the record was made at the vertical dimension of occlusion.

18. Remove the lower bow, mix the artificial stone

---

*Super-Sep, Kerr Manufacturing Co., Romulus, Mich.

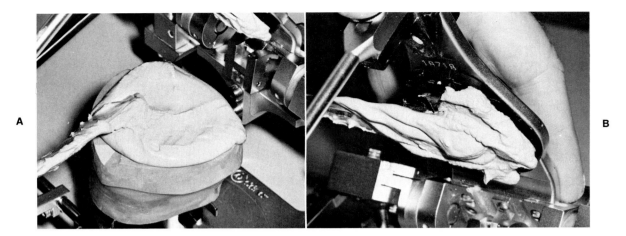

Fig. 5-17. A, Artificial stone is placed on base of maxillary cast. Make certain to fill indexing notches or grooves with stone. B, Stone is placed also in indexes of mounting plate.

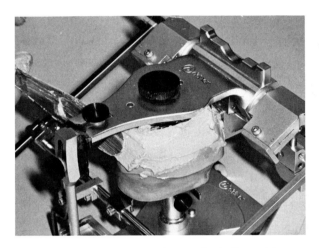

Fig. 5-18. Mounting stone is smoothed with spatula.

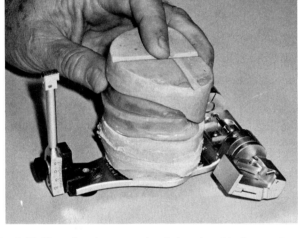

Fig. 5-19. Upper bow is removed and placed upside down on bench. Mandibular cast and occlusion rim are positioned according to jaw relation record.

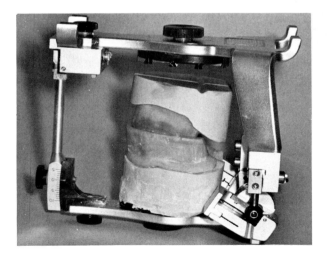

Fig. 5-20. Lower bow is replaced, and space between cast and mounting plate is checked.

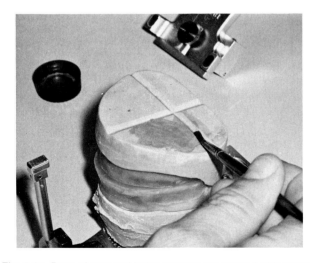

Fig. 5-21. Base of cast and index grooves are painted with separating medium.

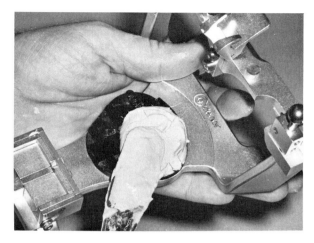

Fig. 5-22. Stone is placed on mounting plate on lower bow.

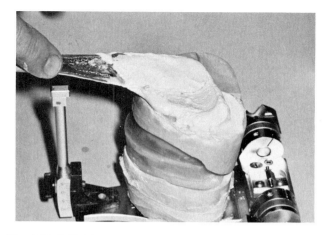

Fig. 5-23. Artificial stone is placed on base and in indexing grooves of lower cast.

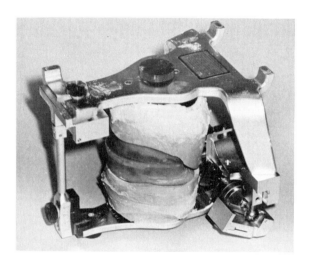

Fig. 5-24. Lower bow is positioned, and care is exercised to see that condyles are seated in their fossae and contact is made between incisal pin and incisal table.

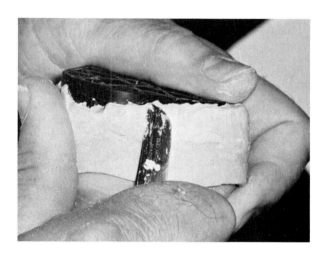

Fig. 5-25. Mounting stone is smoothed with knife.

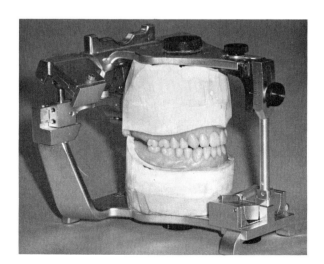

Fig. 5-26. Mounted casts are ready for setting teeth.

with slurry concentrate, and fill all recesses of the mounting plate on the lower bow with stone (Fig. 5-22). Place more stone on the mandibular cast base, and make certain to put stone in the indexing grooves (Fig. 5-23). Turn the lower bow upside down, and seat it on top of the upper bow (Fig. 5-24). See that the condyles remain in the fossae and that the incisal pin contacts the incisal table. Lock the centric latch at this time, and smooth the stone that attaches the mandibular cast to the lower bow of the instrument for a neat appearance (Fig. 5-25). Now the mounting is complete (Fig. 5-26).

Dentatus ARH articulator and face-bow registration

The Dentatus ARH articulator is a superbly constructed semiadjustable articulator that is ideal for construction of a complete denture. Because it is machined

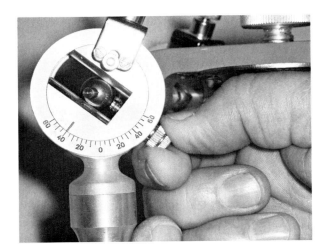

Fig. 5-27. Condylar spheres of articulator should make contact with anterior stops. Then anterior stopscrews are tightened on both sides of articulator.

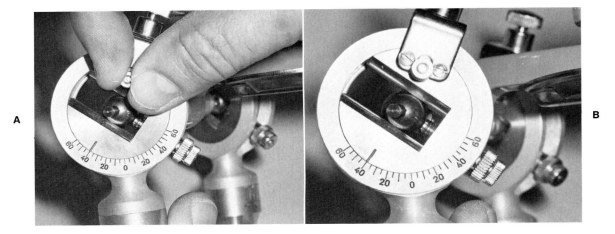

A

B

Fig. 5-28. A, Tightening condylar lockscrews will maintain position of condylar sphere against anterior stop. **B,** Note condylar sphere in contact with anterior stop.

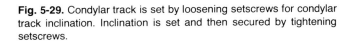

Fig. 5-29. Condylar track is set by loosening setscrews for condylar track inclination. Inclination is set and then secured by tightening setscrews.

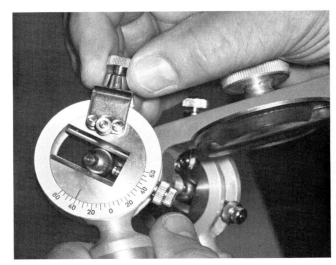

accurately and has an anodized surface, this articulator functions smoothly, creates an excellent appearance, and removal of plaster of Paris or dental stone from articulator surfaces is facilitated.

PROCEDURE

1. Tighten the anterior stopscrews on both sides of the articulator (Fig. 5-27).

2. Check to make certain that the condylar spheres rest against the anterior stopscrews and that they are secure after tightening the condylar lockscrews (Fig. 5-28).

3. Set the condylar track at 40 degrees and secure it (Fig. 5-29).

4. Set the incisal guide pin at 0 (Fig. 5-30).

5. Set the incisal guide table flat (Fig. 5-31).

6. Attach a mounting plate to the upper bow of the articulator, and tighten the lockscrew (Fig. 5-32).

7. Set the condylar posts at 15 degrees (Fig. 5-33).

8. Adjust the calibrations on the face-bow slide until it is possible to obtain the same reading on both sides. Adjust them until there is a slight tension or spring effect with the face-bow to maintain contact between the

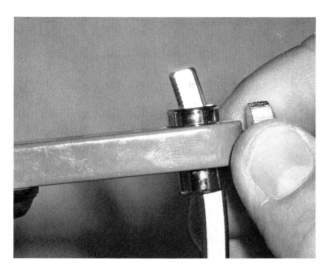

Fig. 5-30. Incisal pin lockscrew is loosened, and pin is set at 0. Lockscrew is tightened after pin is set.

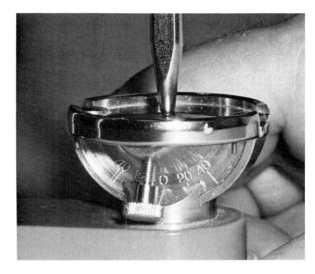

Fig. 5-31. Incisal table is set flat, and locknut for incisal table is tightened to maintain setting.

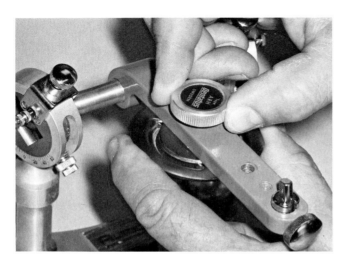

Fig. 5-32. Mounting plate is attached to upper bow of articulator.

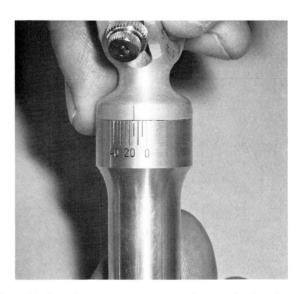

Fig. 5-33. Condylar posts are set at 15 degrees. Locknut for condylar post at base of articulator is loosened, post is set at 15 degrees, and locknut is tightened. Adjustment must be made on both sides of articulator.

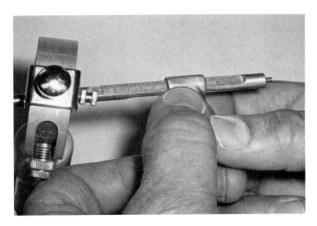

Fig. 5-34. Face-bow slides are adjusted until equal on both sides. This action is predicated on assumption that face-bow record was made in same manner, with same setting on both sides.

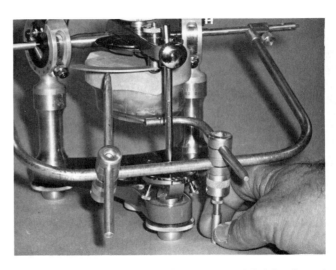

Fig. 5-35. When third point of reference is used, height of cast is adjusted until orbital pointer tip is at same level as orbital axis plane indicator.

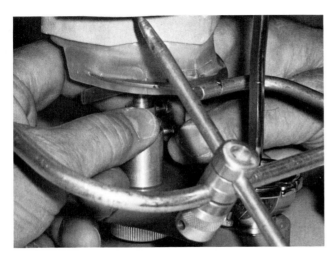

Fig. 5-36. After height is adjusted, maxillary cast support is attached to lower bow of articulator. Cast support is adjusted to contact maxillary occlusion rim and is locked securely.

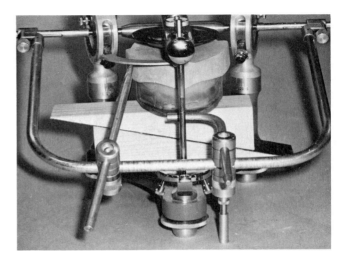

Fig. 5-37. Wooden wedges can be used to support maxillary cast if cast support is unavailable.

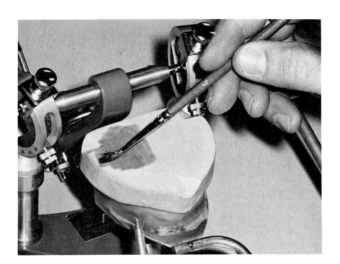

Fig. 5-38. Base of maxillary cast is painted with separating medium.

condylar rods and the condylar axis of the articulator (Fig. 5-34).

9. Place the maxillary cast in the face-bow record, and adjust the height of the face-bow by turning the anterior jackscrew. If using a third point of reference, adjust the height until the orbital pointer touches the movable orbital axis plane indicator (Fig. 5-35).

10. After determining the height, it is possible to place a maxillary cast support or wooden wedges on the articulator to support the maxillary cast (Figs. 5-36 and 5-37). Coat the base of the upper cast with a separating medium (Fig. 5-38). Mix artificial stone with slurry concentrate to lute the maxillary cast to the upper bow of the articulator. The mounting plate and articulator surfaces contacting the stone may be lightly coated with silicone lubricant to facilitate cleanup later.

11. Place stone from this mix on the cast and in the upper mounting plate to assure the flow of stone into all recesses of the mounting plate and a firm attachment of the maxillary cast on the articulator (Fig. 5-39).

12. Close the articulator slowly until the stone on the upper part of the cast joins with the stone in the mounting plate, and tap it gently (Fig. 5-40).

13. Place additional stone wherever required to complete the mounting and fill the voids. It is possible to remove excess stone with a spatula at this time (Fig. 5-41). Allow the stone to set before attaching the mandibular cast. Attach a mounting plate to the lower bow, and invert the articulator.

14. Relate the mandibular cast to the maxillary cast according to the jaw relation record, and lute them together with tongue blades and sticky wax. Close the ar-

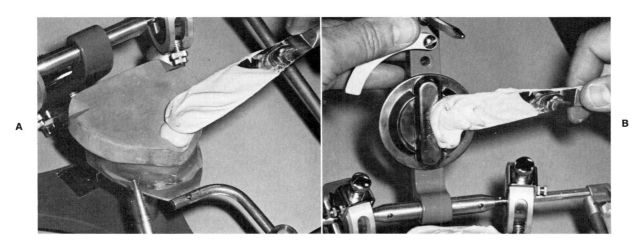

Fig. 5-39. A, Place stone into index notches. **B,** Additional stone is worked into undercuts of upper mounting plate.

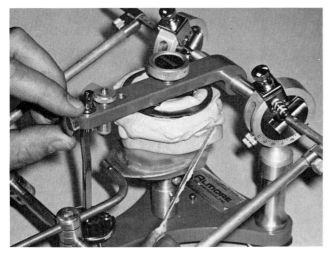

Fig. 5-40. Articulator is closed and tapped until contact is made between incisal guide pin and incisal guide table. Then stone mounting is smoothed with spatula.

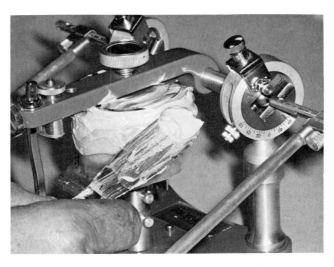

Fig. 5-41. Additional stone can be added to fill voids.

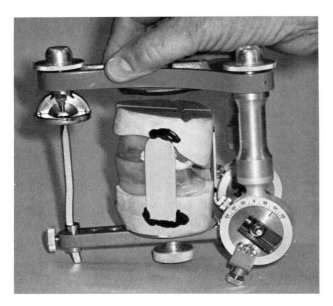

Fig. 5-42. Articulator is closed to evaluate space between mandibular cast and articulator. This procedure will indicate how much stone is needed to mount cast.

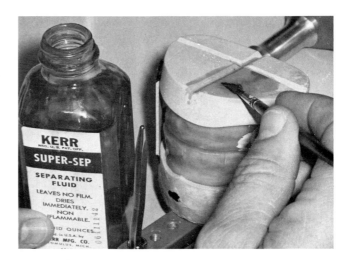

Fig. 5-43. Base of mandibular cast is painted with separating medium.

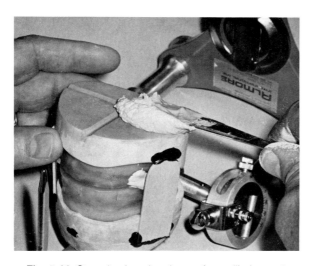

Fig. 5-44. Stone is placed on base of mandibular cast.

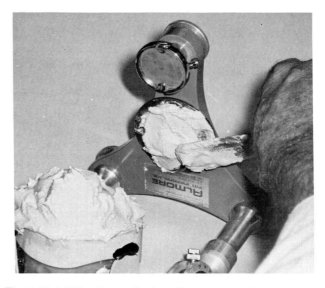

Fig. 5-45. Additional stone is placed in recesses of lower mounting plate.

ticulator to check the clearance between the mandibular cast and articulator and to estimate the amount of stone required for mounting the cast (Fig. 5-42).

15. Paint the base of the mandibular cast with a separating medium* (Fig. 5-43).

16. Mix artificial stone with slurry concentrate, place

it on the base of the lower cast, and make certain that the indexing grooves are full (Fig. 5-44).

17. Place additional stone in the mounting plate on the lower bow of the articulator (Fig. 5-45).

18. Close the articulator, and remove the excess or add stone wherever necessary to fill voids. While the stone is soft, tap the articulator lower bow several times to make certain that the incisal guide pin touches the incisal guide table (Fig. 5-46).

---

*Super-Sep, Kerr Manufacturing Co., Romulus, Mich.

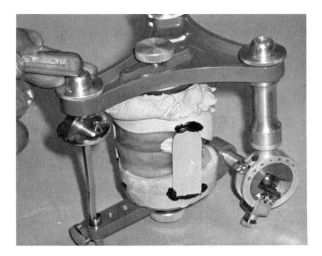

Fig. 5-46. Articulator is closed and tapped gently to obtain contact between incisal guide pin and incisal guide table.

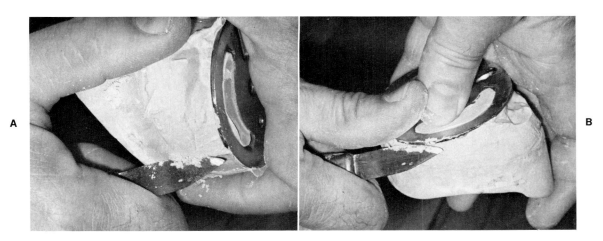

Fig. 5-47. A, When trimming mounting stone, blade is held perpendicular to junction of stone and cast. **B,** Separation of mounting plate from stone can result from trimming stone in this manner.

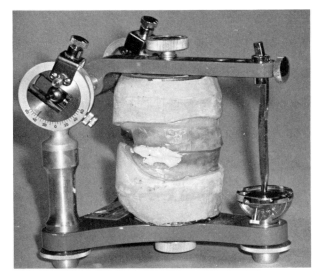

Fig. 5-48. Mounted casts ready for setup.

19. After the stone has set, remove the attached cast from the articulator, and trim and smooth the mounting stone. When trimming the casts, it is best to move the edge of the knife perpendicular to the border of the base of the cast and mounting plates (Fig. 5-47, *A*). Moving the edge parallel, instead of perpendicular, to the border can cause separation of the cast or mounting plate (Fig. 5-47, *B*). Now the mounted casts are ready for setting the denture teeth (Fig. 5-48).

Hanau 130-28 articulator and arbitrary mounting

Various models of Hanau articulators have been in use many years for constructing complete dentures. Therefore probably the majority of articulators used are Hanau articulators. In this series, an arbitrary mounting method and mounting casts with a face-bow record for the Hanau 130-28 articulator will be described.

This method requires positioning the casts in an arbi-

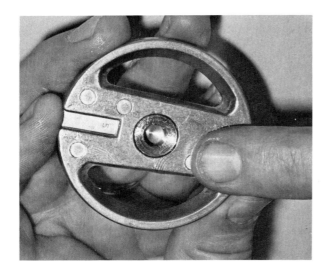

Fig. 5-49. Mounting plates and articulator bows are lubricated with petroleum jelly or Masque.

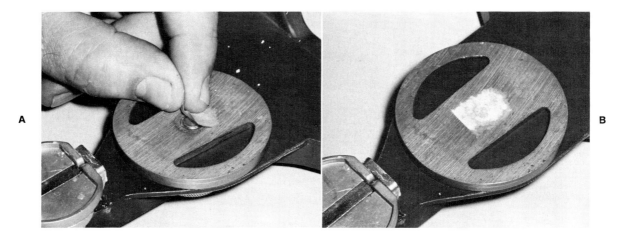

A

B

Fig. 5-50. A, Small piece of paper is placed over threaded hole of older type mounting plates to aid in preventing stone from penetrating threads and act as spacer when removing mounting and replacing it on articulator. It can prevent separation of mounting plate from stone if particle of stone or wax gets in threaded hole. **B,** Lubricant helps hold paper in place.

trary or average position in relation to the opening axis of the articulator. It requires no face-bow registration.

PROCEDURE

1. Coat the mounting plate and articulator member with petroleum jelly or Masque* before attaching the plate to the articulator (Fig. 5-49). This procedure helps keep the articulator free of stone and aids in retrieving the plate from the mounting stone after completion of the denture.

2. Attach the mounting plates to the articulator and, if using the older Hanau mounting plate, place a small square of paper over the threaded hole (Fig. 5-50). It is

---

*Masque, The Harry J. Bosworth Co., Chicago, Ill.

unnecessary to use this paper with new-model Hanau mounting plates (Fig. 5-51).

3. Adjust the incisal guide table to its flat or horizontal position. Set the adjustable incisal guide pin at No. 5 (Fig. 5-52).

4. Set the horizontal condylar inclination at the appropriate setting (usually 0 degrees when using 0-degree teeth or 30 degrees or another inclination, as desired, if using anatomic teeth), and lock the condylar elements in contact with the condyle stopscrews (Fig. 5-53).

5. Place a rubber band on the articulator, extending from the lower annular mark of the incisal guide pin around each condyle support post. Adjust the rubber band to form a plane that divides the space between the upper and lower members of the articulator (Fig. 5-54).

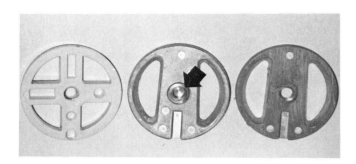

Fig. 5-51. Three types of mounting plates: plastic mounting plate *(left)*, new closed center mounting plate (arrow, *center*), and open center mounting plate *(right)*.

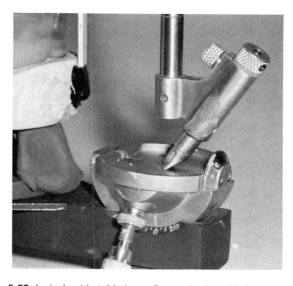

Fig. 5-52. Incisal guide table is set flat, and adjustable incisal guide pin is placed at fifth ring.

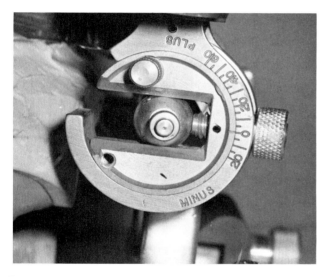

Fig. 5-53. Horizontal condylar inclination is set at 0 degrees. However, setting will vary with type of teeth.

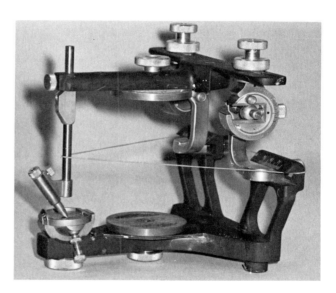

Fig. 5-54. Rubber band aids in orienting plane for casts mounted arbitrarily.

6. Place three lumps of modeling clay on the lower mounting plate to serve as an adjustable cast support (Fig. 5-55).

7. With the baseplate and the occlusion rims luted together, place the maxillary and mandibular casts in correct relationship on the three clay supports in the articulator. Then align them until the occlusal plane of the occlusion rims is parallel to the plane established by the rubber band (Fig. 5-56).

8. Open the articulator, and paint the base of the maxillary cast with a separating medium (Fig. 5-57).

9. Mix artificial stone with slurry concentrate and, using a spatula, add stone to the base of the cast and mounting plate (Fig. 5-58).

10. Close the articulator until the incisal guide pin touches the incisal guide table, and add stone as needed to fill voids (Fig. 5-59).

11. After the stone has set, invert the articulator. Remove the modeling clay cast supports, paint a separating medium on the base of the cast, and attach the lower cast to the articulator with stone (Fig. 5-60).

12. Permit the stone to set, then remove the tongue

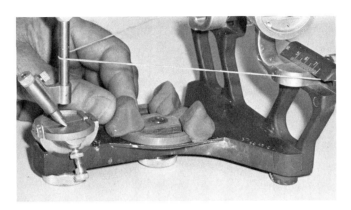

Fig. 5-55. Three lumps of modeling clay are used to orient and support casts during mounting procedure. Clay can be molded to raise or lower casts as needed.

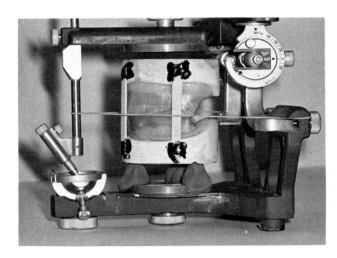

Fig. 5-56. Rubber band serves as reference plane to which occlusal plane of occlusion rims is aligned.

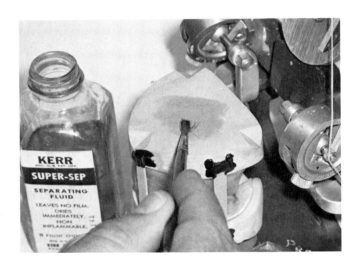

Fig. 5-57. Base of cast is painted with separating medium.

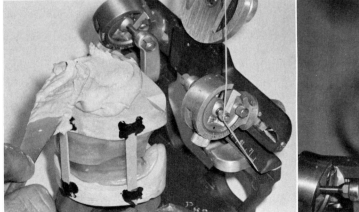

A

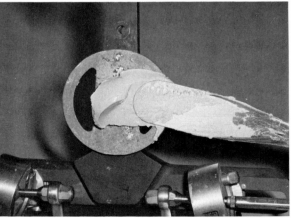

B

Fig. 5-58. A, Place stone onto base of cast and into index notches. **B,** Additional stone is placed in mounting plate.

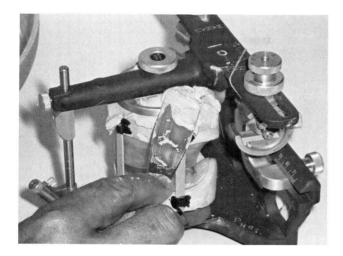

Fig. 5-59. Articulator is closed, and stone is added as needed to fill voids.

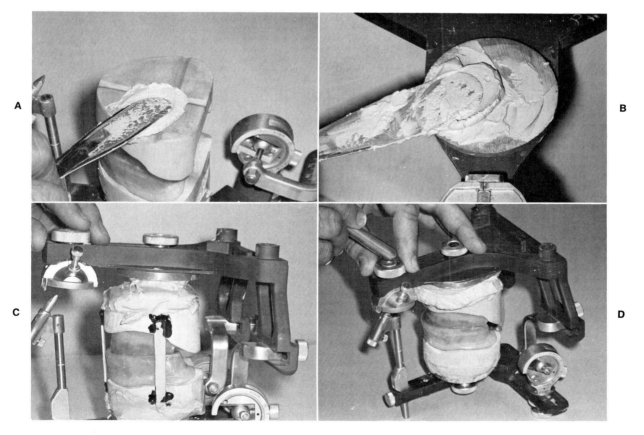

Fig. 5-60. A, Stone is placed on base of cast that has been painted with separating medium. Care is exercised to fill index grooves. **B,** Stone is placed also in mounting plate. **C,** Articulator is closed to join stone on cast with stone on mounting plate. **D,** Lower member is tapped lightly to bring incisal guide pin into contact with incisal guide table.

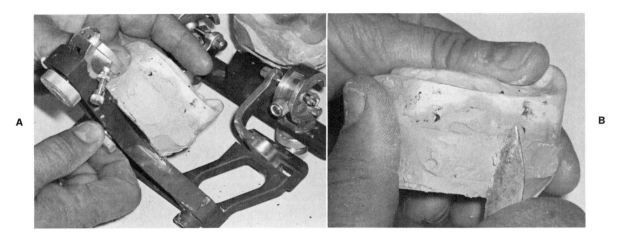

Fig. 5-61. A, Casts are removed from articulator. **B,** Mounting stone is trimmed to create neat smooth appearance.

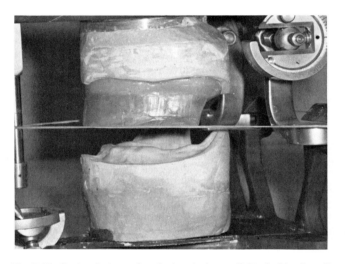

Fig. 5-62. Occlusal plane of occlusion rim is parallel to "rubber band" plane.

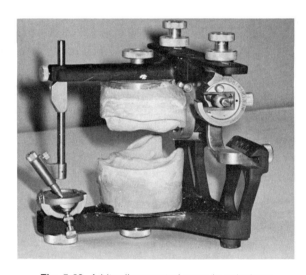

Fig. 5-63. Arbitrarily mounted casts in articulator.

blades, casts, and mountings from the articulator, and trim (Fig. 5-61).

13. Properly mounted casts illustrate the parallelism of the occlusion rim to the plane established by the rubber band (Fig. 5-62). The mounted casts are ready for positioning the denture teeth (Fig. 5-63).

Hanau 130-28 articulator and face-bow registration

After accomplishing a face-bow registration, it is used to mount the maxillary cast in the articulator. After mounting the maxillary cast, orient the mandibular cast to the mounted maxillary cast, according to the centric relation record, and attach it to the lower member of the articulator with artificial stone.

PROCEDURE

1. Adjust the articulator as described for the arbitrary method; however, the horizontal condylar inclination is generally set at 30 degrees instead of 0 degrees.

2. Lubricate the mounting plates and articulator bows with petroleum jelly or Masque as described previously.

3. Place the assembled face-bow and cast on the articulator carefully. Adjust the face-bow condylar slide registrations until they are the same on both sides (Fig. 5-64).

4. Whenever a third point-of-reference record is available, attach the orbital plane indicator to the articulator (Fig. 5-65).

5. Attach a maxillary cast support to the lower mem-

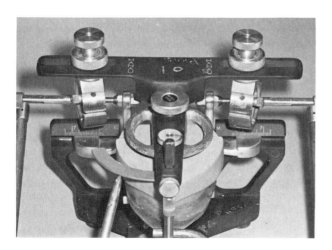

Fig. 5-64. Face-bow is assembled on articulator, and face-bow slide registrations are kept equal.

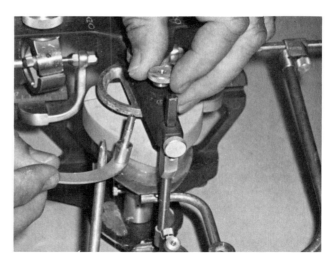

Fig. 5-65. If third point of reference is used, orbital plane indicator is placed on articulator if not already in place.

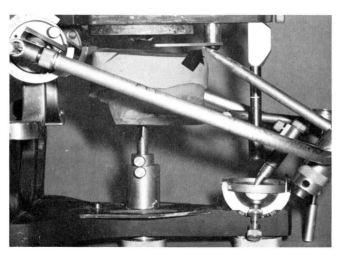

Fig. 5-66. Maxillary cast support is adjusted to maintain cast at correct height. Orbital point tip touches orbital plane indicator (arrow).

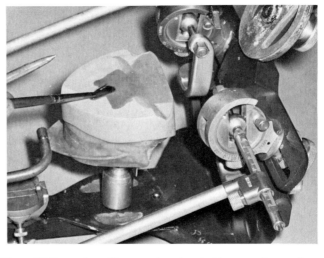

Fig. 5-67. Base of maxillary cast is painted with separating medium.

ber of the articulator, and adjust the height of the face-bow by way of the anterior jackscrew until the orbital pointer touches the orbital plane indicator (Fig. 5-66).

6. Paint the maxillary cast base with a separating medium (Fig. 5-67).

7. Mix artificial stone, and attach the maxillary cast to the articulator as described previously (Fig. 5-68).

8. After the stone has set, release the face-bow from the condylar extensions of the articulator (Fig. 5-69, *A*), and then remove the face-bow fork from the face-bow (Fig. 5-69, *B*).

9. Remove the mounted maxillary cast from the articulator; then remove the baseplate and the occlusion rim from the cast (Fig. 5-70).

10. The face-bow fork is removed from the occlusion rim by warming it over a burner. When the wax has softened, withdraw the fork (Fig. 5-71). Make certain to avoid distorting the record.

11. Replace the baseplate and occlusion rims on their casts, invert the articulator, and assemble the casts according to the jaw relation record (Fig. 5-72). If the centric relation record was made at the vertical dimension of occlusion, no compensating adjustment of the incisal pin is necessary. If the record was made at an increased vertical dimension, the incisal pin should be lengthened by the estimated or measured thickness of the record. Failure to observe this step may result in altering the vertical dimension of occlusion.

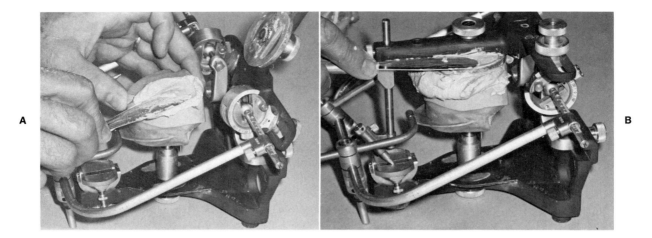

Fig. 5-68. A, Stone is placed on base of cast coated with separating medium and on mounting plate. **B,** Articulator is closed, and stone is added and smoothed wherever required.

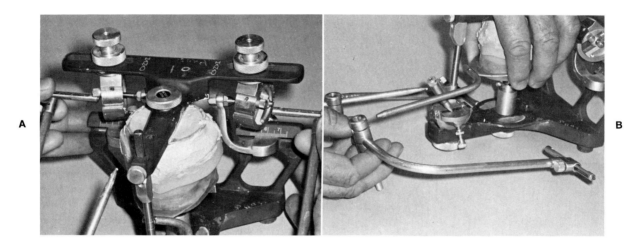

Fig. 5-69. A, Face-bow is removed from articulator after stone is set. **B,** Then face-bow is removed from face-bow fork.

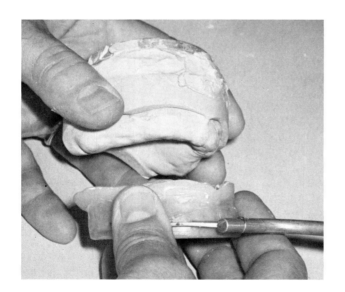

Fig. 5-70. Occlusion rim and face-bow fork are removed from maxillary cast.

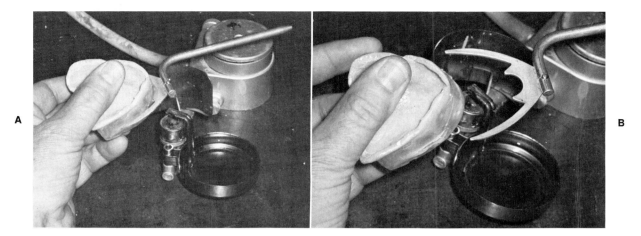

Fig. 5-71. A, Face-bow fork is warmed over burner. *Avoid overheating.* **B,** Warmed face-bow fork is pulled from occlusion rim.

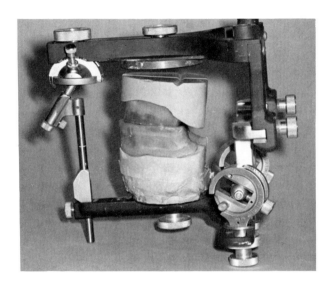

Fig. 5-72. Casts joined together according to jaw relation record are assembled in inverted articulator. This procedure makes it possible to estimate volume of stone needed to attach mandibular cast.

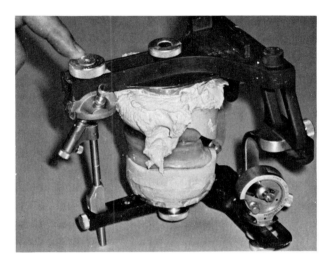

Fig. 5-73. Lower cast is attached to articulator as described previously. Too much stone was used in this instance.

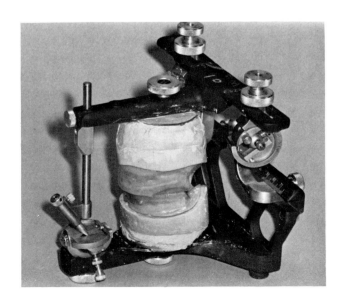

Fig. 5-74. Mounted casts in articulator.

12. Paint the base of the lower cast with a separating medium, and attach the cast of the articulator with artificial stone (Fig. 5-73).

13. Trim the mounting stone with a knife to give a neat appearance (Fig. 5-74).

Hanau H2 Arcon Series articulator and ear-bow record

The Hanau H2 Arcon Series articulator is especially suitable for construction of a complete denture. Mounting casts in this articulator using an ear-bow record to orient the maxillary cast will be described.

PROCEDURE

1. Adjust the horizontal inclination of both condylar guides until they are vertical, approximately 90 degrees, and tighten the thumbnuts (Fig. 5-75).

2. Adjust the lateral indication of both condylar guides to 0 degrees, and tighten their thumbnuts (Fig. 5-76).

3. Adjust the incisal guide to 0 degrees, and tighten the locknut (Fig. 5-77).

4. Adjust the incisal pin to align the median registration groove with the underside of the upper member, and tighten the thumbscrew (Fig. 5-78).

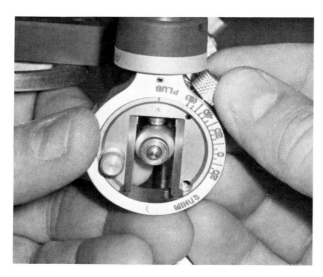

Fig. 5-75. Horizontal condylar inclinations are set at vertical, and thumbnuts are tightened.

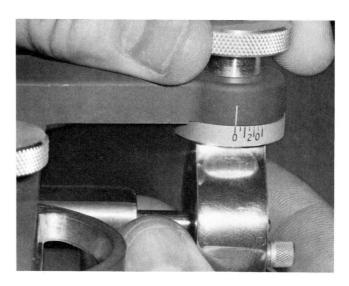

Fig. 5-76. Lateral indications of both condylar guidances are set at 0 degrees.

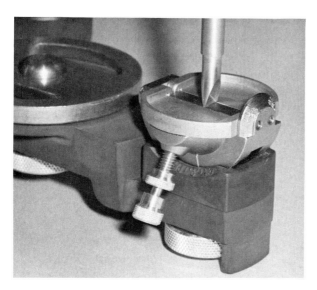

Fig. 5-77. Incisal guide table is set at 0 degrees.

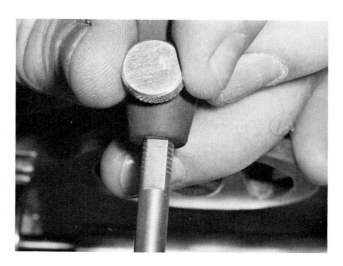

Fig. 5-78. Incisal pin is set so that median registration groove of pin is aligned with underside of upper member.

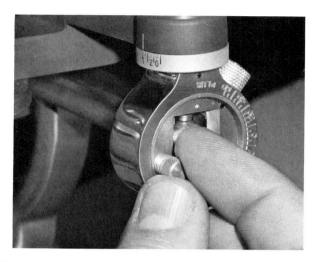

Fig. 5-79. Centric locknut is tightened to allow articulator to operate as hinge.

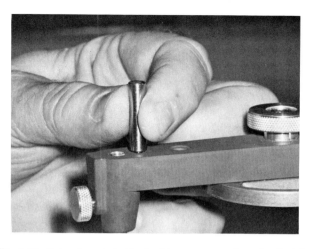

Fig. 5-80. Extension stud attached to upper member of articulator permits articulator to be inverted on bench top without special support.

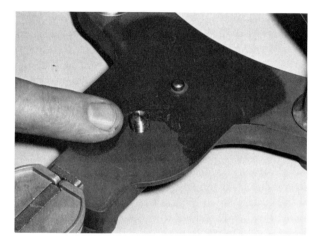

Fig. 5-81. Articulator surfaces that will be exposed to stone are coated with thin layer of petroleum jelly.

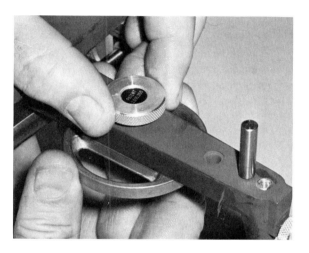

Fig. 5-82. Mounting plate coated with petroleum jelly is attached to upper member of articulator.

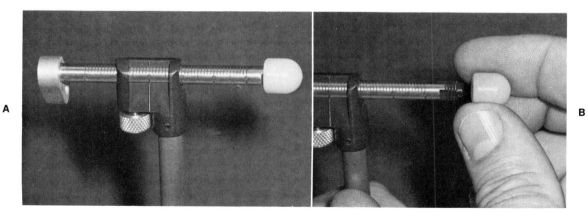

Fig. 5-83. A, Ear-bow with nylon earpiece in place. **B,** Nylon earpiece is removed from ear-bow.

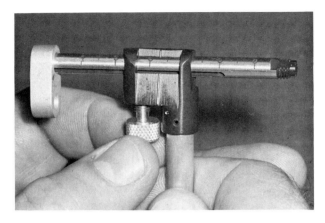

Fig. 5-84. Frame screws are released to permit withdrawal of scales.

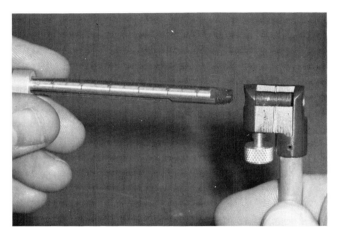

Fig. 5-85. Scales are withdrawn.

5. Tighten the centric lock to restrict the articulator to opening and closing movements only (Fig. 5-79).

6. Attach the extension stud (Fig. 5-80).

7. Apply a thin coating of petroleum jelly to all surfaces of the articulator that will be exposed to the stone mounting medium (Fig. 5-81).

8. Apply a thin coating of petroleum jelly to the mounting plate, and attach it to the upper member firmly (Fig. 5-82).

9. Remove the nylon earpiece from the ear-bow (Fig. 5-83). Fully release the frame screws (Fig. 5-84). Withdraw the scales from their frames (Fig. 5-85).

10. Reverse the scales, and place the condyle compensator right (R) and left (L) at the inside of the bow (Fig. 5-86).

11. Engage the frame thumbscrews in the keyway, and adjust the scales laterally to 6.8 mm for each side. Tighten the frame thumbscrews to maintain this symmetrical adjustment (Fig. 5-87).

12. Attach the mounting jig with the horizontal stud extending forward and in line with the sagittal plane. Loosen the thumbscrew to lower the pivot of the mounting jig (Fig. 5-88).

13. Flex the bow slightly to engage the condyle compensators over the condylar shafts on the articulator. The condyle compensators make the average distance from the condyle center to the patient's external auditory meatus center 12 mm (Fig. 5-89).

14. Lower the anterior portion of the bow assembly to rest the aluminum frontal portion of the bite plane on the horizontal stud of the mounting jig. This position makes it possible to align the incisal edge of the maxillary occlusion rim imprint at a level with the average incisal reference notch in the incisal pin, that is 47 mm below the condylar plane (Fig. 5-90).

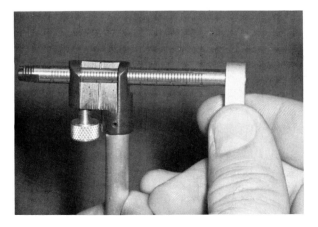

Fig. 5-86. Scales are reversed, and condylar compensator is placed toward articulator. Same procedure is used on both sides.

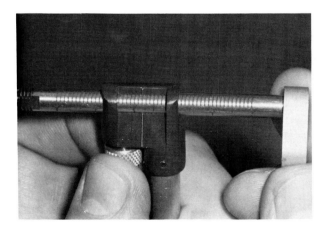

Fig. 5-87. Scales are adjusted symmetrically, for example, 6.8 mm on each side, and frame thumbscrews are tightened.

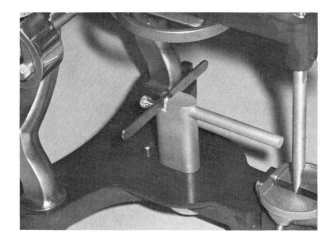

Fig. 5-88. Mounting jig is secured in place in articulator. Loosening thumbscrew allows pivot to be raised or lowered.

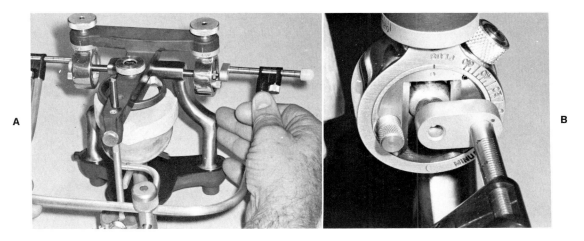

Fig. 5-89. A, Bow is flexed slightly to engage condyle compensators over condyle shafts. Flexing helps to keep bow in position. **B,** Note how condyle compensators are positioned.

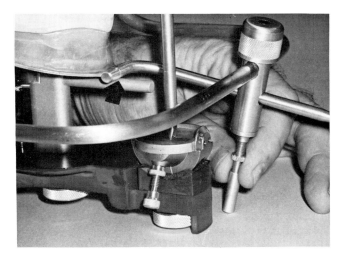

Fig. 5-90. Bow assembly is lowered to allow bite plane (bite fork) to rest on horizontal stud of mounting jig (arrow).

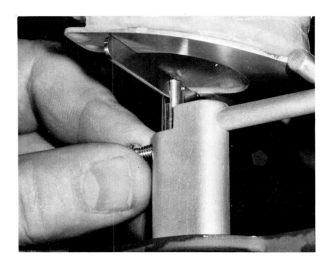

Fig. 5-91. Pivot is raised to contact undersurface of bite plane, and thumbscrew is tightened. Mounting jig supports maxillary cast.

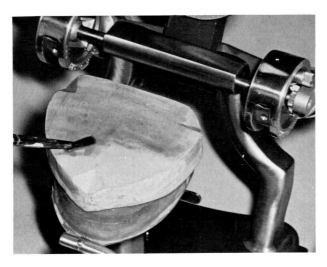

Fig. 5-92. Base of maxillary cast is painted with separating medium.

15. Raise the pivot of the mounting jig to contact the underside of the bite plane, and lock it in position with the thumbscrew to stabilize it and carry the weight of the maxillary cast and stone mounting medium (Fig. 5-91).

16. Paint the base of the cast with a separating medium (Fig. 5-92).

17. Mount the maxillary cast in the articulator with a mixture of stone and slurry concentrate. Smooth the mounting with a spatula, and remove excess stone to expose the top surface of the mounting plate. This action permits convenient removal and accurate reattachment to the articulator (Fig. 5-93). If the jaw relation record is made by a conventional interocclusal record method, and not a wafer technique, it is probably better for the maxillary cast to be mounted in the articulator before making the centric jaw relation record. After mounting the maxillary cast in the articulator, then place the indexing grooves in the wax occlusion rim and record the

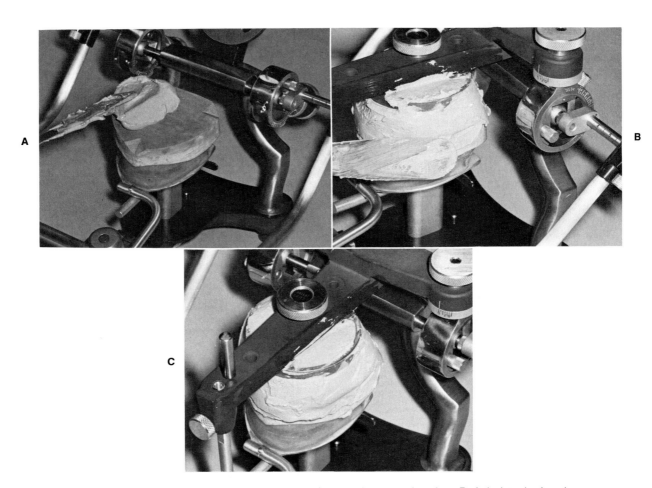

Fig. 5-93. A, Artificial stone is placed on base of cast and on mounting plate. **B,** Articulator is closed, and sides of mounting stone are smoothed. **C,** Mounting stone is allowed to set. With top of mounting plate ring visible, it is easy to retrieve plate later.

jaw relation. If using the wafer technique to record the jaw relationship, it is unnecessary to mount the maxillary cast before obtaining the jaw relation record. However, in this situation it is extremely important to avoid distorting the wax occlusion rim, since this distortion could produce an error in the centric jaw relation record.

18. Remove the mounting jig, and attach the mounting plate to the lower member of the articulator (Fig. 5-94).

19. Invert the articulator, and place the mandibular occlusion rim and cast on the maxillary rim by using the centric jaw relation record to orient the cast (Fig.

5-95). If the centric relation record was made at a slightly increased vertical dimension because of the thickness of the wafer, first measure the distance between the top of the mandibular cast and the articulator ("X" dimension). Then take a second measurement from the same point with the centric relation record in place. Raise the incisal pin to this difference, or X dimension. Failure to observe this step may result in altering the vertical dimension.

20. Paint the base of the cast with a separating medium, and mount the mandibular cast in the articulator (Fig. 5-96). This step completes the procedure.

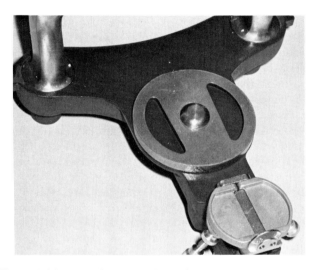

Fig. 5-94. Mounting plate is attached to lower member of articulator.

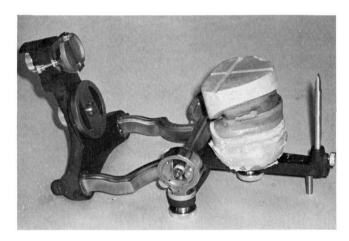

Fig. 5-95. Articulator is inverted, and casts are assembled according to jaw relation record. Note how extension stud supports articulator.

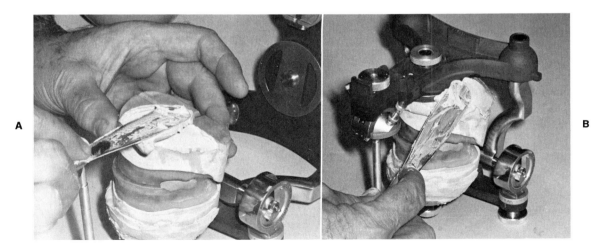

Fig. 5-96. **A,** Artificial stone is mixed and placed on base of cast. It is essential to apply separating medium first. **B,** Articulator is closed, and mounting is completed by adding or removing stone and by smoothing with spatula.

Whip-Mix articulator and unique quick-mount face-bow

The Whip-Mix articulator,* an instrument in widespread use, facilitates mounting casts for complete dentures both quickly and easily, and uses a unique quick-mount face-bow.

PROCEDURE

1. Adjust the intercondylar distance between the two condylar elements on the lower frame of the articulator until it is the same as the condylar width of the patient,

---

*Whip-Mix Corp., Louisville, Ky.

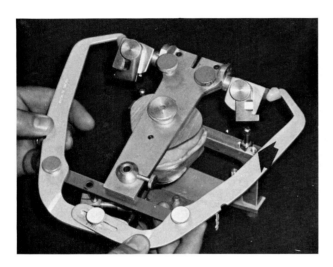

Fig. 5-97. Intercondylar distance is set by removing condylar elements and replacing them in position (arrow) corresponding with index on frame of face-bow.

such as small, medium, or large, as recorded on the face-bow (Fig. 5-97). Set the upper frame at the same width. Add or remove the number of spacers on the shafts of the condylar guides required for the correct adjustment of the intercondylar distance on the upper frame (Fig. 5-98).

2. Set the condylar inclination at 30 degrees (Fig. 5-99).

3. Attach the mounting plates securely to the upper and lower frames of the articulator (Fig. 5-100).

4. Place the plastic incisal guide table on the lower frame of the articulator (Fig. 5-101). Remove the incisal guide pin at this time.

5. Remove the plastic nasion relator assembly from the crossbar of the face-bow, and loosen the three thumbscrews slightly (Fig. 5-102). While holding one arm of the face-bow against the body, place first one pin and then the other on the outer flanges of the condylar guide in the holes on the medial side of the plastic earpieces (Fig. 5-103).

6. Press the face-bow arms against the body.

7. Tighten the three thumbscrews while pressing the face-bow arms against the body.

8. Replace the upper frame of the articulator, with attached face-bow, onto the lower frame of the articulator to permit the fork toggle of the face-bow to rest on the plastic incisal guide table (Fig. 5-104).

9. Place the maxillary cast and occlusion rim in the face-bow registration. A maxillary cast support will prevent displacement of the maxillary cast (Fig. 5-105).

10. Mix artificial stone with slurry concentrate, and add stone to the base of the cast. Exercise care in filling all indentations or indexing grooves (Fig. 5-106).

11. Place additional stone on the mounting plate on

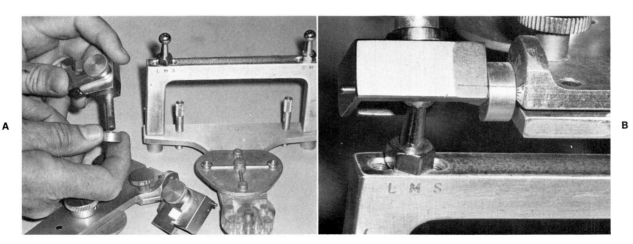

Fig. 5-98. A, One spacer is used on upper frame to set intercondylar distance at medium, two spacers are used on each side to set distance at large *(L),* and no spacers are used to set distance at small *(S).* **B,** Medium *(M)* spacer is in place.

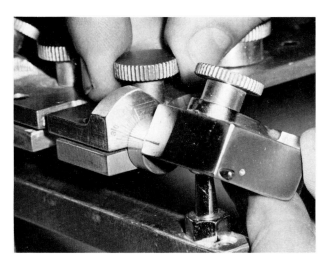

Fig. 5-99. Condylar inclination is set at 30 degrees, and thumbscrew is tightened.

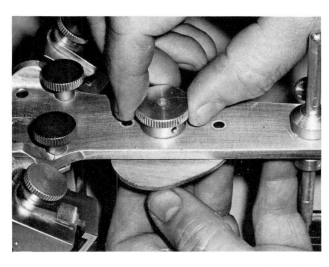

Fig. 5-100. Mounting plates are secured to upper and lower frames of articulator.

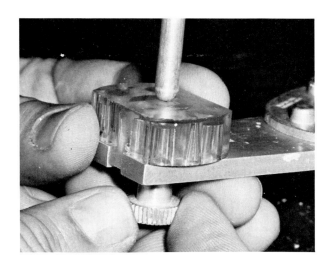

Fig. 5-101. Incisal guide table is placed on lower frame of articulator.

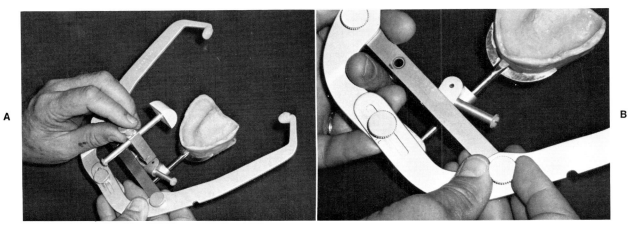

Fig. 5-102. A, Nasion relator assembly is removed from crossbar of face-bow. **B,** Thumbnuts are loosened slightly.

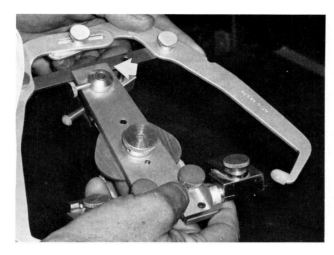

Fig. 5-103. One pin and then other pin on outer flanges of condylar guide are placed in holes on medial side of plastic earpieces, while one arm of face-bow is held against body. Note that upper frame of articulator rests on crossbar of face-bow (arrow).

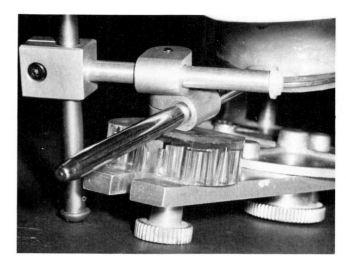

Fig. 5-104. Upper frame of articulator and face-bow are replaced on lower frame to permit fork toggle of face-bow to rest on plastic incisal guide table.

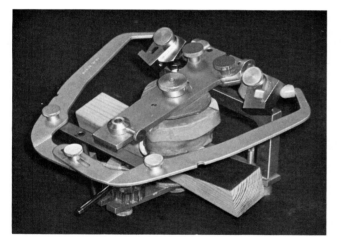

Fig. 5-105. Maxillary cast and occlusion rim are placed in face-bow registration. Wooden wedges can be used to support maxillary cast although adjustable cast support is more convenient.

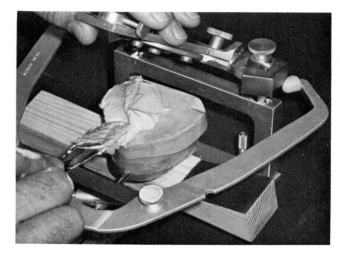

Fig. 5-106. Base of cast is painted with separating medium, artificial stone is placed on base of cast, and care is exercised to fill index grooves or notches.

the upper frame of the articulator, and close the upper frame of the articulator gently until it touches the crossbar of the face-bow again. *Caution:* Do not use too thick a mix of mounting stone because it can cause displacement of the cast as the upper frame is closed in position.

12. Allow the stone mounting the maxillary cast to set, and then remove the face-bow from the articulator (Fig. 5-107).

13. Replace the incisal guide pin in the articulator with the rounded end down, and set it at an opening of 5 mm (by aligning the top edge of the bushing on the pin with the fifth line above the line that encircles the pin) (Fig. 5-108). Optionally, it is possible to lock the upper

and lower bows of the articulator into a hinge rotation by moving the side-shift guides to the extreme negative position, which is as far out as possible. When locking them, see that the articulator is not opened too far, and modify the mounting instructions for the mandibular cast in accordance with the hinge action of the locked articulator.

14. Invert the upper frame of the articulator, thereby positioning the maxillary cast with its occlusion rim surface up, and lute the mandibular cast to the maxillary cast according to the centric jaw relation record (Fig. 5-109).

15. Paint the mandibular cast with a separating medi-

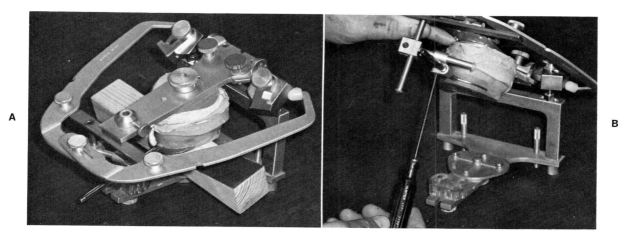

Fig. 5-107. A, Artificial stone is allowed to set. **B,** Face-bow is removed from articulator by loosening setscrew on fork toggle.

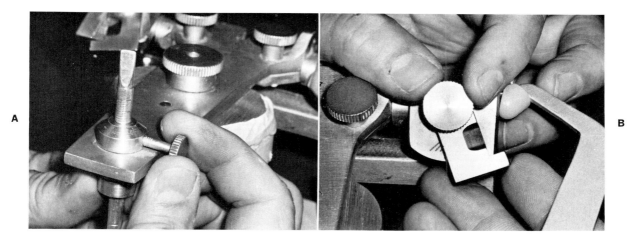

Fig. 5-108. A, Incisal guide pin is replaced with rounded end down, and set at 5-mm opening. **B,** Articulator is locked into hinge rotation by moving side-shift guides out as far as possible.

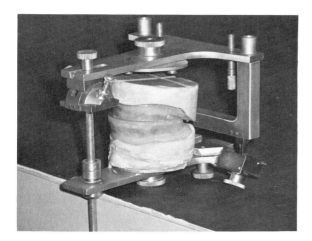

Fig. 5-109. Articulator is placed upside down on bench, and cast is assembled according to centric jaw relation record and luted together.

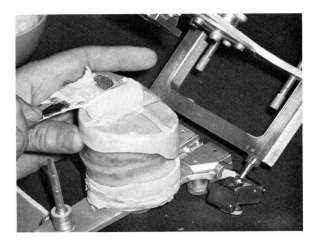

Fig. 5-110. Artificial stone is placed in base of mandibular cast that has been painted with separating medium.

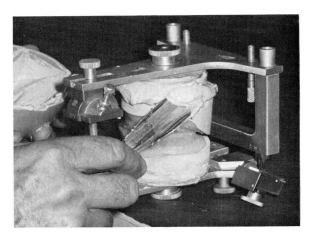

Fig. 5-111. Lower frame is seated in position. Make certain that condylar elements are in position and incisal guide pin touches incisal guide table.

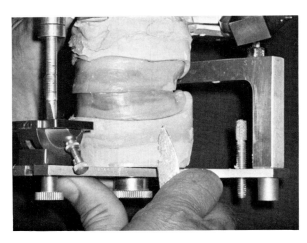

Fig. 5-112. Mounted casts trimmed.

um to permit separation of the cast from the mounting stone later. Mix artificial stone with slurry concentrate to form a smooth consistency. Apply stone to the base of the mandibular cast, and make certain that the indexing grooves or notches contain stone (Fig. 5-110).

16. Place additional stone in the mounting plate on the lower frame of the articulator, and seat the lower frame in position over the upper frame of the articulator (Fig. 5-111). Make certain that the condylar elements are in the correct position and the incisal guide pin contacts the incisal guide table.* Allow the stone to set (Fig. 5-112).

PROBLEM AREAS

The principal problems with mounting casts in articulators are summarized in Table 5-1.

Split remounting plates

The advantages of using split remounting plates† and the procedure for placing split remounting plates in the cast are presented in Chapter 2.

PROCEDURE

1. Assemble the split remounting plate on the cast, and insert the tapered pin (Fig. 5-113).

2. Place the cast in the face-bow registration on the articulator. When using an arbitrary cast mounting, position the casts as described previously. Wrap a strip of masking tape 1½ inches (3.8 cm) wide around the cast to confine the mounting stone (Fig. 5-114).

3. Close the articulator upper bow carefully to see that the tape is not too high. Adjust the height if necessary (Fig. 5-115).

---

*Refer to the Whip-Mix articulator and quick-mount face-bow instruction manual for setting the guidance of the articulator.
†Teledyne Dental Products Co., Hanau Division, Buffalo, N.Y.

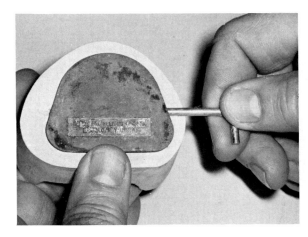

Fig. 5-113. Split remounting plate is assembled on cast, and tapered pin is inserted.

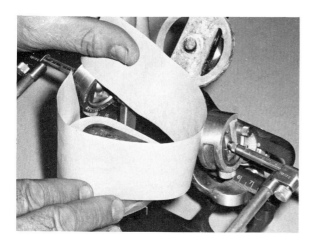

Fig. 5-114. Strip of masking tape is wrapped around cast to confine stone.

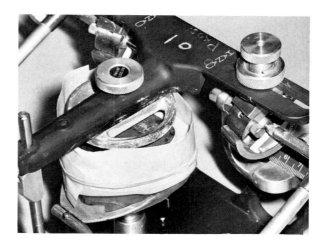

Fig. 5-115. Articulator is closed to make certain that tape is not too high. Note that rubber band helps hold tape in position.

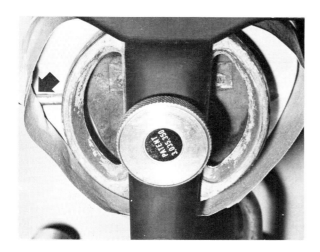

Fig. 5-116. Small hole is placed in tape fcr tapered pin (arrow).

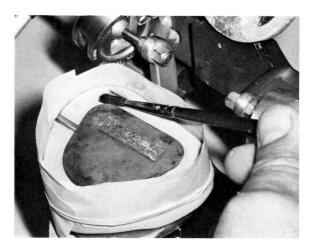

Fig. 5-117. Base of cast is painted with separating medium.

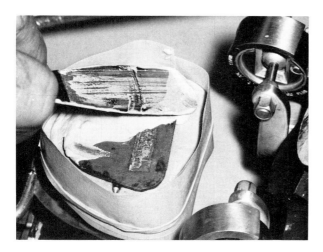

Fig. 5-118. Artificial stone is worked into undercuts of remounting plate.

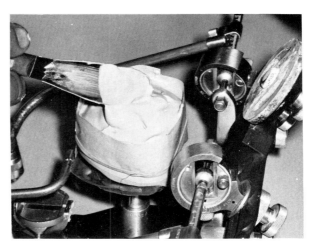

Fig. 5-119. Boxing is filled with artificial stone.

Table 5-1. Mounting casts

Problem	Probable cause	Solution
Articulator settings not adjusted according to specification	Manufacturer's recommendation as to adjustment of articulator not followed	Set instrument according to manufacturer's directions
Relationship of mounted casts incorrect	Incorrect jaw relation record used for mounting	Obtain a new jaw relation record
	Casts not seated accurately in baseplates	Make certain that casts are completely seated in baseplates and that baseplates are not warped
	Occlusion rims not seated accurately in jaw relation record	Check that occlusion rims are joined accurately, according to jaw relation record
	Cast relationship changed by jostling casts when mounting	Add mounting stone carefully to avoid moving casts out of position
	Vertical dimension altered	Incisal pin not changed to X dimension with centric relation record in place when mounting mandibular cast
Casts unable to be separated from mounting stone	Failure to paint base of cast with separating medium	Paint base of cast and index grooves with separating medium

4. Cut a small slit or hole in the tape to permit the tapered pin to extend (Fig. 5-116).

5. Paint the stone cast base with a separating medium (Fig. 5-117).

6. Mix artificial stone with slurry concentrate, and work the stone into the undercuts of the remounting plate carefully (Fig. 5-118). Fill the boxed cast with stone (Fig. 5-119).

7. Add stone to the upper mounting plate. Close the articulator and smooth the stone over the mounting plate (Fig. 5-120).

8. Allow the stone to set, remove the tapered pin, and separate the cast from the mounting stone (Fig. 5-121). It is possible to reattach the cast quickly by assembling it and securing it with the tapered pin.

The principal advantages of the split remounting plate are quick removal and replacement from the articulator and precise adaptation through the metal plates (Fig. 5-122). The principal disadvantage is the extra time required to place the plate in the cast and to retrieve it after completion of the denture.

Retrieving mounting plates

Bange* has developed a mounting plate ejector for quick retrieval of Hanau mounting plates from the mounting stone. The ejector works only on older mounting plates that are through-threaded. It is impossible to

_____
*Bange, A. A.: Personal communication, 1977.

separate the new plates, which are closed on the cast surface by this method.

Conventional separation methods often are time consuming, laborious, and harmful to the mounting plates. One method requires the use of a dental laboratory knife placed at the junction of the gypsum and mounting plate. It is necessary to strike the knife with a hammer to cleave the mounting gypsum from the mounting plate. Tapping the remaining mounting gypsum with a hammer releases it from retention areas of the mounting plate. This method, which defaces the metal mounting plate with dents and nicks, affects the precision fit of the mounting plate to the Hanau articulator.

The mounting plate ejector rapidly and efficiently separates dental gypsum products used in mounting casts on Hanau articulators from Hanau mounting plates (rings). Its use avoids damage to Hanau mounting plates, maintains their accuracy, and greatly increases their longevity. It is useful also in cleaning and truing the threads of mounting plates damaged by other methods of separation.

To construct the mounting plate ejector, attach a knurled metal knob to a $5/16$ inch (0.8-cm) twenty-four–threaded bolt (Fig. 5-123). Extend the bolt ¾ inch (1.91 cm) beyond the knob. Drill and tap a metal pressure plate 2¼ inch (5.72 cm) long, ⅝ inch (1.6 cm) wide and ¼ inch (0.64 cm) thick to allow screwing of the knurled knob and bolt through it. Slots placed in the ends of the metal pressure plate and rubber or plastic tips inserted

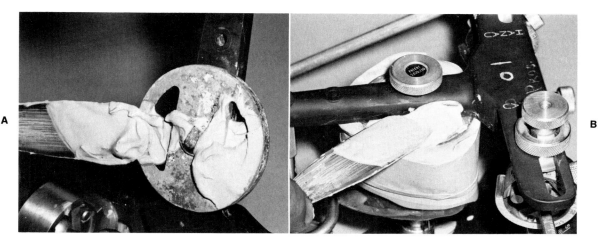

Fig. 5-120. A, Stone is added to upper mounting plate. **B,** Articulator is closed, and stone is smoothed over mounting plate.

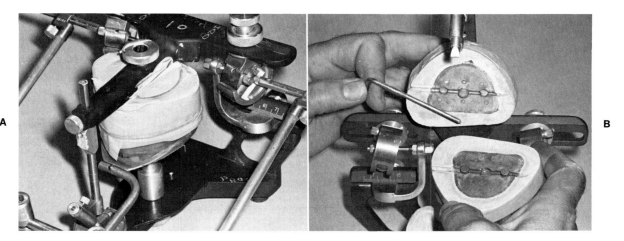

Fig. 5-121. A, Mounting stone is allowed to set. **B,** Tapered pin is removed, and cast is separated from mounting stone.

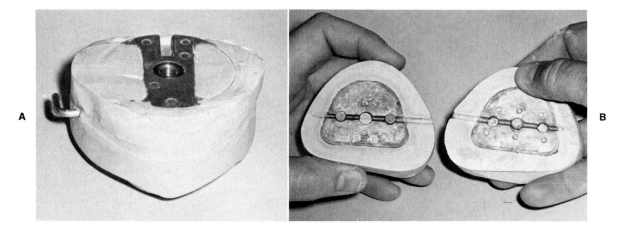

Fig. 5-122. A, Cast can be removed from mounting stone and reattached quickly. **B,** Metal plates make adaptation precise and positioning of cast on mounting stone accurate.

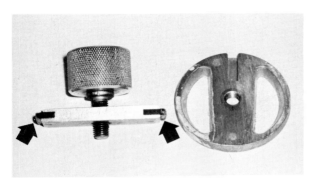

Fig. 5-123. Mounting plate ejector *(left)* and older style mounting plate *(right)*. Plastic tips are placed on ejector to prevent damage to mounting plate (arrows).

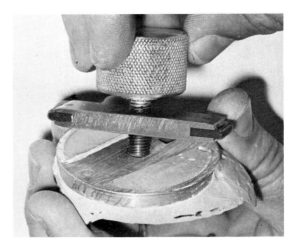

Fig. 5-124. Ejector bolt is screwed into mounting plate until pressure from stone is felt.

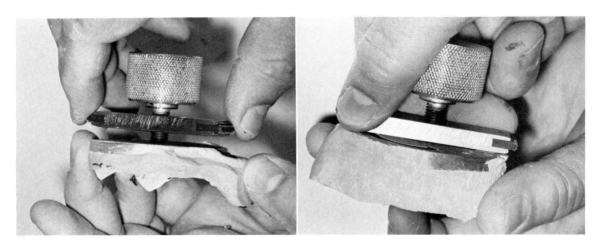

Fig. 5-125. Pressure plate is turned down to contact mounting plate.

A

B

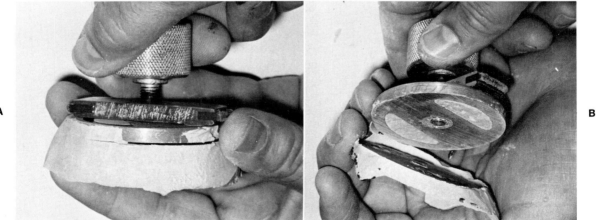

Fig. 5-126. A, Knurled knob is turned to apply pressure. Note stone separating from mounting plate.
B, Stone is separated from mounting plate.

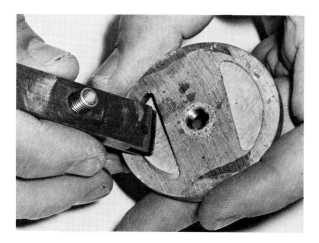

Fig. 5-127. Remaining stone is tapped from mounting plate.

in these slots will prevent damage to the softer metal of the mounting plate.

PROCEDURE

1. Thread the ejection bolt into the mounting plate until pressure is felt against the mounting stone (Fig. 5-124).

2. Turn the pressure plate down snugly against the mounting plate (Fig. 5-125).

3. Apply pressure by turning the knurled knob clockwise until the mounting plate ejects from the mounting stone (Fig. 5-126).

4. Turn the mounting plate over, and tap out any stone remaining in the retentive areas of the mounting plate. The rubber or plastic tip prevents damage to the mounting plates during tapping (Fig. 5-127).

An alternate conventional method of separation is to place a small piece of carding wax in the threaded hole of the mounting plate and tighten the mounting plate onto the threaded lockscrew of the Hanau articulator until the mounting gypsum pops out of the mounting plate. This method can damage the threads of the mounting plate if it is not perpendicular to the pressure plate; it also can damage the Hanau articulator. However, use of this method has led to development of the mounting plate ejector.

SUMMARY

In this chapter methods for mounting casts in several different articulators were described, as well as the use of split remounting plates and the mounting plate–ejector method for retrieving mounting plates from mounting stone.

BIBLIOGRAPHY

Air Force Manual 160-29: Dental laboratory technicians' manual, Washington, D.C., 1959, United States Air Force, pp. 101-102.

Boucher, C. O., Hickey, J. C. and Zarb, G. A.: Prosthodontic treatment for edentulous patients, ed. 7, St. Louis, 1975, The C. V. Mosby Co., pp. 295-312.

Sharry, J. J.: Complete denture prosthodontics, ed. 3, New York, 1974, McGraw-Hill Book Co., pp. 211-240.

Sowter, J. B.: Dental laboratory technology: prosthodontic techniques, Chapel Hill, N.C., 1968, The University of North Carolina Press, pp. 49-50.

CHAPTER 6

ARTIFICIAL TEETH AND GOLD OCCLUSALS

KENNETH D. RUDD, ROBERT M. MORROW, CLARENCE L. KOEHNE,
and WILLIAM B. AKERLY

artificial teeth Teeth fabricated for a prosthesis: usually made of porcelain or plastic.

anatomic teeth Artificial teeth that closely resemble the anatomic form of natural unabraded teeth.

nonanatomic teeth Artificial teeth in which the occlusal surfaces are not copies from natural forms, but are given forms that, in the opinion of the designer, seem more nearly to fulfill the requirements of mastication, tissue tolerance, etc.

cuspless teeth Teeth designed without cuspal prominences on the masticatory surfaces.

zero-degree teeth Prosthetic teeth having no cusp angles in relation to the horizontal plane: cuspless teeth.

metal-insert teeth Artificial teeth, usually of acrylic resin, containing an inserted ribbon of metal or a cutting blade in their occlusal surface, with one edge of the blade exposed. Sometimes they are used in removable dentures.

There are an estimated 20 million edentulous Americans and an additional 10 million who are edentulous in one arch. Additional millions have various missing natural teeth that are in many instances replaced with removable partial dentures. Obviously, a considerable number of artificial teeth are required to restore esthetics and function for these patients.

MATERIALS FOR ARTIFICIAL TEETH

Artificial teeth are made of porcelain, resin, and resin-metal combinations. More porcelain teeth are used than plastic teeth in the United States where plastic teeth consist of about 30% of the market (Encyclopedia Britannica, 1969).

Porcelain teeth

Advantages of porcelain teeth include greater wear resistance than plastic and better retention of surface polish and finishing. Polishing of the denture base is facilitated because porcelain is not easily marred or abraded during routine polishing procedures.

Disadvantages of porcelain teeth include difficulty in restoring surface polish after grinding. These teeth may weaken the denture, since they do not bond to the denture base resin. They are prone to chip or break if dropped on a hard surface, and they cannot be used in some instances where available denture space is minimal. In addition, porcelain teeth may produce a noticeable click in function and can accumulate stain around the gingival margin because of a difference in thermal expansion between porcelain and denture base resin. Porcelain teeth may also abrade opposing natural teeth or teeth restored with resin or metal restorations.

Resin teeth

Advantages of plastic teeth include natural appearance and sound, ease in adjustment, restoration of surface polish, break and chip resistance, and most importantly the capability to bond to most heat-cured denture base resins. This bonding capability can result in a strong break-resistant denture and is a particularly important consideration when constructing overdentures.

Disadvantages of resin teeth include less wear resistance, which can result in a reduced vertical dimen-

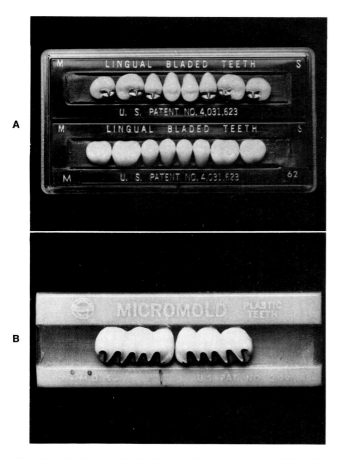

Fig. 6-1. A, Lingual bladed teeth. (Manufactured by U.S. Shizai Corp., Los Angeles, Calif.) Metal blades on mesiolingual cusp of first and second maxillary molars and on lingual cusp of second bicuspid may provide improved chewing efficiency and esthetics. **B,** Micromold M/O posterior teeth have metal ribbon embedded in resin. (Denture teeth manufactured by Howmedica, Inc., Chicago, Ill.)

sion of occlusion and the tendency to dull in appearance during use as a result of loss of surface luster. Care must be taken when polishing the denture to preclude undesirable modifications in tooth contour. Placing amalgam restorations in the occlusal surfaces of resin posterior teeth has been advocated as a means of improving occlusal wear characteristics (Sowter and Bass, 1968).

Metal-insert teeth

Advantages of metal-insert teeth include improved occlusal wear resistance, bonding capability with the denture base resin, and possibly, improved masticatory efficiency. Metal-insert teeth are not as noisy as porcelain teeth, and they may strengthen the denture (Fig. 6-1).

Disadvantages include the cost of metal-insert teeth, and they may not be as esthetic as other artificial teeth.

Artificial teeth with metal occlusals

Advantages of artificial teeth with metal occlusals include excellent wear resistance and durability of occlusal contours. They can occlude with natural or restored dentitions, and their use in some instances may effectively disguise the wearing of complete dentures. In addition, teeth with metal occlusals can effectively reinforce the denture, making it more resistant to breakage (Fig. 6-2) (Schultz, 1951; Wallace, 1964; Davies and Pound, 1966; Koehne and Morrow, 1970).

Components of artificial teeth

Porcelain anterior teeth have metal pins embedded into the porcelain for mechanical retention in the denture base resin (Fig. 6-3). Resin anterior teeth do not

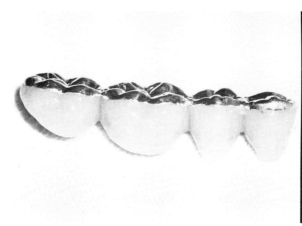
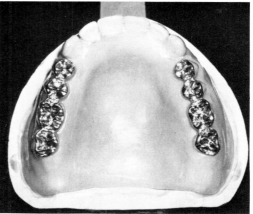

Fig. 6-2. Denture teeth with metal occlusals can effectively strengthen denture.

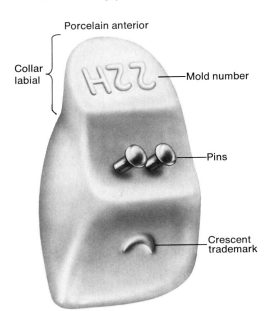

Fig. 6-3. Pins embedded in porcelain retain tooth in denture base resin. (Courtesy Dentsply International, Inc., York, Pa.)

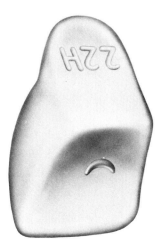

Fig. 6-4. Resin teeth bond chemically to denture base resin, thus pins are not required. (Courtesy Dentsply International, Inc., York, Pa.)

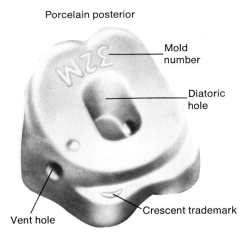

Fig. 6-5. Diatoric holes are filled with resin during packing procedure to retain teeth on denture base. (Courtesy Dentsply International, Inc., York, Pa.)

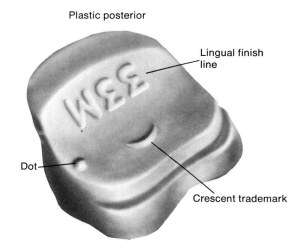

Fig. 6-6. Resin posterior teeth bond chemically to denture base. Grooves or indentations placed in these teeth prior to packing denture base resin can improve attachment of tooth to denture base. (Courtesy Dentsply International, Inc., York, Pa.)

have retention pins, since resin teeth bond chemically to the denture base resin (Fig. 6-4). Porcelain posterior teeth have retentive recesses (diatorics) in the ridge laps that, when filled with denture base resin, retain the teeth in the denture base (Fig. 6-5). Resin posterior teeth do not have diatorics because they are similar to resin anterior teeth and bond chemically to the denture base (Fig. 6-6). Recesses can be placed in resin teeth ridge laps when the denture is packed to improve the bond between the tooth and denture.

MOLD AND SHADE IDENTIFICATION

Artificial teeth are available in numerous molds and shades. Mold and shade identifying codes are not standard throughout the industry. Thus is is necessary to maintain appropriate mold and shade data in the office or laboratory for each manufacturer's teeth.

Mold numbering systems

Some manufacturers have a system-logic mold identification; however, all systems are not standard.

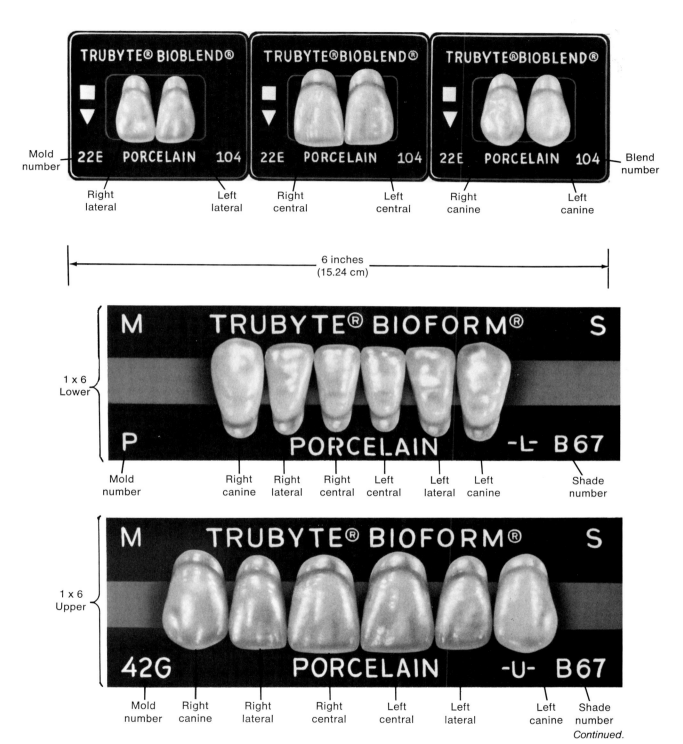

Fig. 6-7. Representative selection of teeth manufactured by Dentsply International, Inc. (Courtesy Dentsply International, Inc., York, Pa.)

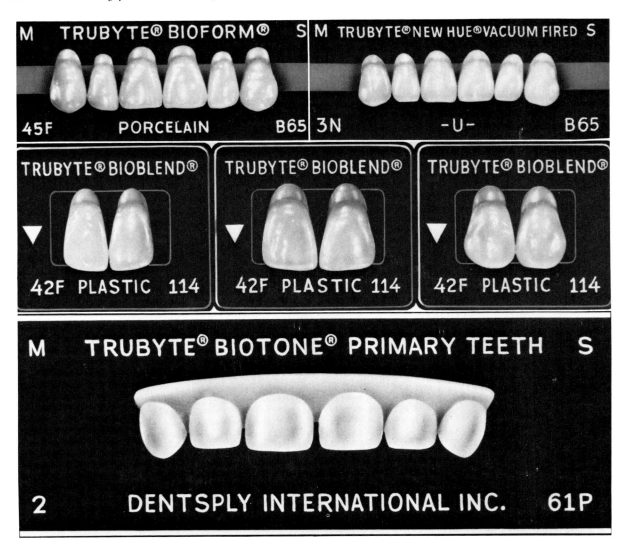

Fig. 6-7, cont'd. For legend see p. 179.

Dentsply International, Inc., has the Trubyte Bioform mold numbering system, which uses two numbers and one letter on the lower left of the tooth mounting card (Fig. 6-7). The first number indicates the classification of the mold: 1, square; 2, square tapering; 3, square ovoid; 4, tapering; 5, tapering ovoid; 6, ovoid; and 7, square tapering ovoid.

The second number indicates whether the tooth is long, medium, or short and whether the labial surface is straight or convex incisogingivally: 1, long, straight; 2, medium, straight; 3, short, straight; 4, long, curved; 5, medium, curved; and 6, short, curved.

The letter indicates the width of all six anterior teeth set on a curve: B, less than 44 mm; C, 44 to 46 mm; D, 46 to 48 mm; E, 48 to 50 mm; F or X, 50 to 52 mm; G, 52 to 54 mm; H, 54 to 56 mm; and J above 56 mm.

The Lincoln Dental Supply Company has suggested a system-logic coding system in which universal coded numbers would be provided for the shade and mold of artificial teeth. The four- to five-digit system is derived from approximate measurements of the teeth. The first two numbers in the code would indicate the combined width of the six anterior teeth on a curve. The third number would be the width of the central incisor, and the last one or two numbers would indicate central incisor length (Fig. 6-8). This system would seem to have merit and be a positive step toward standardization. The system could be expanded to include appropriate identifiers for other characteristics such as typal form (square, tapering, ovoid, etc.).

The Myerson Tooth Corporation identifies molds with numbers and letters. "A" molds have subtle labial

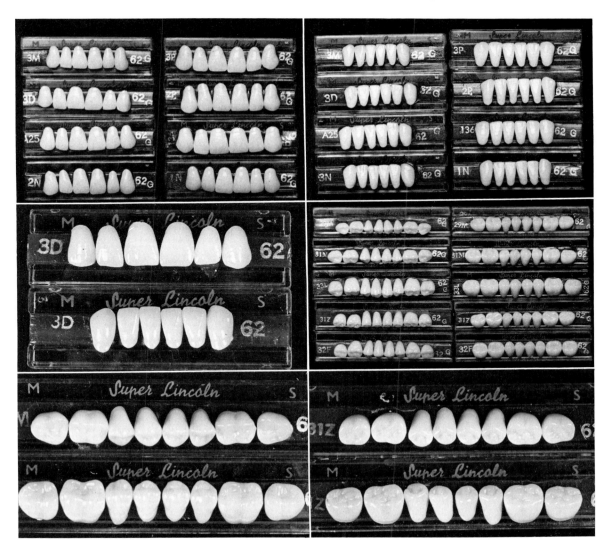

Fig. 6-8. Representative group of teeth marketed by Lincoln Dental Supply Co., Philadelphia, Pa.

carvings, slender forms, and excellent balance between the ridge lap and bite. "Y" molds are similar to "A" molds, but have shorter ridge laps. "P" molds have shorter, less sloping, ridge laps and are well suited for "butting" (Fig. 6-9). A more comprehensive system is used for Myerson Special teeth. The width of the six anterior teeth, suggested lower molds, posterior combinations, and central incisor width and length are all indicated on the tooth card, which appears to be an excellent aid for tooth selection.

Universal teeth are available in a wide range of molds and shades in plastic (Verident) and porcelain (Univac). Shades are indicated by a letter and number (P1-P6, B1, Y1-Y6, R1-R5) and molds are identified by letters and numbers (M45) (Fig. 6-10).

Unitek Vita teeth are available in resin and porcelain in a variety of shades identified by a letter and a number (A-1, A-2, B-2, etc.). Mold selections are related to facial shapes (square, tapering, ovoid, etc.) (Fig. 6-11). Unitek also publishes a convenient tooth shade comparison chart (pp. 186 and 187) for porcelain and acrylic teeth.

Posterior teeth

The posterior teeth are often identified by the name of the particular tooth form. Specific molds and shades are identified by numbers that represent the combined mesiodistal width of the four posterior teeth and a letter to indicate the occlusogingival height of the tooth, S, short; M, medium; and L, long (Figs. 6-12 and 6-13).

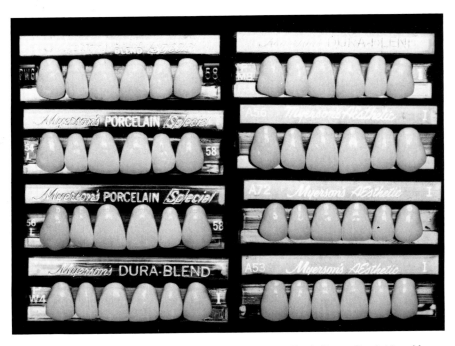

Fig. 6-9. Representative teeth manufactured by Myerson Tooth Corp., Cambridge, Mass.

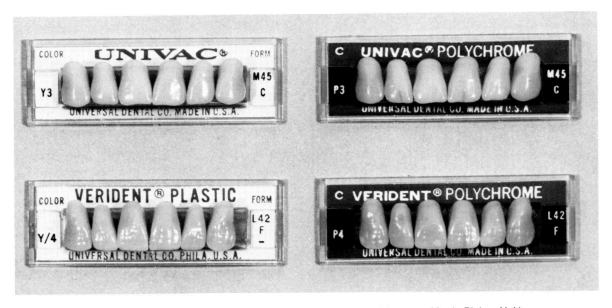

Fig. 6-10. Representative molds of teeth. (Courtesy Universal-Lactona, Morris Plains, N.J.)

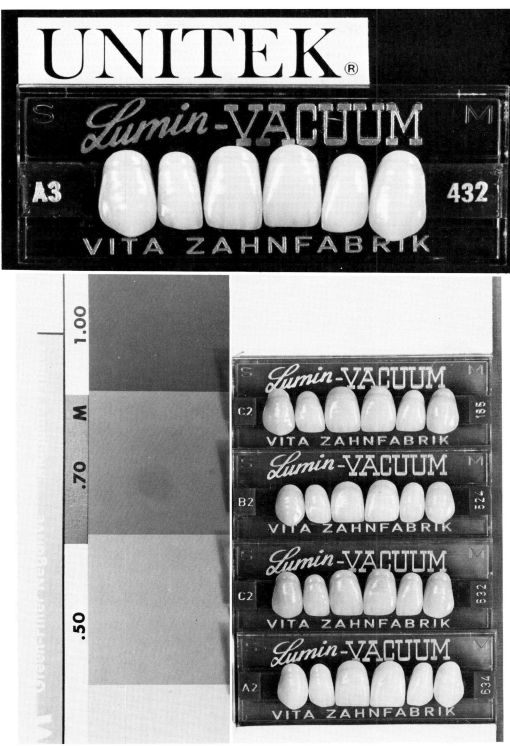

Continued.

Fig. 6-11. Vita teeth manufactured by Unitek Corporation. (Courtesy Unitek Corp., Monrovia, Calif.)

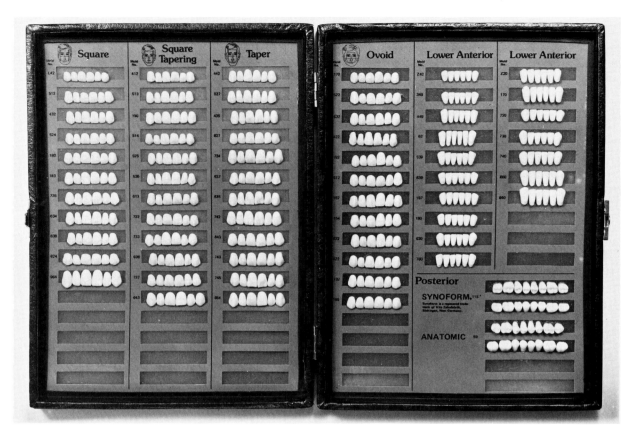

Fig. 6-11, cont'd. For legend see p. 183.

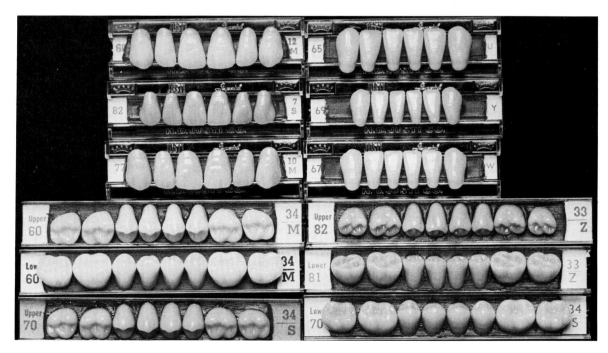

Fig. 6-12. Representative molds of teeth from H. D. Justi Co., Philadelphia, Pa.

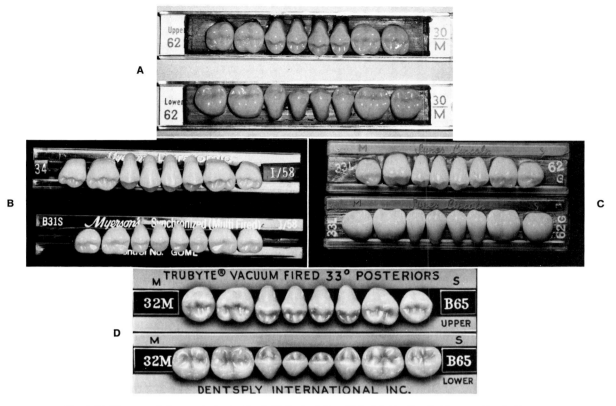

Fig. 6-13. Representative posterior teeth. **A,** H. D. Justi Co., Philadelphia, Pa. **B,** Myerson Tooth Corp., Cambridge, Mass. **C,** Lincoln Dental Supply Co., Philadelphia, Pa. **D,** Courtesy Dentsply International, Inc., York, Pa.

CONSTRUCTING METAL OCCLUSALS

Unquestionably, the use of metal occlusal surfaces on prosthetic teeth can contribute to their clinical success (Koehne and Morrow, 1970). Metal occlusal surfaces may be indicated (1) when constructing a denture that is to be opposed by a reconstructed dentition with gold occlusal surfaces; (2) when constructing a complete denture, removable partial denture, or overdenture with a functionally generated path concept in which considerable modification of the denture teeth is necessary to place the occlusal surfaces and core in harmony, (3) when special wax carving techniques are completed on a fully adjustable articulator, and (4) when their use is indicated to reinforce and strengthen the denture or overdenture.

PROCEDURE

The procedure described is for constructing gold occlusals for complete dentures. The method can be easily modified for removable partial dentures or overdentures.

1. After the jaw relation recording appointment, anterior and posterior teeth are positioned for try-in. Resin posterior teeth are selected, since these teeth will be cut down prior to waxing the occlusion (Fig. 6-14).

2. Reduce the resin teeth to create space for carving wax. Reduce the central region of the tooth somewhat more than the cusps (Fig. 6-15).

3. Reduce maxillary and mandibular teeth to provide approximately 4 mm of interocclusal space. Move articulator into lateral and protrusive positions to verify space adequacy (Fig. 6-16).

4. Add inlay wax to the prepared teeth, and contour the occlusal surfaces of the individual teeth (Fig. 6-17).

5. Carve secondary anatomic details, and check the waxed occlusion in centric, lateral, and protrusive positions (Fig. 6-18). Note particularly that adequate horizontal overlap has been provided to minimize cheek biting.

6. Wash the wax occlusal surfaces gently with green soap, rinse them in cool water, and remove excess water with an air syringe.

7. Mix the casting investment compatible with the metal alloy to be used, and paint it on the occlusal

Text continued on p. 190.

Tooth shade comparison chart (PORCELAIN)*

Note: Due to the distinctive shade characteristics of Vita* Teeth, exact comparison is not possible. This chart is only to be used as a relative guide. (For example, Lumin Vacuum Shade C-1 is somewhat darker than Bioblend Shade 100.)

Unitek	Justi	Dentsply	Myerson's	Universal	Universal	Swissdent	Swissdent	Dentsply
Vita Lumin Vacuum	Vivostar	Bioblend	Aesthetic M.F.	Univac Polychrome	Univac	Swissdent Candulor	Swissdent 900	Bioform
A-1	Lighter than 17 J	100	Lighter than 1	None	None	Lighter than 84	Lighter than A 902	Closest to 51
A-2	Lighter than 17 M	104	H	Lighter than P 1	B 1	86	A 902	Closest to 62
A-3	17 S 27 J	106	66 M	Closest to P 3	Lighter than Y 2	90	901	65
A-4	29 M	Closest to 118	D	P 9	Closest to Y 5	97	Darker than B 903	Less yellow than 82
B-2	17 J	Closest to 104	Closest to 1	Lighter than P 1	Closest to B 1	87	A 902	Darker & less pink than 62
B-3	19 M	108	Closest to E	Closest to P 3	Closest to Y 3	Lighter than 91	A 901	Closest to 68
B-4	27 S 27 M	Closest to 116	Lighter than D	More yellow than P 3	Closest to Y 4	Closest to 92	902	Closest to 56
C-1	17 J	Darker than 100	1	P 1	Less pink than B 1	Darker than 86	Less yellow than A 902	Closest to 91
C-2	Darker than 37 M	Darker than 106	G	Greyer than P 2	More yellow than R 2	90	None	Lighter than 94
C-3	39 M	113	69 M	Greyer than P 4	Closest to R 4	98	904	Closest to 95
C-4	Lighter than 39 S	Darker than 113	More orange than 69 M	P 6	R 5	Darker than 99	None	Closest to 96
D-2	37 J	None	None	P 1	Y 1	None	None	Closest to 92
D-3	17 M	Closest to 108	Lighter than G	P 2	R 2	90	Darker than A 902	Closest to 93

*Courtesy Unitek Corp., Monrovia, Calif.

Tooth shade comparison chart (ACRYLIC)*

Note: Due to the distinctive shade characteristics of Vita* Teeth, exact comparison is not possible. This chart is only to be used as a relative guide. (For example, Lumin Acryl-V Shade D-3 is between Bioblend Shades 100 and 102.)

Unitek	Justi	Dentsply	Dentsply	Dentsply	Universal	Universal	Swissdent	Myerson's
Vita Lumin Acryl-V	Imperial	Bioblend	Bioform	Biotone	Polychrome	Verident	Swissdent 900	Durablend Durablend Special
A-1	None	Lighter than 100	Lighter than 91	None	None	B-1	None	None
A-2	None	104	62	59	Darker than B-1	Slightly darker than Y-1	Lighter than A-902	I
A-3	60	102	52	61	Darker than Y-1	Y-2	901	H
B-2	None	Closest to 104	59	Lighter than 59	Y-1	Slightly lighter than Y-3	None	58 (Special)
B-3	62	108	64	Little more yellow than 61	None	Closer to Y-2	Lighter than 904	None
B-4	64	116	56	None	Y-5	None	903	E
C-1	None	100	91	Slightly more grey than 59	Lighter than R-1	R-1	None	Greyer than I
C-2	69	Darker than 104	94	None	R-2	R-2	Closest to A-902	H (Special)
C-3	Darker than 66	113	95	Lighter than 69	Closest to Y-3	R-3	Closest to 904	G (Special)
C-4	70	Closest to 113	Between 95-96	69	Y-6	Y-4	903	69 (Special)
D-3	Lighter than 60	Between 100-102	92	Closest to 59	R-1	Lighter than Y-1	None	Lighter than 60 (Special)
D-4	65	Between 104-106	69	67	Y-3	Closest to Y-2	B-902	Lighter than 69
D-5	82	114	81	Darker than 77	Closest to Y-6	Y-6	B-903	C (Special)
E-2	Closest to 62	Lighter than 104	53	None	B-1	Lighter than R-2	Lighter than 900	Between H and I
E-3	More orange than 60	109	65	62	R-3	None	B-901	Lighter than H (Special)

*Courtesy Unitek Corp., Monrovia, Calif.

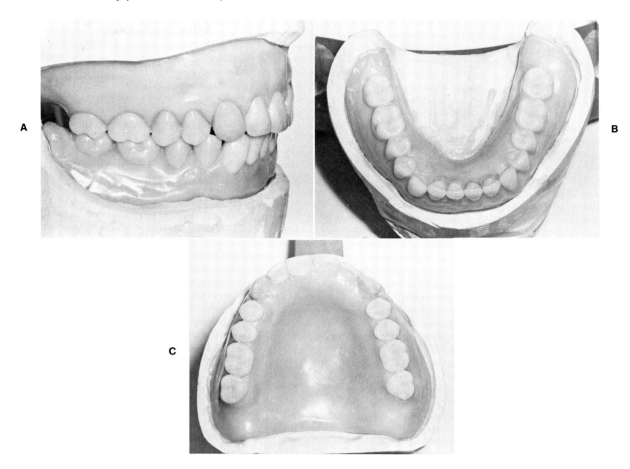

Fig. 6-14. **A,** Resin posterior teeth are set up and waxed for try-in in usual manner. **B,** Occlusal view of mandibular resin tooth setup. **C,** Occlusal view of maxillary setup.

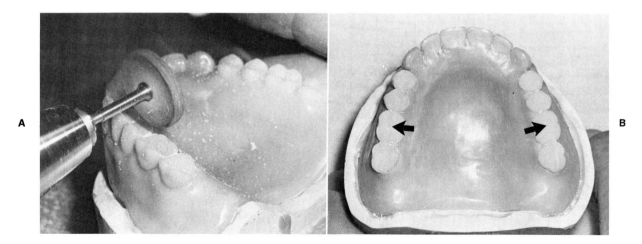

Fig. 6-15. **A,** Resin teeth are reduced to create space for carving wax. **B,** Teeth are reduced somewhat deeper in central portion (arrows) than over cusp.

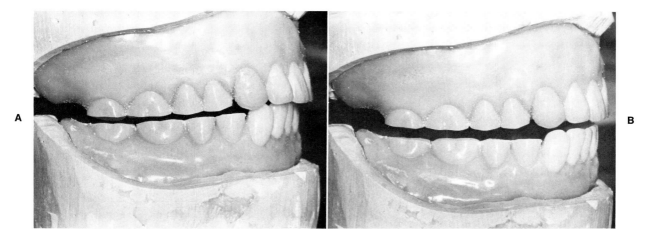

Fig. 6-16. A, There should be approximately 3 to 4 mm of space between upper and lower teeth when casts are in centric jaw relation position. **B,** Articulator is moved into eccentric positions, and space between reduced teeth checked.

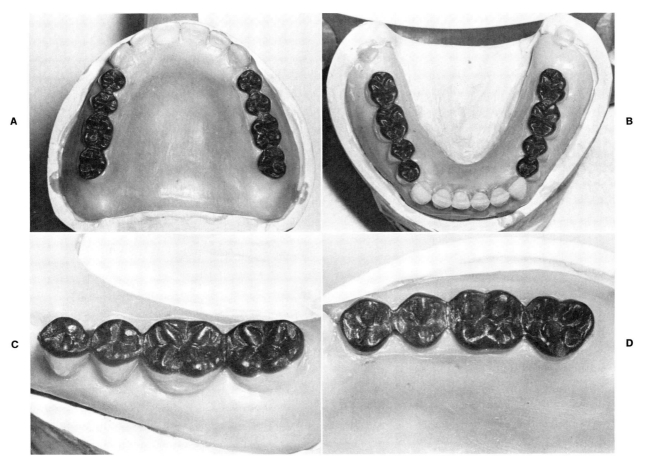

Fig. 6-17. A, Inlay wax is flowed on reduced resin teeth, and occlusal surfaces are contoured. **B,** Wax patterns carved on mandibular denture teeth. **C,** Secondary anatomic details are placed in wax patterns. **D,** Wax pattern occlusion should be checked in centric position as well as functional eccentric position.

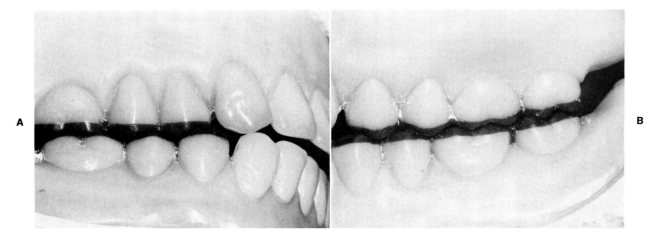

Fig. 6-18. A, Lateral positions are checked while carving wax patterns. **B,** Adequate horizontal overlap of at least 1 mm should be provided to prevent possible cheek biting.

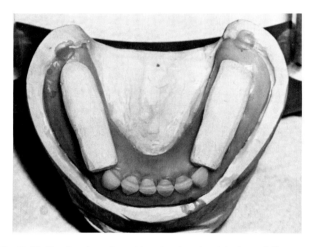

Fig. 6-19. Casting investment is mixed and painted carefully on occlusal surfaces of wax carving.

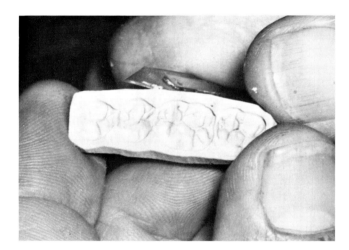

Fig. 6-20. Investment index should be reduced by carving with sharp knife.

surfaces of the wax carvings (Fig. 6-19). Take care to paint the investment in the grooves of the wax-up to assure faithful reproduction of the contours.

8. After the investment has set, carefully lift it from the waxed occlusals. Trim the investment with a sharp No. 25 blade to reduce excess bulk (Fig. 6-20).

9. Control the thickness of the castings by trimming the investment occlusogingivally to produce a casting thickness of 1 to 2 mm. Reduction is accomplished in such a manner as to make the gold the same thickness over the occlusobuccal line angles. This results in a minimum gold display with an outline that resembles a three-quarter cast crown (Fig. 6-21).

10. Flow casting wax into the resultant mold to completely fill it (Fig. 6-22).

11. After the wax has cooled, attach a length of 14-gauge half-round casting wax, flat surface up, to the wax

pattern. The 14-gauge wax should be 2 to 3 mm short of the total pattern length at each end (Fig. 6-23). Paint clear fingernail polish on the wax, and place small resin-retention crystals or beads on the tacky surface.

12. Select a large paper clip, bend it to shape, and sprue the wax pattern (Fig. 6-24).

13. Add an additional 10-gauge round sprue to the central portion of the wax pattern (Fig. 6-25).

14. Reinforce the sprue/pattern junctions with wax (Fig. 6-26).

15. Seal the sprued pattern into an appropriate sprue former (Fig. 6-27).

16. Flow additional wax over the metal sprue to ease its withdrawal later (Fig. 6-28).

17. Securely wax the sprues to the sprue former (Fig. 6-29).

18. Place the sprued pattern in the casting ring, and

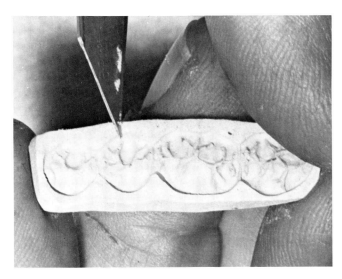

Fig. 6-21. Occlusal gingival thickness of investment index is reduced to provide for thickness of 1 to 2 mm in casting. Carving should be contoured to produce outline form on casting that resembles three-quarter cast crown.

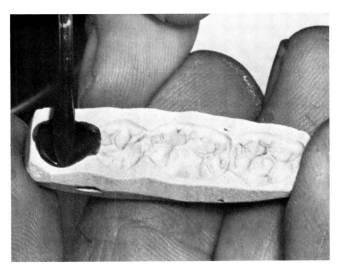

Fig. 6-22. Casting wax is flowed into index to make wax pattern.

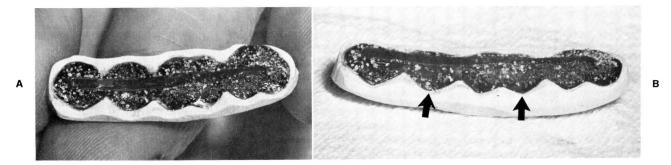

Fig. 6-23. A, Strip of 14-gauge half-round wax is placed on wax pattern, flat surface up, to provide retention for acrylic resin. Small crystals or beads are also placed on wax pattern to provide additional resin retention. **B,** Note how investment index has been carved (arrows) to simulate outline of three-quarter crown on metal occlusals.

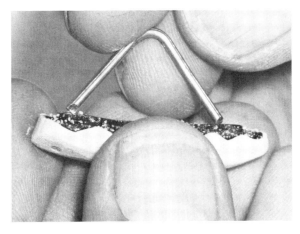

Fig. 6-24. Large paper clip is shaped and used to sprue wax pattern.

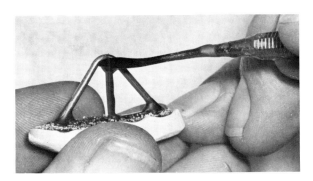

Fig. 6-25. Additional 10-gauge round sprue is extended from bend of paper clip to central portion of wax pattern and sealed in position.

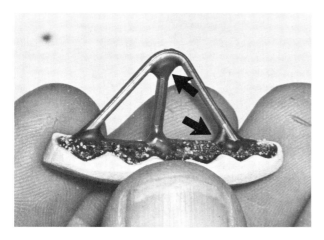

Fig. 6-26. Junctions (arrows) are smoothed with wax to provide smooth flow of gold into mold with minimal turbulence.

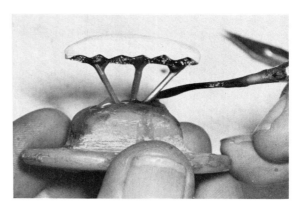

Fig. 6-27. Sprued pattern is sealed to sprue former.

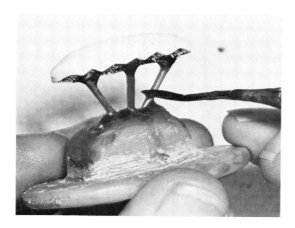

Fig. 6-28. Additional wax is flowed over metal sprue to facilitate removal of sprue from casting ring later.

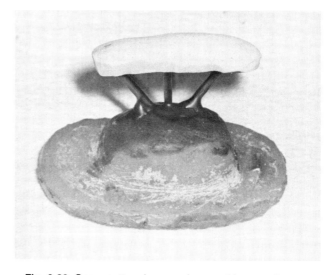

Fig. 6-29. Sprue pattern is securely waxed to sprue former.

fill with cool water. The investment is thoroughly soaked to contribute to a smooth juncture with the refractory investment to be added (Fig. 6-30). After soaking for a few minutes, pour the water from the ring, and remove excess water by gently shaking. Mix the investment, and invest the pattern.

19. Complete the burnout and casting procedure in accordance with the alloy used. Type III gold alloys are satisfactory. Clean and examine the completed casting (Fig. 6-31).

20. Carefully check and remove any nodules on the casting (Fig. 6-32).

21. Cut off sprues flush with the underside of the casting (Fig. 6-33).

22. Polish the casting to a high luster (Fig. 6-34).

23. Remove the inlay wax from one upper posterior quadrant, and place the upper gold occlusal unit in position. Check the occlusion with the opposing wax occlusals (Fig. 6-35). Usually the occlusion will be high and upper resin teeth will need further reduction to accommodate the 14-gauge half-round retentive strip (Fig. 6-36).

24. After the vertical dimension of occlusion has been restored, seal the upper gold occlusal unit to the upper teeth with ivory wax (Fig. 6-37, *A*).

25. Remove the wax from the lower teeth, replace it with the gold occlusal unit, and adjust the resin teeth as necessary to restore the occlusal vertical dimension. Seal the lower gold occlusal to the lower resin teeth with ivory wax (Fig. 6-37, *B*).

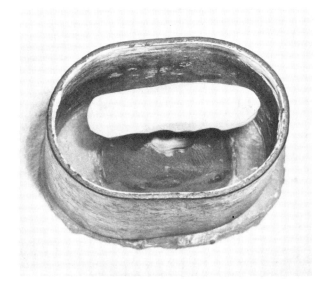

Fig. 6-30. Sprued pattern and investment index are placed in casting ring and filled with cool water. Investment is thoroughly soaked prior to filling ring with refractory investment.

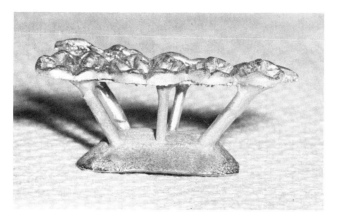

Fig. 6-31. Casting is examined carefully to determine that it is satisfactory.

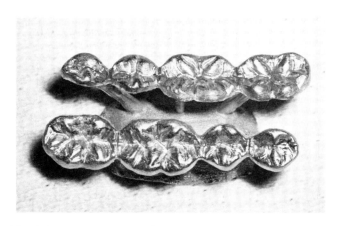

Fig. 6-32. Note particularly if occlusal carvings have been reproduced faithfully.

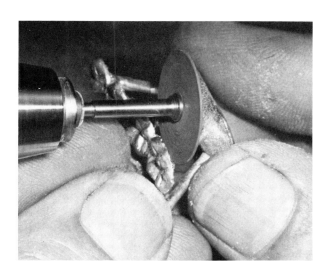

Fig. 6-33. Sprues are cut off flush with underside of casting.

A

B

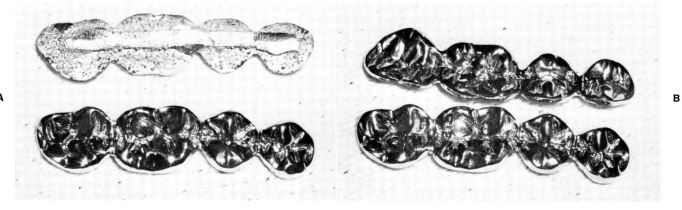

Fig. 6-34. A, Casting should be highly polished. **B,** Occlusal view of polished gold occlusal.

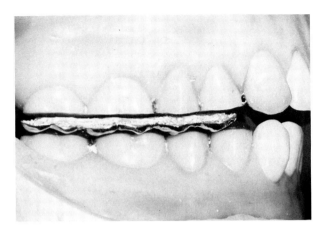

Fig. 6-35. Maxillary gold occlusal has been placed in position, and occlusion with opposing wax pattern checked. In this situation vertical dimension of occlusion has been increased, and maxillary resin teeth will require further reduction to restore vertical dimension of occlusion.

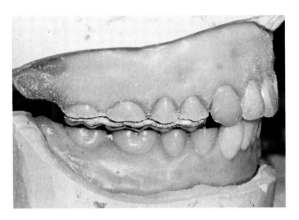

Fig. 6-36. Reduction of posterior resin teeth has resulted in restoration of original vertical dimension of occlusion.

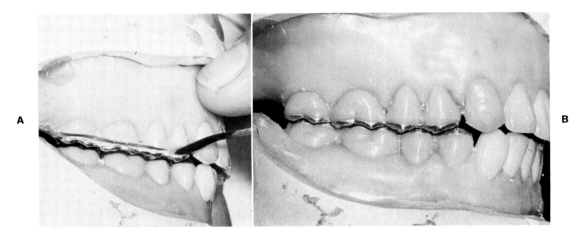

Fig. 6-37. A, Upper gold occlusal is sealed to resin teeth with ivory wax. **B,** Upper and lower gold occlusal units have been sealed to upper and lower teeth with ivory wax.

26. Remove the denture teeth with gold occlusals from the articulator. Ivory wax can be added at this time to modify the buccal and lingual resin contours if desired (Fig. 6-38). Addition of wax facilitates removal of the resin teeth after the boilout.

27. Flask the teeth with gold occlusal surfaces in the usual manner. When flasking, depress the buccal surfaces in the mold slightly toward the occlusal surface. This facilitates positive retention of the gold occlusals in the mold and permits easier removal of the resin teeth after the boilout (Fig. 6-39).

28. Complete the boilout procedure, and remove the resin denture teeth from the mold. Resin teeth can be removed easier if wax was flowed on the ridge lap and

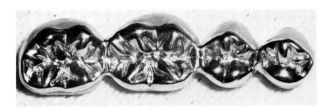

Fig. 6-38. Occlusal units are removed from articulator, and ivory wax added where needed to modify buccal and lingual resin contours.

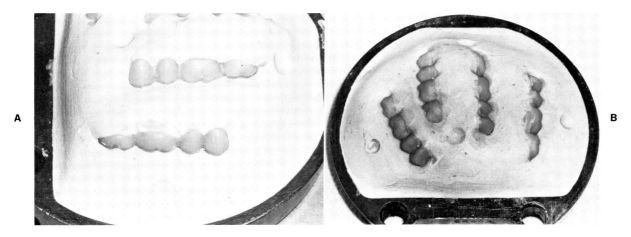

Fig. 6-39. A, Teeth are flasked with buccal surfaces facing upward. Buccal surfaces of teeth are depressed slightly toward occlusal surface to facilitate retention of gold occlusal in mold during packing. **B,** Note depression of occlusal surfaces that facilitates retention of gold occlusal in mold.

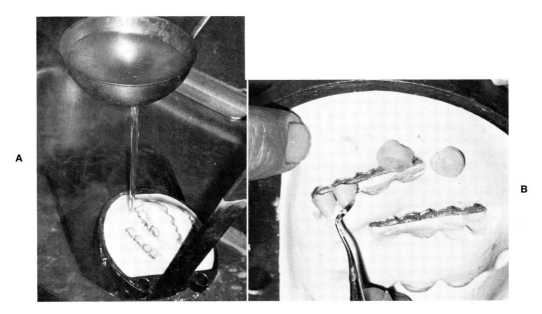

Fig. 6-40. A, Wax is boiled out in usual manner. **B,** Wax flowed over ridge laps and onto lingual aspects of resin teeth before flasking facilitates removal of teeth after boilout procedure.

lingual aspect of the teeth before flasking (Fig. 6-40). Space created by wax removal greatly simplifies removing the teeth.

29. Scrub the mold with detergent solution to thoroughly remove wax residue (Fig. 6-41).

30. Flush the mold with clean boiling water (Fig. 6-42).

31. Paint tinfoil substitute on the stone mold. Avoid coating the gold with tinfoil substitute (Fig. 6-43).

32. Add heat-curing tooth-shaded resin to the mold by the sifting technique (Fig. 6-44). Powder of the appropri-

ate body shade is placed first and saturated with heat-curing monomer (Fig. 6-45).

33. Fill the mold with resin, and keep surface moist with monomer (Fig. 6-46).

34. Sift in the incisal shade last to simulate incisal translucency (Fig. 6-47). Normally the gold is not opaqued.

35. Place a plastic sheet over the resin, and close the flask in a bench press (Fig. 6-48).

36. Remove the flask from the press, open it, and remove the plastic sheet (Fig. 6-49).

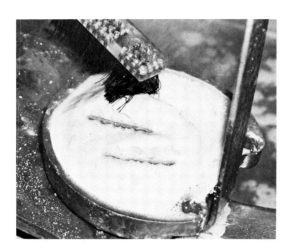

Fig. 6-41. Mold is thoroughly cleaned with detergent solution to remove all traces of wax residue.

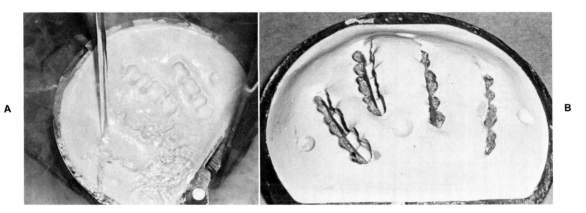

A

B

Fig. 6-42. A, Mold is flushed with final rinse of clean boiling water. **B,** Mold is permitted to cool prior to painting with tinfoil substitute.

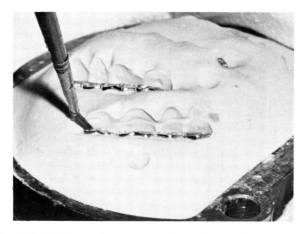

Fig. 6-43. Tinfoil substitute is painted on all parts of gypsum mold that will contact resin. Take care to avoid coating gold with tinfoil substitute.

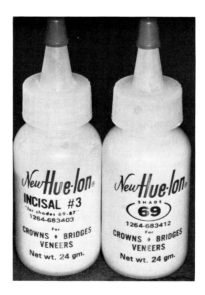

Fig. 6-44. Heat-curing tooth-shaded resins are used to construct gold occlusal units.

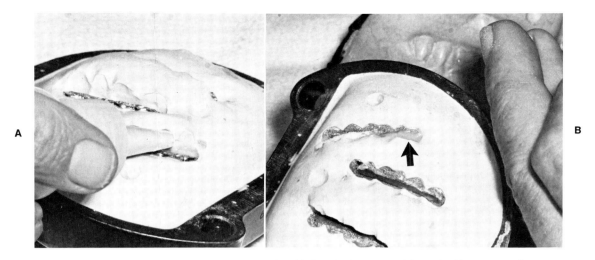

Fig. 6-45. A, Body shade is sifted into mold first. **B,** Powder is saturated (arrow) with monomer from dropper.

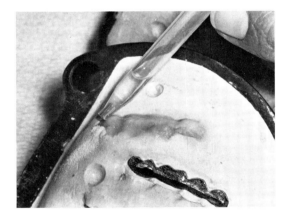

Fig. 6-46. Mold is filled with appropriate body shade resin, and surface is kept moist with monomer.

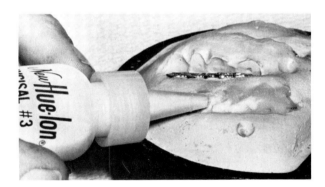

Fig. 6-47. Incisal shade is sifted in last to simulate incisal translucency and moistened with monomer.

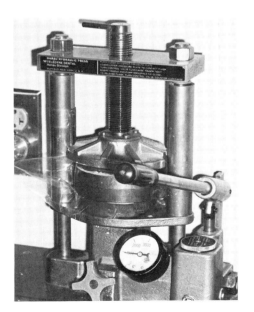

Fig. 6-48. Plastic sheet is placed over resin; flask is closed and trial packed in bench press.

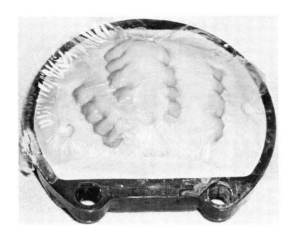

Fig. 6-49. Flask is removed from press, opened, and plastic sheet removed.

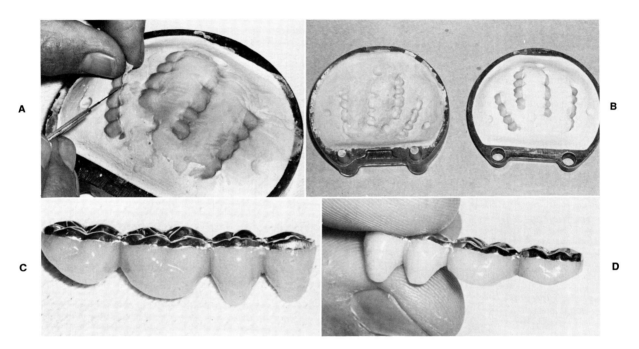

Fig. 6-50. A, Flash is removed by trimming carefully around teeth with No. 25 blade in Bard-Parker handle. **B,** After curing gold occlusal unit, flask is opened, and teeth are removed and polished. **C,** Polished gold occlusal unit is ready for repositioning in articulator. **D,** Gold occlusal unit demonstrating contour that resembles a three-quarter crown.

37. Trim the excess flash with a knife, and continue trial packing until no flash is apparent (Fig. 6-50, *A*). Repaint the upper flask with tinfoil substitute, close the flask in the compress, and cure it according to the manufacturer's recommendations.

38. After curing, open the flask, remove the occlusal units, and polish them (Fig. 6-50, *B*, *C*, and *D*).

39. Place the gold occlusal units on the baseplates in the articulator, and wax them for try-in (Fig. 6-51).

40. Process the denture in the usual manner, and pol-ish it (Fig. 6-52). Processing errors should be minimal, since the occlusal discrepancy will require grinding of the gold.

PROBLEM AREAS

Principal problems associated with making gold occlusals are related to incorrect cast relationships on the articulator; failure to carve the wax occlusal surfaces to harmonize with functional movements; failure to reduce the investment index to control thickness and the buccal

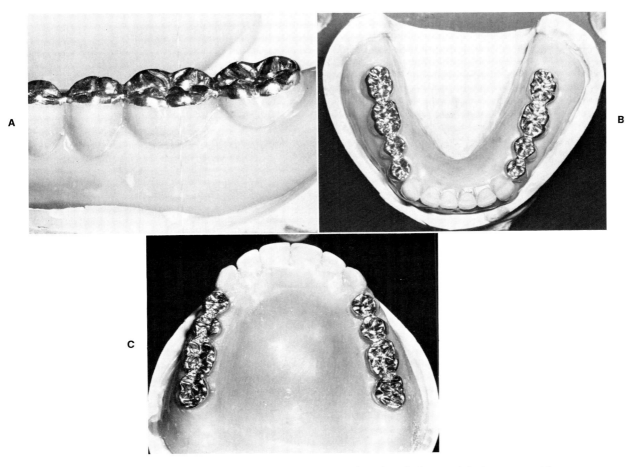

Fig. 6-51. A, Gold occlusal units are repositioned on baseplates in articulator and denture rewaxed for try-in. **B,** Mandibular denture waxed gold occlusal units ready for try-in. **C,** Maxillary denture with gold occlusal units waxed for try-in.

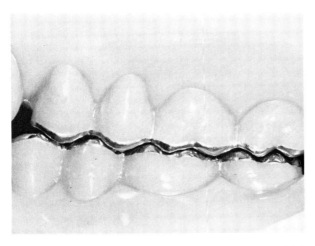

Fig. 6-52. Denture is processed in usual manner; then, it is finished and polished.

outline of the gold casting; failure to place retention wax on the underside of the casting (crystals and 14-gauge half-round wax form); overcarving the investment index, resulting in a thin casting; failure to place wax on the resin teeth to permit removal from the mold after block-out; and packing the occlusal units in the incorrect shade or with autopolymerizing resin (Table 6-1). Wax carvings for gold occlusals must be completed on casts mounted properly in the articulator. It could be difficult and expensive to extensively modify gold occlusals after processing because of a faulty cast mounting. The occlusal anatomy in the wax pattern should harmonize with functional movements of the patient. Trimming the investment index correctly is critical to success, since it controls casting occlusogingival thickness and buccal outline form. Thin castings, as a result of excessive trimming, may not permit occlusal correction without perforation after the denture is processed. If a thin layer of wax is not flowed on the ridge laps and lingual surfaces of the

Table 6-1. Gold occlusal units

Problem	Probable cause	Solution
Occlusion of gold occlusal units incorrect on insertion of denture	Jaw relationship and original cast mounting in error Articulator settings were disturbed after mounting	Make certain that jaw relation record and articulator mounting are correct before sending to laboratory Check articulator settings periodically when constructing gold occlusals
Gold occlusal units do not function properly in functional positions on articulator	Wax-up not checked in lateral and protrusive positions	Carefully adjust wax patterns to accommodate functional positions
Gold castings too thick, and buccal outline is in a straight line	Investment index was not trimmed properly to produce casting approximately 2 mm thick with buccal outline that resembles three-quarter cast crown	Reduce depth of index with sharp knife to produce casting thickness of approximately 2 mm; buccal outline must be scalloped to resemble three-quarter cast crown
Casting too thin	Investment index overtrimmed occlusogingivally	Do not overtrim; maintain approximately 2 mm thickness
Resin teeth cannot be removed from mold after boilout	Wax not flowed on ridge laps and lingual surfaces of resin teeth before flasking	Flow wax on ridge laps and lingual surfaces of resin teeth prior to flasking; resultant space after boilout facilitates removal of teeth from mold
Completed gold occlusal units are of incorrect shade	Body shade selection incorrect Too much incisal shade used	Compare shade selector with anterior teeth on articulator Do not use excessive amounts of incisal shade

resin teeth before flasking, it may be difficult to remove them after the boilout without breaking the mold. Gold occlusal units should be processed in heat-curing resin of the proper shade if maximum esthetics are to be achieved.

Fabrication of metal occlusal denture teeth
PROCEDURE

1. Select the type of resin posterior tooth desired for the metal occlusal form.

2. Rub the teeth lightly on a metal file to flatten the occlusal surface if monoplane teeth are to be used (Fig. 6-53).

3. Align the teeth as desired on a flat surface such as a glass slab. Lute the teeth together with autopolymerizing resin* (Fig. 6-54).

4. Modify the teeth, if desired, with inlay wax (Fig. 6-55).

5. Lightly rub them on the flat file to ensure flatness of the modified composite form (Fig. 6-56).

6. Apply beading wax around the composite form 0.5 mm from the occlusal surface (Fig. 6-57).

Fig. 6-53. Flat plane teeth should be rubbed lightly against metal file to flatten occlusal surface.

---

*DuraLay acrylic, Reliance Dental Manufacturing Co., Chicago, Ill.

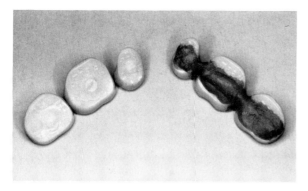

Fig. 6-54. Teeth are aligned on flat surface such as glass slab. Aligned teeth are luted together with DuraLay.

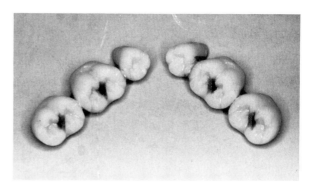

Fig. 6-55. Occlusal surfaces of teeth can be modified, if desired, with inlay wax.

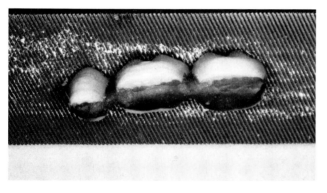

Fig. 6-56. Surfaces are again rubbed against file to ensure flatness of modified form.

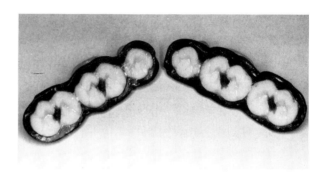

Fig. 6-57. Beading wax is applied around composite form 1.5 mm from occlusal surface.

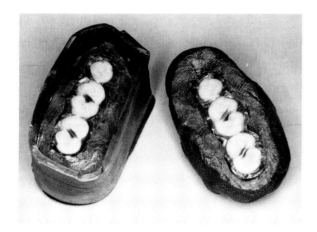

Fig. 6-58. Clay or wax is added around beading wax to enlarge base for boxing with boxing wax.

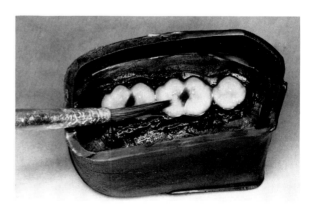

Fig. 6-59. Occlusal form is lubricated with debubblizer solution.

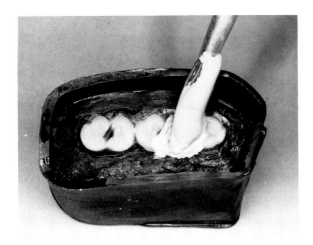

Fig. 6-60. Improved stone is mixed in mechanical spatulator under reduced atmospheric pressure and brushed in mold, taking care to not incorporate air that will result in voids.

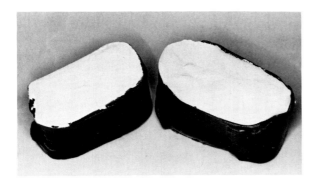

Fig. 6-61. Mold is filled with improved stone.

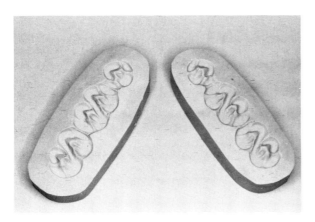

Fig. 6-62. Stone impression of occlusal form is trimmed and smoothed in preparation for boxing.

7. Add clay or wax around the beading wax to enlarge the base, and box it with boxing wax (Fig. 6-58).

8. Lubricate the occlusal form with a debubblizer solution* and remove the excess with a stream of air (Fig. 6-59).

9. Brush a vacuumed mix of improved stone in the mold, making sure not to incorporate air (Fig. 6-60).

10. Fill the mold with improved stone (Fig. 6-61).

11. Trim and smooth the stone impressions of the occlusal forms to prepare to be boxed for making the flexible mold (Fig. 6-62). The flexible mold will yield multiple replicas poured in the investment material.

12. Spray the stone impressions with clear lacquer, which will serve as a separating medium (Fig. 6-63).

13. Allow the lacquer to dry, and spray lightly once again (Fig. 6-64).

14. Glue the stone impressions on a flat piece of cardboard with Super-glue. Box the impressions with cardboard, leaving at least ¼ inch (0.64 cm) distance from the stone forms. Seal the cardboard boxing securely with sticky wax (Fig. 6-65).

15. Assemble the silicone mold-making materials. Follow the manufacturer's directions and weigh the components accurately in paper cups (Fig. 6-66). Weigh the base material first, reset the scales, and add the thinner. Mix thoroughly for 1½ to 2 minutes. Reset the scale and add the catalyst. Mix thoroughly for 2½ minutes or until there are no streaks in the material.

16. Pour into the mold and onto the model just short of covering the stone (Fig. 6-67).

17. Place the mold in a vacuum, preferably under a

---

*Debubblizer, Kerr Manufacturing Co., Romulus, Mich.

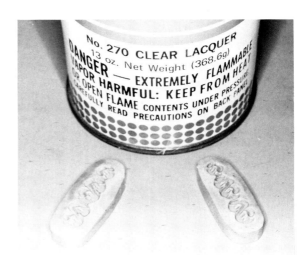

Fig. 6-63. Stone impression is sprayed with clear lacquer that serves as separating medium.

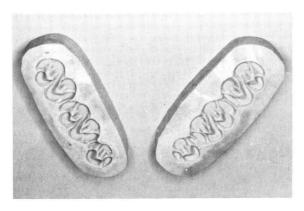

Fig. 6-64. First coat of lacquer is permitted to dry, and impression is sprayed again.

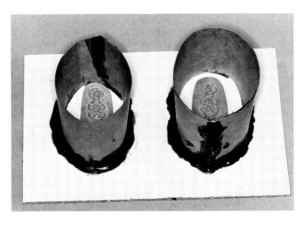

Fig. 6-65. Cardboard boxing is securely sealed with sticky wax.

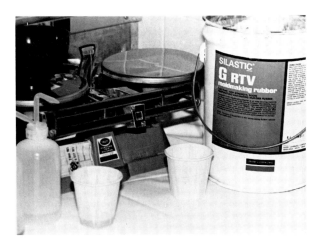

Fig. 6-66. Material is proportioned according to manufacturer's recommendations, and components weighed accurately in paper cups.

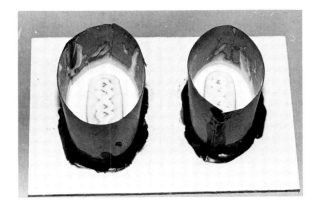

Fig. 6-67. Material is poured into mold and onto model just short of covering stone.

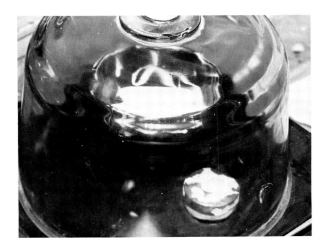

Fig. 6-68. Mold is placed under reduced atmospheric pressure until all air has been eliminated from silicone.

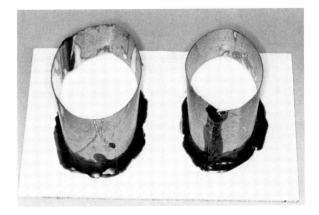

Fig. 6-69. Silicone material is poured into mold until layer of ¼ inch (0.64 cm) is achieved.

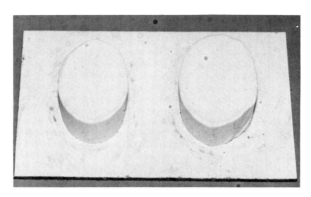

Fig. 6-70. Boxing material is removed from sides of silicone.

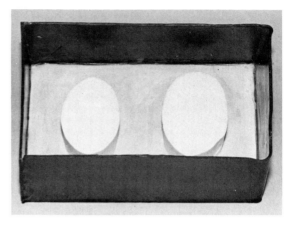

Fig. 6-71. Cardboard base is boxed with boxing wax.

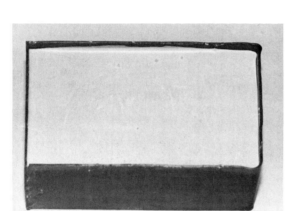

Fig. 6-72. Improved stone is poured around silicone molds to provide additional support and maintain accuracy.

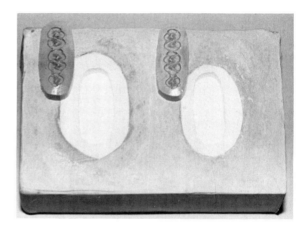

Fig. 6-73. Boxing material and stone impressions are removed from silicone mold.

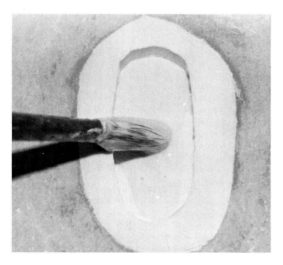

Fig. 6-74. Investment, suitable for metal to be used, is flowed into silicone mold.

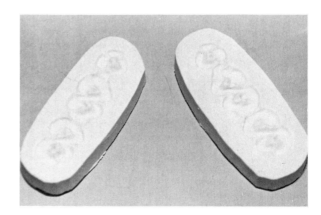

Fig. 6-75. Investment dies are removed from silicone mold and inspected for accuracy.

bell jar–vacuum machine, until all air has been eliminated from the silicone material (Fig. 6-68).

18. Pour more silicone material in the mold until ¼ inch (0.64 cm) of silicone has covered the stone (Fig. 6-69).

19. Remove the boxing material from the sides of the silicone after 24 hours (Fig. 6-70).

20. Box the cardboard base with boxing wax (Fig. 6-71).

21. Pour improved stone around the silicone mold to provide support and maintain accuracy (Fig. 6-72).

22. Remove the boxing materials and stone impressions from the silicone mold (Fig. 6-73).

23. Flow an investment* into the silicone mold, using a soft-bristle artist's brush (Fig. 6-74).

24. Remove the investment dye from the silicone mold and inspect for accuracy of detail (Fig. 6-75).

25. Flow casting wax onto the investment model to the desired thickness of the occlusal form (Fig. 6-76).

---

*Select an investment compatible with metal alloy, such as Investic for Ticonium.

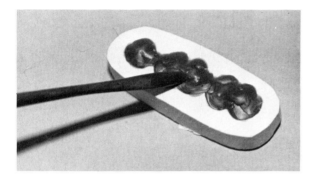

Fig. 6-76. Casting wax is flowed into investment model to create desired thickness of occlusal casting.

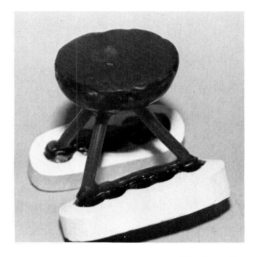

Fig. 6-79. Wax patterns are sprued for investing.

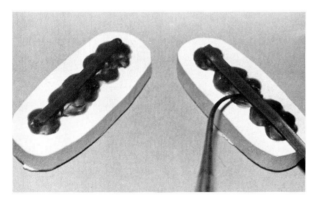

Fig. 6-77. A 14-gauge half-round wax form is luted to previously applied wax to provide retention for resin.

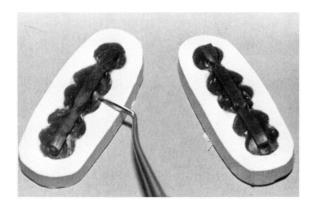

Fig. 6-78. Excess wax is removed from margins of wax pattern.

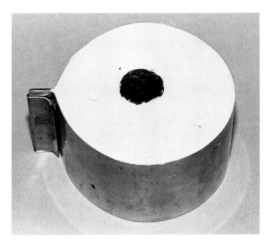

Fig. 6-80. Investment index is soaked in cool water for several minutes prior to filling ring.

26. Lute a half-round wax form onto the previously applied wax. This bar of wax will provide retention for resin (Fig. 6-77).

27. Remove excess wax from the margins of the wax patterns (Fig. 6-78).

28. Sprue the wax patterns for investing (Fig. 6-79).

29. Soak the investment for several minutes in water that is room temperature, and paint investment around the wax and into a suitable size investing ring (Fig. 6-80).

30. After 1 hour, place the investment in a burnout oven at less than 900° F (482° C). Elevate the tempera-

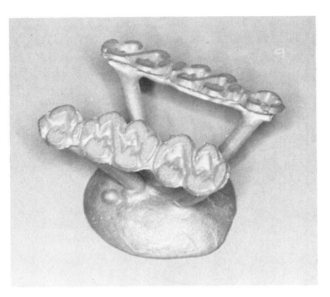

Fig. 6-81. Gold occlusals are cast after wax has been burned out.

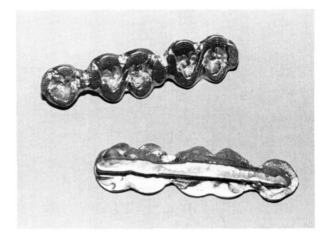

Fig. 6-82. Casting is cleaned, and sprues removed.

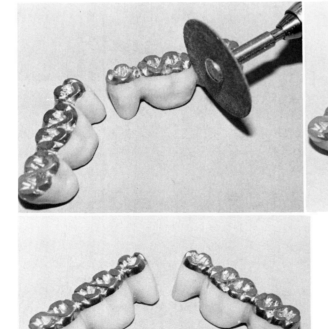

Fig. 6-83. Occlusal units are finished with disks, pumice wheels, and polished on lathe with pumice followed by a high shine polishing material.

ture to 1300° F (141° C), and cast after 1½ hours (Fig. 6-81).

31. Clean the casting, and remove the sprues and trim (Fig. 6-82). Grind the borders smooth and flat.

32. Wax up the metal forms to the desired tooth contours. Invest them in a flask, and process them with acrylic resin of the desired shade. Finish the forms with disks, pumice wheels, and finally, polish them on a lathe with pumice and a high shine polishing material (Fig. 6-83).

PROBLEM AREAS

Problems particular to this procedure are shown in Table 6-2.

Technique for silicone mold for multiple waxing of similar tooth contours
PROCEDURE

1. Wax the metal form to the desired contour (Fig. 6-84, *1*). Make a stone index with keyed sides (Fig. 6-84, *2*). Apply clay or boxing wax several millimeters thick to collars of the wax tooth forms (Fig. 6-84, *3*). Box and pour silicone around the waxed form as previously described (Fig. 6-84, *4*).

2. Place the metal occlusal forms in the indexes, and reposition the silicone to form a mold (Fig. 6-85).

3. Flow molten wax into the silicone mold. Allow the

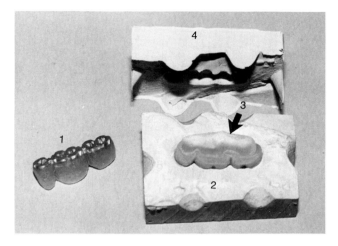

Fig. 6-84. Metal form is waxed to create desired contour *(1)*. Stone index is made with keyed sides *(2)*. Clay or boxing wax is applied to collars of wax tooth forms *(3)*. Silicone material is poured around waxed form as previously described *(4)*.

Table 6-2. Fabrication of metal occlusal denture teeth

Problem	Probable cause	Solution
Improper arch form	Teeth not set up properly or not arranged properly on glass slab	Set up teeth properly before making impression for mold investment cast
Occlusal surfaces not flat or even	Manufacturing defects or processing changes in luting medium	Rub teeth lightly on fine emery or metal file
Metal occlusals too thick and not esthetic	Improper beading; can also cause investment to fracture on separation	Apply beading 1 to 1.5 mm from occlusal surface
Voids or nodules in metal occlusals	Failure to apply debubblizer or vibrate stone or silicone properly	Reduce surface tension with debubblizer and vibrate stone using soft brush
Silicone rubber material sticks to stone	Failure to apply clear lacquer to stone before covering with silicone rubber	Apply two coats of clear lacquer as separating medium
Silicone rubber does not set up properly	Materials improperly measured or mixed	Measure and mix materials according to manufacturer's directions
Metal occlusal has ragged finishing line	Investment material and wax not trimmed properly	Trim investment prior to waxing; trim wax back to margin
Resin body has voids or porosity	Improper packing or processing of acrylic resin	Mix, pack, and process acrylic according to manufacturer's directions

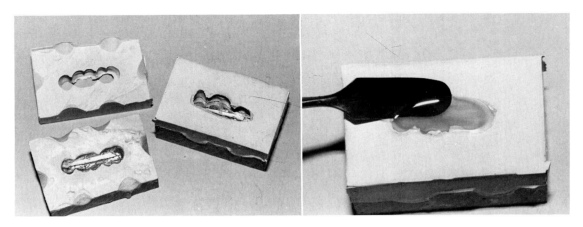

Fig. 6-85. Metal occlusal forms are placed in indexes, and silicone is repositioned to form mold.

wax to harden. Remove and trim the waxed form, and invest and process it with acrylic resin of the desired shade.

SUMMARY

Artificial teeth have been discussed in this chapter. Methods used by manufacturers to identify their various molds and shades were considered briefly; however, it seems that a uniform system for mold and shade identification would benefit the consumer. Methods for constructing artificial teeth with metal occlusals were also presented.

REFERENCES

Davies, H. G., and Pound, E.: Metal cutting surfaces aid denture function, Dent. Surv. **42**:47-53, Oct., 1966.
Encyclopedia Britannica. **21**:759, 1969.
Koehne, C. L., and Morrow, R. M.: Construction of denture teeth with gold occlusal surfaces, J. Prosthet. Dent. **23**:449-455, 1970.
Schultz, A. W.: Comfort and chewing efficiency in dentures, J. Prosthet. Dent. **1**:38-48, Jan.-March, 1951.
Sowter, J. B., and Bass, R. E.: Increasing the efficiency of resin posterior teeth, J. Prosthet. Dent. **19**:465-468, 1968.
Wallace, D. H.: The use of gold occlusal surfaces in complete and partial dentures, J. Prosthet. Dent. **14**:326-333, 1964.

CHAPTER 7

ARRANGING AND ARTICULATING ARTIFICIAL TEETH

RICHARD A. SMITH, A. ANDERSEN CAVALCANTI, and HUGH E. WOLFE

Arranging and articulating artificial teeth are critical elements in constructing removable dental restorations. The purpose of this chapter is to describe the methods of arranging and articulating anterior teeth, 33-degree anatomic posterior teeth, 20-degree posterior teeth, Pilkington-Turner* 30-degree posterior teeth, and Rational* 0-degree posterior teeth to produce optimal treatment results for edentulous and partially edentulous patients. Troubleshooting information relative to preventive and corrective measures is given in Table 7-1 on p. 248.

NATURAL ANTEROPOSTERIOR PLACEMENT OF MAXILLARY ANTERIOR TEETH

Anteroposterior positioning of anterior teeth is extremely important in esthetics and phonetics because of the support that teeth give to lips, cheeks, and other tissues of the oral cavity. Since it is necessary to maintain proper support of these tissues for natural esthetics, it is important to place artificial teeth in essentially the same position as natural teeth. This consideration must not be overlooked when using a resorbed residual maxillary ridge as the primary control for tooth position.

Extreme changes in shape and/or size make a resorbed ridge a questionable landmark to use as a positive control for tooth position. Setting artificial teeth directly over the center of (resorbed) residual ridges has been quite common; however, this practice makes the

---

*Dentsply International Inc., York, Pa.

development of natural esthetics practically impossible or, at best, extremely difficult because the natural teeth seldom occupy the so-called *over-the-ridge* position.

No dental restoration, particularly a complete denture, can be truly esthetic or functional if it fails to position teeth in their proper natural place in the mouth. Properly positioned teeth give support to the lips, cheeks, and other tissues of the oral cavity that is vital to a natural appearance.

After the removal of teeth, the loss of bone structure is usually greater on the buccolabial aspect of the maxillary ridge than on the palatal aspect. As a result, the center of the residual ridge is more palatal and therefore somewhat smaller and different in shape than it was prior to removal of the teeth.

If artificial teeth are to have the best and/or most natural esthetic and functional qualities, it is essential to place them in a position as close as possible to that occupied by the natural teeth, providing these were acceptable esthetically and functionally.

Ridge resorption can have a major effect on the position of the anterior teeth. Fig. 7-1, *A*, illustrates the position of the natural central incisor and its relationship to the ridge. Fig. 7-1, *B*, illustrates the same ridge immediately after removal of the tooth; dotted lines indicate the position of the natural root. In Fig. 7-1, *C*, the direction of resorption is up and back; the solid line identifies the resorbed ridge; the dotted line, the original contour of the ridge. One of the most common errors in tooth positioning, setting the teeth over the ridge with-

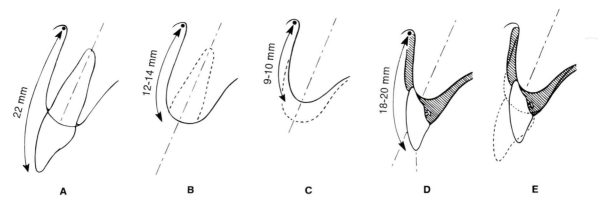

Fig. 7-1. Ridge resorption affects considerably position of anteriors. **A,** Natural central incisor in relation to ridge. **B,** Same ridge after removal of tooth. **C,** Direction of resorption is up and back. Solid line indicates resorbed ridge, and dotted line indicates original contour. **D,** Placing teeth directly over resorbed ridge is common error in tooth positioning. **E,** Dotted line indicates original position of natural tooth for comparison with improper setting of artificial tooth.

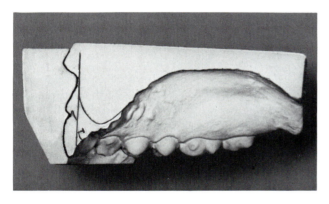

Fig. 7-2. Sectioned cast of natural teeth with labial matrix in position.

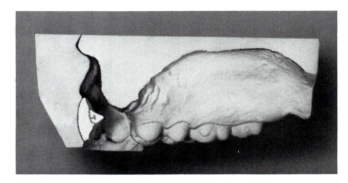

Fig. 7-3. Cast has been trimmed to simulate normal ridge resorption.

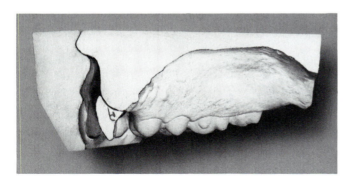

Fig. 7-4. Artificial tooth that has deviated considerably from position of natural tooth after being set on resorbed ridge.

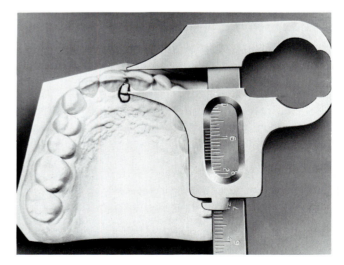

Fig. 7-5. Distance from center of incisive papilla to labial surface of central incisors.

out consideration of the original positioning of the natural teeth, is shown in Fig. 7-1, *D*. In Fig. 7-1, *E*, the denture with teeth set over the ridge, as shown in *D*, is superimposed over the original position of the natural central incisor as shown in *A*. The loss of vertical dimension and lip support, as well as the inevitable resultant loss in esthetics, is readily apparent. Figs. 7-2, 7-3, and 7-4 are another series of matrix studies showing the relationship between tooth position and ridge resorption. Fig. 7-2 shows a cross section of the matrix and cast made before the natural teeth were removed. The cast has been trimmed to simulate a normal amount of ridge resorption in the anterior area in Fig. 7-3. Fig. 7-4 shows what happens to tooth positioning when the teeth are set "up and back" on the resorbed ridge. For natural esthetics and phonetics, the artificial teeth should be of the same length and in the same position anteroposteriorly as the original natural teeth. An artificial tooth set on the ridge may deviate considerably from its true natural position (Fig. 7-4). This "on-the-ridge" position of the teeth *cannot* afford the lip the proper support.

In determining the forward position of the maxillary central incisor, a useful guide is the relationship in natural dentitions between the upper central and the incisive papilla. After outlining the papilla in pencil and bisecting it, the procedure is to measure the distance from the center of the papilla to the labial surface of the tooth (Fig. 7-5). The average distances for the three basic arch forms, square, ovoid, and tapering, differ (Fig. 7-6). Although these distances may vary, the averages serve as reasonable guides and starting points when finding out how far forward to set a central incisor.

Relationship of arch form to tooth arrangement

Nature tends to harmonize not only the form of the maxillary central incisors with the form of the face; but also with the form of the arch and arrangement of the teeth. Persons with predominantly square faces often have mainly square arrangements of teeth. In general, these same principles of harmony apply to the square tapering, tapering, and ovoid types.

Although loss of teeth and consequent resorption of the labial and buccal alveolar processes can change the original form of the maxillary arch, nature leaves a guide to tooth arrangement in the form of the mandibular arch. Even though resorption can and does occur, usually the direction is downward, primarily toward the body of the mandible, and often the lower arch tends to preserve its outline form. Frequently, the mandibular ridge is a fairly reliable guide to tooth arrangement for the edentulous patient.

Tooth arrangement in square arch

Usually the arrangement is to set the two central incisors to almost a straight line across the front of the square arch. Then the lateral incisors are placed with a nearly full labial aspect so that they show little rotation in at the distal aspect. This positioning of the central and lateral incisors gives width to the positioning of the canines and prominence to these teeth. The four incisors tend to have little rotation, and the radius of the square arch tends to be wider than that of the tapering arch.

The larger radius of this arch allows sufficient room for placing the incisors without crowding or lapping. Overall, in the typal square arrangement the visual effect is fairly straight from canine to canine. In addition, teeth arranged in a typal square-arch configuration tend to be

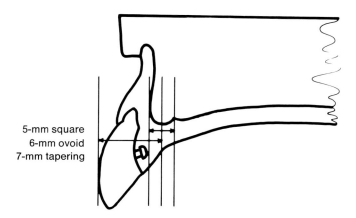

Fig. 7-6. Average distances from center of papilla to labial surface of central incisor are shown for three types of arch forms.

5-mm square
6-mm ovoid
7-mm tapering

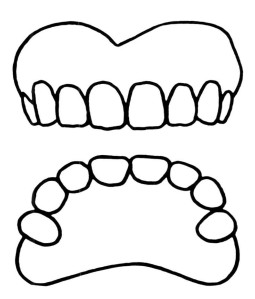

Fig. 7-7. Common configuration for square arch form from labial and incisal aspects.

more or less straight up and down, rather than sloping. The full or nearly full labial surface presented by the six anterior teeth gives a broad effect that is in harmony with the broad square face (Fig. 7-7).

Tooth arrangement in tapering arch

In the tapering arch, the central incisors are often farther forward of the canines than in other types of arches (Fig. 7-8). A characteristic of the tapering arrangement is the rotation of the central incisors on their long axes inward at the distal aspect. This rotation more or less sets the two teeth at an angle, thereby creating a pointed effect to the arrangement.

In the tapering arch, considerable rotating and lapping of teeth are often evident because this arch has less space than any other type, and crowding is inevitable. Crowding and rotation of the teeth reduce the amount of labial surface visible anteriorly. The typal tapering arrangement does not look as wide as other setups. Usually this narrowing is in harmony with the narrowing effect visible in the lower third of the tapering face.

Other typical characteristics of arrangements of this type are the raising of the lateral incisors from the occlusal plane and the depressing of them at the gingival plane. In addition, the necks of the canines at the gingival area are usually quite prominent, and the incisal tips of the canines are often at the same height or slightly above the incisal edges of the lateral incisors. In a typal tapering arrangement, the teeth exhibit some slope; for example, one may project the incisal edges of the central and lateral incisors forward and bring out the cervical area of the canines, leaving their incisal tips in harmony with the central and lateral incisors.

Tooth arrangement in square tapering arch

The square tapering arrangement combines characteristics of the square and the tapering forms, but modifies both. It has characteristic square placement of the central incisors, such as little or no rotation, with the typical tapering effect or rotation of the lateral incisors and canines. However, the square tapering arrangement does not exhibit the illusion of fullness or width like the square arrangement; the canines often show more distal rotation than in a square arrangement (Fig. 7-9).

Tooth arrangement in ovoid arch

The ovoid arrangement has a definite curvature. The central incisors in the ovoid anterior arch usually set well forward of the canines. They are usually in a position between that of the square arch and that of the tapering arch. In the ovoid arrangement, there is seldom rotation. As a result, a typical alignment shows fullness of the labial surface from canine to canine. This align-

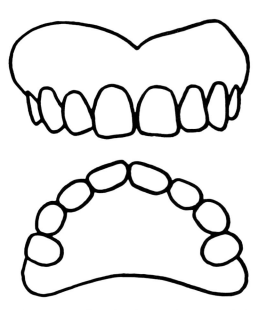

Fig. 7-8. Common configuration for tapering-type arch form from labial and incisal aspects.

ment and the setting to the curved arch give a broad, rounding effect that harmonizes with a round ovoid face (Fig. 7-10).

Considerations affecting placement and positioning of anterior teeth

In placing and positioning the maxillary anterior teeth, the objective is to provide a balance between maximum esthetics and proper phonetics. As seen previously, anterior teeth set directly over the ridges are not in the position formerly occupied by the natural teeth. Therefore these anterior teeth fail to provide support for the musculature of the lower third of the face, and they interfere with proper phonetics. Without the proper support, these facial muscles tend to sag into unnatural positions. In positioning the maxillary anteriors, their relationship to the occlusal and sagittal planes is important.

Occlusal plane

Generally the central incisor, when set at approximately the same angle as the natural tooth, is at an inclination slightly offset from the vertical edge, and the incisal edge touches the occlusal plane. The lateral incisor often has a slightly more accentuated slope than that of the central incisor. The incisal edge of the lateral incisor may be raised slightly, approximately 0.5 mm from the occlusal plane. The canine usually sets more prominently and to a line at right angles to the occlusal plane, with the incisal edge set on that plane (Fig. 7-11).

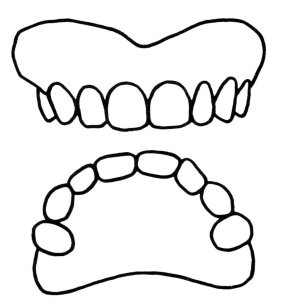

Fig. 7-9. Common configuration for square tapering arch form from labial and incisal aspects.

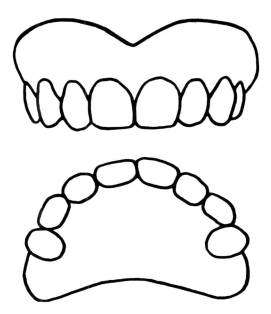

Fig. 7-10. Common configuration for ovoid-type arch form from labial and incisal aspects.

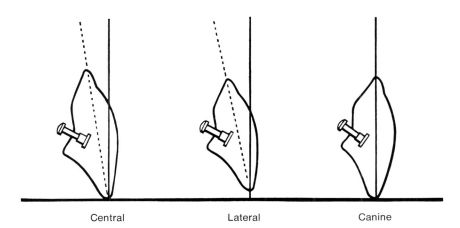

Central   Lateral   Canine

Fig. 7-11. Inclination of central, lateral, and canine teeth and their average relation to occlusal plane.

Sagittal plane

The sagittal plane divides the body vertically into halves. In the dental arch, this plane approximates the median line. The desirable angulation to the sagittal plane or median line can be correlated to the form of both the arch and the tooth. Generally, the square arch form and tooth, as well as the ovoid arch form and tooth, can be set to approximately the same angulations. The tapering forms desirably should be set to a slightly greater angulation.

It is essential to realize that any technique for the preliminary arrangement of teeth, both anteriors and posteriors, is based on average, or so-called normal, conditions. Many times practical considerations dictate modifications of these methods to cope most effectively with the multitude of individual differences in the oral and facial anatomy. However, basic principles that apply to average situations will serve as a workable foundation on which to base necessary modifications. After placement of the six maxillary anterior teeth in position with due regard to the requirements of vertical dimension, vertical overlap, and horizontal overlap, the remaining considerations that affect their arrangement in the arch are essentially esthetic (Fig. 7-12).

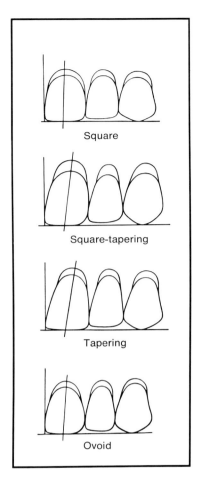

Fig. 7-12. Average relation of anterior teeth to sagittal plane and occlusal plane for square, square-tapering, tapering, and ovoid tooth-arch configurations.

Factors of softness and vigor

Some conditions directly affect the individual arrangement and esthetic appearance of a natural dentition. Softness in tooth arrangement depends on the selection of harmonious forms of teeth as a prerequisite and the use of smaller lateral and central incisors wherever indicated. With respect to tooth arrangement and selection, softness can also mean a reduction of the labial surface in terms of its visual appearance.

A rounded mesiodistal curvature of the tooth in combination with an ovoid outline of the tooth appears softer than a flat mesiodistal tooth with more angularity in its outline. A rounded form or a curved form is much softer to the eye than a straight line or a flat plane.

On the other hand, a characteristic of the bold, vigorous face is the dominant size and alignment of the teeth. The relatively larger size of the lateral incisors and canines and their straight bold arrangement are important considerations in achieving the effect of strength.

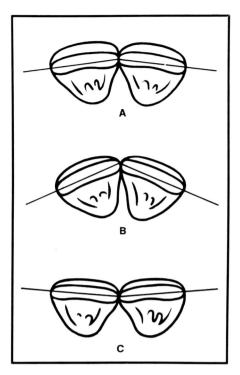

Fig. 7-13. Tooth positioning for visual effect. **A,** Appear normal. **B,** Central incisors appear smaller. **C,** Teeth appear larger, creating effect of boldness and strength.

However, vigor, boldness, and strength are not necessarily solely or primarily masculine characteristics because many female patients also have strong, bold faces.

Softening, or the alternate, vigor, depends on the size and shape of teeth in relationship to the face, as well as the positioning of the teeth in the arch. The more labial surface of the teeth that is visible, particularly in the lateral incisors, the stronger the tooth arrangement appears.

Examples of the application of the principle of tooth positioning for visual effect are shown in Fig. 7-13. Positioning the two central incisors normally makes the front view of these teeth look normal in size or in relation to each other (Fig. 7-13, *A*). In another arrangement, positioning the two central incisors with the mesial edges slightly more prominent and with the distal edges rotated inwardly makes them appear smaller (Fig. 7-13, *B*).

From a straight front view, the teeth in the latter arrangement look smaller than those in the first one. This illusion results from merely rotating the teeth to give them a somewhat smaller and softer look. Rounding the distoincisal surface of each tooth slightly with a rubber wheel softens this effect still more. It is essential to avoid rounding all teeth exactly alike to maintain a slight degree of asymmetry in this arrangement.

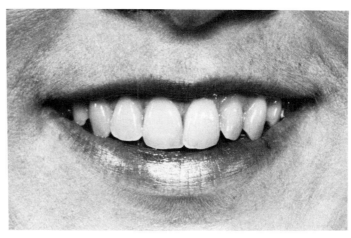

Fig. 7-14. Asymmetry of natural teeth. Patient's right central incisor has mesial surface slightly turned in and its distal aspect prominent. Right lateral incisor has distal surface turned out, giving tooth broad appearance. Right canine has prominent cervical area. Left central incisor has distal surface turned inward, and mesial surface slightly overlapping right central. Left lateral incisor has slight overlap over central incisor, and distal surface is depressed. Left canine has mesial surface turned out and prominent cervical area.

In the third arrangement (Fig. 7-13, *C*), placing the same two central incisors to make the teeth look larger creates the illusion of boldness or strength. This effect is the result of merely rotating the mesial edges in and the distal edges out to show more facial surface. Also, depressing the lateral incisors slightly behind the central incisors accentuates the boldness and strength of the tooth arrangement more. Grinding the teeth incisally, thereby leaving the distoincisal area prominent, and grinding toward the mesioincisal area make this illusion even stronger.

Influence of asymmetry on tooth arrangement

Another point of interest in tooth arrangement is the relationship between facial asymmetry and the associated asymmetry in tooth arrangement. Few faces have true symmetry in terms of a precise left- and right-side balance. Many faces that appear to be symmetrical on initial observation display a variety of subtle or minute differences on closer observation.

Similarly, subtle and minute differences exist in the arrangement of natural teeth. Conversely, asymmetry may be apparent to a marked degree in many faces; the left and right sides may show considerable variance. In instances when asymmetry in the face is pronounced, asymmetry may also be seen in the tooth arrangement.

Asymmetry determines the relative vigor or softness of either side of the face. The size and position of the anterior and posterior teeth in the arrangement produce the asymmetry. It is an extremely subtle factor, and as minor a variation as the depression and/or rotation of either the left or right canine at the gingival surface is sufficient to create this effect. At times also the lateral incisors may differ slightly in size, such as a reduction in the size of a lateral incisor on one side of the mouth to make it smaller than the corresponding one on the opposite side. Perhaps even positioning one central incisor

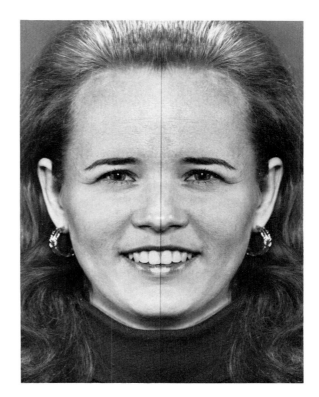

Fig. 7-15. Two right sides of face put together by split photography, making face and dental arch look wider.

slightly anterior to the other may produce the same effect (Fig. 7-14).

In the human anatomy, asymmetry is far more prevalent than perfect symmetry. Natural teeth generally reflect the asymmetry seen in the face. The conventional method of split photography best illustrates asymmetry of facial form and tooth arrangement. This technique compares an original photograph with two composites, one made up from two right sides (Fig. 7-15)

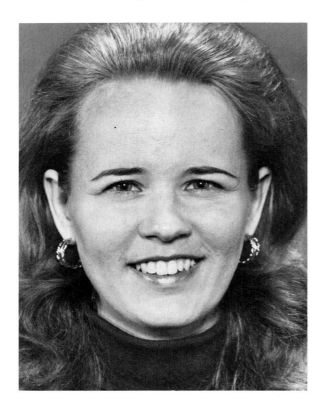

Fig. 7-16. Original photograph of natural face showing pleasing asymmetry of face and teeth.

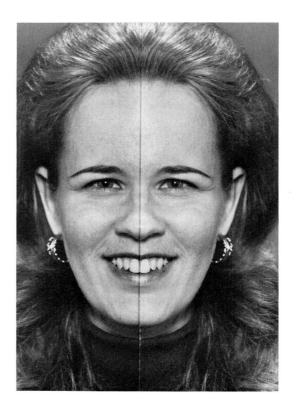

Fig. 7-17. Two left sides of face put together by split photography, making face and dental arch look smaller.

and the other from two left sides of the face (Fig. 7-17). The original photograph is that of a young woman with natural dentition (Fig. 7-16).

From a careful examination of the photograph showing the natural face form of the patient (Fig. 7-16), it is apparent that the malar (cheek) area of the right side is more developed than this area on the left side. The dental arch form is wider on the right side, and the arrangement and size of the teeth on both sides differ. However, these features combine to create a pleasing overall composition.

In a split photograph, using two right sides of the patient (Fig. 7-15), the face and dental arch appear to be wider. In a photograph of two left sides of the patient (Fig. 7-17), the face and dental arch appear to be smaller. In both instances, it is apparent that the face form, arch form, and tooth arrangement no longer have the natural, pleasing asymmetry observed in the original photograph.

Spacing of anterior teeth

When developing more characterization in a denture, spacing the teeth is another important consideration, but one that requires caution. Although spacing of teeth may be one of the many irregularities in nature, it is less no-

ticeable in a natural dentition than generally believed. Dentitions with a noticeable degree of spacing between the maxillary central incisors occur rather infrequently, and spacing between two or more teeth in the maxillary arch appears only slightly more frequently.

Overall spacing usually results from drifting of the teeth. In addition, patients with an abnormally large arch in which the size of the teeth is in proportion to the size of the face also show spacing because the teeth are too small to fill the arch properly. Preoperative records, such as casts or photographs, are excellent guides to natural spacing between central incisors or to overall spacing, rather than arbitrary rules.

It is possible to introduce esthetic spacing into a denture (Fig. 7-18). The inverted type of spacing shown at the top may be difficult for the patient to keep clean. On the lower left is a straight up-and-down vertical space between the two central incisors. In the lower right illustration is a conical type space; the space is larger at the incisal opening than toward the gingival opening. To be classified as a true diastema, the space should be completely open, and the adjacent teeth should make no contact. As noted previously, preoperative records are a preferred guide to spacing.

Modification of an embrasure produces another type

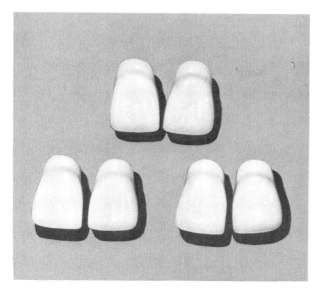

Fig. 7-18. Types of diastemas to be used judiciously between central incisors.

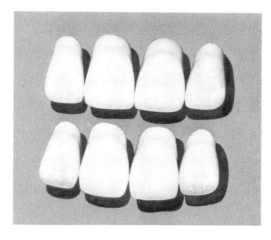

Fig. 7-19. Embrasure modification. Teeth in top row make normal contact. Teeth in lower row have been ground slightly with rubber wheel to modify and enlarge embrasures.

of relationship (Fig. 7-19). Here the teeth are in contact, in contrast to the diastema in which the abutting teeth make no contact. The upper illustration shows the amount of space present after setting up the teeth to make normal contact in the incisal third area. In the lower illustration, slight grinding of the teeth and modification with a rubber wheel have enlarged the embrasures and moved the contact toward the middle third of the teeth.

Natural dentitions that have a pleasing appearance often may have slight spacing, diastema, between the lateral incisors and canines. This effect may be incorporated judiciously in a denture tooth arrangement to improve the appearance of the patient.

Crowding and lapping

Crowding or lapping of the teeth in a natural dentition often is present in abnormally small arches. The size of the teeth is often proportionate to the size of the face, but too large for the amount of space in the arch. Crowding or lapping is the method that nature uses to deliver the full complement of natural teeth in an arch that is too small to accommodate them.

Crowded and lapped conditions sometimes appear in various facial forms and typal tooth arrangements, but most frequently in the tapering classification. The crowded, lapped, and considerably rotated arrangement is typical of the narrow tapering arch, and often is present when the vault is quite high.

It is possible to place lateral incisors in a variety of treatments (Fig. 7-20). In the upper left, the extreme

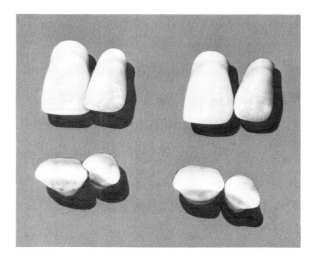

Fig. 7-20. Typical examples of crowding and lapping. Teeth on right create visual effect of lapping without actually lapping.

lapping of a lateral over a central incisor ties the teeth together too closely and can make them look like a solid band of color in the mouth. An incisal view of the same position of these teeth is in the lower left. The lateral incisor is too far ahead of the central incisor to give a pleasing esthetic effect. This position also can cause irritation to the lip and may exert a dislodging pressure on the denture.

The upper right shows the results of a suggested method for improvement. The mesial aspect of the lateral incisor and the distal aspect of the central incisor have slight embrasures ground on them. The central and lateral incisors still maintain contact; however, the lateral incisor is not as far forward, and the teeth make contact at a slightly different angle.

Slight grinding has softened even more the outline form of the lateral incisor on the distal aspect. In the lower right, the suggested position of the central and lateral incisors, in addition to the enlarged embrasure and slight change in outline form, creates the visual effect of a lapped lateral incisor without actually lapping.

Arranging maxillary anterior teeth

These suggestions for arranging anterior teeth presuppose the selection of artificial teeth that are suitable to the patient in form, size, shade, or blend. The procedures used for arranging anterior teeth differ. The usual method is to place each tooth individually. As each tooth is set, it is customary to check the alignment of its incisal edge in relation to both the maxillary and mandibular occlusion rims (Fig. 7-21).

Following are five considerations in positioning or setting anterior teeth:

1. Anteroposterior positioning
2. Anterior slope
3. Mesiodistal inclination
4. Inferosuperior positioning to a horizontal plane (incisal length)
5. Rotation on long axis

PROCEDURES

1. Place the central incisors in position with the incisal edges touching the mandibular occlusion rim (Fig. 7-21) or, the occlusal plane selected (Fig. 7-22).

2. Position the lateral incisors with the incisal edge raised approximately 1 mm from this plane (Fig. 7-23).

3. Place the canines with the incisal tip touching the occlusal plane or mandibular occlusion rim, and tilt the cervical third buccally to give it prominence. Normally, when positioned properly, the mesiolabial aspect of these teeth will be visible from the anterior view (Fig. 7-24).

The position of canine teeth plays an important role in the esthetic appearance of natural dentition. In a denture it plays an equally important role because it influences both the anterior and posterior tooth arrangement.

Positioning of maxillary canines

Proper positioning of the upper canines is highly important: the rotation showing the mesiolabial portion of the tooth (Fig. 7-25), the vertical long axis (Fig. 7-26), and the prominent gingival area with the incisal edge "tucked in" to harmonize with adjacent incisal areas (Fig. 7-27).

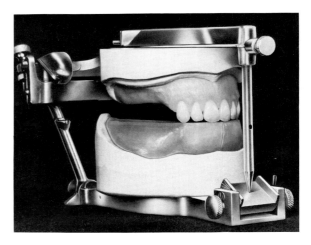

Fig. 7-21. Maxillary anterior teeth are arranged carefully in relation to properly contoured occlusion rim.

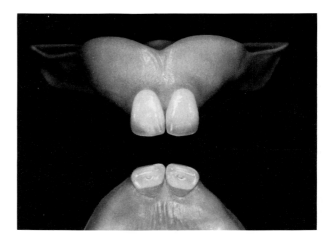

Fig. 7-22. Typical positioning for maxillary central incisors.

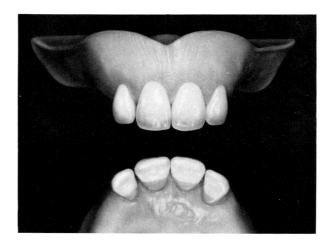

Fig. 7-23. Lateral incisors are positioned slightly shorter than centrals.

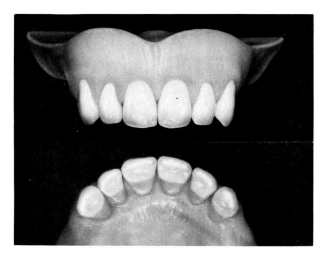

Fig. 7-24. Canines, like central incisors, usually touch occlusal plane.

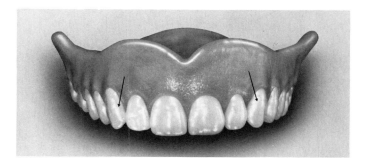

Fig. 7-25. Correct positioning of canines (arrows) viewed from front with mesiolabial surface prominent.

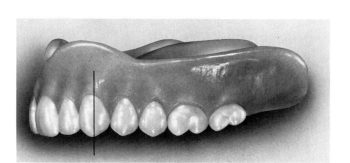

Fig. 7-26. Profile or side view emphasizing almost vertical long axis or position of canine.

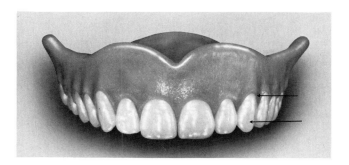

Fig. 7-27. Desirable prominent setting of canine at gingival portion (top arrow) rather than at incisal edge (bottom arrow).

Personalization of setup by selective grinding

One of the most important considerations in producing a natural appearing denture is personalization, which is possible to introduce by carefully performed, selective grinding procedures. Two molds of artificial anterior teeth illustrate this observation (Fig. 7-28). Grinding has altered both molds, *left*, and the teeth are as carded, *right*. Alterations in the top mold, *left*, are for vigor and strength. By comparison, alterations in the lower mold, *left*, project an image of delicacy, softness, and youthfulness. A natural overall appearance results from careful modification of the six teeth of each set to bring about the given effects (Fig. 7-29).

Fig. 7-30 illustrates how to progressively make a square tapering mold into a stronger appearing tooth, *top*. The central incisor, *top left*, is as it comes from the card. The same tooth, *top center*, is shown after slight, but relatively straight, grinding on the incisal edge. Although it is possible to make many changes in this tooth,

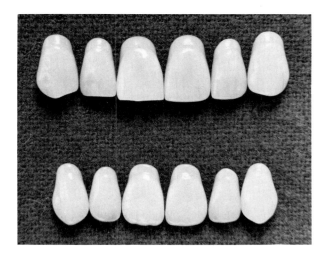

Fig. 7-28. Halves of two molds of teeth personalized by selective grinding. Top mold after alterations to project image of vigor and strength, and bottom mold after grinding to create image of delicacy and softness.

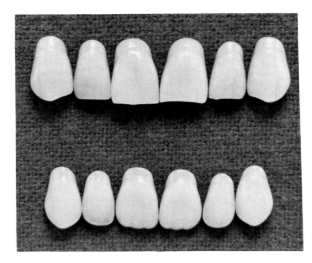

Fig. 7-29. Natural overall appearance obtained by careful grinding of six teeth of each set to create desired effects.

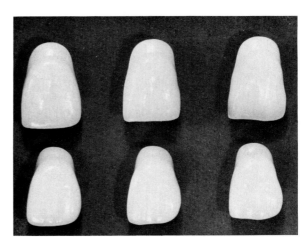

Fig. 7-30. *Top row,* square tapering tooth can be modified progressively into stronger appearing tooth. *Bottom row,* ovoid mold can be modified into vigorous and stronger appearing form.

its big strong square look creates the illusion of strength and vigor as long as it remains square and blocky in appearance. The next tooth, *top right,* shows how to increase the vigorous appearance more. Grinding the labial surface has increased the height of the mesial and distal lobes. Further modification of the incisal edge has strengthened and matured its appearance.

Modification of a typically soft or delicate ovoid tooth form is shown in Fig. 7-30, *bottom.* In a female patient of somewhat vigorous appearance, the desire is not only to retain the essential softness of the teeth, as emphasized by their curvature and ovoid influence, but also to introduce a slightly more vigorous factor. Slight grinding on the incisal edge of the center tooth, *bottom row,* has increased its vigorous appearance and strength. Next to this tooth is an even more vigourous tooth form developed for the patient, with additional characterizing on the labial and incisal surfaces.

A similar example of the same type of treatment on lateral incisors is shown in Fig. 7-31. The upper teeth are the same square tapering mold as the central teeth shown in Fig. 7-30. This tooth is strong and vigorous, and it is possible to increase the illusion of strength and vigor by modifying the incisal edge, *top right.* Below this is an alternate treatment in which the tooth has a much softer and more delicate appearance than the original mold as a result of slight rounding of the mesial and distal aspects, *bottom right.*

Special treatment of a lateral incisor can change its appearance (Fig. 7-32). The tooth on the left is as manufactured, whereas the tooth on the right is the same one after narrowing at the incisal surface. Now the tooth appears to be wider through the midsection. This treatment helps strengthen the lateral incisor and gives it a

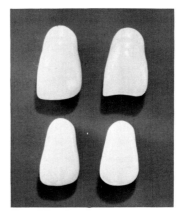

Fig. 7-31. Square tapering lateral incisor, *top row,* as it comes from tooth card and after modification for strength and vigor *(right).* Lateral incisor, *bottom row,* before and after *(right)* modification for softer appearance.

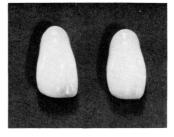

Fig. 7-32. Lateral incisor unmodified, *left.* Same tooth narrowed at incisal edge to strengthen overall impression, *right.*

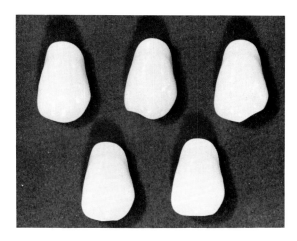

Fig. 7-33. *Upper left,* stock canine as manufactured. Others have been modified to look like natural canines. *Lower right,* unnatural pattern, canine with incisal edge straight.

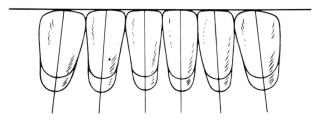

Fig. 7-34. Frontal view of mandibular anterior teeth with average positioning, which does not produce good esthetic effect.

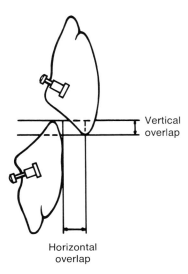

Fig. 7-35. Vertical overlap or overbite in which horizontal plane used for relating mandibular anterior teeth is above occlusal plane.

suggestion of almost primitive strength. Used with discretion, this treatment can improve denture esthetics.

There are several interesting treatments to use on the incisal edge of canine teeth. Fig. 7-33 shows a stock tooth as manufactured, *upper left;* an example of concave grinding on the mesial angle of the tooth, simulating natural abrasion, *center;* an example of grinding to simulate distal abrasion, *upper right;* and an example of incisal modification, simulating the incisal abrasion in a young patient, *lower left.* An example of what not to do with the canine is shown on the *lower right;* nature seldom abrades natural canines in a straight line.

Considerations affecting arrangement of mandibular anterior teeth

A front view of the lower anterior teeth shows them arranged in average horizontal alignment of their incisal edges (Fig. 7-34). The long axes of the central incisors are perpendicular to the plane. The long axes of the lateral incisors incline slightly distally at the neck. The long axes of the canines incline still more distally at the neck. Such an even "picket-fence" arrangement will not create a natural esthetic appearance, although it is possible to use it as a starting point of reference.

The horizontal plane used for aligning lower anterior teeth may be above the actual occlusal plane, a distance usually described as the vertical overlap or overbite (Fig. 7-35). Esthetic and phonetic needs of a patient affect the amount or degree of vertical overlap of the teeth and, consequently, the degree of incisal guide-table angulation. It is possible to arrange teeth in harmony with various degrees of incisal guide-table angulation.

Some prefer to position both the maxillary and mandibular anterior teeth prior to setting the posterior teeth. In such instances, the position of the anterior teeth, the amount of vertical and horizontal overlap (overbite and overjet), and other factors, such as the condylar guidance, plane of occlusion, and degree of compensating curve desired, may affect the choice of posterior teeth for a harmonious occlusion.

As a rule, incisal guide-table angulations of more than 20 degrees may indicate the use of 33-degree anatomic teeth or Pilkington-Turner 30-degree posterior teeth. Incisal guide-table angulations of 20 degrees or less may call for the use of 20-degree posterior teeth. A flat incisal guide table may indicate 0-degree Rational posterior teeth. It also affects the anteroposterior compensating curve.

A proximal view of the mandibular anterior teeth indicates average anteroposterior inclinations to a horizontal plane (Fig. 7-36). Mandibular anterior teeth are an integral part of the esthetics and phonetics for complete dentures. Crowding and/or irregularity in the position of the lower anterior teeth generally mirror condi-

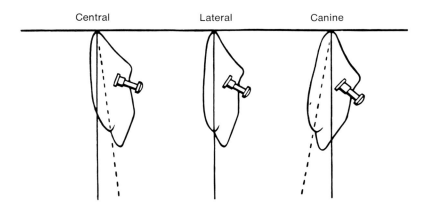

Fig. 7-36. Proximal view of lower anteriors showing average anteroposterior inclinations to horizontal plane.

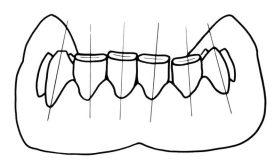

Fig. 7-37. Diagram of lower anteriors set correctly with long axes *not* projecting to common center.

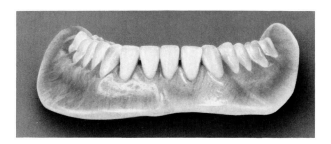

Fig. 7-38. Denture with teeth as in Fig. 7-37 rotated, lapped, or spaced with no two long axes parallel.

tions that exist in the upper arch. However, lower anterior teeth are usually more crowded and irregular than upper anterior teeth with a similar condition.

By careful rotation and inclination and, on occasion, slight proximal grinding and polishing, it is possible to crowd and lap mandibular teeth, thereby creating a natural esthetic appearance. In some instances, the lower teeth are much more conspicuous than the upper teeth; particular attention to their arrangement is essential.

It is necessary to avoid setting the mandibular anterior teeth with their long axes projecting to one common center. This type of arrangement develops a symmetrical, even, and unnatural appearance. Rotation of the lower anterior teeth and lapping them produce more characterization if no two long axes of the teeth are parallel to each other (Figs. 7-37 and 7-38).

Overall evaluation of anterior tooth arrangement

Although there are many methods and guides for arranging artificial anterior teeth, the overall visual effect of teeth in the mouth of the patient resulting from their shape, size, color, and position determines their acceptance or rejection. The teeth also must fulfill the physiologic, phonetic, and emotional requirements of the individual patient.

This area of dentistry is truly as much an art as a science. In any given situation, experience and judgment are the final determinants as to whether a given arrangement of teeth is usable in completing the denture to the satisfaction of those involved.

POSTERIOR TOOTH ARRANGEMENT
Selection of posterior molds

Many types of posterior tooth forms are available for the prosthodontic treatment of patients. Needs of individual patients and the preference of the dentist performing the treatment determine the selection of the various tooth types. Making a recommendation for the use of one type over another is beyond the scope of this chapter.

To fulfill the needs of various treatment philosophies and techniques, a wide range of posterior tooth forms is available. This chapter describes some of the most popular types, such as, the 33-degree anatomic posterior teeth, 20-degree posterior teeth, Pilkington-Turner* 30-

degree posterior teeth, and Rational* 0-degree posterior teeth. Another workable posterior tooth form available from the manufacturer of the teeth described in this text is the Functional* posterior tooth form. It is similar to the 33-degree anatomic posterior tooth form, but with somewhat less cuspal "rise."

The dentist should select the type of posterior tooth form to be used and indicate it on the work authorization form. If the upper anterior mold used in the tooth arrangement is in harmony esthetically with the size and shape of the patient's face, it is easy to select an appropriate posterior tooth mold from the mold charts published by a given manufacturer. The charts list numbered molds in the types of posterior teeth described in this chapter. They also show the lines of anterior teeth made by this same manufacturer and the posterior teeth that harmonize with them. Therefore selection of a posterior tooth mold of a given type for use with a given anterior tooth mold is a relatively simple procedure.

Selections from mold charts are not infallible; however, they usually provide workable combinations of posterior and anterior teeth. In instances of clearly limited space between the maxillary and mandibular ridges, it may be preferable to use a medium or short version of a given mold instead of a long or medium mold, although the mold chart may indicate one of the latter. For example, if a dentist uses an upper anterior mold 22E and wishes to use a 33-degree anatomic posterior tooth, the mold chart of the manufacturer indicates that 30L is the harmonizing posterior mold. However, if the interridge space is limited, a posterior mold 30M or even a 30S might be substituted in extreme instances.

As a general rule, for esthetic and functional reasons, it is usually preferable to use the posterior molds recommended by the manufacturer on the mold chart if feasible. Using significantly smaller posterior molds may create the possibility of an unsightly "stair-step" appearance between the canine and first premolar.

If there is a marked lack of interridge space, particularly in the tuberosity area, it is possible to leave the second molar out of the setup. Some prefer to leave out a premolar, but usually the esthetic appearance is better with the use of both premolars and elimination of the second molar.

Although there may be sufficient space vertically for a given posterior mold, one should consider leaving out the second molars (or setting them slightly out of occlusion) if they extend distally past the area in which the mandibular ramus begins its upward curve. Artificial teeth in occlusion, distal to the horizontal area of the mandibular ridge, may contribute to instability of the dentures.

---

*Dentsply International Inc., York, Pa.

Surveying the mandibular cast (to aid in determining position for posterior teeth)
PROCEDURE

1. With a pencil, mark the crest of the mandibular ridge from the base of the retromolar pad to the canine area (Fig. 7-39).
2. Using a straightedge, extend this line to the land area of the cast at the anterior and posterior borders (Fig. 7-40).
3. Repeat this procedure for the other side.
4. Place the occlusion rim on the lower cast.
5. Align a straightedge with each of the marks on the land area of the cast (Fig. 7-41).
6. Scribe a line on the occlusion rim corresponding to the line drawn on the crest of the ridge. This line serves as an aid in checking the alignment and position when setting maxillary posterior teeth on the baseplate.

Arranging 33-degree anatomic maxillary posterior teeth

The procedures described here are the usual methods. Often the existing conditions warrant changes for mechanical reasons. For example, it may be necessary to alter the basic position of the posterior teeth to create the required tongue room. Various cusps of the maxillary posterior teeth may be related to a flat occlusal plane in a generally easy and highly adaptable manner. This method simplifies the initial positioning and improves the later occlusion (Figs. 7-42 and 7-43).

When using a fully adjustable articulator, set to a given patient's needs, the starting plan is the same. However, it may be necessary to alter the basic design of the occlusal surfaces by selective grinding and milling to conform to the given articulator settings.

PROCEDURE

1. Place the maxillary first premolar with its long axis at right angles to the occlusal plane. Then place the buccal and lingual cusps on the plane.
2. Place the maxillary second premolar in like manner. Align the facial surfaces of the premolars and the canine with a straightedge (Fig. 7-44).
3. Have the mesiobuccal and mesiolingual cusps of the maxillary first molar touch the occlusal plane. Raise the distobuccal cusp approximately 0.5 mm and the distolingual cusp approximately 0.5 to 0.75 mm.
4. Raise all cusps of the second molar from the lower occlusal plane after the positioning and angulation of the first molar. See that the mesiobuccal cusp is approximately 1 mm from the occlusal plane.
5. Follow the same procedure in placing the posterior teeth on the opposite side. Fig. 7-44 shows an occlusal

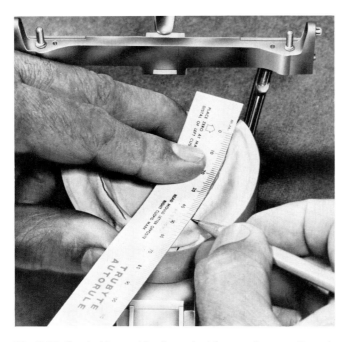

Fig. 7-39. Crest of lower ridge is marked from canine area through center of retromolar pad.

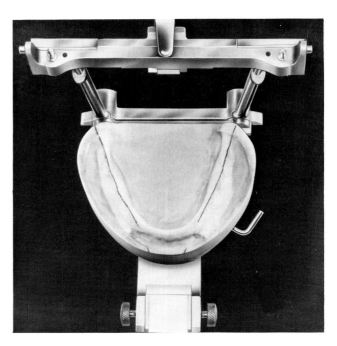

Fig. 7-40. Same surveying procedure as in Fig. 7-39 has been used on both sides and extended onto land area of cast.

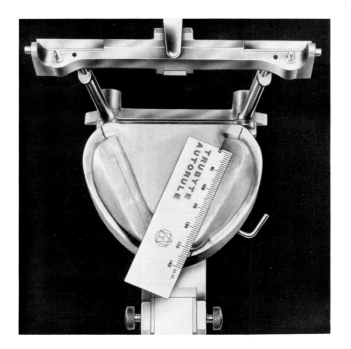

Fig. 7-41. With straightedge, this line is related to and scribed onto lower wax rim to aid in aligning maxillary posterior teeth.

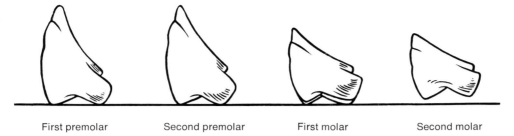

First premolar   Second premolar   First molar   Second molar

Fig. 7-42. Typical cusp relationships of 33-degree anatomic teeth to flat occlusal plane.

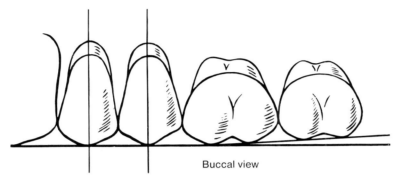

Buccal view

Fig. 7-43. Buccal view of same cusp relationships as in Fig. 7-42 shows distobuccal cusp of first molar approximately 0.5 mm from this plane. Distolingual cusp is raised approximately 0.50 to 0.75 mm from this plane. Cusps of second molar are raised from occlusal plane after positioning of first molar. Mesiobuccal cusp should be approximately 1 mm from occlusal plane.

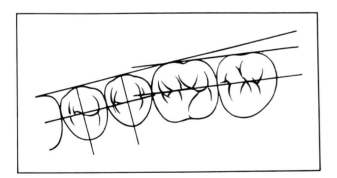

Fig. 7-44. Buccal ridges of molars are angled slightly inward from line extending along facial surfaces of canine and two premolars.

view of the setting of 33-degree maxillary posterior teeth.

A straightedge may be used to align the labial ridge of the canine with the buccal ridge of the first and second premolars and with the mesiobuccal ridge of the first molar. The procedure for aligning the buccal ridges of molars is similar, but it is necessary to angle them slightly inward. This is the usual arrangement, but modifications for individual conditions are possible (Fig. 7-44).

Articulation of 33-degree anatomic mandibular posterior teeth
Articulation of mandibular first molar

The mandibular first molar is a key tooth in articulation. If careful attention is paid to setting this tooth, it will facilitate considerably articulation of the remaining posterior teeth.

PROCEDURE

1. With the articulator open, use wax to attach the mandibular first molar to the baseplate in an approximately correct position, but slightly high.

2. Close the articulator carefully to bring the mandibular molar to its proper position.

3. Guide it to the correct occlusal relationship with the maxillary first molar and maxillary second premolar.

4. Check to ensure that the incisal guide pin remains in contact with the incisal table during all excursions.

The mesiolingual cusp of the upper first molar seats squarely in the central fossa of the lower first molar. This position establishes the proper buccal overjet. From the buccal aspect (Fig. 7-45), the ridge of the mesiobuccal cusp of the upper first molar rests in the

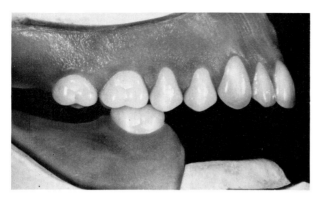

Fig. 7-45. Buccal view of 33-degree anatomic mandibular first molar in centric occlusion.

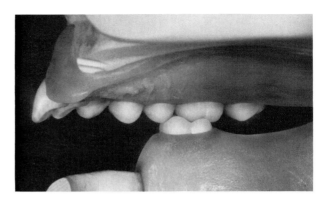

Fig. 7-46. Mandibular first molar in centric occlusion, lingual view.

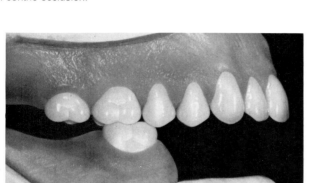

Fig. 7-47. Mandibular first molar in working occlusion, buccal view.

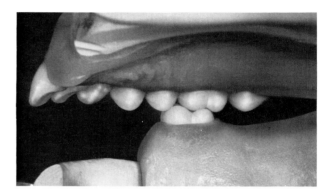

Fig. 7-48. Mandibular first molar in working occlusion, lingual view.

buccal groove of the lower first molar in centric occlusion.

Fig. 7-46 shows a lingual view of the lower first molar in relation to the upper first molar and second premolar. The mesiolingual cusp of the upper first molar is well seated in the central fossa of the lower, and the mesiolingual cusp of the lower first molar fills the embrasure between the upper second premolar and the first molar.

In Fig. 7-47, the working relationship of the lower first molar, articulating with the upper first molar and second premolar, is apparent, and the buccal cusps of the upper and lower first molars are in contact. The distal facet of the upper second premolar is in contact with the mesiobuccal marginal ridge of the lower first molar. The interrelationship of the lower first molar to the upper second premolar and first molar is seen from the lingual view in working occlusion in Fig. 7-48 and from the buccal view in balancing contact in Fig. 7-49.

Articulation of mandibular second molar

The mesiobuccal inclined plane of the lower second molar contacts the marginal ridge of the distobuccal cusp of the upper first molar (Fig. 7-50) in centric occlusion.

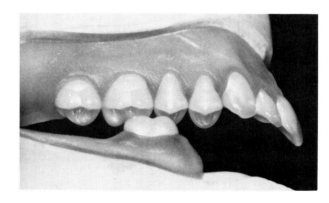

Fig. 7-49. Mandibular first molar in balancing contact, buccal view.

Note the position of the lingual cusp of the upper second molar in relation to the central fossa of the lower second molar in centric occlusion (Fig. 7-51). The position of the lower second molar as it moves into working relationship with the upper first and second molar is seen in Fig. 7-52. Note the cuspal contact of the mesiobuccal cusp of the lower second molar with the distal slope of the cusp

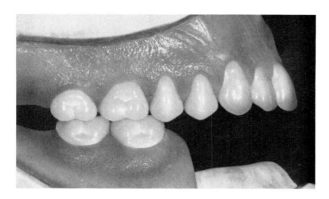

Fig. 7-50. Mandibular second molar in centric occlusion, buccal view.

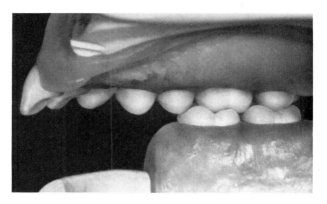

Fig. 7-51. Mandibular second molar in centric occlusion, lingual view.

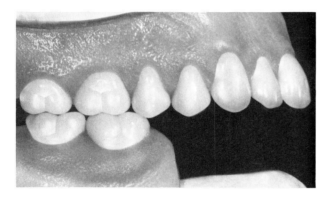

Fig. 7-52. Mandibular second molar in working occlusion, buccal view.

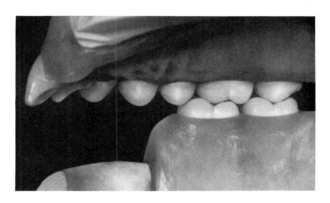

Fig. 7-53. Mandibular second molar in working occlusion, lingual view.

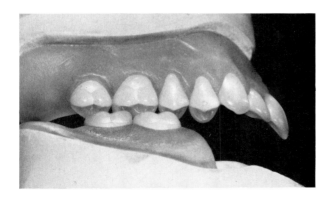

Fig. 7-54. Mandibular second molar in balancing contact, buccal view.

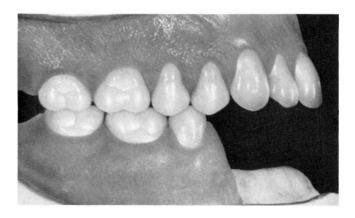

Fig. 7-55. Mandibular second premolar in centric occlusion, buccal view.

of the upper first molar. The buccal cusps of the upper and lower second molars are in contact with each other.

Fig. 7-53 illustrates a lingual view of the relationship of the second molars in working occlusion, and a buccal view of their relationship in balancing contact is seen in Fig. 7-54.

Articulation of mandibular second premolar

The lower second premolar buccal cusp rests between the upper first and second premolars. The tip of the buccal cusp contacts the mesial marginal ridge of the upper second premolar (Fig. 7-55). The lingual aspect of the lower second premolar in centric occlusion shows its lingual cusp between the upper first and second premolars. The mesiolingual ridge of the lower second premolar engages the distal slope of the lingual cusp of the upper first premolar (Fig. 7-56).

In working occlusion, the distobuccal slope of the lower second premolar contacts the mesiobuccal slope of the upper second premolar. The mesiobuccal slope of

the lower second premolar contacts the distobuccal slope of the upper first premolar (Fig. 7-57). The lingual cusp of the lower second premolar contacts the distolingual area of the upper first premolar and the mesiolingual area of the upper second premolar in working occlusion (Fig. 7-58). The mesial slope of the buccal cusp of the lower second premolar is in contact with the distal slope of the lingual cusp of the upper first premolar in balancing occlusion (Fig. 7-59).

Articulation of mandibular first premolar

In centric occlusion, the lower first premolar is positioned with the tip of the buccal cusp in contact with the mesial marginal ridge of the upper first premolar (Figs. 7-60 and 7-61). The distobuccal slope of the lower first premolar contacts and glides over the mesiobuccal slope of the upper first premolar in working occlusion (Figs. 7-62 and 7-63). The mandibular first premolar is shown in balancing contact (Fig. 7-64).

In some instances there may not be sufficient space

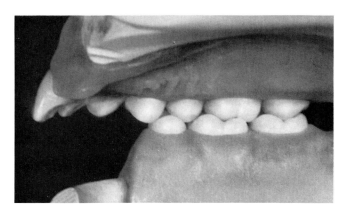

Fig. 7-56. Mandibular second premolar in centric occlusion, lingual view.

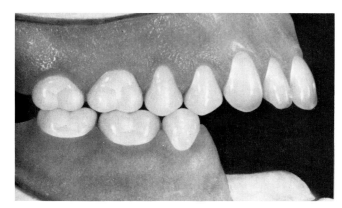

Fig. 7-57. Mandibular second premolar in working occlusion, buccal view.

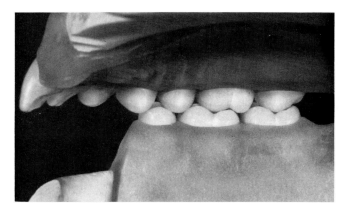

Fig. 7-58. Mandibular second premolar in working occlusion, lingual view.

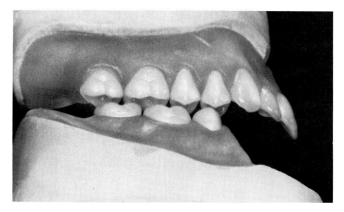

Fig. 7-59. Mandibular second premolar in balancing contact, buccal view.

for the mandibular first premolar. For esthetic reasons it is often advisable to grind the mandibular first premolar rather than alter the anterior teeth. Therefore many do not set the mandibular first premolar until the mandibular anterior teeth are in position.

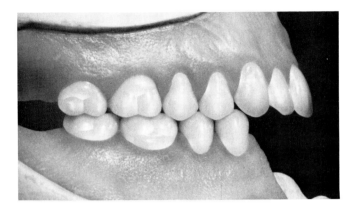

Fig. 7-60. Mandibular first premolar in centric occlusion, buccal view.

Checking completed setup of 33-degree anatomic posterior teeth

After completion of the setup of the 33-degree anatomic posterior teeth, it is essential to check it in all relationships: centric occlusion (Figs. 7-65 and 7-66), working occlusion (Figs. 7-67 and 7-68), and balancing contact (Figs. 7-69 and 7-70). Fig. 7-71 provides an anterior view of the completed tooth arrangement, and a view of it on the articulator is given in Fig. 7-72.

Alternate method of articulation of 33-degree anatomic maxillary posteriors to mandibular posteriors

An alternate method of arranging and articulating teeth for complete dentures preferred by some is to relate the mandibular teeth to a predetermined occlusal plane first, in a manner similar to that shown in Fig. 7-125. Then it is necessary to articulate the maxillary teeth with the mandibular teeth. Articulation of 33-

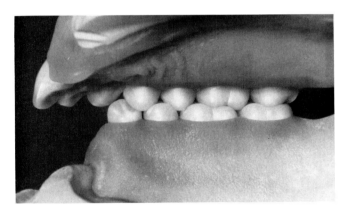

Fig. 7-61. Mandibular first premolar in centric occlusion, lingual view.

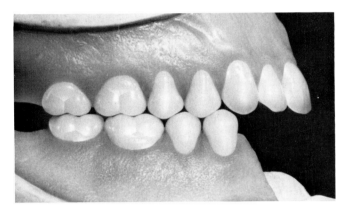

Fig. 7-62. Mandibular first premolar in working occlusion, buccal view.

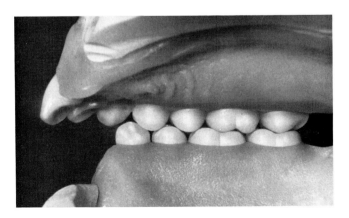

Fig. 7-63. Mandibular first premolar in working occlusion, lingual view.

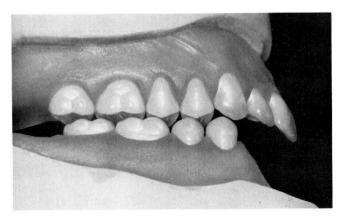

Fig. 7-64. Mandibular first premolar in balancing contact, buccal view.

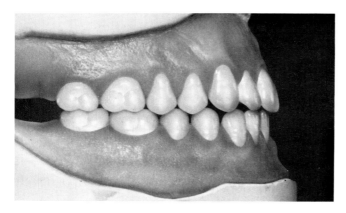

Fig. 7-65. Completed setup of 33-degree anatomic posteriors in centric occlusion, buccal view.

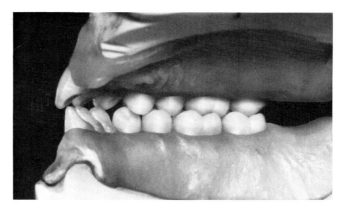

Fig. 7-66. Completed setup in centric occlusion, lingual view.

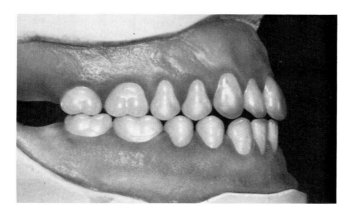

Fig. 7-67. Completed setup in working occlusion, buccal view.

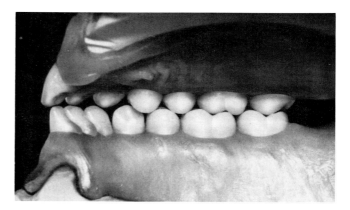

Fig. 7-68. Completed setup in working occlusion, lingual view.

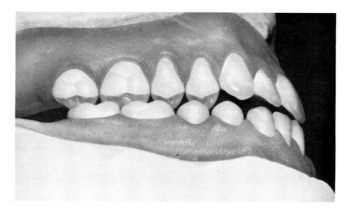

Fig. 7-69. Completed setup in balancing contact, buccal view.

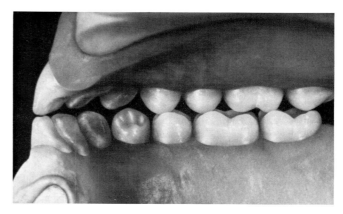

Fig. 7-70. Completed setup in balancing contact, lingual view.

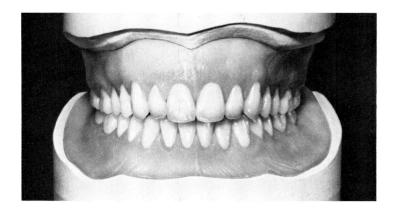

Fig. 7-71. Anterior view of completed setup.

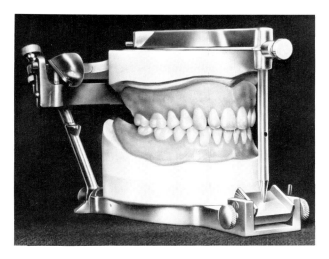

Fig. 7-72. Completed tooth arrangement on articulator.

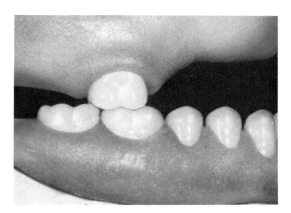

Fig. 7-73. Upper 33-degree anatomic first molar in centric occlusion, buccal view.

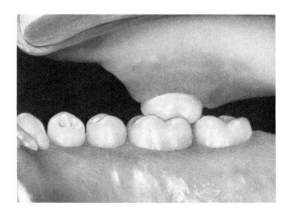

Fig. 7-74. Upper first molar in centric occlusion, lingual view.

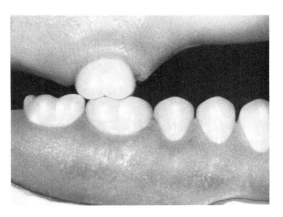

Fig. 7-75. Upper first molar in working occlusion, buccal view.

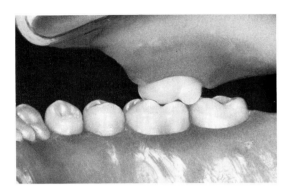

Fig. 7-76. Upper first molar in working occlusion, lingual view.

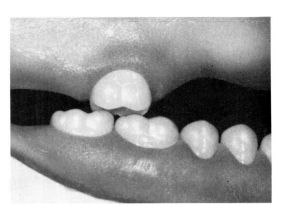

Fig. 7-77. Upper first molar in balancing contact, buccal view.

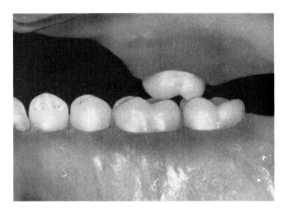

Fig. 7-78. Upper first molar in balancing contact, lingual view.

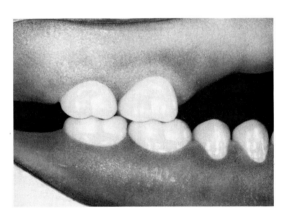

Fig. 7-79. Upper second molar in centric occlusion, buccal view.

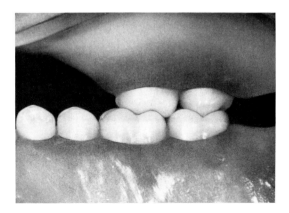

Fig. 7-80. Upper second molar in centric occlusion, lingual view.

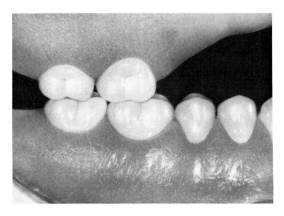

Fig. 7-81. Upper second molar in working occlusion, buccal view.

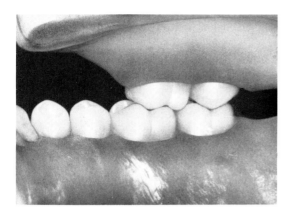

Fig. 7-82. Upper second molar in working occlusion, lingual view.

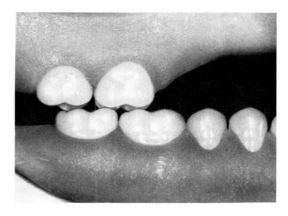

Fig. 7-83. Upper second molar in balancing contact, buccal view.

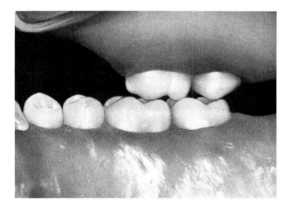

Fig. 7-84. Upper second molar in balancing contact, lingual view.

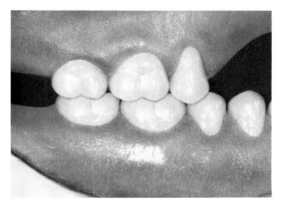

Fig. 7-85. Upper second premolar in centric occlusion, buccal view.

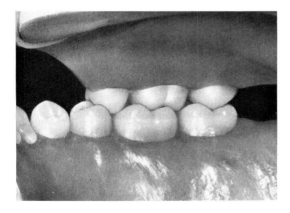

Fig. 7-86. Upper second premolar in centric occlusion, lingual view.

degree anatomic maxillary posterior teeth to mandibular posterior teeth is shown in a series of illustrations. Articulation of the 33-degree anatomic maxillary first molar in its various positions is shown in Figs. 7-73 to 7-78. Articulation of the 33-degree anatomic maxillary second molar is shown in Figs. 7-79 to 7-84. Articulation of the 33-degree anatomic maxillary second premolar is shown in Figs. 7-85 to 7-90. Articulation of the maxillary first premolar is shown in Figs. 7-91 to 7-96.

Arranging 20-degree maxillary posterior teeth
PROCEDURE

1. Place the maxillary first premolar with its long axis at right angles to the occlusal plane. Place the buccal and lingual cusps on the plane (Fig. 7-97).

2. Place the maxillary second premolar in like manner. Align the facial surfaces of the premolars and the canine with a straightedge (Fig. 7-98).

3. Have the mesiobuccal and mesiolingual cusps of the upper first molar touch the occlusal plane. Raise the

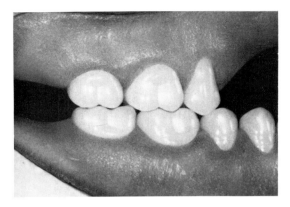

Fig. 7-87. Upper second premolar in working occlusion, buccal view.

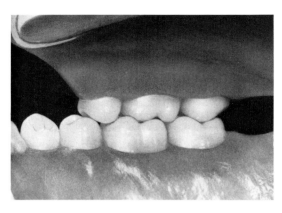

Fig. 7-88. Upper second premolar in working occlusion, lingual view.

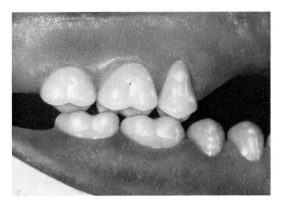

Fig. 7-89. Upper second premolar in balancing contact, buccal view.

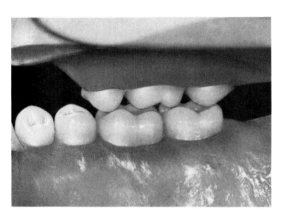

Fig. 7-90. Upper second premolar in balancing contact, lingual view.

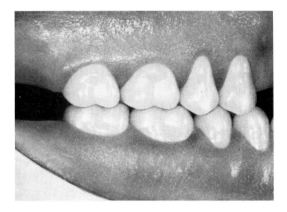

Fig. 7-91. Upper first premolar in centric occlusion, buccal view.

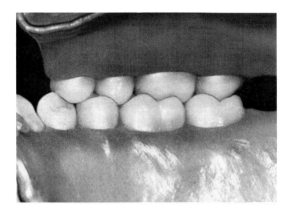

Fig. 7-92. Upper first premolar in centric occlusion, lingual view.

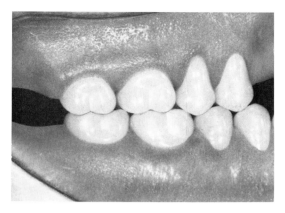

Fig. 7-93. Upper first premolar in working occlusion, buccal view.

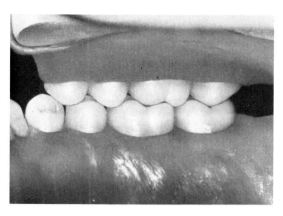

Fig. 7-94. Upper first premolar in working occlusion, lingual view.

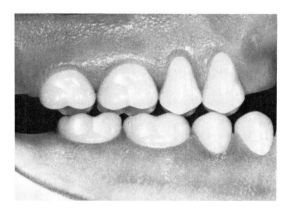

Fig. 7-95. Upper first premolar in balancing contact, buccal view.

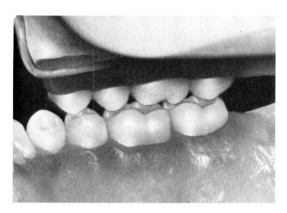

Fig. 7-96. Upper first premolar in balancing contact, lingual view.

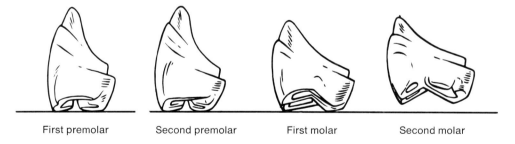

First premolar   Second premolar   First molar   Second molar

Distal view

Fig. 7-97. Typical cusp relationships of 20-degree posterior teeth to flat occlusal plane.

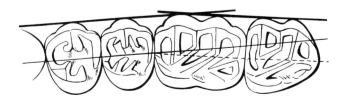

Fig. 7-98. Buccal ridges of molars are angled slightly inward from line extending along facial surfaces of canine and two premolars.

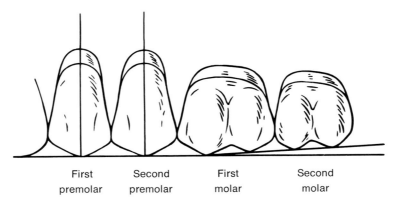

First premolar Second premolar First molar Second molar

Buccal view

Fig. 7-99. Buccal view of the same cusp relationships as in Fig. 7-97 shows distal cusps of first molar raised approximately 0.5 mm. All cusps of second molar are raised from occlusal plane after positioning of first molar. Mesiobuccal cusp of second molar should be approximately 1 mm from occlusal plane.

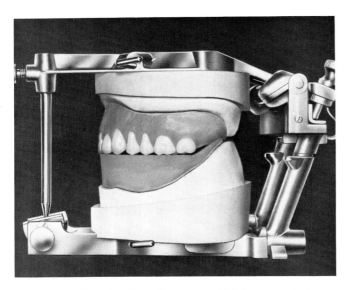

Fig. 7-100. Completed maxillary setup of 20-degree posteriors.

distobuccal cusp approximately 0.5 mm and raise the distolingual cusp accordingly (Fig. 7-99).

4. Raise all cusps of the second molar from the lower occlusal plane after positioning the first molar. Place the mesiobuccal cusp approximately 1 mm from the occlusal plane (Fig. 7-99).

5. Follow the same procedure in placing the posteriors on the opposite side.

6. As shown in Fig. 7-98, use a straightedge to align the labial ridge of the canine, buccal ridges of the first and second premolars, and mesiobuccal ridge of the first molar. Align the buccal ridges of the molars similarly, and angle them slightly inward (palatally).

The maxillary arrangement is complete (Fig. 7-100). The buccal and lingual cusps of the upper first and second premolars should touch the occlusion rim. The mesiobuccal and mesiolingual cusps of the first molar should touch the occlusion rim. The distobuccal cusp should be raised approximately 0.5 mm from the occlusion rim, and the distolingual cusp raised accordingly. All cusps of the second molar are raised from the occlusal plane after positioning the first molar. The mesiobuccal cusp should be approximately 1 mm from the occlusal plane.

Articulation of 20-degree posterior mandibular teeth
Articulation of first molar

The ridge of the mesiobuccal cusp of the upper first molar rests in the anterior buccal groove of the lower first molar in centric occlusion (Fig. 7-101). The mesiolingual cusp of the upper first molar fits into the central fossa of the lower first molar (Fig. 7-102).

The buccal cusps of the lower molar are in contact with the buccal cusps of the upper first molar and the distal slope of the buccal cusp of the upper second premolar in working occlusion (Fig. 7-103). Also in working occlusion, the mesiolingual cusp of the upper first molar is in contact with the ridges formed by the protrusive and retrusive lingual planes of the lower first molar (Fig. 7-104). When the teeth of the opposite side move into working position, the mesiolingual cusp of the upper first molar slides through the distobuccal groove of the lower first molar. The lingual cusp of the upper second premolar is in contact with the protrusive plane of the mesiobuccal cusp of the lower first molar (Figs. 7-105 and 7-106).

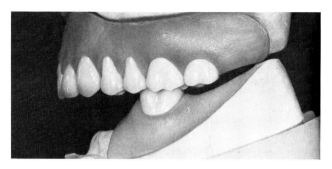

Fig. 7-101. Mandibular 20-degree first molar in centric occlusion, buccal view. NOTE: Camera angle exaggerates horizontal overlap of maxillary anterior teeth in relation to mandibular residual ridge.

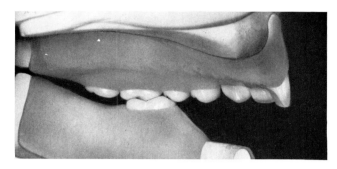

Fig. 7-102. Mandibular first molar in centric occlusion, lingual view.

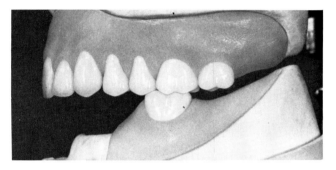

Fig. 7-103. Mandibular first molar in working occlusion, buccal view.

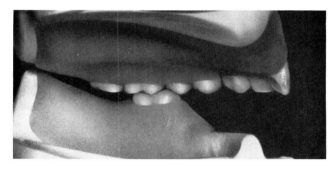

Fig. 7-104. Mandibular first molar in working occlusion, lingual view.

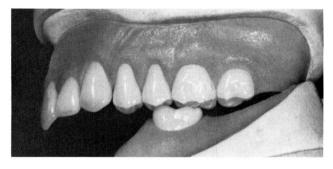

Fig. 7-105. Mandibular first molar in balancing contact, buccal view.

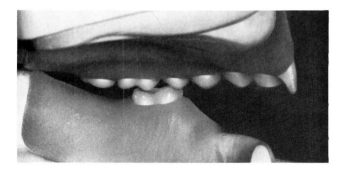

Fig. 7-106. Mandibular first molar in balancing contact, lingual view.

Articulation of mandibular second premolar

In centric occlusion, the tip of the lower buccal cusp contacts the mesial marginal ridge of the upper second premolar as well as the distal marginal ridge of the upper first premolar (Fig. 7-107). Also in centric occlusion, the lingual cusp is at the embrasure between the upper first and second premolars. The mesiolingual ridge contacts the distal slope of the lingual cusp of the upper first premolar (Fig. 7-108).

In working occlusion, the distobuccal slope of the lower premolar contacts the mesiobuccal slope of the upper second premolar. The mesiobuccal slope of the lower second premolar contacts the distobuccal slope of the upper first premolar (Fig. 7-109). Also in working occlusion, the lingual cusp of the lower second premolar closes the embrasure formed by the upper first and second premolars (Fig. 7-110). In balancing contact, the mesial slope of the buccal cusp of the lower second premolar is in contact with the distal slope of the lingual cusp of the upper first premolar (Figs. 7-111 and 7-112).

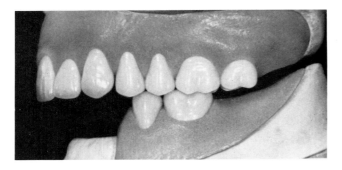

Fig. 7-107. Mandibular second premolar in centric occlusion, buccal view.

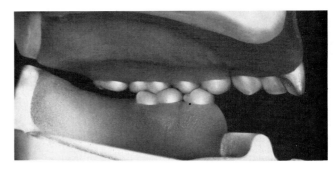

Fig. 7-108. Mandibular second premolar in centric occlusion, lingual view.

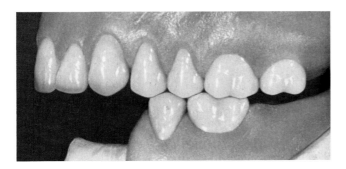

Fig. 7-109. Mandibular second premolar in working occlusion, buccal view.

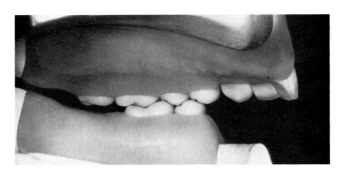

Fig. 7-110. Mandibular second premolar in working occlusion, lingual view.

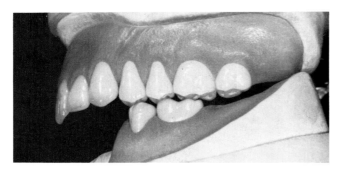

Fig. 7-111. Mandibular second premolar in balancing contact, buccal view.

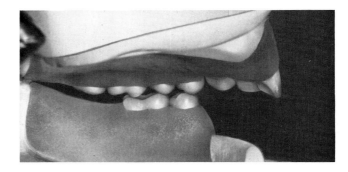

Fig. 7-112. Mandibular second premolar in balancing contact, lingual view.

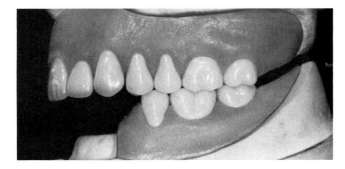

Fig. 7-113. Mandibular second molar in centric occlusion, buccal view.

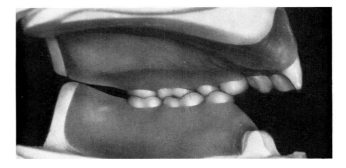

Fig. 7-114. Mandibular second molar in centric occlusion, lingual view.

Articulation of mandibular second molar

In centric occlusion, the ridge of the mesiobuccal cusp of the upper second molar rests in the buccal groove of the lower second molar (Fig. 7-113). Also in centric occlusion, the mesiolingual cusp of the upper second molar fits squarely into the central fossa of the lower second molar (Fig. 7-114).

In working occlusion, the buccal cusps of the lower second molar are in contact with the buccal cusps of the upper second molar and with the distal slope of the upper first molar (Fig. 7-115). Also in working occlusion, the mesiolingual cusp of the upper second molar is in contact with the ridges formed by the protrusive and retrusive lingual planes of the lower second molar. The mesiolingual slope of the lower second molar touches the distolingual cusp of the upper first molar (Fig. 7-116).

In balancing contact, the mesiolingual cusp of the upper second molar slides through the distobuccal groove of the lower second molar. The distolingual cusp of the upper first molar contacts the mesiobuccal protrusive plane of the lower second molar (Figs. 7-117 and 7-118).

Articulation of mandibular first premolar

The relationships of the mandibular first premolar in centric occlusion, working occlusion, and balancing position are shown in Figs. 7-119 to 7-124.

Alternate method of articulation of 20-degree maxillary posterior teeth to mandibular posterior teeth

As noted previously (p. 229), a method of arranging and articulating artificial teeth preferred by some is to complete the mandibular setup first. In this instance, position the mandibular teeth in relation to a predetermined occlusal plane (Fig. 7-125). As shown in Fig. 7-125, it may consist of a carefully formed maxillary occlusion rim.

The buccal and lingual cusps of the lower first and second premolars should touch the maxillary occlusion rim. The mesiobuccal and mesiolingual cusps of the lower first molar touch the occlusion rim, and the distal cusps fall slightly below the rim. Elevating the mesiobuccal cusp of the lower second molar slightly places the mesial slope in alignment with the protrusive inclination of the distal cusp of the lower first molar. After the

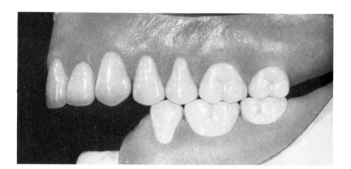

Fig. 7-115. Mandibular second molar in working occlusion, buccal view.

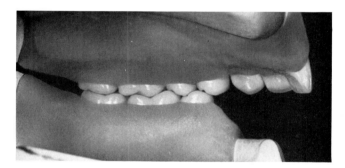

Fig. 7-116. Mandibular second molar in working occlusion, lingual view.

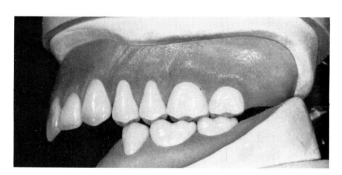

Fig. 7-117. Mandibular second molar in balancing contact, buccal view.

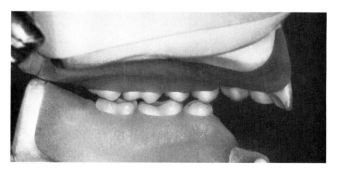

Fig. 7-118. Mandibular second molar in balancing contact, lingual view.

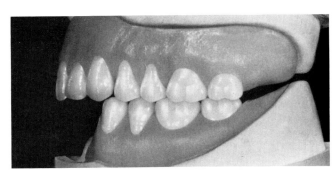

Fig. 7-119. Mandibular first premolar in centric occlusion, buccal view.

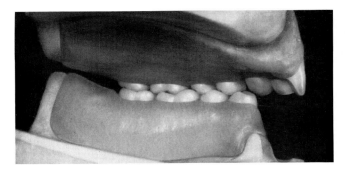

Fig. 7-120. Mandibular first premolar in centric occlusion, lingual view.

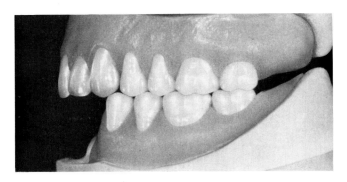

Fig. 7-121. Mandibular first premolar in working occlusion, buccal view.

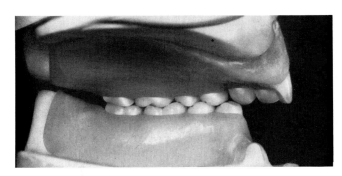

Fig. 7-122. Mandibular first premolar in working occlusion, lingual view.

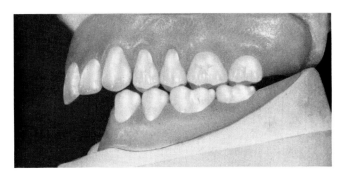

Fig. 7-123. Mandibular first premolar in balancing relation, buccal view.

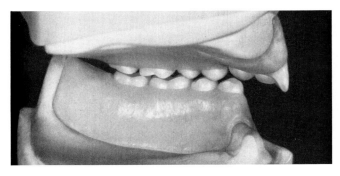

Fig. 7-124. Mandibular first premolar in balancing relation, lingual view.

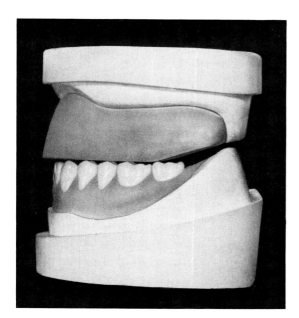

Fig. 7-125. Mandibular 20-degree posterior teeth have been positioned in relation to predetermined occlusal plane.

mandibular teeth are in position, articulate the maxillary teeth with them.

Articulation of maxillary first molar

In centric occlusion, the ridge of the mesiobuccal cusp of the upper first molar rests in the anterior buccal groove of the lower first molar. The distal inclined plane of the upper first molar touches the mesiobuccal cusp of the lower second molar (Fig. 7-126). Also in centric occlusion, the mesiolingual cusp of the upper first molar fits squarely into the central fossa of the lower first molar. The distolingual cusp of the upper first molar touches the mesial ridge of the lower second molar (Fig. 7-127).

In working occlusion, the buccal cusps of the upper first molar are in contact with the buccal cusps of the lower first molar and the mesial slope of the lower second molar (Fig. 7-128). Also in working occlusion, the mesiolingual cusp of the upper first molar is in contact with ridges formed by protrusive and retrusive lingual planes of the lower first molar. The distal slope of the upper distolingual cusp touches the mesial slope of the mesiolingual cusp of the lower second molar (Fig. 7-129).

When the teeth of the opposite side go into working

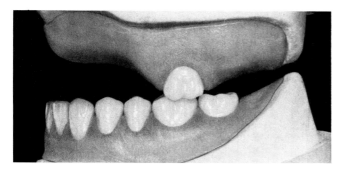

Fig. 7-126. Maxillary 20-degree first molar in centric occlusion, buccal view.

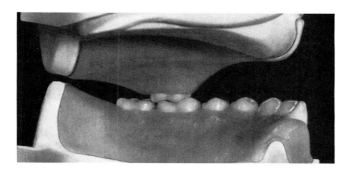

Fig. 7-127. Maxillary first molar in centric occlusion, lingual view.

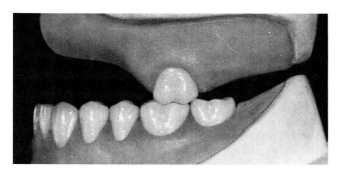

Fig. 7-128. Maxillary first molar in working occlusion, buccal view.

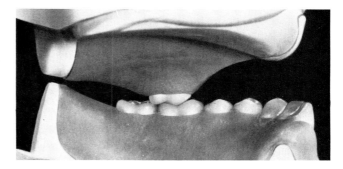

Fig. 7-129. Maxillary first molar in working occlusion, lingual view.

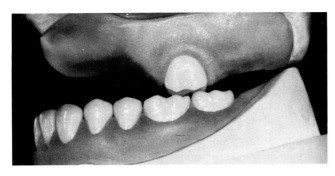

Fig. 7-130. Maxillary first molar in balancing contact, buccal view.

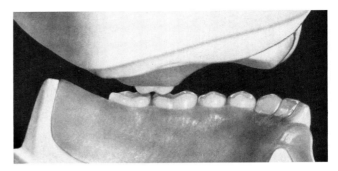

Fig. 7-131. Maxillary first molar in balancing contact, lingual view.

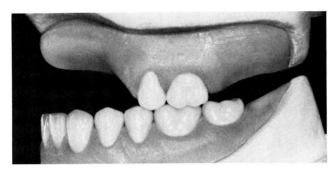

Fig. 7-132. Maxillary second premolar in centric occlusion, buccal view.

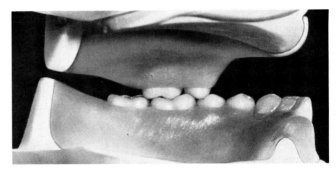

Fig. 7-133. Maxillary second premolar in centric occlusion, lingual view.

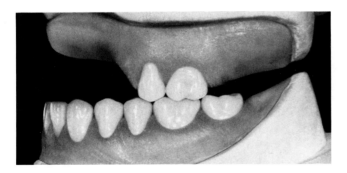

Fig. 7-134. Maxillary second premolar in working occlusion, buccal view.

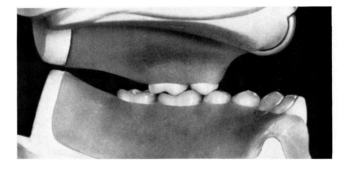

Fig. 7-135. Maxillary second premolar in working occlusion, lingual view.

occlusion, the mesiolingual cusp of the upper first molar slides through the distobuccal groove of the lower first molar (Fig. 7-130). The distolingual cusp of the upper first molar contacts the mesiobuccal cusp of the lower second molar (Fig. 7-131).

Articulation of maxillary second premolar

In centric occlusion, the tip of the buccal cusp of the upper second premolar contacts the mesiobuccal ridge of the buccal cusp of the lower first molar and the distobuccal ridge of the lower second premolar (Fig. 7-132).

Also in centric occlusion, the lingual cusp of the upper second premolar is at the embrasure between the lower first molar and lower second premolar. The distal ridge contacts the mesiolingual cusp of the lower first molar, and the mesial ridge contacts the distal slope of the lower second premolar (Fig. 7-133).

In working occlusion, the distobuccal slope of the upper second premolar contacts the mesiobuccal slope of the lower first molar. The mesiobuccal slope of the upper second premolar contacts the distobuccal slope of the lower second premolar (Fig. 7-134). Also in working

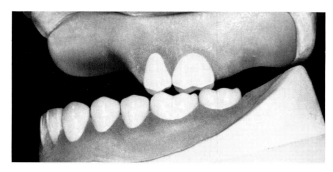

Fig. 7-136. Maxillary second premolar in balancing contact, buccal view.

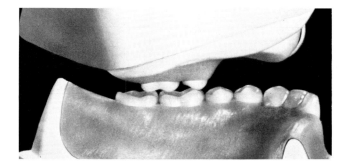

Fig. 7-137. Maxillary second premolar in balancing contact, lingual view.

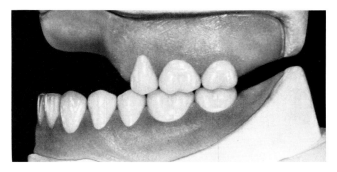

Fig. 7-138. Maxillary second molar in centric occlusion, buccal view.

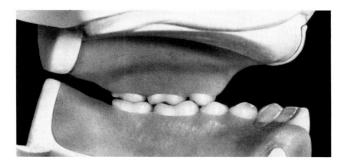

Fig. 7-139. Maxillary second molar in centric occlusion, lingual view.

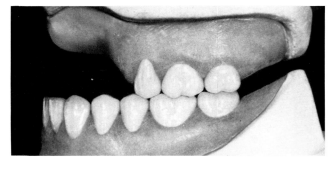

Fig. 7-140. Maxillary second molar in working occlusion, buccal view.

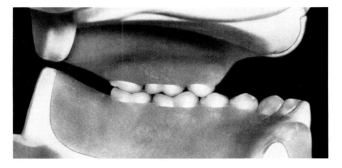

Fig. 7-141. Maxillary second molar in working occlusion, lingual view.

occlusion, the lingual cusp of the upper second premolar closes the embrasure formed by the lower first molar and lower second premolar (Fig. 7-135).

In balancing contact, the lingual cusp of the upper second premolar contacts the mesiobuccal cusp of the lower first molar (Figs. 7-136 and 7-137).

Articulation of maxillary second molar

In centric occlusion, the ridge of the mesiobuccal cusp of the upper second molar rests in the buccal groove of the lower second molar (Fig. 7-138). Also in centric oc-

clusion, the mesiolingual cusp of the upper second molar fits squarely into the central fossa of the lower second molar (Fig. 7-139).

In working occlusion, the buccal cusps of the upper second molar are in contact with the buccal cusps of the lower second molar (Fig. 7-140). Also in working occlusion, the mesiolingual cusp of the upper second molar contacts ridges formed by the protrusive and retrusive lingual cusp planes of the lower second molar (Fig. 7-141).

In balancing contact, the mesiolingual cusp of the

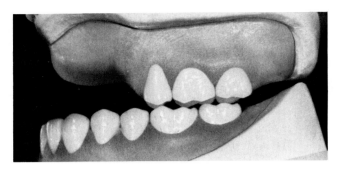

Fig. 7-142. Maxillary second molar in balancing contact, buccal view.

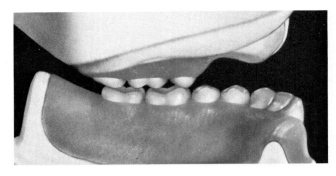

Fig. 7-143. Maxillary second molar in balancing contact, lingual view.

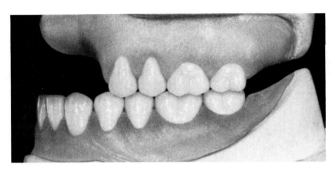

Fig. 7-144. Maxillary first premolar in centric occlusion, buccal view.

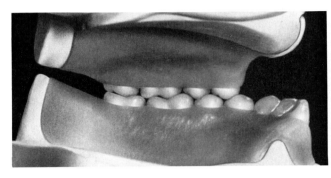

Fig. 7-145. Maxillary first premolar in centric occlusion, lingual view.

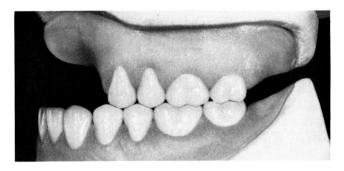

Fig. 7-146. Maxillary first premolar in working occlusion, buccal view.

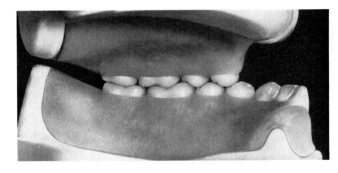

Fig. 7-147. Maxillary first premolar in working occlusion, lingual view.

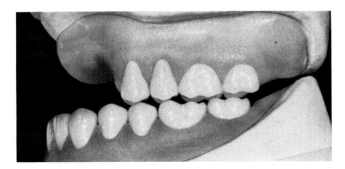

Fig. 7-148. Maxillary first premolar in balancing contact, buccal view.

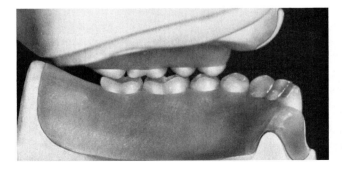

Fig. 7-149. Maxillary first premolar in balancing contact, lingual view.

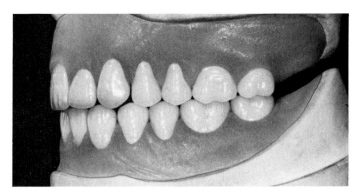

Fig. 7-150. Completed setup of 20-degree posteriors in centric occlusion, buccal view.

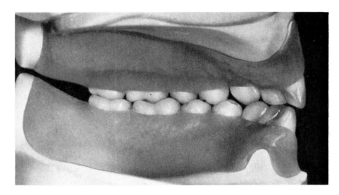

Fig. 7-151. Completed setup in centric occlusion, lingual view.

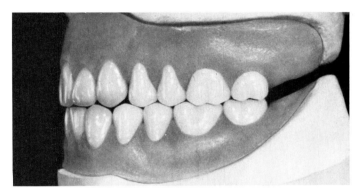

Fig. 7-152. Completed setup in working occlusion, buccal view.

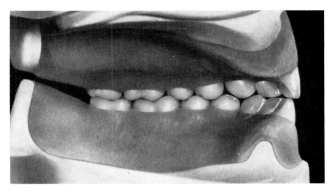

Fig. 7-153. Completed setup in working occlusion, lingual view.

upper second molar slides through the distobuccal groove of the lower second molar (Figs. 7-142 and 7-143).

Articulation of maxillary first premolar

In centric occlusion, the tip of the buccal cusp of the upper first premolar contacts the distobuccal ridge of the lower first premolar and the mesiobuccal ridge of the lower second premolar (Fig. 7-144). Also in centric occlusion, the lingual cusp of the upper first premolar is at the embrasure between the lower first and second premolars. The mesial ridge of the upper first premolar contacts the distal slope of the lower first premolar, and the distal ridge contacts the mesial slope of the lower second premolar (Fig. 7-145).

In working occlusion, the distobuccal slope of the upper first premolar contacts the mesiobuccal slope of the lower second premolar. The mesiobuccal slope of the upper first premolar contacts the distobuccal slope of the lower first premolar (Fig. 7-146). Also in working occlusion, the lingual cusp of the upper first premolar closes the embrasure formed by the lower first and second premolars (Fig. 7-147).

In balancing contact, the lingual cusp of the upper first premolar contacts the buccal cusp of the lower second premolar (Figs. 7-148 and 7-149).

Checking completed setup of 20-degree posterior teeth

After completion of the setup of the 20-degree posterior teeth, it is essential to check it in all relationships: centric occlusion (Figs. 7-150 and 7-151), working occlusion (Figs. 7-152 and 7-153), and balancing contact (Figs. 7-154 and 7-155). An anterior view of the completed tooth arrangement is shown in Fig. 7-156.

Arranging Pilkington-Turner 30-degree posterior teeth

The individual relationship of each Pilkington-Turner maxillary posterior tooth to an occlusal plane is shown in Fig. 7-157. Note that the lingual cusp of the first and second premolars should touch the occlusal plane. The buccal cusps are raised approximately 0.5 mm.

NOTE: Diagrams can exaggerate the positions of teeth in relation to a flat plane. "Average" dentures do not normally require a distance of more than 2 mm from the

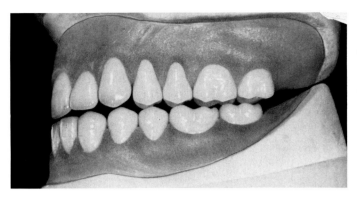

Fig. 7-154. Completed setup in balancing contact, buccal view.

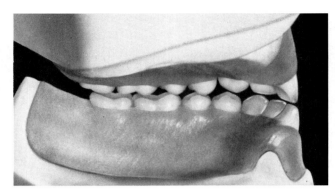

Fig. 7-155. Completed setup in balancing contact, lingual view.

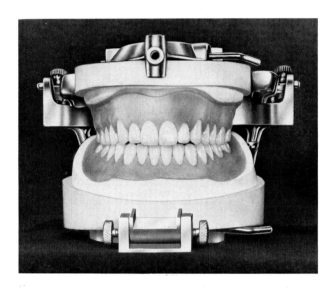

Fig. 7-156. Anterior view of completed tooth arrangement.

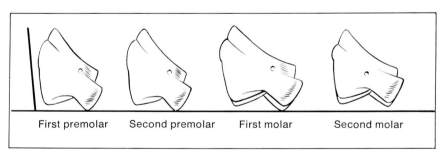

Fig. 7-157. Cusps of Pilkington-Turner posterior teeth are shown in relation to flat occlusal plane. Lingual cusps of premolars touch, and buccal cusps are approximately 0.5 mm from plane. Mesiolingual cusp of first molar touches plane. Second molar follows alignment of first molar. Distobuccal cusp of second molar normally is not more than 2 mm from plane.

distobuccal cusp of the second molar to the occlusal plane. The arrangement of posterior teeth in this manner forms a compensating curve (the counterpart of the curve of Spee in natural dentitions).

NOTE: This positioning of the maxillary teeth is an "average" positioning. The ridge relations, condylar guidance, and incisal guidance may make it necessary to increase or decrease the degree of the compensating curve to effect a balanced occlusion.

The long axes of the premolars should be at right angles to the occlusal plane, whereas the molars may incline slightly toward the mesial surface (Fig. 7-158). The mesiobuccal cusp of the first molar is raised approximately 0.5 mm to place it out of contact with the occlusal

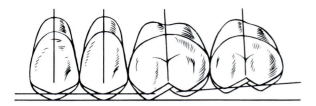

Fig. 7-158. From buccal view, premolars are vertical to plane. Cervical area of molars incline slightly toward mesial line.

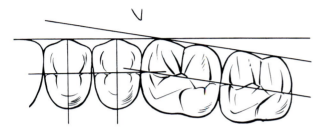

Fig. 7-159. Positioning of Pilkington-Turner molars in relation to line along facial surface of canine and premolars.

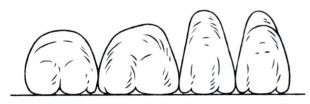

Fig. 7-160. Rational 0-degree posterior teeth are set contacting flat plane.

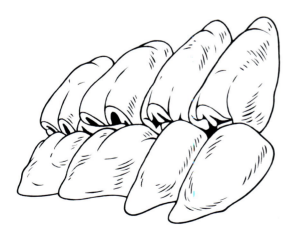

Fig. 7-161. Buccal overjet of upper Rational 0-degree teeth in "normal" jaw relation.

plane. The mesiolingual cusp touches the plane, and the distobuccal cusp is raised approximately 1 mm. The mesiobuccal cusp of the second molar is raised approximately 1 mm; the distobuccal cusp approximately 1.5 mm. An occlusal view of the setting of these maxillary posteriors is shown in Fig. 7-159.

The mandibular tooth arrangement is completed and checked in a manner similar to that shown in the section on the 33-degree anatomic posterior teeth (Figs. 7-45 to 7-72).

Arranging Rational 0-degree posterior teeth

Rational 0-degree posterior teeth may be used for complete denture construction when a preference for a flat occlusal form or conditions indicate their use. The purpose of this chapter is not to discuss indications or contraindications of flat teeth in comparison with teeth that have cusps of varying degrees of steepness.

However, some consider flat tooth forms useful in so-called problem cases, such as those with malrelation of the jaws; crossbites; flat or heavily resorbed ridges, making denture bases less stable; and those persons with uncoordinated jaw movements for whom it is difficult to obtain a valid centric relation record.

It is possible to set flat teeth to a curve or to a flat plane. This chapter will describe the latter procedure, which is more common.

NOTE: Set the anterior teeth so that the degree of vertical overlap (overbite) is 0 degrees or nearly so. After positioning the maxillary and mandibular anterior teeth, shape the lower wax occlusion rim to form a flat occlusal plane extending from the tips of the lower canines through the centers of the retromolar pads. Make the right and left sides the same height and have them parallel laterally and anteroposteriorly. This plane also should be roughly parallel to the mean foundation plane of the mandibular ridge, as viewed from the side. Mark the center of the mandibular ridge on the top of the lower wax occlusion rim by surveying the mandibular cast and marking the rim, as shown in Figs. 7-39 to 7-41.

Rational 0-degree posterior teeth are available as single teeth, or in solid quadrant blocks of four teeth each for setting up as a unit. The principles of positioning both types are the same. Set the maxillary teeth so that their centers (from anterior to posterior) lie approximately over the line scribed on the mandibular wax rim. This position can vary as individual situations indicate. The teeth, as viewed from the side, form a flat surface against this plane (Fig. 7-160). Then set the mandibular teeth to occlude with the maxillary teeth. In a "normal" jaw-relation situation, there will be a buccal overjet of the upper teeth (Fig. 7-161).

However, in some situations in which there is a small upper arch and a large lower arch, it is possible to posi-

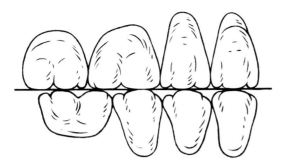

Fig. 7-162. Premolars can be set to oppose molars if needed because there is no interdigitation of cusps.

Table 7-1. Arrangement and articulation of artificial teeth

Problem	Probable cause	Solution
Lack of vertical space to set anterior teeth	Recent extractions with large unresorbed ridges present	Grind ridge lap area of teeth carefully (do not impinge on pins in porcelain teeth) Use plastic teeth if heavy ridge-lap reduction required; leave labial collar if possible
Lack of space to set posterior teeth	Small interridge space	Grind ridge lap carefully (do *not* grind away vent holes on porcelain teeth), leave off second molar, or use shorter posterior mold
Lack of space (anteroposterior) to set mandibular first premolar	Often a Class II (retrusive) jaw relation	Leave 1 mm diastema between upper canine and first premolar (giving more space for lower), or grind lower premolar carefully on mesial and distal surfaces to narrow it, or leave out lower central or lateral (in extreme conditions)
Movement of teeth because of wax shrinkage	Excess heat applied during setup and/or wax-up	Do not overheat wax
	Undue time elapsed before investing	Invest for processing as soon as practical after wax-up
Chipping of porcelain teeth	Thermal shock during wax-up	Avoid direct flame on teeth
	Too much pressure during packing of compression-molded denture-base resin	Avoid excess pressure when using compression-molded denture-base materials
	Undue leverage during deflasking procedures	Deflask carefully
	Leave ground porcelain tooth surfaces unpolished	Polish teeth carefully after grinding (p. 249)

tion the posterior teeth in an "end-to-end" occlusal surface relationship, or even a crossbite. As mentioned previously, some believe that flat posteriors are preferable in such situations. Additionally, if the upper and lower space available for setting teeth anteroposteriorly is mismatched, it is possible to set premolars to oppose molars, since there is no interdigitation of cusps (Fig. 7-162).

It is advisable when using 0-degree posterior teeth to select or modify the canines, so that they tend to have a blunt incisal edge rather than a pointed one. Usually optimal contact and/or embrasure between a canine and a 0-degree premolar can be obtained more readily with a somewhat blunted canine than with a pointed one.

The proper setting of flat teeth requires attention to detail comparable to that used in arranging cusp teeth. It is important to pay special attention to see that there is good occlusal contact in the setup when viewed from different sides, especially the lingual aspect.

TRY-IN

The try-in is the time for the dentist to determine the esthetics of the restoration and to write the final instructions to the dental laboratory about these considerations.

The tooth arrangement should be carefully waxed to produce a natural anatomic form and appearance, and rough or sharp edges should be removed from the baseplates. The color of the wax should be pleasing, and it should approximate the color of the finished dentures.

The dentist may wish to check the following aspects at the time of try-in:

1. Midline harmony
2. Relation of anterior teeth to lips
3. Prominence of cervical area of canines
4. Anteroposterior position of anterior teeth
5. Occlusal plane
6. All original esthetic considerations, such as shape, size, and color of teeth
7. Phonetic acceptability
8. Vertical dimension
9. Occlusal relations
10. Overall patient comfort and acceptance

GRINDING PORCELAIN TEETH

After processing, remounting, and modifying the tooth form by selective grinding procedures, it is strongly recommended that ground surfaces of porcelain teeth be repolished. Rough surfaces, which may tend to collect stain and debris, are a major cause of chipping and flaking. Smooth porcelain surfaces "glide" smoothly over each other; however, rough, unpolished surfaces "catch" and "trip," thereby causing discomfort and ultimately resulting in chipping and flaking of the porcelain. A few moments of polishing at this time can prevent potential problems and later embarrassment.

In addition, it is necessary to polish porcelain teeth highly if they occlude with plastic teeth and grinding has penetrated the glaze of the porcelain teeth. Prosthodontic authorities recognize the need in some instances to give consideration to the advisability of occluding porcelain teeth against plastic teeth. In this instance, porcelain teeth must present a smooth surface to avoid undue wear of the resin teeth. When feasible, avoid grinding porcelain when it opposes plastic teeth.

Four easy steps are essential in reshaping and polishing porcelain teeth:

1. Grind and reshape porcelain with fairly soft, fine, uniform grit stones.

2. Smooth ground surfaces with a rubber wheel to remove stone marks and to round sharp or square corners.

3. Pumice the rubber-wheeled areas to smooth the porcelain even more and to impart an initial polish.

4. Apply a commercially available porcelain polish* to develop a final polish with a high luster.

SUMMARY

This chapter has described methods of arranging and articulating anterior teeth, 33-degree anatomic posterior teeth, 20-degree posterior teeth, Pilkington-Turner 30-degree posterior teeth, and Rational 0-degree posterior teeth. These methods may be used to produce optimal treatment results for edentulous and partially edentulous patients.

---

*Trupolish or Dentsply Porcelain Tooth Finishing Kit, Dentsply International, Inc., York, Pa.

CHAPTER 8

WAXING AND PROCESSING

KENNETH D. RUDD, ROBERT M. MORROW, EARL E. FELDMANN,
and AMBROCIO V. ESPINOZA

waxing (wax-up) The contouring of a wax pattern or the wax base
   of a trial denture into the desired form.
flasking The act of investing a pattern in a flask. The process of investing the cast and a wax denture in a flask preparatory to molding the denture base material into the form of the denture.
processing The procedure of bringing about polymerization of appliances; processing of dentures.
denture processing The conversion of a wax pattern of a denture,
   or trial denture, into a denture with a base made of another material, such as acrylic resin.

WAXING FOR TRY-IN

The wax try-in is an important appointment for the
dentist and patient. Preparation of the trial denture for
try-in involves contouring the wax on the trial denture to
produce a denture base form that reproduces the contours of the original tissues in the dentulous mouth. If
carving and contouring are accomplished skillfully, it is
much easier to evaluate the appearance and speech of
the patient during the try-in appointment.

Waxing the maxillary trial denture
PROCEDURE

1. Adapt a softened roll of baseplate wax about 6 mm
wide and 5 cm long to the facial surface of one side of the
trial denture, and contour with the fingers while the
wax is soft (Fig. 8-1).

2. Adapt the wax to cover the necks of the teeth, and
extend it on the flanges of the trial denture (Fig. 8-2).

3. Contour the baseplate wax immediately above the
necks of the anterior teeth to produce a gingival bulge,
or fullness, simulating the attached gingiva (Fig. 8-3).

4. Contour the wax above the canine tooth to simulate
the canine eminence found in the dentulous mouth. The
waxed canine eminence should blend into the peripheral
border without producing additional thickness of that
border (Fig. 8-4).

5. Develop a slight root prominence over the maxillary central incisors. The prominence should not be as
definite as the canine eminence and should fade out
before the border is reached.

6. Carve a slight depression, or fossa, between the
root of the central incisor and the canine eminence (Fig.
8-5). This should be a very slight depression and not
hollowed out to any extent.

7. Contour the anterior flange of the trial denture to
produce a slightly convex effect overall.

8. Wax a gingival bulge immediately above the necks
of posterior teeth. This convexity should resemble the
gingival bulge placed in the anterior region, although
in the case of the posterior teeth it may be somewhat
more accentuated. The gingival bulge area should be
almost nonexistent in the first premolar area, becoming
progressively more prominent in the second premolar
and molar region (Fig. 8-6). Vertically the gingival bulge
should be approximately 5 to 6 mm wide over the second
molar.

9. Extend the gingival bulge distal to the second
molar, and blend it in with the wax, forming the maxillary tuberosity distal to the second molar.

10. Carve a slight depression above the premolar
teeth, extending it from the canine eminence posteriorly
to the molar process (Fig. 8-7). This depression is the
canine fossa and is important if normal facial expression
is to be obtained.

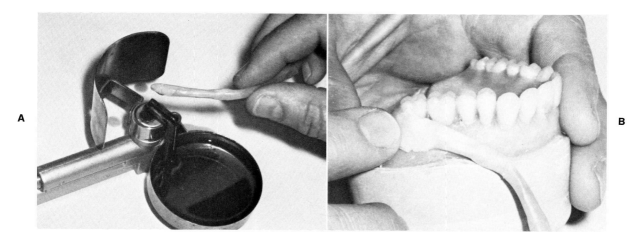

Fig. 8-1. A, Roll of baseplate wax is softened. **B,** Softened wax is adaptec to flange of baseplate.

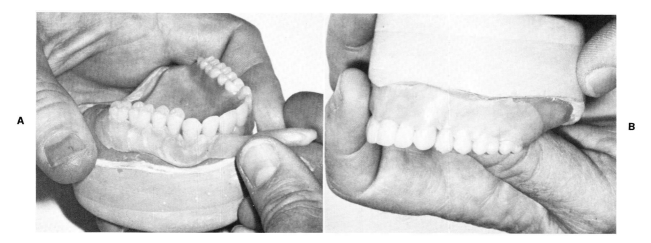

Fig. 8-2. A, Necks of teeth are covered with softened wax. **B,** Adapted wax extends over most of buccal surface.

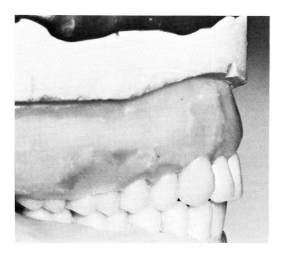

Fig. 8-3. Wax is contoured to form fullness or convexity above anterior teeth.

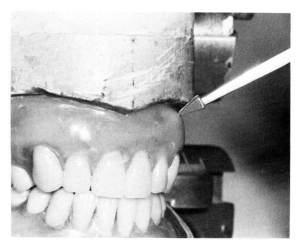

Fig. 8-4. Canine eminence should *not* extend to border.

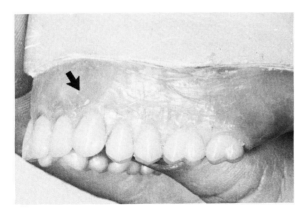

Fig. 8-5. Slight depression is created between roots of central incisor and canine tooth (arrow).

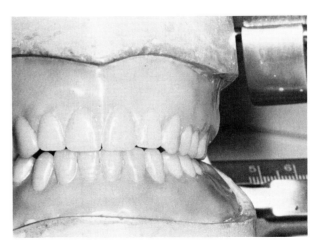

Fig. 8-6. Buccal gingival bulge becomes progressively more prominent in second premolar and molar region.

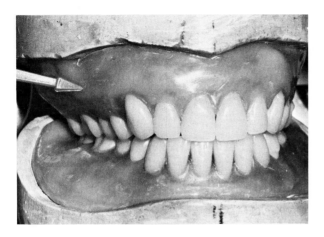

Fig. 8-7. Slight depression is carved above premolars.

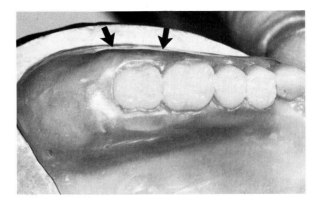

Fig. 8-8. Region above gingival roll is slightly concave (arrows).

11. Carve the area above the posterior gingival bulge to produce a slightly concave surface (Fig. 8-8). This extends from the peripheral roll superiorly, to the gingival bulge inferiorly.

12. After adapting and contouring wax on the facial surfaces of the trial denture, seal the baseplate wax around the necks of each tooth with a wax spatula (Fig. 8-9).

13. Use a roach carver, or a No. 7 spatula, to remove excess wax from the facial surfaces of the denture teeth until the finish lines on the necks of the teeth are barely exposed (Fig. 8-10).

14. Use a roach carver, or a No. 7 spatula, held at approximately a 60-degree angle, to carve the gingival margin around the anterior teeth (Fig. 8-11).

15. Carve the gingival margin around the posterior teeth with a roach carver, or No. 7 spatula, held at a 45-degree angle. Follow the finish lines around the

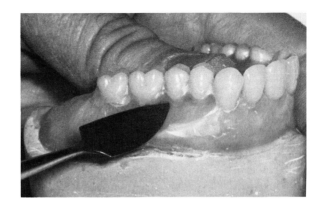

Fig. 8-9. Hot wax spatula is used to seal around neck of each tooth.

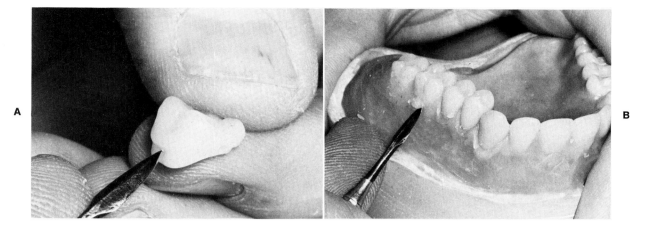

Fig. 8-10. A, Finish line on denture tooth is indicated by roach carver. **B,** Wax is removed from denture teeth at level of finish line.

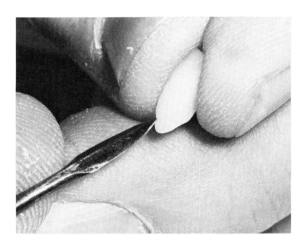

Fig. 8-11. Carver should be held at approximately 60-degree angle when trimming around anterior teeth.

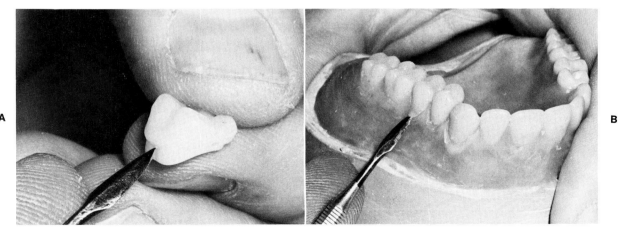

Fig. 8-12. A, Carver is held at 45-degree angle when carving around necks of posterior teeth. **B,** Wax is removed at level of finish line.

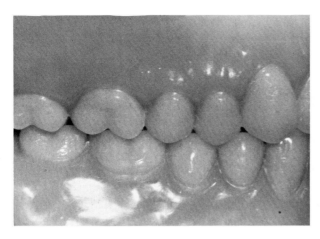

Fig. 8-13. Gingival papillae are carved so that they will be convex mesiodistally and occlusogingivally in completed denture.

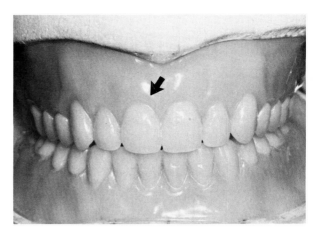

Fig. 8-14. Subtle gingival roll can be placed above anterior teeth (arrow).

necks of the teeth, removing all wax remaining on the teeth above the finish line (Fig. 8-12).

16. Carve the wax to produce a convex gingiva papilla. The gingival papilla of the denture should be convex, both occlusogingivally and mesiodistally (Fig. 8-13).

17. Carve the width of the gingival margin around all teeth until it is approximately 0.5 mm in width.

18. Use an alcohol torch to flame the wax surface, taking care to not overheat the wax, thereby obliterating the carved contours.

19. As an option, a subtle gingival roll may be carved above the anterior teeth (Fig. 8-14). Use a roach carver, a Woodson No. 1 plastic instrument, or small Kingsley scraper, to remove approximately 0.5 mm of wax about 1 to 1.5 mm above the necks of the teeth following the contour of the gingival margin. Use care when flaming the gingival roll, otherwise, the wax will be melted, and the roll destroyed. Polish this area with a piece of damp nylon stocking.

20. Use the tip of a No. 23 explorer, held perpendicular to the tooth, and carefully follow the gingival margin outline around each tooth, without creating an undercut, to remove any wax (Fig. 8-15). The explorer produces a clear separation between the wax and tooth and will result in a more esthetic denture.

21. If desired, the wax denture may be stippled at this time with a modified bristle brush or toothbrush (Fig. 8-16, *A* and *B*). Stipple the region of the attached gingiva. It is usually more effective if the stippling is confined to the interproximal areas of the teeth (Fig. 8-16).

22. Flame the stippling very lightly, taking care to not melt the wax (Fig. 8-17).

23. Seal the baseplate wax of the palate to the lingual surfaces of the denture teeth.

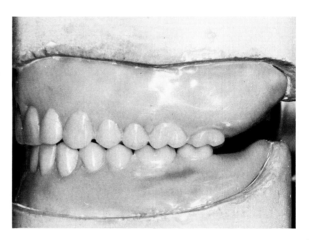

Fig. 8-15. There should be sharp delineation between denture tooth and wax.

24. When the wax is cool, use a roach carver, or No. 7 spatula, in a vertical position to remove a sufficient amount of wax in a vertical direction. This will expose the finish line on the lingual surfaces of the teeth.

25. Trim the wax around the necks of the teeth with a No. 7 spatula from a palatal direction at approximately a 20-degree angle below the horizontal (Fig. 8-18). In this manner, the wax is carved to form a slight obtuse angle, and a smooth junction with the lingual surfaces of the teeth at the finish line is assured.

26. Flame the wax lightly with an alcohol torch, and again trim around the necks of the teeth to remove all traces of wax.

27. Polish the wax with a piece of damp nylon stocking until it presents a smooth shiny surface. Check the entire maxillary denture carefully, flame it lightly, and

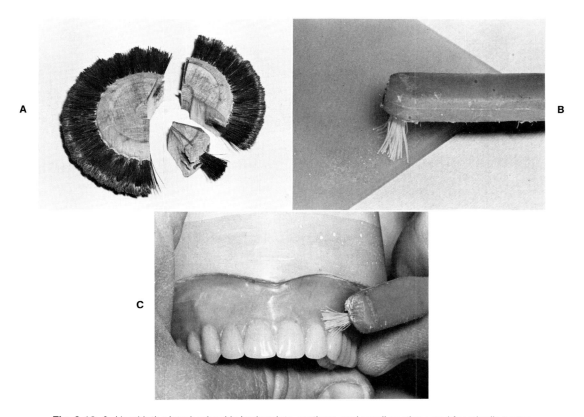

Fig. 8-16. A, Used lathe brush wheel is broken into sections, and small section used for stippling wax. **B,** Toothbrush, modified by removing all except one row of bristles, makes excellent stippling brush. **C,** Stippling is placed in region of attached gingiva and is usually more prominent between teeth rather than directly over roots.

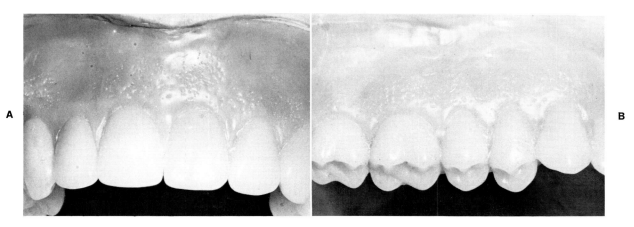

Fig. 8-17. A, Do not overflame stippling. **B,** Light flaming imparts realism to stippling.

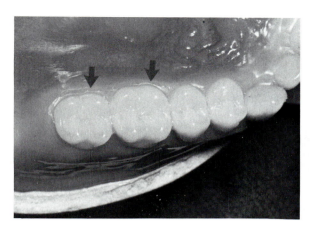

Fig. 8-18. Wax on palatal side is trimmed from teeth at obtuse angle (20 degrees below horizontal plane, arrows).

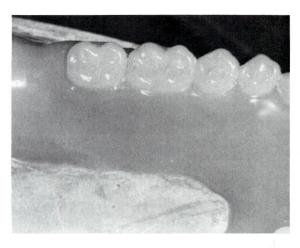

Fig. 8-19. Lingual gingival margins of mandibular denture are carved similar to maxillary denture.

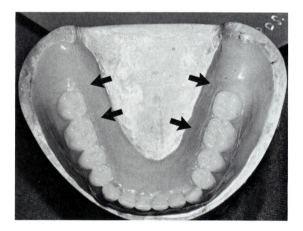

Fig. 8-20. Lingual surfaces of posterior flanges should not be convex. They may be slightly concave, though not too deep (arrows).

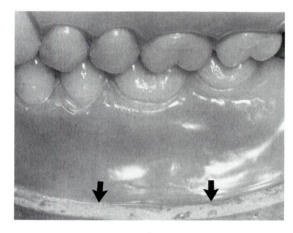

Fig. 8-21. Peripheral roll of wax denture completely fills cast border (arrows).

polish any rough areas with a piece of damp nylon stocking. Check the waxed denture carefully for pits. These must be filled with wax using a spatula rather than flaming with a torch. The maxillary waxed denture is now ready for try-in.

Waxing the mandibular trial denture
PROCEDURE

1. Flow wax on the lingual surfaces of the lower trial denture and carve the gingival margins to produce a gingival margin angle of approximately 20 degrees below the horizontal (Fig. 8-19).
2. Wax the lingual flanges of the lower denture from the posterior teeth to the peripheral roll to produce an inclined plane that slopes toward the tongue. The contour of the posterior lingual flange should not be convex, but in some instances may be slightly concave. The

concavity should not be deep, or the tongue can fill the concavity and dislodge the denture during tongue movement (Fig. 8-20).
3. Contour and wax the distal lingual area of the lingual flange so that it blends into the retromylohyoid space (Fig. 8-20).
4. Wax the peripheral roll to completely fill the peripheral roll outline on the cast. The wax should be contoured to produce a rounded border as will be required in the finished denture (Fig. 8-21).
5. On the labial surface, wax a small gingival bulge just below the gingival margins of the four incisor teeth, similar to that in the maxillary teeth.
6. Develop a canine eminence below each canine tooth.
7. The gingival bulge should be convex in shape; however, no extreme root prominences should be present.

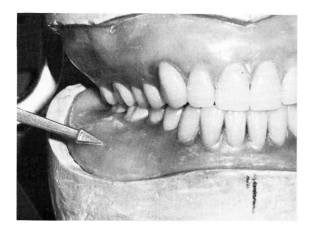

Fig. 8-22. Area between posterior gingival bulge and denture border should be slightly concave.

Table 8-1. Waxing the trial denture

Problem	Probable cause	Solution
Denture teeth not exposed to cervical finish line	Wax placed above finish line and not carved properly	Use roach carver and trim wax to expose denture tooth
Denture too thick, not contoured to simulate dentulous mouth	Too much wax added during wax-up Failure to carve anatomic contour in wax	Do not overwax Carve anatomic contours in wax-up
Denture wax-up unsightly because of discoloration	Wax was overflamed	Do not overheat wax when flaming with torch
	Wax in waxing tray is old and discolored	Use fresh wax in waxing tray to preserve color
	Incorrect type of alcohol used in torch, causing smoke discoloration	Use proper alcohol in torch

8. Contour the area between the gingival bulge and the peripheral roll to produce the concavity. As in the case of the maxillary denture, carve the canine eminences so that they blend with the contour of the peripheral border.

9. Carve the interproximal papilla to completely fill the interproximal space. It should be full bodied and convex mesiodistally and incisogingivally.

10. The free gingival margin, gingival bulge, and interproximal papilla are contoured similarly to that of the maxillary trial denture.

11. Contour the space between the posterior gingival bulge and the peripheral border so that it is slightly concave (Fig. 8-22). Overcarving this area, producing a pronounced concavity, could cause food to be retained on the finished denture.

12. Carve around the individual teeth to produce a slight gingival crevice between the wax and denture teeth.

13. Before the trial dentures are tried in the mouth, check the occlusion on the articulator to be sure that the teeth have not moved during the waxing procedure.

PROBLEM AREAS

The principal problems associated with waxing a trial denture for try-in are related to covering up too much of the denture teeth with too much wax, failure to develop anatomic contours, and using wax that may be discolored from overheating (Table 8-1). All of these errors contribute to a trial denture that is not esthetic and should be avoided. Add only enough wax to develop the desired contours, and carefully trim excess wax from the trial denture. Be sure that the denture teeth are exposed properly by trimming the wax to the level of the gingival margin on the denture teeth. On the trial dentures, carefully establish anatomic contours that simulate those of a normal dentulous mouth. Avoid overcontouring that can be garish and unrealistic. Use new wax when waxing the denture, and do not overheat the wax when flaming

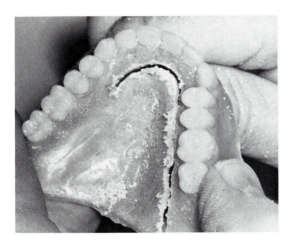

Fig. 8-23. Palate is removed from resin baseplate with handpiece-mounted fissure bur.

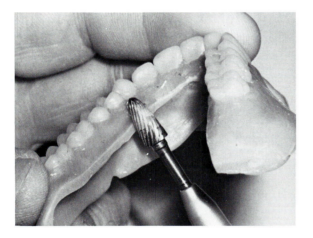

Fig. 8-24. Bevel can be smoothed and perfected with large acrylic bur.

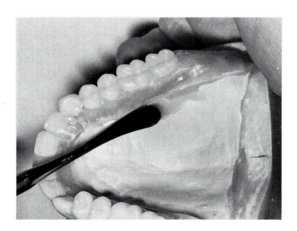

Fig. 8-25. Trial denture sealed to cast with baseplate wax.

it, because it will produce unsightly discolorations. The trial denture should simulate the appearance of the finished denture as closely as possible.

WAXING FOR FLASKING

A plastic palate form can be used to replace the smooth palate of the baseplate. It will provide anatomic detail for the palate of the maxillary denture and permit better control of palate thickness. The baseplate itself may not have a uniform thickness and, as a result the completed denture, will require additional finishing time. An anatomic palate may be freehand waxed, in which case the plastic palate form is omitted. In this case, baseplate wax is adapted to the cast in place of the baseplate palate and carved to the desired contour.

Adding a plastic palate form
PROCEDURE

1. Remove the maxillary trial denture from the cast, and cut out the palate section using a No. 701 or 702 fissure bur in a handpiece (Fig. 8-23). Cut the palate approximately 5 to 6 mm from the denture teeth, inclining the cut to produce an upward-facing bevel on the resin baseplate. The bevel may be smoothed and perfected by using an acrylic bur (Fig. 8-24). A shellac baseplate palate may be removed with a hot spatula or a bur and should be beveled in the same manner.

2. Brush away all resin debris from the cutting procedure, and replace the maxillary denture on the cast.

3. Wax the trial denture to the cast around the entire border of the trial denture (Fig. 8-25). Check the thickness of the palate form with a Boley gauge before adapting it to the cast. It is important that the finished denture have an approximate palate thickness of 2 mm. Since some plastic palate forms may not be this thick, additional wax can be flowed onto the cast before adapting

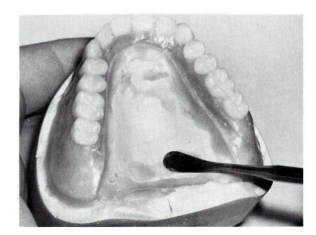

Fig. 8-26. Baseplate wax is flowed onto cast to thicken resultant denture palate.

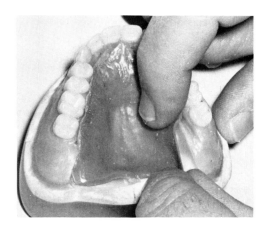

Fig. 8-27. Plastic form is adapted to cast using care to avoid wrinkles or air bubbles.

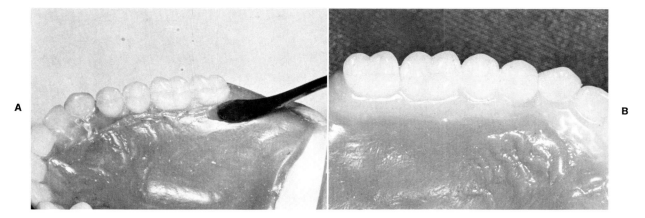

Fig. 8-28. A, Palate form is waxed to trial denture. **B,** There should be no sharp ledge at junction between palate form and wax.

the palate form to produce the desired thickness (Fig. 8-26).

4. Place the palate form on the cast to check the overall fit. Shape the palate form with scissors, or a sharp No. 25 blade in a Bard-Parker handle, so that it closely conforms to the outline of the resin section removed from the baseplate.

5. Beginning in the anterior portion, adapt the plastic palate to the cast, aligning the incisive papilla area in position behind the maxillary central incisor teeth. Continue the adaptation posteriorly, taking care to avoid entrapment of air, which produces air bubbles beneath the palate and creates localized thickened areas in the denture (Fig. 8-27).

6. Use care when adapting the palate to avoid wrinkels. Trim the palate form posteriorly so that it ends at the posterior extent of the maxillary denture.

7. Add wax to the bevel to produce a smooth junction between the wax overlying the resin baseplate and the plastic palate form (Fig. 8-28, *A*). There should be no sharp ledge or thick border between the palate form and

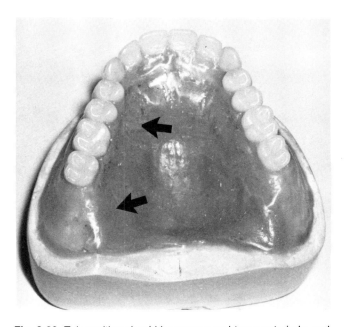

Fig. 8-29. Tuberosities should be convex and taper anteriorly, ending in region of second premolar (arrows).

wax (Fig. 8-28, *B*). Smooth the wax junction with a piece of damp nylon stocking material.

8. Add wax in the tuberosity area to produce a slight convexity lingual to the second molars. This convexity should taper anteriorly and end in the area of the first or second premolar. Viewed from above, the narrowest part of the maxillary arch should be in the first premolar region, and it should widen progressively posteriorly (Fig. 8-29).

9. Seal the posterior border of the palate form to the cast with a spatula and baseplate wax. Smooth the wax to produce a smooth junction between the palate form and wax. Optionally, a smooth palate can be obtained by adapting a sheet of baseplate wax to the cast (Fig. 8-30). A layer of baseplate wax forming the palate gives good palate thickness control, and if rugae or other anatomic forms are desired, they can be waxed in at this time (Fig. 8-31). The waxed denture should exhibit those contours desired in the finished denture (Fig. 8-32).

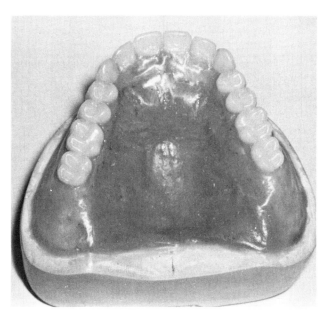

Fig. 8-30. Smooth palate can be obtained by adapting sheet of baseplate wax to cast. Additions of wax beneath baseplate wax may be necessary to achieve adequate palate thickness.

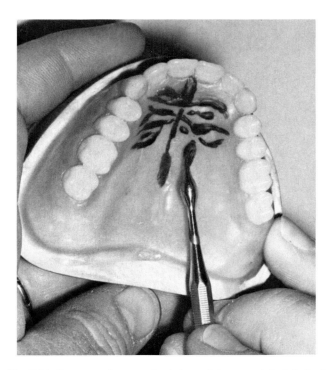

Fig. 8-31. Rugae can be waxed onto baseplate wax palate if desired.

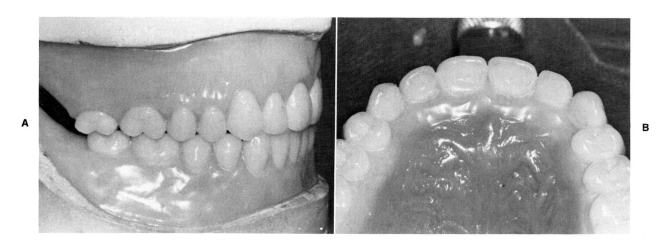

Fig. 8-32. **A,** Waxed denture should simulate contours desired in completed denture. **B,** Note smooth borders of palate wax-up.

PROBLEM AREAS

The principal problems associated with placing a palate form are related to failure to establish a proper bevel, failure to align the palate form correctly, and trapping air beneath the palate form during adaptation (Table 8-2). Placing an upward-facing bevel on the plastic baseplate with a bur, correctly aligning the palate form so that the rugae are in proper position, and carefully adapting the palate form with finger pressure will usually prevent these problems.

Flasking the denture
PROCEDURE

1. Check the seal of the trial denture to the cast, and fill in deficient areas with baseplate wax. Take care to completely fill the peripheral border; however, do not overflow wax onto the cast borders (Fig. 8-33).

2. Check the occlusion with tissue paper or plastic tape (Fig. 8-34). Adding wax, cutting out the palate section, and removing and replacing the denture on the cast may produce occlusion errors that should be corrected before flasking the denture.

3. Select flasks that fit together accurately without rocking (Fig. 8-35). Lubricate the flasks with silicone lubricant* to facilitate cleanup after processing (Fig. 8-36).

4. Remove the waxed denture and cast from the articulator, and paint the cast with a separating medium† (Fig. 8-37).

5. Place the dentures and casts in the flask to check the height of denture teeth in the flask.

6. Soak the wax dentures on their casts in clear slurry water for a few minutes. The casts will take up slurry

---

*Masque, The Harry J. Bosworth Co., Chicago, Ill.
†Super-Sep, Kerr Manufacturing Co., Romulus, Mich.

Table 8-2. Adding a plastic palate form

Problem	Probable cause	Solution
Palate of finished denture has thick ledge at junction of palate form and baseplate	Baseplate not beveled when palate form was adapted	Bevel baseplate to make smooth junction between palate form and baseplate
Midline of palate form, or rugae, not in correct position	Palate form not aligned properly when adapted	Position palate form so that rugae, incisive papilla, midline are located in area of natural counterpart
Palate of finished denture has thick areas not evenly distributed	Air bubble trapped under palate form during adaptation	Use care when adapting to minimize air entrapment Puncture air bubbles with sharp instrument; express air

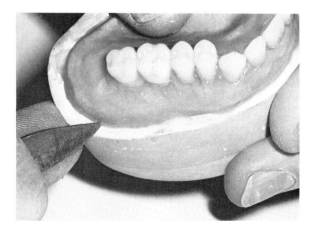

Fig. 8-33. Wax extending onto cast border is removed before flasking.

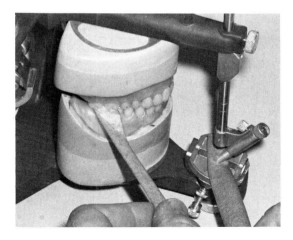

Fig. 8-34. Occlusion is checked before removing casts for flasking.

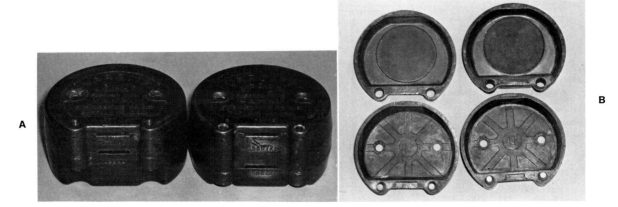

Fig. 8-35. A, Flasks should fit together without rocking. Be certain that numbers match. **B,** Flasks should be clean and free of plaster.

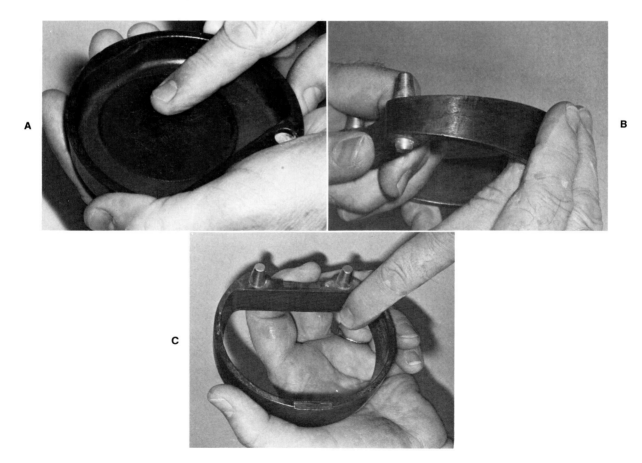

Fig. 8-36. A, Interior of flask is lubricated with silicone lubricant. **B** and **C,** Exterior and joining surfaces are coated with silicone lubricant.

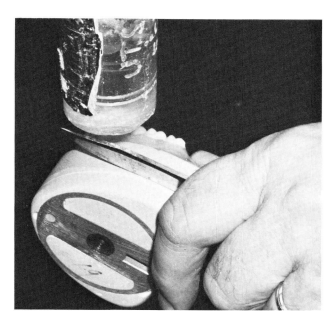

Fig. 8-37. Wax denture and cast are removed from mounting stone.

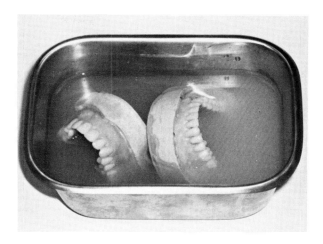

Fig. 8-38. Waxed denture and cast are soaked in clear slurry water for few minutes.

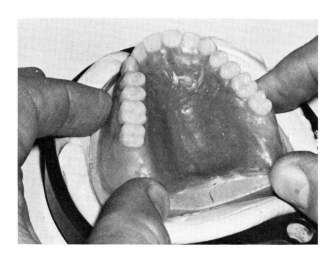

Fig. 8-39. Denture and cast are settled into stone mix.

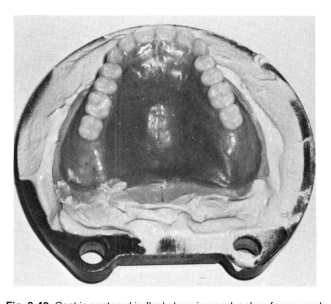

Fig. 8-40. Cast is centered in flask, keeping occlusal surfaces parallel to bench top.

water and, as a result, remove less water from the investing stone mix (Fig. 8-38).

7. Proportion artificial stone by weight (usually 200 gm is adequate for half-flasking a denture), and mix it with the recommended volume of water. Artificial stone is recommended for flasking because of its superior compression strength.

8. Place the stone mix in the flask, and settle the wax denture and cast into the mix (Fig. 8-39). Center the cast in the flask, keeping the occlusal plane approximately parallel to the base of the flask (Fig. 8-40).

9. Smooth the stone around the cast with a spatula (Fig. 8-41). Remove stone as necessary, and fill any deficient areas (Fig. 8-42).

10. Allow the stone to complete the initial set, and trim and smooth it with a sharp plaster knife (Fig. 8-43).

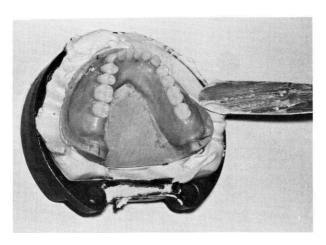

Fig. 8-41. Stone is smoothed with spatula.

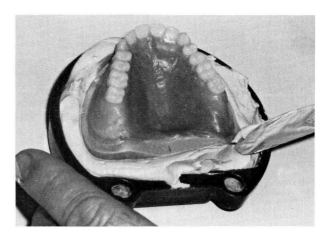

Fig. 8-42. Areas are filled where needed to eliminate undercuts.

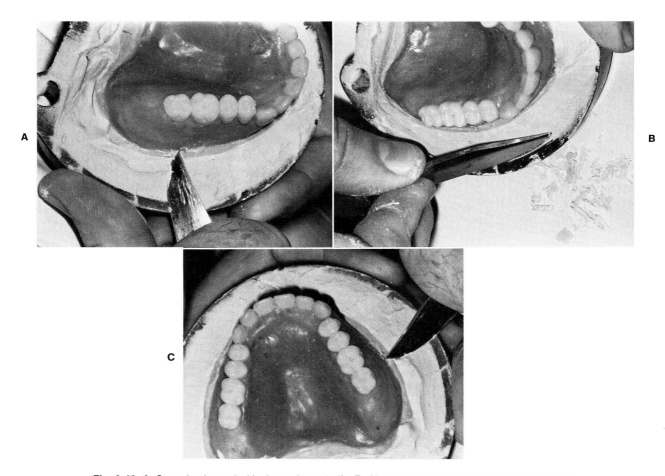

Fig. 8-43. A, Stone is trimmed with sharp plaster knife. **B,** All stone is removed on flask rims. **C,** Avoid gouging or cutting wax denture. Note curved blade, which is recommended for trimming flasking stone.

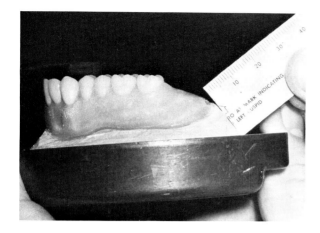

Fig. 8-44. Flasking stone is examined for undercuts, which must be removed or filled in before top half of flask is poured.

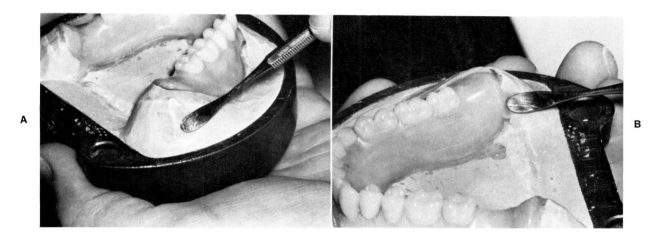

A

B

Fig. 8-45. A, Heel undercuts are blocked out with baseplate wax. B, Distolingual region is frequently undercut and should be blocked out.

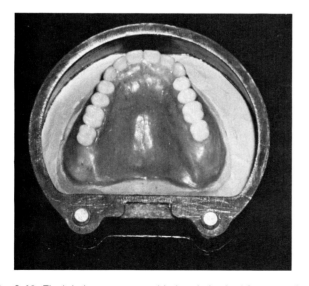

Fig. 8-46. Flask halves are assembled and checked for stone that could prevent accurate seating.

A blade with a curved end is recommended to prevent damage to the wax denture.

11. Remove all stone undercuts that would prevent separation of the flask halves (Fig. 8-44). Undercuts occur commonly in the posterior lingual region of mandibular dentures. Undercuts can be blocked out with wax before pouring the upper half of the flask to prevent heel breakage on opening of the flask (Fig. 8-45).

12. Place the top half of the flask into position on the lower half to determine that no stone remains on the rim to prevent complete seating (Fig. 8-46).

13. Paint all stone surfaces in the lower half of the flask with a separating medium* (Fig. 8-47, A). Take care not to place the separating medium on the wax denture or teeth. This is particularly true if the denture teeth are plastic, since some separating media can stain

---

*Super-Sep, Kerr Manufacturing Co., Romulus, Mich.

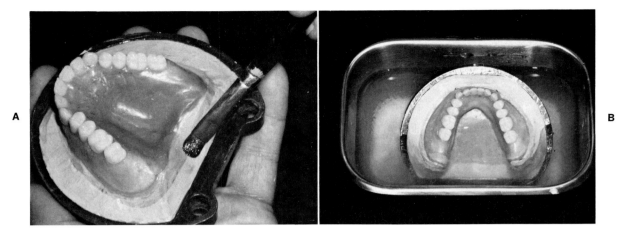

Fig. 8-47. A, All stone surfaces are painted with separating medium. **B,** Flask is soaked in clear slurry water for few minutes before second pour is added.

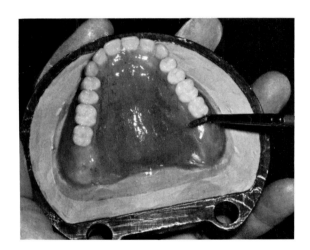

Fig. 8-48. Wax is painted with surface tension–reducing agent to minimize bubbles.

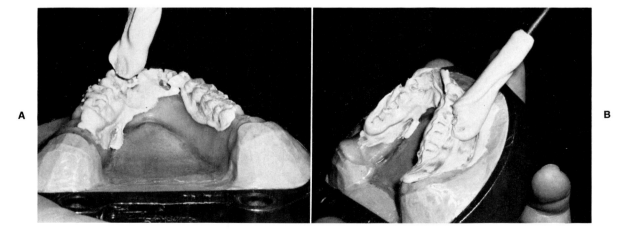

Fig. 8-49. A, Stone is painted on occlusal surfaces with stiff brush. **B,** Stone is painted on wax surfaces to minimize voids.

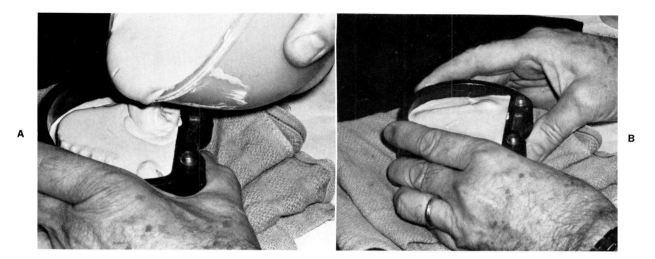

Fig. 8-50. A, Stone is poured into flask slowly while on vibrator to reduce air entrapment. **B,** If vibrator is not available, flask can be tapped against towel on bench top, using care to hold flask halves together.

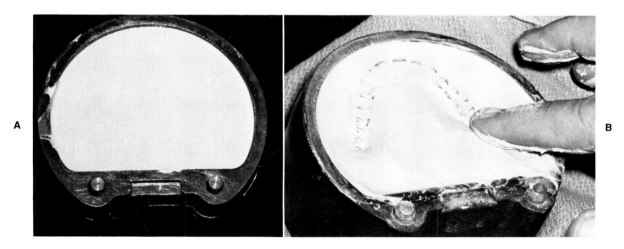

Fig. 8-51. A, Flask is filled to within ¼ inch (0.64 cm) of top. **B,** Stone is removed from occlusal surfaces of teeth.

resin denture teeth. Soak the lower half of the flask and invested cast in clear slurry water before pouring stone into the top half of the flask (Fig. 8-47, *B*).

14. With the upper half of the flask in position, make a mix of artificial stone as previously described. Mixing the stone in a mechanical spatulator under reduced atmospheric pressure results in minimal air inclusion and fewer nodules on the processed denture, materially reducing the finishing time.

15. Paint the wax surface with a surface tension reducer* (Fig. 8-48), and place stone on the occlusal surfaces of the denture teeth and into the interproximal

areas with a stiff bristle brush or finger (Fig. 8-49). This procedure reduces voids or bubbles and materially reduces the amount of time required to finish the denture. It can be done while the flask is being held on a vibrator operating at low speed.

16. Pour stone into the flask, allowing time for the stone to flow over the denture and in the lower half of the flask. Take care to avoid air entrapment, which can produce voids (Fig. 8-50, *A*). In the absence of a vibrator, the stone may be settled by bouncing the flask on a bench covered with a folded towel (Fig. 8-50, *B*). Care must be taken to hold the flask halves firmly together.

17. Fill the flask to within approximately ¼ inch (0.64 cm) of the top (Fig. 8-51, *A*). Remove the stone with a

---

*Debubblizer, Kerr Manufacturing Co., Romulus, Mich.

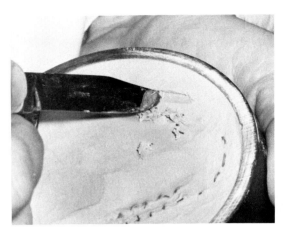

Fig. 8-52. Small retentive grooves are placed in set stone to maintain cap in position.

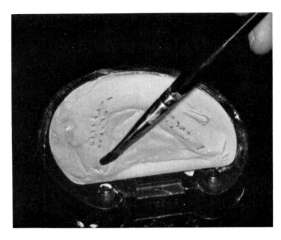

Fig. 8-53. Stone surface is painted with separating medium. Do not permit separating medium to contact resin denture teeth.

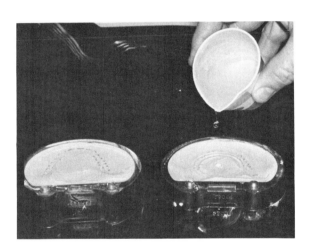

Fig. 8-54. Clear slurry water is poured on stone and allowed to remain while stone for cap is mixed.

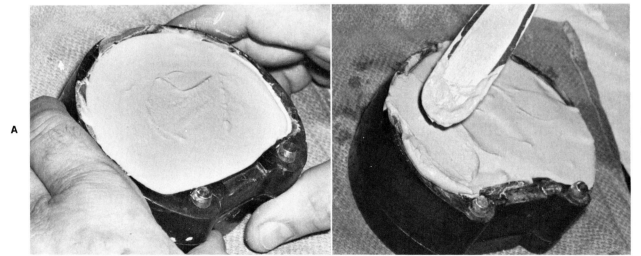

Fig. 8-55. A, Slurry water is poured off, and flask is filled with stone. B, Flask is completely filled with stone.

finger to expose the occlusal surfaces of the teeth in preparation for pouring a stone cap later (Fig. 8-51, *B*).

18. Permit the stone to set before pouring the stone cap.

19. After the stone has set, it is sometimes desirable to cut small retentive grooves in the stone to prevent premature separation of the cap (Fig. 8-52). Carefully paint the stone surface with a separating medium (Fig. 8-53). Do not allow the separating medium to contact the occlusal surfaces of the incisal edges of teeth. This is particularly important when resin teeth are used, because they may become stained.

20. Pour clear slurry water onto the stone surface, and allow it to remain while the stone is being mixed for the stone cap (Fig. 8-54).

21. Pour the slurry water off, and vibrate the stone onto the surface, filling the flask (Fig. 8-55).

22. Place the lid on the filled flask, and tap it gently to be sure that the flask has been completely filled (Fig. 8-56).

23. Allow the stone to set before the wax is eliminated.

PROBLEM AREAS

Problems associated with flasking are related to failure to identify and block out undercuts in the flasking stone; incorporating air inclusions in the investing stone, resulting in nodules on the denture; and failure to paint a separating medium on the investing stone (Table 8-3). Undercuts on the flasking stone should be identified and eliminated by trimming it with a knife or by filling it in with baseplate wax. Failure to do this may result in a broken cast when separating the flask halves. Investing stone should be brushed on the denture during flasking to reduce air inclusions. Better yet, the investing stone should be mixed in a mechanical spatulator under reduced atmospheric pressure.* Be sure to paint a separating medium on the stone in the lower half of the flask before pouring the upper half, otherwise, separation will be difficult, if not impossible.

---

*Combination Vac-U-Vester Power Mixer, Whip-Mix Corp., Louisville, Ky.

Table 8-3. Flasking the denture

Problem	Probable cause	Solution
Flask halves cannot be separated after removal from boiling water	Undercuts exist in flasking stone or on casts Separating medium not painted on stone in lower half of flask	Examine casts and flasking stone carefully to locate and block out undercuts Paint separating medium on stone in lower half of flask before pouring upper half
Heel broken on mandibular cast on flask separation	Undercut on cast not blocked out with wax	Check heel area of mandibular denture after half flasked to locate and block out undercuts
Denture has many nodules of acrylic attached when removed from flask	Investing stone not painted on denture during flasking Investing stone not vacuum spatulated	Paint investing stone on teeth; wax denture with stiff brush Mix investing stone in mechanical spatulator under reduced atmospheric pressure

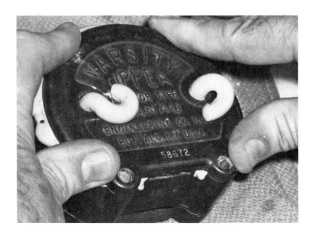

Fig. 8-56. Lid is placed on flask and tapped to determine that flask is filled.

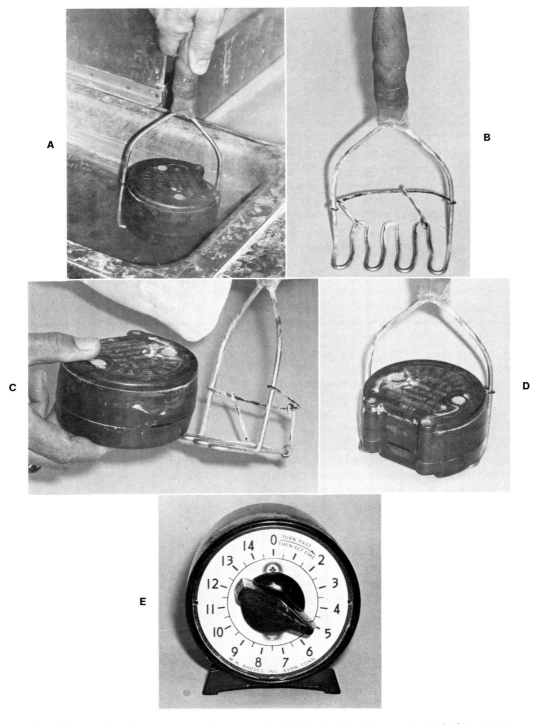

Fig. 8-57. A, Flask immersed in boiling water. **B,** Suitable flask holder can be made from potato masher. **C,** Wires added to potato masher prevent flask from slipping. **D,** Flask in modified potato masher. **E,** Timer is used to assure adequate wax softening.

Wax elimination

After the stone has set, the flask is placed in boiling water to soften the wax.

PROCEDURE

1. The flask, in a suitable holder, is placed in boiling water for approximately 5 minutes (Fig. 8-57, *A*). A suitable flask holder can be made from a potato masher (Fig. 8-57, *B*). It is essential that a timer be used to prevent liquefying the wax (Fig. 8-57, *E*).

2. Remove the flask, and pry it open with a plaster knife. Be sure to pry on the side opposite any potential undercuts (Fig. 8-58).

3. Discard the softened wax and plastic denture base, and check that no denture teeth have been dislodged on opening the flask (Fig. 8-59).

4. Place half of the flask in a holder, and flow clean boiling water, to which detergent has been added, over the surface of the teeth, cast, and stone to eliminate all traces of wax (Fig. 8-60).

5. A brush and soap, or detergent solution, can be used to clean the cast and stone, followed with a clean boiling water flush (Fig. 8-61). Place the flask aside to cool.

6. Flush the flask with clean boiling water to remove all traces of detergent water (Fig. 8-62).

7. Place the half flask in an upright position, and allow it to drain and cool (Fig. 8-63).

8. The lower half of the flask is treated in the same manner.

Painting the tinfoil substitute

Tinfoil substitute is applied to all stone surfaces of the cast after the flasks have cooled so that they can be handled comfortably.

PROCEDURE

1. Pour enough tinfoil substitute into a small container for use on the flasks at hand (Fig. 8-64). Never dip a brush into the main container because it is very easily contaminated and its effectiveness destroyed.

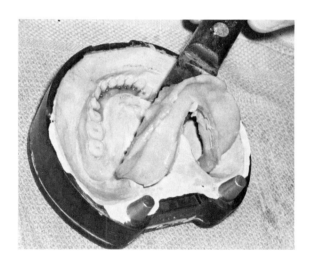

Fig. 8-59. Baseplate and softened wax are removed. Check for dislodged denture teeth at this time.

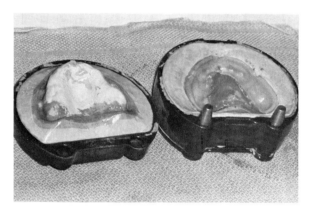

Fig. 8-58. Flask halves separated.

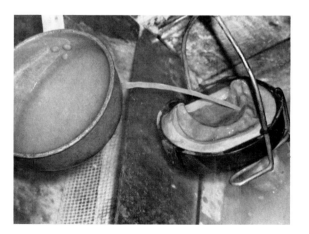

Fig. 8-60. Mold is flushed with hot water to which detergent has been added.

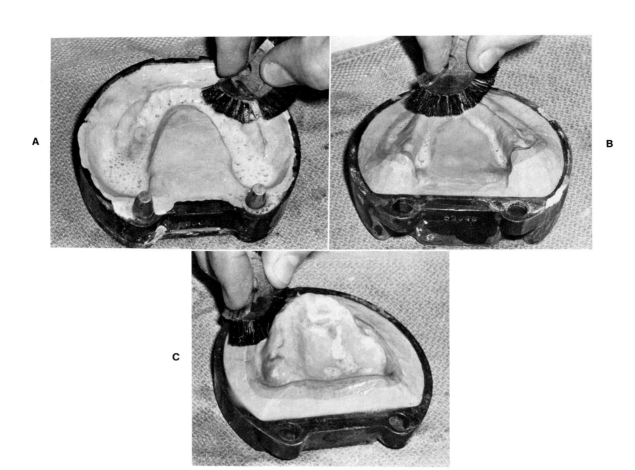

Fig. 8-61. **A,** Worn-out lathe brush wheel can be used to scrub cast to eliminate all traces of wax. **B** and **C,** Molds should be thoroughly cleansed.

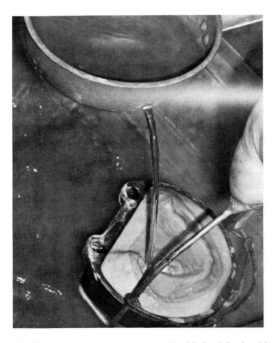

Fig. 8-62. Detergent solution is removed with final flush with clean boiling water.

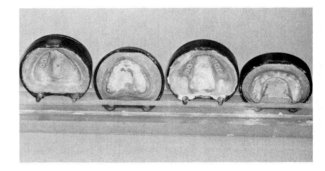

Fig. 8-63. Flasks are allowed to drain and cool in upright position. Note grooved plastic holder used to hold casts upright.

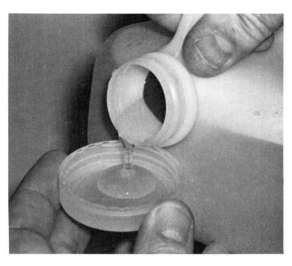

Fig. 8-64. Tinfoil substitute is poured in small container for immediate use. Any tinfoil substitute remaining after using should be discarded and not returned to storage container.

2. Carefully paint the tinfoil substitute on the stone surfaces in the flask (Fig. 8-65). Do not paint tinfoil substitute on the ridge laps of the teeth.

3. Certain tinfoil substitutes are quite thick and can be diluted by adding water. Take care, however, to not overdilute, since the effectiveness of the tinfoil substitute may be compromised.

4. After the stone in the flask has been coated with tinfoil substitute, place it aside, and allow it to dry (Fig. 8-66). Be sure that all areas of stone have been painted with tinfoil substitute, or the denture base resin will adhere to the stone, making a difficult finishing problem.

PROBLEM AREAS

Principal problems associated with applying tinfoil substitute to the flasking stone and cast are related to omitting the tinfoil substitute, using contaminated tinfoil substitute, overdiluting the tinfoil substitute, and inadvertently coating the ridge laps of resin teeth with tinfoil substitute when applying it to the stone (Table 8-4). Tinfoil substitute should be carefully painted on the

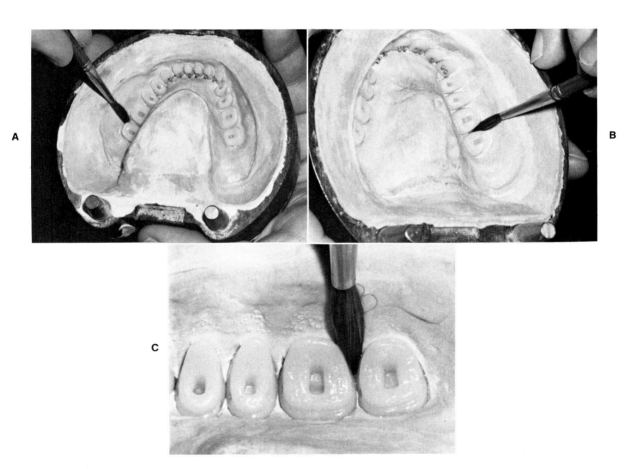

Fig. 8-65. A, Tinfoil substitute is carefully painted on stone. **B,** Do not allow tinfoil substitute to puddle in interproximal areas. **C,** Do not place tinfoil substitute on ridge laps of teeth.

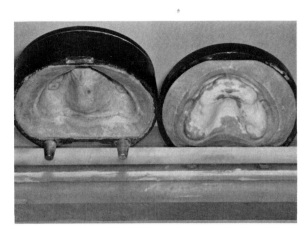

Fig. 8-66. Coated flasks are allowed to drain and dry.

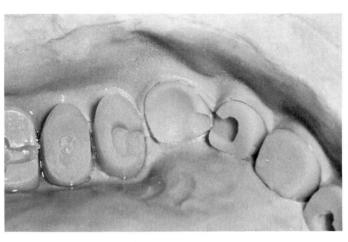

Fig. 8-67. Small recesses placed in ridge laps of resin denture teeth facilitate stronger attachment between teeth and denture base.

Table 8-4. Painting the tinfoil substitute

Problem	Probable cause	Solution
Flasking stone sticks tenaciously to cured denture surface	Tinfoil substitute not applied to cast or flasking stone	Paint stone and cast with tinfoil substitute
	Tinfoil substitute contaminated with stone	Pour fresh tinfoil substitute in small container for immediate use; do not dip brush in principal storage container
	Tinfoil substitute too diluted as a result of thinning	Do not add too much water to thin tinfoil substitute
	Wax elimination not completed during boilout, rendering tinfoil substitute ineffective	Cleanse interior of mold and cast surface thoroughly with boiling water to which detergent has been added; flush with clean boiling water
Resin teeth fail to bond to denture base resin	Tinfoil substitute painted on ridge laps of denture teeth	Remove any tinfoil substitute that contacts ridge laps of resin teeth
	Wax residue remains on ridge laps of denture teeth	Cleanse interior of mold, denture teeth, and cast thoroughly with boiling water to which detergent has been added; flush with clean boiling water

flasking stone and cast, leaving no areas uncoated. Fresh tinfoil substitute should be used, and the applying brush never dipped in the principal storage bottle. A sufficient volume of tinfoil substitute should be poured into a secondary container for use. Some tinfoil substitutes are viscous and difficult to paint. The thick material can usually be diluted with water to a more usable consistency; however, it should not be overdiluted, or a poor separating effect will result. Ridge laps of resin denture teeth should not be coated with tinfoil substitute. If tinfoil substitute is painted on the ridge laps it should be removed, or the bond between the tooth and denture base may be compromised.

Preparing ridge laps

When resin teeth are used in the denture, it is advisable to roughen the ridge laps or make diatorics in these teeth with a bur to provide additional area for bonding between the denture base resin and denture tooth. This is particularly true when highly cross-linked denture base resins are used. A No. 4 or 6 round bur can be used to place indentations in anterior teeth. Grooves or indentations can be placed in resin posterior teeth in order to materially improve the attachment between the denture teeth and denture base resin (Fig. 8-67). After the indentations have been placed, be sure to remove all traces of acrylic grindings from the flask.

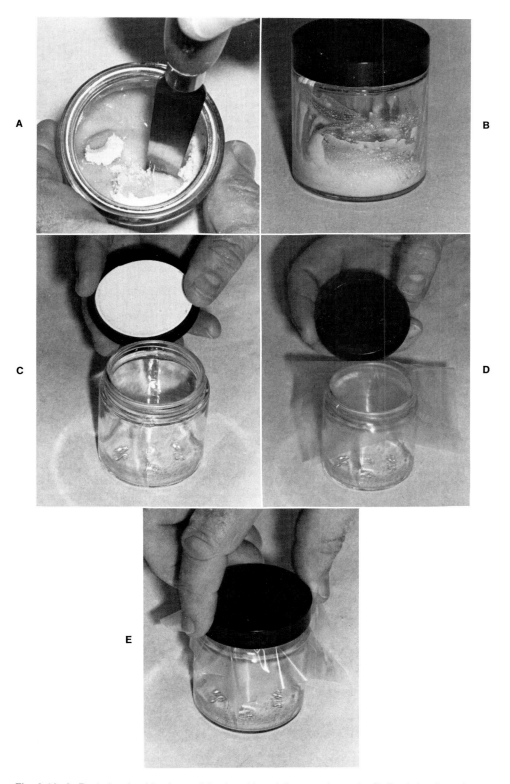

Fig. 8-68. A, Resin is mixed in clean mixing jar with stainless steel spatula. **B,** Resin is allowed to set in closed jar until dough stage is reached. **C,** Mixing jar lid should form tight seal when in place. **D,** Lid does not provide good seal, thus plastic sheet is placed over jar before lid is screwed on. **E,** Plastic serves as gasket, forming tight seal.

Packing the denture
PROCEDURE

1. Choose an appropriate shade denture base resin to meet the needs of the patient, and proportion it according to the manufacturer's instructions.

2. Mix the resin in a clean mixing jar with a stainless steel spatula (Fig. 8-68, *A*). Place it aside until the resin reaches the proper stage (dough) for packing (Fig. 8-68, *B*). It is important that the mixing jar be airtight to prevent evaporation of the acrylic monomer, which will cause the mix to be grainy (Fig. 8-68, *C*). If the lid does not seal well, a sheet of thin plastic can be used to gain a seal (Fig. 8-68, *D* and *E*).

3. Handle the resin with plastic gloves to prevent contaminating the resin with skin oils and to prevent

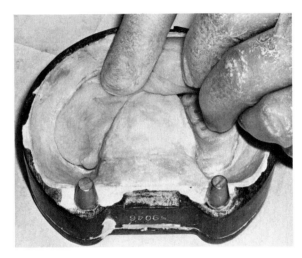

Fig. 8-69. Resin is handled with plastic gloves to prevent contamination.

possible development of contact dermatitis through repeated contacts with the resin (Fig. 8-69).

4. After the resin has reached the dough stage, remove it from the jar, form it into a roll, and adapt it to the flask (Fig. 8-70).

5. Place plastic sheets over the resin, place the flask halves in position, and close it slowly in a bench compress (Fig. 8-71) to permit the flow of acrylic resin into the minute intricacies of the mold.

6. Open the denture flask, and cut away excess resin flash, replace the plastic sheets, and trial pack the flask again (Fig. 8-72).

7. Continue trial packing until no more flash is apparent on opening the flask (Fig. 8-73).

8. At this time, when the flask is opened, the resin should exhibit a shiny surface (Fig. 8-74).

9. After the final trial pack, repaint the cast portion of the flask with tinfoil substitute, and allow it to dry (Fig. 8-75). Place a sheet of plastic over the denture base resin to minimize monomer evaporation.

10. Assemble the flask, and close it until metal-to-metal contact between the flask rims is achieved (Fig. 8-76).

11. Place the denture in a compress, and bench cure it, if specified by the manufacturer, before curing it in a curing unit.

PROBLEM AREAS

Principal problems associated with packing the denture are related to failure to adequately fill the mold with resin, packing the resin at the wrong stage, failure to bench cure the packed denture prior to curing, and failure to achieve metal-to-metal contact of the flask (Table 8-5). The mold should be completely filled and flash extruded during initial trial packing. Failure to fill

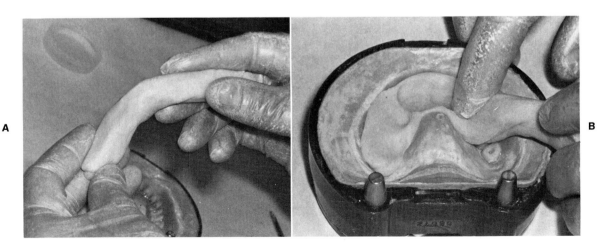

Fig. 8-70. A, Resin dough is removed and formed into roll. **B,** Resin adapted in flask.

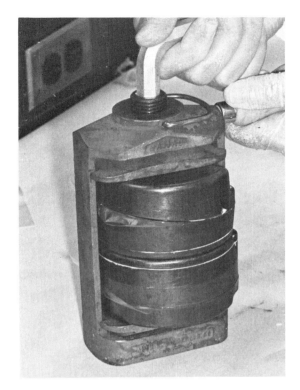

Fig. 8-71. Flask is closed slowly in compress.

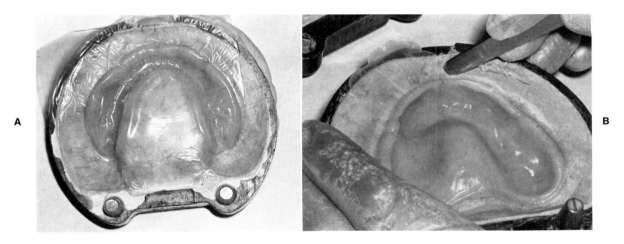

A   B

Fig. 8-72. A, Plastic sheet removed, and resin flash trimmed. B, Dull spatula is used to trim flash. Sharp knife can cut stone, allowing stone particles to be incorporated in resin.

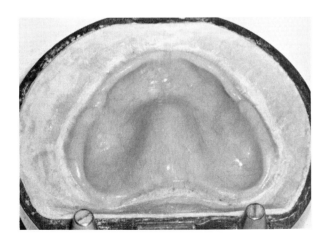

Fig. 8-73. Trial packing is continued until no flash is apparent on opening flask.

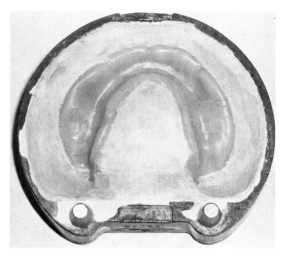

Fig. 8-74. Resin surface is glossy when flask is opened; however, it dulls rapidly.

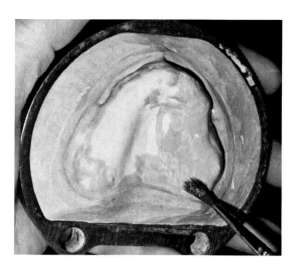

Fig. 8-75. Cast is again coated with tinfoil substitute and allowed to dry before final closure.

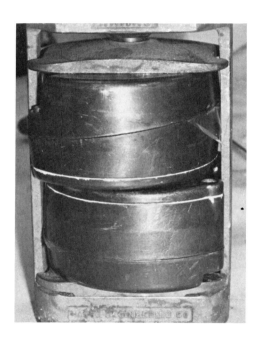

Fig. 8-76. Flask rims contact, indicating flask is closed.

Table 8-5. Packing the denture

Problem	Probable cause	Solution
Cured denture has porosity	Flask underpacked with resin	Fill mold completely before curing; properly packed resin should exhibit glossy surface when flask is first opened
	Thick denture base heated too rapidly	Bench cure, followed by long curing cycle
Cured denture has increased processing error	Denture resin packed at late, or rubbery, stage	Pack resin during dough stage
	Flask not properly closed prior to curing	Make certain metal-to-metal contact of flask rims is achieved before curing

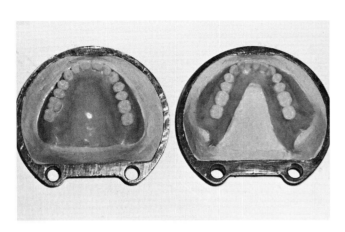

Fig. 8-77. Waxed dentures are half-flasked in usual manner.

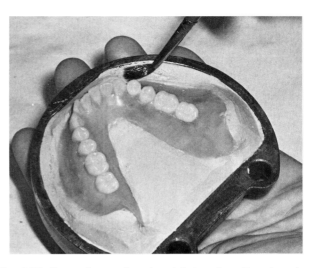

Fig. 8-78. Separating medium is painted on investing stone from denture border to flask rim.

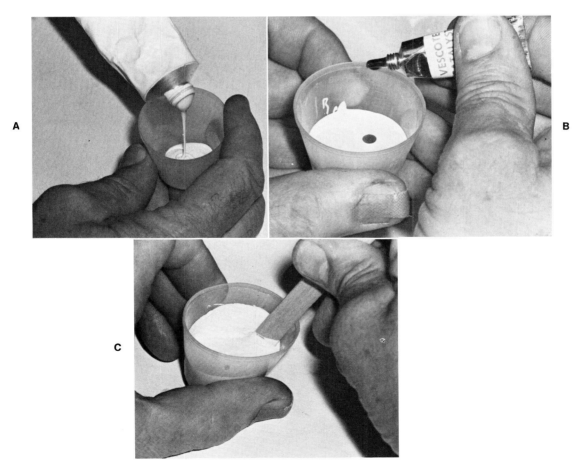

Fig. 8-79. A, Investment coating material is proportioned according to size of denture: 5 ml of base for small dentures, 10 ml for larger dentures. **B,** Catalyst is added to base: 1 drop for each 5 ml of base. **C,** Catalyst is thoroughly mixed with base for 15 to 20 seconds.

the mold, or underpacking, can result in a denture with porosity. Attempting to pack the denture resin too soon may result in the resin being too sticky to handle properly. Resin should be packed at the dough stage. Packing the resin at a late stage, such as the rubbery stage, can require excessive force to close the mold. This can produce tooth movement in the mold and increase processing error. Thick dentures should be bench cured before being subjected to increased temperature. The long curing cycle, starting at room temperature and rising to 165° F (74° C) is recommended for thick dentures to prevent porosity. In any instance the manufacturer's instructions should be closely followed. Failure to achieve metal-to-metal contact of the flask rims during packing can also contribute to increased processing error.

ALTERNATE FLASKING PROCEDURE

Various silicone mold, or investment coating, materials have been used to flask complete dentures. The resultant flexible mold facilitates rapid retrieval of the cured denture from the flask, reduces the finishing time required to remove investing plaster or stone from the denture, serves as a moisture barrier, and does not require application of tinfoil subsitute to the mold material. Disadvantages include cost of material and the tendency for denture teeth to be occasionally dislodged from the flexible mold.

PROCEDURE

1. Dentures, waxed in the usual manner, are half flasked in stone (Fig. 8-77).

2. Paint a separating medium on the investing stone in the lower half of the flask from the denture border to the flask rim (Fig. 8-78).

3. Proportion the investment coating material* ac-

---

*Vescote, Teledyne Dental Products Co., Getz-Opotow Division, Elk Grove Village, Ill.

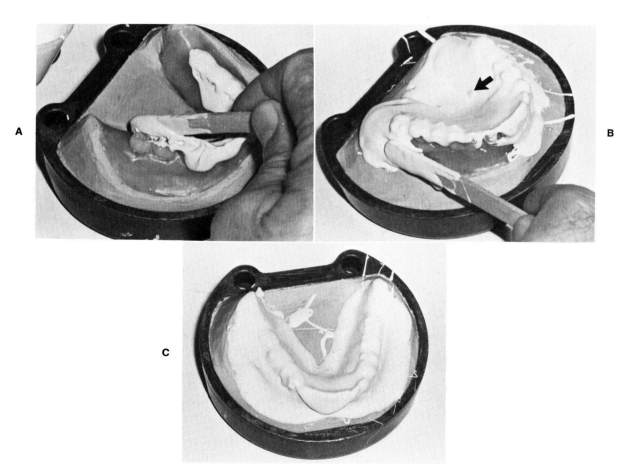

Fig. 8-80. **A,** Silicone investment coating is painted on dry denture. Avoid entrapment of air, which results in resin nodules on cured denture. **B,** Entire denture is covered with investment coating. Air bubble (arrow) in material should be punctured. **C,** Investment coating extends onto investing stone surface.

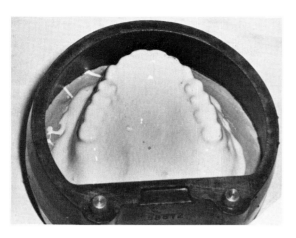

Fig. 8-81. Upper half of flask is placed in position. Make certain that flask rims contact.

cording to the manufacturer's recommendations (Fig. 8-79).

4. Paint the mixed mold material over the waxed denture with a spatula (Fig. 8-80), using care to thoroughly coat the entire denture surface and teeth.

5. Place the upper half of the flask in position on the lower half (Fig. 8-81). Remove any mold material from between the flask rims that could prevent accurate seating.

6. Add stone to fill the flask while the surface of the investment coating is still tacky (Fig. 8-82).

7. Place the lid in the flask, and tap to determine that the flask is completely filled (Fig. 8-83).

8. After the stone has set, immerse the flask in boiling water for 5 minutes to soften the wax. The mold is then flushed with a detergent solution and clean boiling water (Fig. 8-84).

9. Place small recesses in the ridge laps of plastic den-

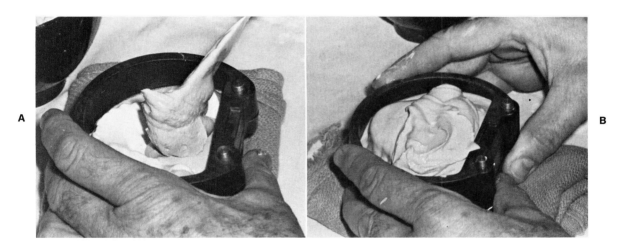

Fig. 8-82. A, Stone mix is vibrated into flask. Investment coating should have tacky surface. **B,** Flask is tilted while vibrating to allow stone to flow into all portions of flask. Large void produced by air entrapment could change contour of denture surface.

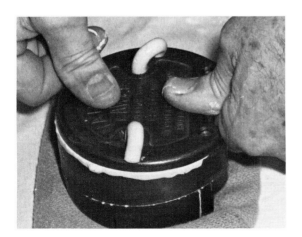

Fig. 8-83. Stone extrudes through holes in flask lid, indicating that flask is full.

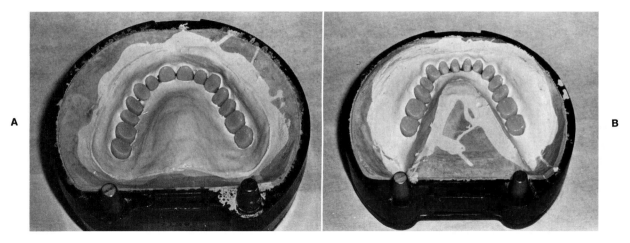

Fig. 8-84. A, All traces of wax are removed from upper flask. Note smooth, bubblefree surface of mold. **B,** Lower mold is also bubble free and ready for packing.

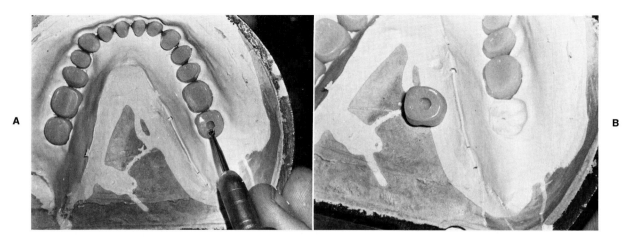

Fig. 8-85. A, Grinding ridge laps of plastic denture teeth can contribute to stronger attachment between teeth and denture base. **B,** Flexibility of mold allows removal of denture tooth for ridge-lap preparation. Tooth is then easily replaced in indentation. Same flexibility, however, can also lead to inadvertent dislodgment of teeth during boilout and packing.

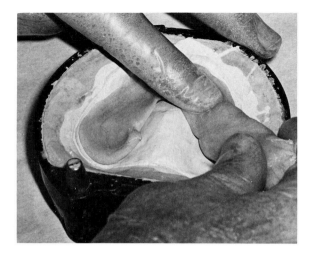

Fig. 8-86. Denture resin is packed in mold and trial packed in usual manner.

ture teeth to facilitate a stronger union between the denture tooth and denture base (Fig. 8-85).

10. Mix the denture base resin according to the manufacturer's recommendations, and pack the mold in the usual manner. The denture is then cured and polished (Fig. 8-86).

Curing the denture

After bench curing the denture for 1 or more hours, place the denture in water at room temperature, and program the curing temperatures according to the manufacturer's recommendations. It is helpful to place a small ball of excess resin around the handle of the compress if the dentures are to be cured overnight in the laboratory. The resin ball is checked the next morning to assure that the power has not been inadvertently turned off during the night, leaving the denture undercured. Cured resin on the handle of the compress, though not infallible, is an indicator that the curing unit performed its function.

Deflasking the denture

After the denture has been cured, it is removed from the curing unit and allowed to bench cool. The denture is then ready for deflasking, finishing, and polishing.

SUMMARY

Waxing, flasking, and processing procedures for complete dentures have been described in this chapter. These are important steps in complete denture construction. Esthetics, function, and patient satisfaction depend on a skillfully waxed and properly processed prosthesis. As is the case with most dental laboratory procedures, careful attention to detail and skill achieved through experience invariably contribute to a superior prosthesis.

BIBLIOGRAPHY

Boucher, C. O., Hickey, C., and Zarb, G. A.: Prosthodontic treatment for edentulous patients, ed. 7, St. Louis, 1975, The C. V. Mosby Co., pp. 447-460.
Feldmann, E. E., and Calomeni, A. A.: Complete denture laboratory manual, San Antonio, Tex., 1977, The University of Texas Health Science Center.
Martinelli, N.: Dental laboratory technology, ed. 2, St. Louis, 1975, The C. V. Mosby Co., pp. 150-157.
Sharry, J. J.: Complete denture prosthodontics, ed. 3, New York, 1974, McGraw-Hill Book Co.
Sowter, J. B., Dental laboratory technology: prosthodontic technique, Chapel Hill, N.C., 1968, The University of North Carolina Press, pp. 88-95.

CHAPTER 9

FINISHING AND POLISHING

KENNETH D. RUDD, ROBERT M. MORROW, AMBROCIO V. ESPINOZA,
and JESSE S. LEACHMAN

finishing and polishing Removal of excess restoration material
from the margins and contours of a restoration and polishing of
the restoration.
polishing (noun) The art or process of making a denture or casting
smooth and glossy.
polishing (verb) Making smooth and glossy usually by friction: to
give luster.

After the complete dentures have been cured, they
are removed from the curing unit and bench cooled to
room temperature. Then the dentures are removed from
the flask and remounted in the articulator. Occlusion
errors are corrected, a face-bow index is made when
indicated, and the dentures are removed from the cast
and finished and polished. Methods of deflasking complete, dentures, constructing a face-bow index, and
polishing complete dentures will be described in this
chapter.

DEFLASKING

When deflasking complete dentures, it is best to use a
deflasker,* which allows retrieval from the flask without
damage to the dentures or flask (Fig. 9-1). Deflasking
with a hammer can damage the flask and result in unnecessary breakage of the dentures (Fig. 9-2).

PROCEDURE

1. Remove the lid from the flask containing the bench-
cooled denture (Fig. 9-3).
2. Place the flask, bottom side up, in the deflasker,

and tighten the thumbscrew until it contacts the bottom
plate (Fig. 9-4).
3. Place the pry bars through the slots in the side of
the deflasker, and engage the slots in the flask between
both halves of the flask (Fig. 9-5).
4. Press down on the engaged pry bars first (Fig. 9-6),
and then pry up (Fig. 9-7). These movements readily
separate the flask from the stone enclosed denture.
5. Place a knife-blade in contact with the junction between the stone cap and the rest of the stone enclosing
the denture. Tap the back of the knife blade with a plastic mallet to separate the stone cap and to expose the
cusp tips and incisal edges of the denture teeth (Fig.
9-8).
6. Use care in separating the stone cap from dentures
with porcelain teeth (Fig. 9-9).
7. With a saw and a spiral blade, cut through the stone
that encloses the denture opposite the central incisor
teeth (Fig. 9-10). Take care to avoid sawing into the
teeth or denture base.
8. Place more saw cuts at the distobuccal corners of
the flasked denture (Fig. 9-11), so that the stone enclosing the denture has three cuts (Fig. 9-12).
9. Place a knife in the anterior saw cut, and pry gently
to separate the stone from the buccal and anterior
flanges of the denture (Fig. 9-13).
10. Place a knife in the posterior cut, and pry laterally
to separate any posterior section of stone that may have
adhered to the buccal flange of the denture (Fig. 9-14).
11. Remove stone from the palate or tongue area of
the mandibular dentures by first relieving the stone
adjacent to the lingual surfaces of the denture teeth

---

*Teledyne Dental Products Co., Hanau Division, Buffalo, N.Y.

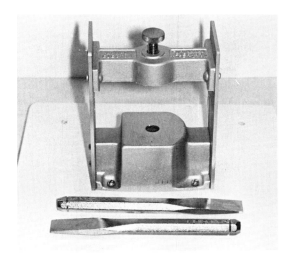

Fig. 9-1. Deflasker and pry bars facilitate quick removal of stone and dentures from flasks without damage to denture or flask.

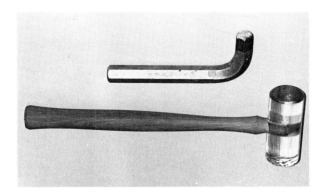

Fig. 9-2. Hammering stone from flask with plastic hammer or metal L wrench eventually ruins flask and often breaks denture base or teeth.

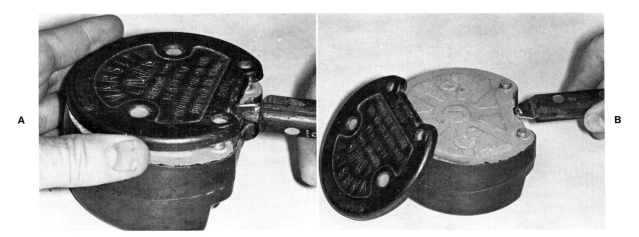

Fig. 9-3. A, Blade of heavy-bladed laboratory knife is placed in slot between top and upper half of flask, and top is lifted off. **B,** Top is removed from flask with knife in position shown.

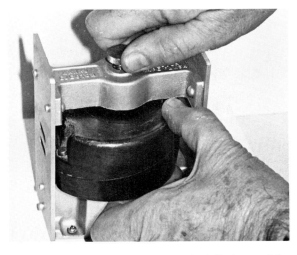

Fig. 9-4. Flask is placed bottom side up in deflasker, and thumb-screw is tightened.

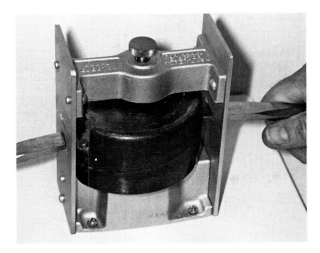

Fig. 9-5. Pry bars inserted through slots in sides of deflasker to engage slots in flask.

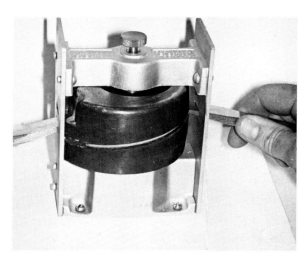

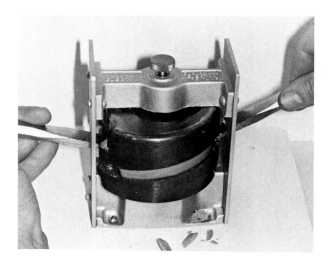

Fig. 9-6. With pry bars engaged, pry down on them to separate bottom half of flask. Thumbscrew contacting bottom circular plate holds stone in position.

Fig. 9-7. Pry bars are lifted up to separate top half of flask. Note that top half is on bottom, since flask is in deflasker, bottom side up.

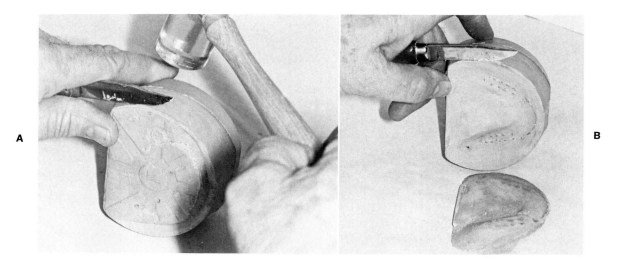

A   B

Fig. 9-8. A, Tap back of knife blade with plastic mallet to separate stone cap. **B,** Separating medium properly applied facilitates separation of stone cap, exposing cusp tips of denture teeth.

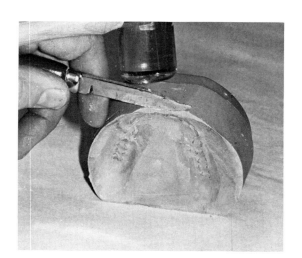

Fig. 9-9. Solid tap with knife held in this position can fracture one or more porcelain anterior teeth. Place knife at side as shown in Fig. 9-8, *B.*

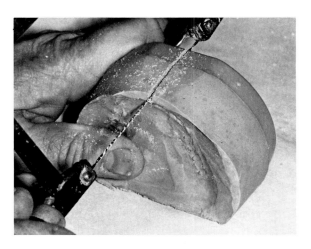

Fig. 9-10. Saw through investing stone, using spiral blade.

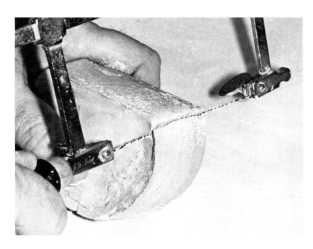

Fig. 9-11. Additional saw cuts are made at distobuccal corners of flasked denture.

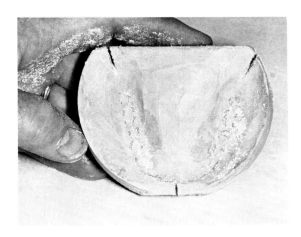

Fig. 9-12. Three saw cuts are made in investing stone.

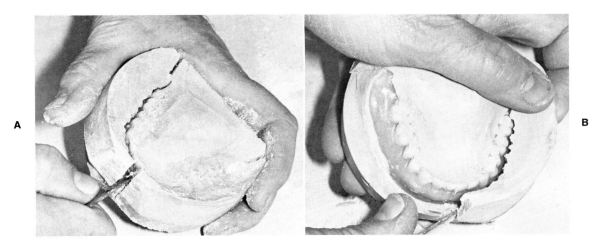

Fig. 9-13. A, Plaster knife blade is placed in anterior saw cut, and stone is pried from buccal contours of denture. **B,** After one section is removed, remaining buccal section is separated.

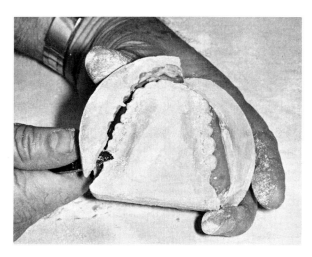

Fig. 9-14. If it is difficult to separate second section, pry in posterior saw cut to break it loose.

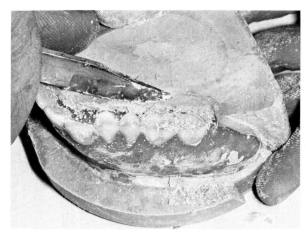

Fig. 9-15. Stone is cut away from lingual surfaces of teeth before attempting to remove it from palate of upper dentures or lingual region of lower dentures. Otherwise, these teeth can be fractured when stone is removed. Shell blaster can be used to expose teeth if care is taken to keep resin from being burned.

with a knife (Fig. 9-15). Take care to avoid cutting the teeth or denture base.

12. After relieving the stone adjacent to the lingual surfaces of the denture teeth, gently pry the stone in the lingual area of the mandibular denture or the palate of the maxillary denture, and lift it away from the denture (Fig. 9-16).

13. Make more cuts lingual to the heel area of the mandibular dentures if necessary (Fig. 9-17).

14. Remove the denture from the investing stone except where it encloses the cast (Fig. 9-18).

15. Protect the teeth with the hand and, with a plastic mallet, carefully tap away the stone enclosing the cast. Exercise care to avoid damaging the teeth by striking them with the mallet (Fig. 9-19).

16. Use a toothbrush to clean out the index grooves on the base of the cast (Fig. 9-20). This cleansing makes it possible to position the cast accurately on the mounting stone for correction of any processing error.

17. After retrieval from the stone, the dentures are ready for remounting on the articulator (Fig. 9-21).

PROBLEM AREAS

Problems that occur during deflasking are (1) breaking of the denture, (2) breaking of the cast, or (3) breaking of both. A secondary problem is damage to the flask as a result of using a hammer to tap the stone from the flask. Attention to the details of flasking to eliminate undercuts, proper use of tinfoil substitute, and careful deflasking procedures minimize breakage of the dentures and facilitate rapid retrieval (Table 9-1).

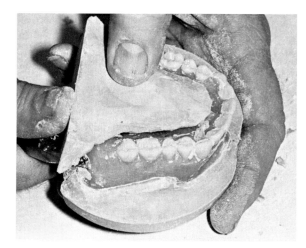

Fig. 9-16. Lift palatal section of stone from denture. Note that lingual surfaces of teeth are cleared first.

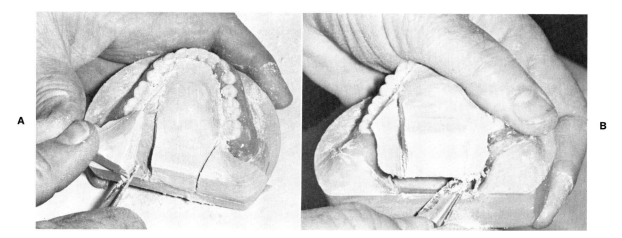

Fig. 9-17. A, It may be necessary to take out more wedges of stone before removing lingual section of stone from mandibular dentures. **B,** Remaining lingual section of stone is pried from denture gently after other wedges are removed. Removal of small wedges can prevent fracturing of mandibular cast.

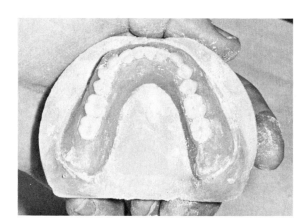

Fig. 9-18. Investing stone was removed except around base of cast.

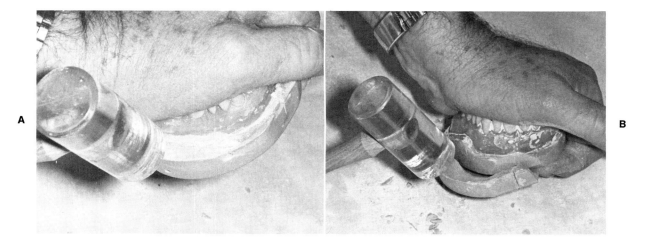

Fig. 9-19. A, Protect denture teeth with hand before tapping away remaining stone. **B,** In this manner, rest of stone is separated from cast, and denture teeth are not struck with mallet inadvertently.

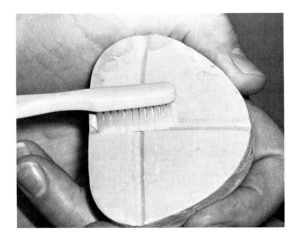

Fig. 9-20. Brush index grooves with toothbrush to remove particles of stone that prevent accurate replacement in articulator.

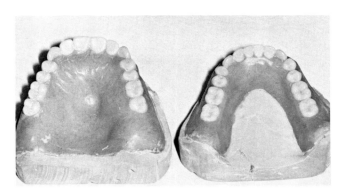

Fig. 9-21. Dentures ready for remounting in articulator to correct any processing error. Some dentists prefer to make this correction after making new jaw relation record and remounting.

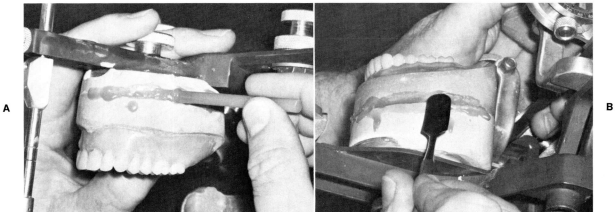

A

B

Fig. 9-22. A, Maxillary cast is sealed to mounting stone with sticky wax. Make certain that cast and mounting stone fit together accurately before sealing. B, Mandibular cast is sealed to mounting stone in similar manner.

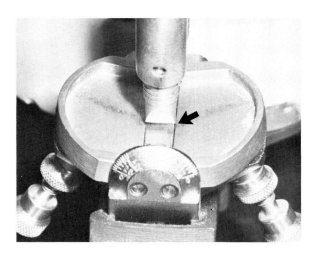

Fig. 9-23. Close articulator, and check incisal pin to determine amount of processing error (arrow).

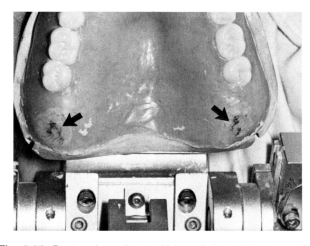

Fig. 9-24. Denture base is too thick as indicated by articulating paper marks (arrows). This problem usually results from removing dentures from articulator for final waxing and not replacing them to check occlusion.

Table 9-1. Deflasking

Problem	Probable cause	Solution
Denture base or denture teeth broken during deflasking	Deflasker not used to deflask denture Knife blade hit teeth when removing stone cap Hammer used to tap denture out of flask	Use deflasker to remove flask from enclosed stone Place knife blade on side of investing stone, not on anterior side; control depth of penetration Do not use hammer to tap stone away from denture
Stone adhering to surface of denture	Failure to place tinfoil substitute on stone prior to packing Tinfoil substitute contaminated with stone Tinfoil substitute diluted too much prior to painting on stone	Paint tinfoil substitute on stone prior to packing denture base resin Use fresh tinfoil substitute poured into small container from storage jar; do not dip directly into storage jar Do not overdilute tinfoil substitute to achieve workable consistency
Casts cracked and distorted and unable to fit together with mounting stone accurately.	Casts distorted by hammering on them when retrieving dentures from flask	Use deflasker to remove flask from stone

REMOUNTING DENTURES

After the index grooves or notches are cleaned, the dentures and casts are sealed to the mounting stone with sticky wax (Fig. 9-22).

PROCEDURE

1. After remounting the dentures in the articulator, check the relationship of the incisal guide pin to the incisal guide table (Fig. 9-23). Often the incisal guide pin does not contact the incisal guide table because of changes during processing. A processing error of 1 mm, though not insignificant, is correctable. However, an error of more than 1 mm, which often requires considerable reduction on the occlusal surfaces of the denture teeth to regain the vertical dimension of occlusion, is undesirable.

2. Check contacts between the heel of mandibular dentures and the tuberosity region of maxillary dentures to make certain that the increase in vertical dimension is not the result of an overly thick denture base resin in these areas (Fig 9-24).

3. Place articulating paper between the teeth, and gently tap the articulator together to indicate deflective occlusal contacts (Fig. 9-25).

4. Adjust these contacts with a stone if the teeth are porcelain or a bur if the teeth are resin (Fig. 9-26). Continue to adjust the occlusion in the centric relation position and in the eccentric positions, according to the rules of selective grinding. Do not adjust the cusps in the centric relation position unless they are high not only in the centric relation position, but also in the right- and left-lateral and protrusive positions. Generally, reduction results in grinding of the fossae rather than the cusp tips. When adjusting the working position, adjust the buccal cusps of the upper teeth and the lingual cusps of the mandibular teeth to eliminate deflective contacts. On the nonworking, or balancing side, deflective contacts are usually on centric holding cusps, and grinding requires a compromise. We prefer to grind the inclines of the maxillary lingual cusps rather than the buccal cusps of the mandibular dentures.

5. Move the articulator into a working position, and examine the relationship of the working cusps (Fig. 9-27). Mark the deflective contacts with articulating paper, and examine the resulting pattern (Fig. 9-28). Eliminate deflective contacts on porcelain teeth by adjusting the buccal cusps of the maxillary teeth and the lingual cusps of the mandibular teeth with a stone.

6. Examine the balancing contacts in a similar manner, and adjust the lingual cusps of the maxillary teeth or the buccal cusps of the mandibular teeth to correct deflective contacts (Fig. 9-29).

7. After completing the selective grinding, move the articulator into the various positions, and check the occlusion with tissue paper strips. Now the incisal guide pin should contact the incisal guide table and, thereby, indicate reestablishment of the original vertical dimension of occlusion (Fig. 9-30). Do not complete definitive polishing of the occlusal surfaces of the teeth at this time because the dentist usually remounts the dentures on the day of insertion.

8. Recheck the occlusion on the articulator in the centric relation position, using articulator paper, and evaluate the pattern of contacts. Equalize the contacts on the right and left sides to assure a uniform distribution (Fig. 9-31).

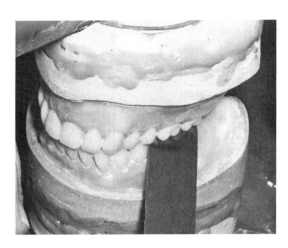

Fig. 9-25. Articulating paper is used to indicate teeth with deflective occlusal contacts. Articulator condylar elements are locked securely in centric position for this check.

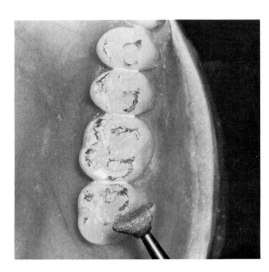

Fig. 9-26. Each mark is analyzed before any decision is made about grinding. In centric relation position, opposing fossa is deepened unless offending cusp is high not only in that position, but also in eccentric positions. Application of this rule *usually* results in deepening of sulci, rather than reduction of cusps when correcting centric relation position. Fine stone is used to modify porcelain teeth, and bur or stone is used for resin teeth.

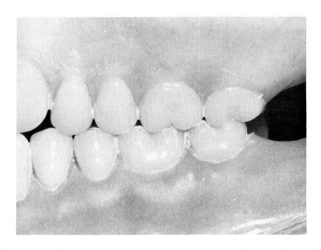

Fig. 9-27. Articulator is moved into working position, and cuspal relationship between maxillary and mandibular teeth is examined.

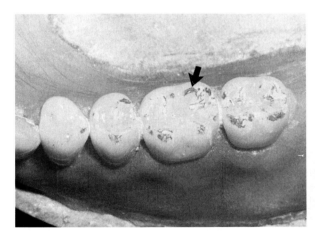

Fig. 9-28. Working contacts are marked with articulating paper and adjusted if necessary. Inclines of buccal cusps of maxillary teeth and inclines of lingual cusps of mandibular teeth are adjusted to provide smooth lateral movements without cuspal interference. Lingual cusps of mandibular molars, indicating heavier contact, will be reduced (arrow).

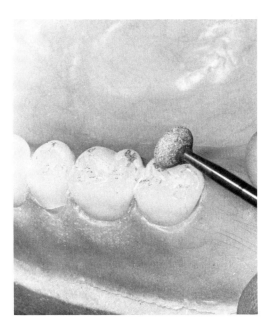

Fig. 9-29. Maxillary lingual cusps were marked by articulating paper as articulator was moved into balancing position for this side. Heavy contacts on lingual cusps were reduced.

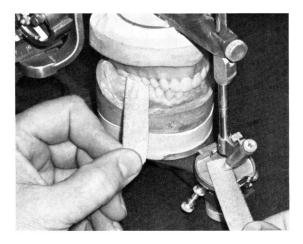

Fig. 9-30. After vertical dimension of occlusion is reestablished, tissue paper strips are used to determine whether contact is equalized on both sides.

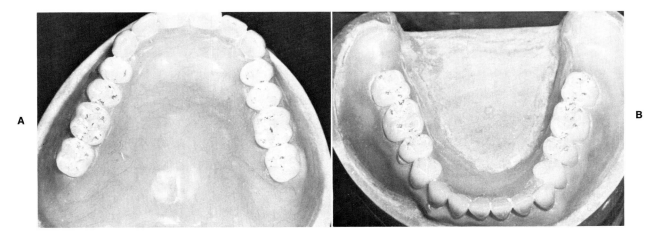

Fig. 9-31. A, Occlusal surfaces of maxillary teeth show numerous contacts with similar pressure marks. **B,** Mandibular occlusal surfaces have similar marks.

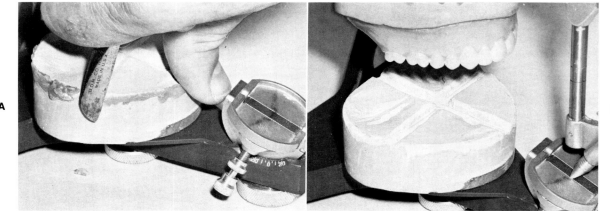

Fig. 9-32. A, Scrape sticky wax from sides of stone mounting. **B,** Sticky wax was removed from lower mounting.

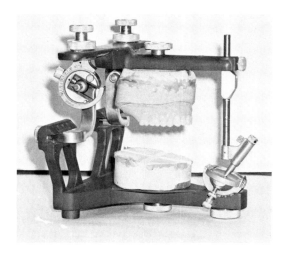

Fig. 9-33. Lower mounting stone is boxed with strip of boxing wax. In other instances, two strips may be required for sufficient height.

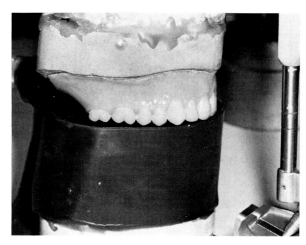

Fig. 9-34. Upper edge of boxing wax is extended 1 or 2 mm above level of occlusal surfaces of teeth to assure adequate imprint.

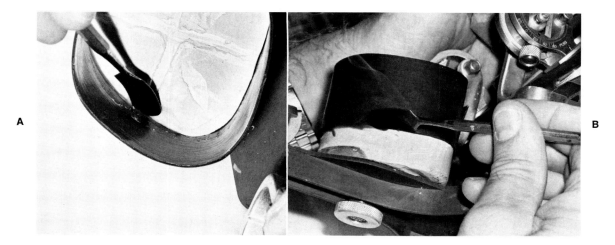

Fig. 9-35. A, Hot spatula is used to seal boxing wax to mounting stone. **B,** Wax is sealed on exterior of boxed mounting to make it watertight.

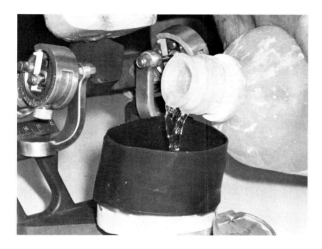

Fig. 9-36. Water poured into boxed mounting will show leaks. Soak mounting stone to assure better sticking of stone to be added.

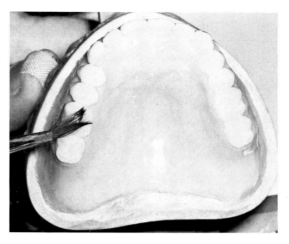

Fig. 9-37. Separating medium assures clean separation of teeth from stone.

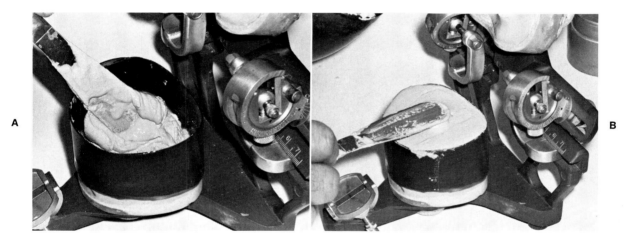

Fig. 9-38. A, Boxed enclosure is filled with stone. **B,** Stone surface is smoothed with spatula.

MAKING A FACE-BOW INDEX

After adjusting the occlusion on the articulator, making a face-bow index preserves the face-bow mounting of the maxillary denture. Unless a face-bow transfer was used for the original mounting, it is unnecessary to make a face-bow index at this time.

PROCEDURE

1. Remove the mandibular denture and cast from the mounting stone, and scrape off any sticky wax used in securing the lower cast to the mounting stone (Fig. 9-32).

2. Box the lower mounting stone with boxing wax (Fig. 9-33). Extend the upper edge of the boxing wax 1 or 2 mm above the level of the occlusal surfaces of the maxillary teeth (Fig. 9-34).

3. Seal the boxing wax to the stone to make it watertight (Fig. 9-35).

4. Pour water into the boxed stone to soak it and facilitate joining of the next pour of stone (Fig. 9-36).

5. Paint the occlusal surfaces of the maxillary teeth with a microfilm* separating medium (Fig. 9-37).

6. Mix the stone, and fill the boxed area (Fig. 9-38).

7. Place additional stone on the occlusal surfaces of the maxillary teeth (Fig. 9-39).

8. Close the articulator to create an indentation in stone of the occlusal surfaces of the maxillary teeth (Fig. 9-40).

9. Allow the stone to set; then remove the boxing

*Kerr Microfilm, Kerr Manufacturing Co., Romulus, Mich.

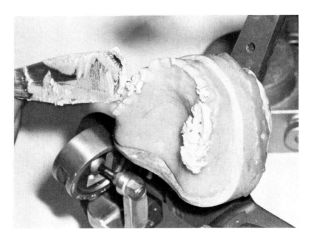

Fig. 9-39. Stone is placed on occlusal surfaces of teeth to minimize voids.

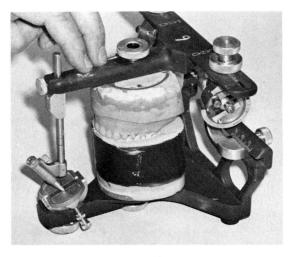

Fig. 9-40. Articulator is closed, pressing occlusal surfaces of denture teeth into stone. Tap articulator until incisal guide pin touches incisal guide table.

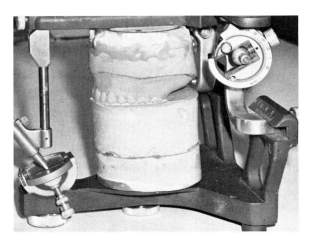

Fig. 9-41. Boxing wax is removed, and articulator opened after stone is set. Trim stone if any imprints are too deep. Face-bow index is complete.

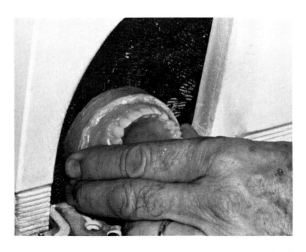

Fig. 9-42. Thickness of cast is reduced on cast trimmer to facilitate recovery of denture.

wax, and trim it. The face-bow index is complete (Fig. 9-41).

REMOVING DENTURES FROM CAST

After correction of the processing error and construction of a face-bow index if required, the dentures are ready for removal from the cast and finishing and polishing.

PROCEDURE

1. Using a cast trimmer, thin the casts with the dentures seated on them, but avoid trimming the denture base (Fig. 9-42).

2. Remove the stone from the denture in small sections (Fig. 9-43, *A*). Use a bur or a saw judiciously in removing the stone in sections without damaging the denture (Fig. 9-43, *B* and *C*).

3. A shell blaster also is useful in removing stone from the interior of the denture (Fig. 9-44).

4. A pneumatic chisel aids in removing stone from the denture; however, great care is essential to prevent damage to the denture, particularly to the denture teeth (Fig 9-45). Do not attempt to pry the denture from the cast because it can result in fracturing the denture. After removal from the cast, the dentures are ready for finishing and polishing.

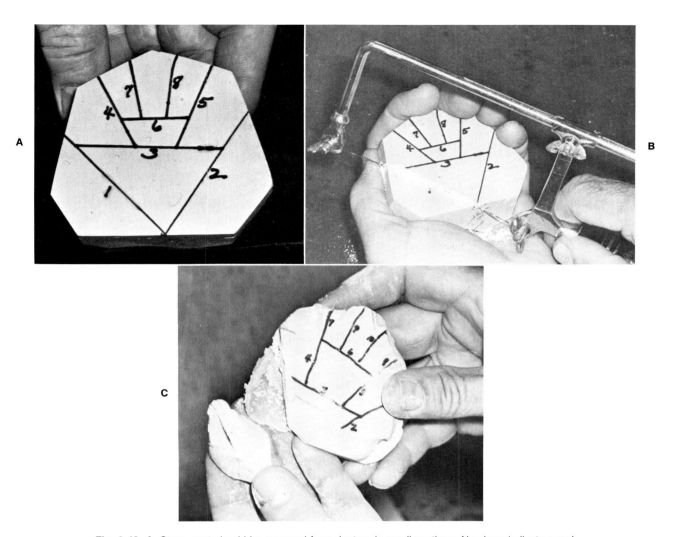

Fig. 9-43. A, Stone cast should be removed from denture in small sections. Numbers indicate usual sequence. **B,** Saw or bur can be used to section stone. Care must be taken to not damage denture base. **C,** Freed section of stone is removed.

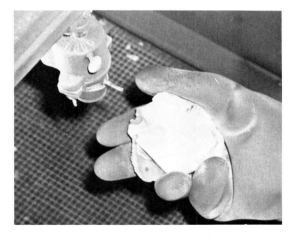

Fig. 9-44. Laboratory shell blaster is very effective for removing stone. Use care to not burn resin.

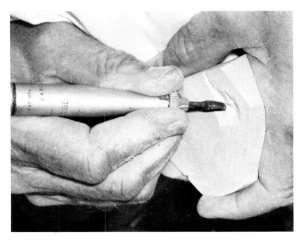

Fig. 9-45. Pneumatic chisel can be used to remove stone.

POLISHING THE COMPLETE DENTURE

Two methods of polishing complete dentures will be presented.

PROCEDURE FOR METHOD ONE

1. After taking the complete denture from the cast, use a shell blaster to remove any stone that adheres to the denture. Take care to avoid burning the surface of the acrylic resin when shell blasting.

2. Trim the flash from the complete denture with an arbor band or a large bur mounted on a laboratory lathe (Fig. 9-46).

3. Finish the frenum attachments with a small carbide bur to create the desired freedom (Fig. 9-47).

4. With a chisel carefully remove stone adhering to the gingival margins (Fig. 9-48). Make a chisel by grinding a broken instrument to form a sharp triangular edge, which facilitates the removal of stone from the gingival margin.

5. Check the interior of the denture carefully with a finger to locate any nodules of acrylic resin, and remove them with a round bur (Fig. 9-49).

6. Complete the relief for the frenum attachments by using a No. 558 or a No. 701 bur to do the final finishing and to open the frenum attachment.

7. Finish the lingual border area of the mandibular complete denture with a handpiece-mounted small carbide bur (Fig. 9-50). Frequently, a standard size arbor band is too large for this area (Fig. 9-51).

8. Thin the palate if necessary. Take care to avoid pro-

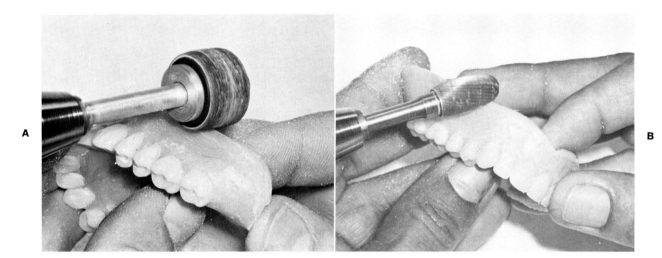

Fig. 9-46. A, Lathe-mounted arbor band is used to trim borders. **B,** Laboratory-size carbide bur is used for trimming borders.

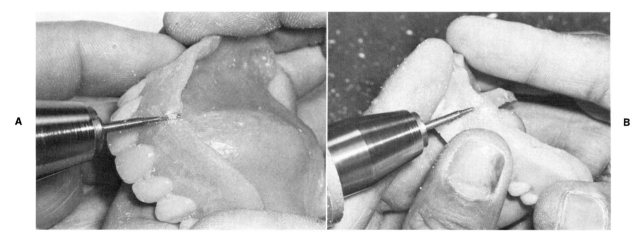

Fig. 9-47. A, Fissure bur mounted in handpiece or lathe is used to deepen frena notches. **B,** Do not make frena relief too deep for proper retention of dentures.

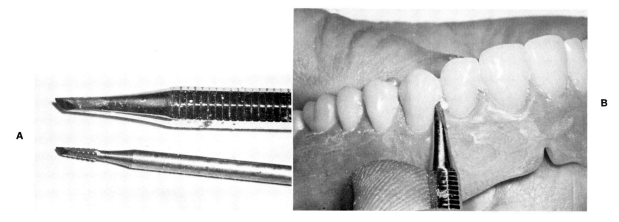

Fig. 9-48. A, Pointed chisel is made by sharpening broken dental instrument or fissure bur, then it is placed in wooden handle. **B,** Chisel is used to remove stone from between teeth or to remove acrylic resin nodules from denture.

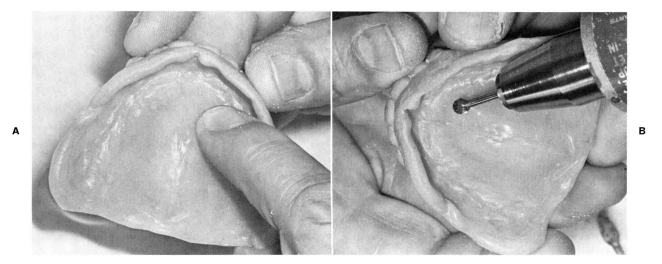

Fig. 9-49. A, Finger is used to check for nodules or sharp feather edges on denture resin. **B,** Nodules are removed with handpiece or lathe-mounted bur.

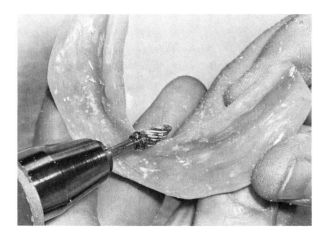

Fig. 9-50. Small handpiece-mounted or lathe-mounted carbide bur is used to finish lingual border of denture.

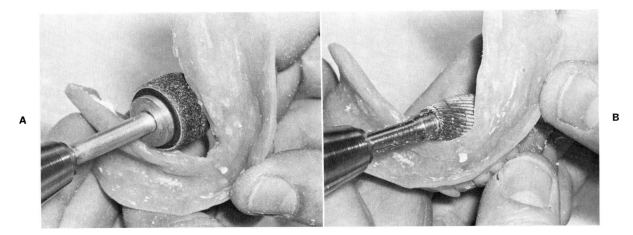

Fig. 9-51. A, Arbor band is too large for finishing this area. If used here, borders of denture can be overthinned. **B,** Laboratory bur of correct diameter for finishing border.

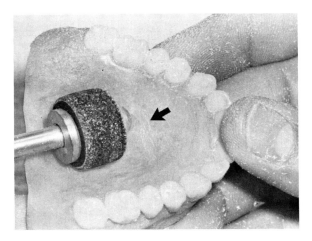

Fig. 9-52. Grooves in palate (arrow) produced by incorrect use of arbor band are difficult to remove.

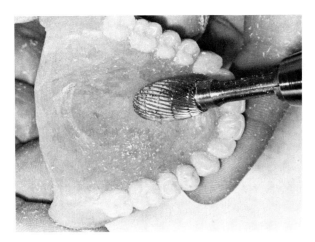

Fig. 9-53. Production of grooves is minimized by using large egg-shaped bur to reduce thickness of palate.

ducing grooves when using an arbor band (Fig. 9-52). A large lathe-mounted laboratory bur also is useful for this procedure (Fig. 9-53).

9. Pumice the dentures with a prepared rag wheel.

Preparing rag wheel

Special preparation of a rag wheel makes it more effective for pumicing and polishing. The procedure described also reconditions used rag wheels by giving them the flexibility and fluffiness necessary to achieve a smooth finish (Fig. 9-54).

PROCEDURE

1. Place the rag wheel on a spiral chuck, run the lathe at low speed, and use a knife to cut the threads holding the rag-wheel plies together. Hold the knife firmly while cutting the threads (Fig. 9-55).

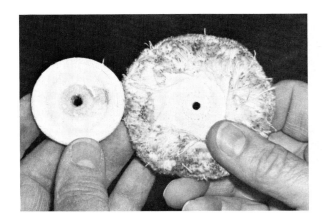

Fig. 9-54. Badly worn rag wheel in need of renovation *(left),* and fluffy wheel after reconditioning *(right).*

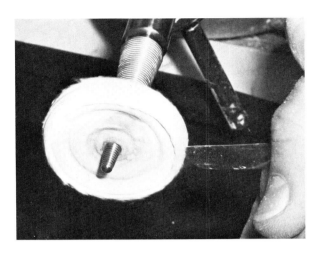

Fig. 9-55. Rotate lathe slowly, and use knife to cut threads holding cloth plies together.

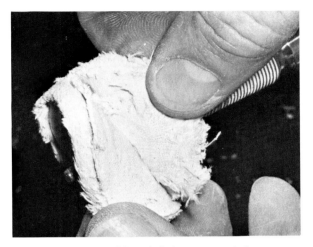

Fig. 9-56. Plies of cloth are separated.

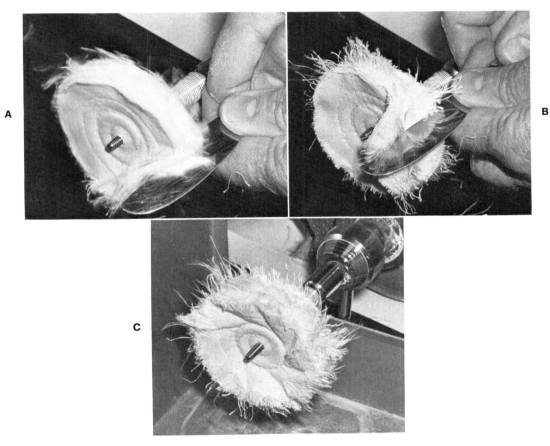

Fig. 9-57. A, Stainless steel plaster spatula or dull dinner knife is held against wheel while running lathe at low speed. **B,** Cloth plies are separated by knife. **C,** Wheel after fluffing on lathe.

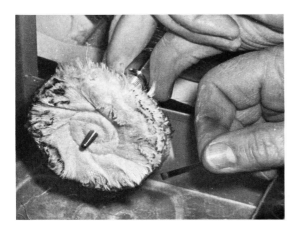

Fig. 9-58. Match used to singe off protruding threads. *Do not singe threads while suction device is in operation, because this will produce draft.* Singe rag wheel in metal pan after removing all flammable material. Have water available to douse wheel. After singeing, place rag wheel in water.

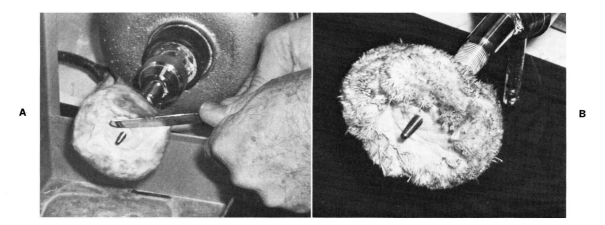

Fig. 9-59. A, Fluff singed wheel on lathe as described previously. **B,** Reconditioned rag wheel is ready for use for pumicing or producing high gloss on acrylic resin.

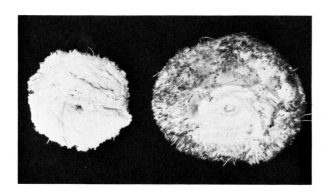

Fig. 9-60. Old rag wheel *(left)* was rehabilitated, and new rag wheel *(right)* was fluffed to improve efficiency.

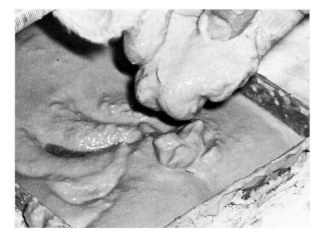

Fig. 9-61. Generous amount of flour of pumice slurry is used for polishing resin. Fine pumice polishes almost as fast as coarser grades and produces smoother surface.

2. Stop the lathe, separate the plies of the rag wheel, and make certain to cut the thread completely (Fig. 9-56).

3. With the rag wheel on the spiral chuck, rotate the lathe at low speed, and hold a stainless steel plaster spatula against the rag wheel to remove the cut threads and make the wheel fluffy (Fig. 9-57).

4. Singe the frayed threads with a lighted match to make the wheel uniform (Fig. 9-58). Place a metal pan beneath the wheel, and have the lathe and any suction device in the nonoperating position. Have a bowl of water available to douse the wheel if it flares.

5. After placing the rag wheel in water, return it to the lathe, and start the lathe at low speed. Rotate the singed wheel against the stainless steel spatula again to fluff it and remove any remaining threads (Fig. 9-59).

6. The modified rag wheel is ready for use (Fig. 9-60).

Pumicing denture
PROCEDURE

1. Make a slurry of fine flour of pumice with water (Fig. 9-61). Using copious amounts of the slurry, wet the rag wheel, and polish the denture at low speed. Move the denture throughout the polishing to prevent formation of plane surfaces. Use a brush or prophy cup with the slurry to polish areas less accessible to the rag wheel (Fig. 9-62).

2. Polish the palate and areas of the denture not

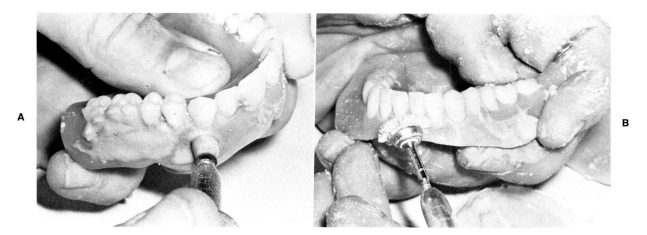

Fig. 9-62. A, Where larger rag wheel might eliminate anatomic details, polish denture with hand-piece-mounted rubber prophy cup and flour of pumice slurry. **B,** Use medium bristle brush in same manner as prophy cup.

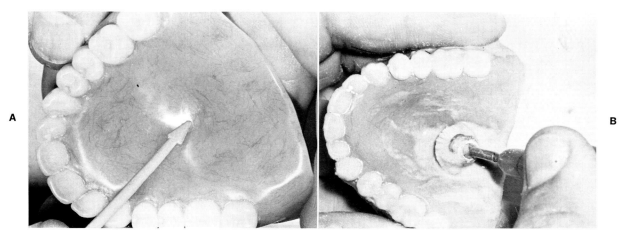

Fig. 9-63. A, Scratches deep in vault of palate are difficult to remove with rag wheel. **B,** Handpiece-mounted brush safely removes scratches or grooves in vault.

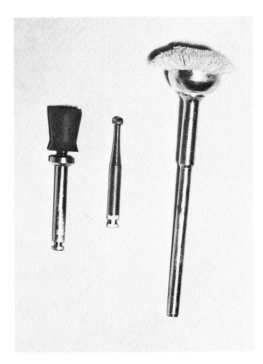

Fig. 9-64. No. 200 finishing bur *(center)*, rubber prophy cup *(left)*, and handpiece-mounted brush *(right)* are used to place stippled or eggshell surface on denture.

readily accessible to the rag wheel by using a prophy cup or a Dixon brush with slurry of flour of pumice. Smooth the denture in this manner because a larger polishing instrument would obliterate anatomic details (Fig. 9-63). After completing the pumicing, wash the denture thoroughly in water, dry it, and examine it for scratches. If any scratches are visible on the pumiced surface, repeat the pumicing, and postpone the high polishing until after removing all scratches.

3. Stipple the denture with a No. 200 finishing bur (Fig. 9-64). Rotate this bur slowly in a handpiece, and hold it in light contact with the surface of the denture to be stippled, that is, the area of the attached gingiva (Fig. 9-65). Use light random circular movements of the bur against the resin surface to produce an eggshell, or stippled, effect that breaks up light reflections and corrects minor imperfections in the resin (Fig. 9-66).

4. Go over the stippled area lightly with a rubber prophy cup and a slurry of flour of pumice (Fig. 9-67).

5. Put a high shine on the denture with No. 341 Ti-Gleam*, or prepared chalk slurry, and a modified rag wheel (Fig. 9-68). Do not use this rag wheel with any other polishing material. Examine the denture carefully for scratches, and polish out any missed previously (Fig. 9-69). Take care when polishing or pumicing the denture to keep from abrading the anatomic details of the plastic teeth.

6. Brush the denture with green soap to remove all traces of polishing material, and examine the denture carefully. Rinse the denture in water, and store it in a plastic container of water until needed (Fig. 9-70).

---

*No. 341 TiGleam, Ticonium, Albany, N.Y., or equivalent.

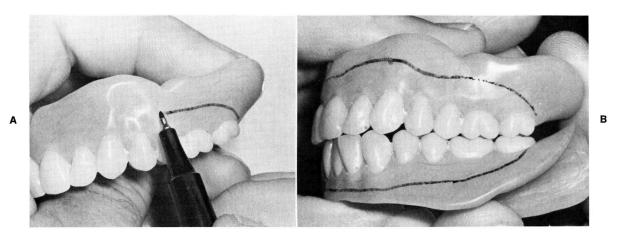

Fig. 9-65. A, Area of denture to be stippled is outlined with felt-tip pen. Stippling or peened surface is confined to area occupied by attached gingiva. **B,** Areas on maxillary and mandibular dentures are outlined for stippling.

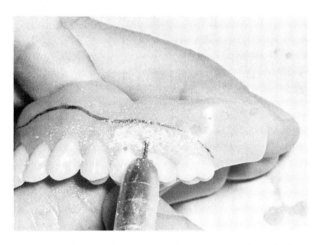

Fig. 9-66. Random circular movements at slow speed with light pressure are used to create stippled surface. Position of denture is changed to facilitate making random swirls.

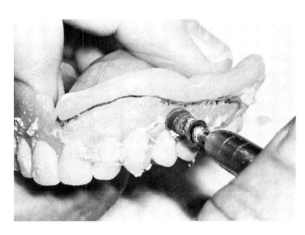

Fig. 9-67. Pumice stippling with flour of pumice slurry and hand-piece-mounted rubber prophy cup. Pumice lightly to avoid polishing away stippled surface.

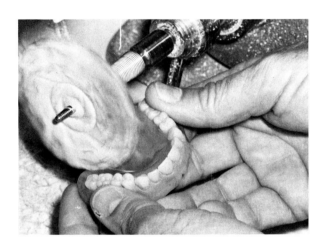

Fig. 9-68. Denture is buffed to high luster. Prepared chalk slurry, No. 341 TiGleam, Shur-shine, rouge, or other high-shine materials can be used to create highly polishing surface.

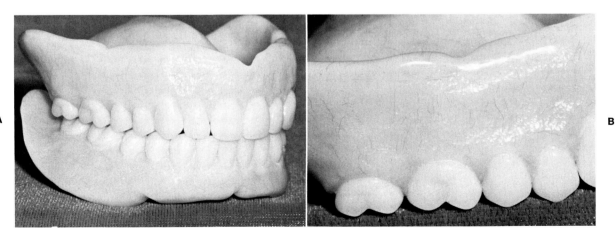

Fig. 9-69. A, Dentures are examined carefully for scratches, and high shine is restored after scratches are removed. **B,** Note effect of stippling.

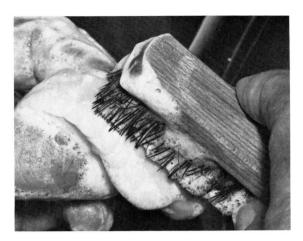

Fig. 9-70. Denture is cleaned thoroughly with brush and soap solution to remove all traces of polishing materials. Completed denture is rinsed and stored in water until needed.

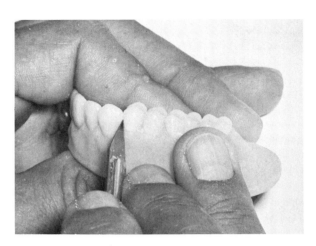

Fig. 9-71. Optional method of removing plaster or stone from denture is to use No. 25 blade in Bard-Parker handle. When using blade, exercise care to avoid cutting fingers or plastic teeth.

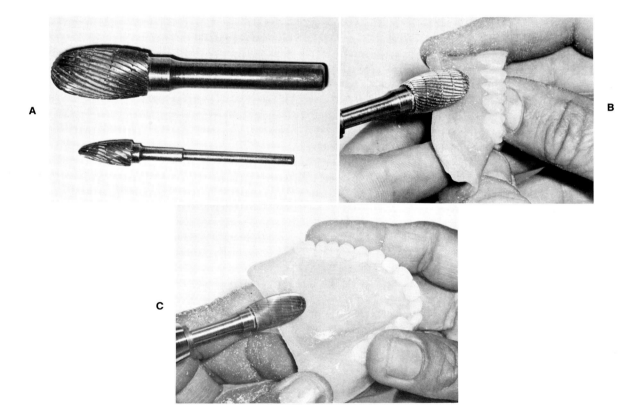

Fig. 9-72. A, Carbide burs for laboratory use are excellent for removing resin flash. Lower bur can be used in lathe or handpiece. **B,** Flash is removed from buccal border. **C,** Flash on posterior border is removed, and area is thinned.

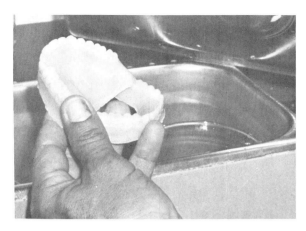

Fig. 9-73. Dentures can be placed in ultrasonic cleaner containing appropriate solution before or after flash is removed. Stone remaining around teeth is removed quickly and easily.

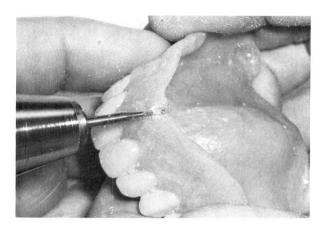

Fig. 9-74. Adjust for frenum clearance with lathe-mounted fissure bur.

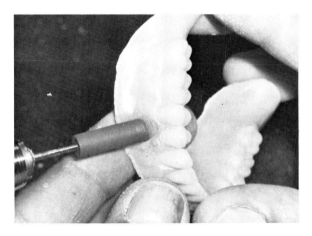

Fig. 9-75. Rubber points can be shaped for particular area to be smoothed. Care is required to avoid damage to plastic teeth.

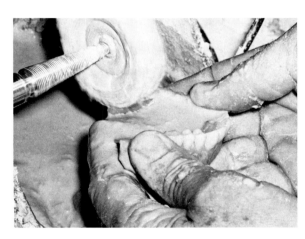

Fig. 9-76. Flour of pumice mixed with water and modified rag wheel are used to polish denture.

PROCEDURE FOR METHOD TWO

1. Remove the denture from the cast as described previously.

2. Remove the stone that adheres to the gingival-margin area of the denture with a Bard-Parker handle and a No. 25 blade (Fig. 9-71). Trim away excess flash with a laboratory lathe-mounted carbide bur (Fig. 9-72). Place the denture in an ultrasonic cleaner, containing a solution for removal of gypsum products (Fig. 9-73). Adjust for frenum clearance with a No. 558 bur mounted in a laboratory lathe (Fig. 9-74).

3. Use a rubber point* mounted on a mandrel and a dental lathe to remove scratches from the denture base

*No. 255 clasp polishers, Ticonium, Albany, N.Y.

in areas inaccessible to the larger pumice wheel (Fig. 9-75). Pumice the denture using flour of pumice or fine pumice mixed with water and a modified rag wheel, as described previously (Fig. 9-76).

4. Polish areas between the teeth with a bristle brush and pumice slurry (Fig. 9-77).

5. Put the initial high shine on the denture with a soft rag wheel and prepared chalk mixed with water (Fig. 9-78).

6. Put the final high shine on the denture with a soft chamois wheel and gold rouge (Fig. 9-79).

7. Stipple the denture with a straight handpiece No. 4 round bur bent slightly to rotate eccentrically (Fig. 9-80).

8. Place the bur in a lathe and, with the lathe running

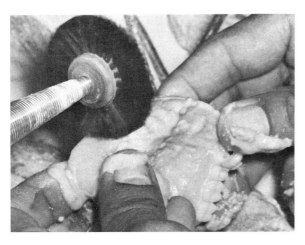

Fig. 9-77. Polish interproximal areas with lathe-mounted brush wheel and flour of pumice slurry. Caution is advised if plastic teeth are used, since anatomic details can be polished away.

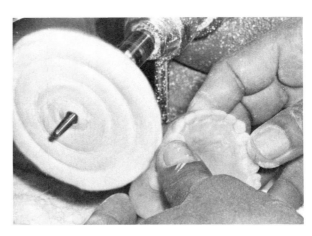

Fig. 9-78. Rag wheel and prepared chalk mixed with water are used for initial high shine. This rag wheel should not be used with other polishing materials.

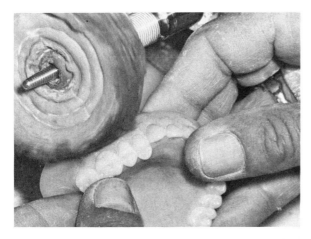

Fig. 9-79. Soft chamois wheel and gold rouge are used for final high shine.

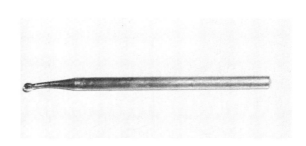

Fig. 9-80. Straight handpiece No. 4 round bur bent slightly for use in stippling.

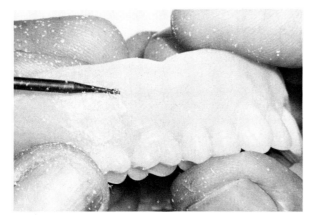

Fig. 9-81. Modified bur produces stippled surface. Do not bend bur too much or use excessive pressure when stippling to avoid creating rough surface.

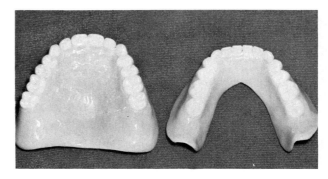

Fig. 9-82. Dentures are examined carefully, touched up wherever necessary, scrubbed thoroughly, and stored in water until needed.

at slow speed, stipple the surface of the denture base in a random motion (Fig. 9-81). Apply a high polish to the dentures again, scrub them with soap and water, and place them in a container of water until ready for use by the dentist (Fig. 9-82).

POLISHING TEETH

Acrylic resin teeth are polished by the same method as the denture base material. A rubber prophy cup and fine pumice or flour of pumice are used to restore the surface luster of acrylic teeth after modification. A high luster is restored to the surface of these teeth with a soft rag wheel and a high-shine material, such as rouge or prepared chalk slurry. Care should be taken when polishing resin teeth to avoid removing too much material from the occlusal surfaces and, thereby, affecting the occlusion. One disadvantage of using plastic teeth is the possibility of altering them during the polishing by inadvertent contact between the teeth and polishing wheel.

Polishing porcelain teeth

Since it is more difficult to polish ground porcelain teeth than acrylic teeth, restoring a satisfactory surface requires more effort.

PROCEDURE

1. Smooth the surface of ground porcelain teeth with a medium polishing wheel.*

2. Smooth the surface again with a fine polishing wheel.†

3. Polish in two directions with a lathe-mounted rag wheel and a slurry of flour of pumice.

4. Do the final polishing with a clean lathe-mounted rag wheel and a slurry of porcelain finishing polish.‡

The procedure described restores an acceptable surface to porcelain teeth, although it is not as smooth as the original glaze.

SUMMARY

Methods for deflasking, finishing, and polishing complete dentures have been described in this chapter. The success of the restoration is often directly related to the quality of the technical procedures involved.

---

*Super-polish wheel No. 37, ⅝ × ⅛ inch (1.6 × 0.32 cm), medium grit, Dental Development and Manufacturing Co., Brooklyn, N.Y.
†Superpolish wheel No. 37, ⅝ × ⅛ inch (1.6 × 0.32 cm), fine grit, Dental Development and Manufacturing Co., Brooklyn, N.Y.
‡Tru-polish No. 3, Dentsply International, Inc., York, Pa.

CHAPTER 10

DUPLICATE DENTURES

KENNETH D. RUDD and ROBERT M. MORROW

duplicate denture A second denture intended to be a copy of the first denture.

A spare or backup denture is a definite advantage for the patient whose original denture requires repair or modification. The laterature contains reports of several methods of duplicating dentures with heat-curing and autopolymerizing resin (Geiger, 1955; Adam, 1958; Shaw, 1962; Manoli and Griffin, 1969; Azarmehr and Azarmehr, 1970; Zoeller and Beetar, 1970; Wagner, 1970; Boos and Carpenter, 1974; Brewer and Morrow, 1975; Singer, 1975).

METHODS

This chapter presents three methods of duplicating dentures with pour-type autopolymerizing resin.* The methods differ principally in the type of flask and the investing medium used. They are (1) the modified–denture flask method (Brewer and Morrow, 1975), (2) the pour-resin–flask method (Boos and Carpenter, 1974), and (3) the cup-flask method (Wagner, 1970; Singer, 1975).

Modified–denture flask method

This method requires the use of a modified denture flask and alginate irreversible hydrocolloid to flask the denture to be duplicated.

PROCEDURE

1. Modify the denture flask by removing a rectangular section from the upper part (Fig. 10-1). This opening will allow access for the sprues. Although it is unnecessary to have a new flask, the parts should fit together accurately without rocking.

2. If the denture to be duplicated has thin areas, add wax to the *exterior* surface of the denture to thicken these areas before flasking (Fig. 10-2).

3. Roll utility wax to form a sprue approximately 75 mm long and 15 mm in diameter (Fig. 10-3).

4. Attach the sprues to the lingual surface of the heels of mandibular dentures and to the palatal surface of the tuberosity region of maxillary dentures (Fig. 10-4).

5. Paint the round plate from the lower part of the flask with an adhesive,* and insert it from the *exterior* surface, rather than from the interior (Fig. 10-5). This insertion prevents distortion of the alginate mold by inadvertent displacement of the plate while handling the flask.

6. Apply the same adhesive* to the interior surface of the flask to facilitate retention of the alginate (Fig. 10-6).

7. Mix eight scoops of regular setting alginate with the recommended volume of water for the first pour. Cooling the water will allow additional working time.

8. Mix the alginate with a mechanical spatulator†

---

*Pronto II, Vernon-Benshoff Co., Inc., Albany, N.Y.; Pour-N-Cure, Coe Laboratories Inc., Chicago, Ill.; or TruPour Fluid Resin System, Dentsply International, Inc., York, Pa.

*Hold, Teledyne Dental Products Co., Getz/Opotow Division, Elk Grove Village, Ill.
†Combination Vac-U-Vestor Power Mixer, Whip-Mix Corp., Louisville, Ky.

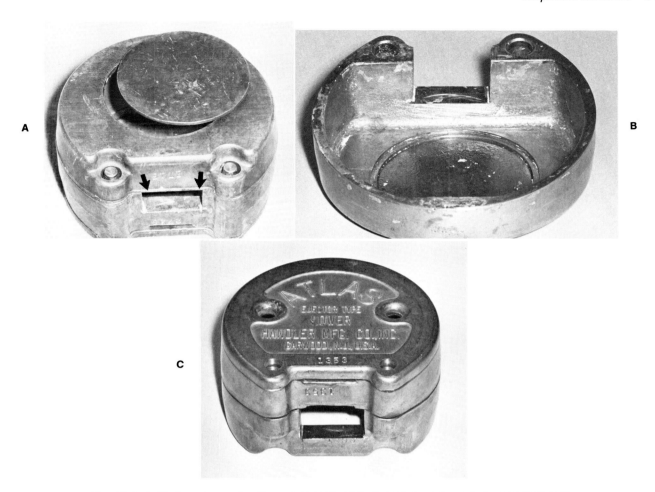

Fig. 10-1. A, Rectangular section (arrows) is removed from cope or upper part of upper flask or **B,** from drag or lower part of lower flask. **C,** Wax sprues will extend through opening.

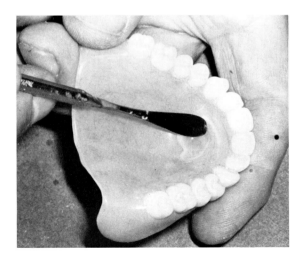

Fig. 10-2. Wax is added to exterior surface of denture where thinness can result in miscast.

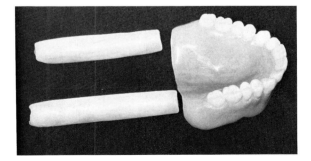

Fig. 10-3. Sprues of utility wax or orthodontic tray wax should be approximately 75 mm long and 15 mm in diameter.

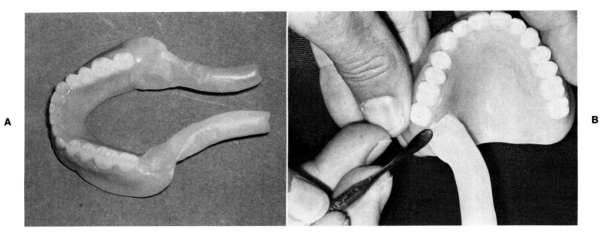

Fig. 10-4. A, Sprues should be added to lingual surfaces of mandibular heel region. Portions of denture should not extend above sprue attachment when held vertically to prevent entrapment of air during pouring of resin and resultant void. B, Sprues are attached to tuberosity regions of maxillary dentures. Seal sprues to denture with wax spatula.

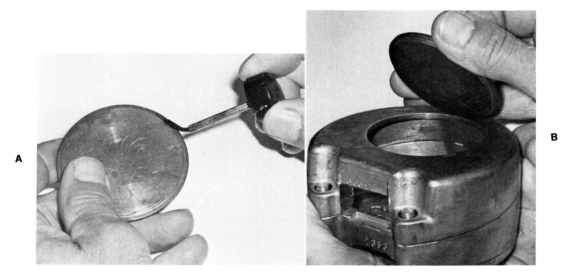

Fig. 10-5. A, Edges of round plate are painted with adhesive (Hold). B, Plate is inserted from exterior surface rather than interior.

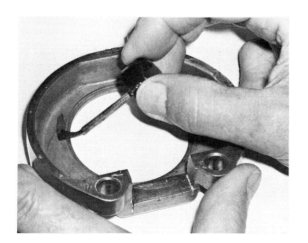

Fig. 10-6. Interior of flask is painted with adhesive (Hold) to maintain alginate in flask when halves are separated.

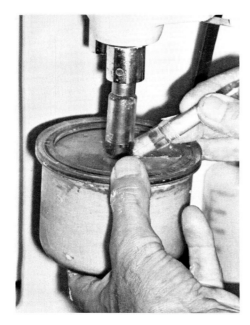

Fig. 10-7. Alginate mixed under reduced atmospheric pressure has fewer air inclusions.

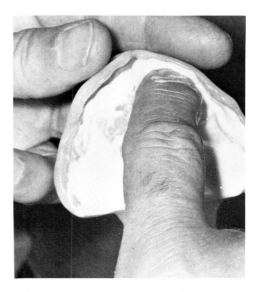

Fig. 10-8. Alginate is painted into interior of denture; care is exercised to minimize voids.

under reduced atmospheric pressure to minimize air inclusions in the material (Fig. 10-7). Hand spatulate thoroughly if a power mixer is unavailable.

9. After mixing, place alginate into the interior of the denture with a finger or a brush, taking care to avoid the entrapment of air and resultant voids (Fig. 10-8). Fill the denture completely (Fig. 10-9).

10. Place the remainder of the alginate mix in the lower part of the flask (Fig. 10-10).

11. Settle the filled denture into the mix, as during a routine flasking procedure (Fig. 10-11). The wax sprues can support the denture, thereby preventing it from sinking into the alginate (Fig. 10-12). The alginate should extend approximately 3 mm onto the exterior surface of the denture.

12. After the alginate has set, trim away any excess that flows over the edges of the flask (Fig. 10-13).

13. Place the upper part of the flask in position, and adapt the wax sprues to seal the rectangular opening (Fig. 10-14).

14. Mix six scoops of alginate with three times the recommended volume of water to make a pourable consistency.

15. Pour the alginate into the flask slowly. Use a finger or brush to wipe alginate onto the teeth of the denture to minimize voids (Fig. 10-15). The second pour will not stick to the first one.

16. Completely fill the flask, and place the top in position (Fig. 10-16). Allow the alginate to set approximately 15 minutes or longer if using cold water.

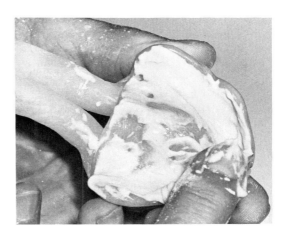

Fig. 10-9. Interior of denture is filled with alginate.

17. After the alginate has set, open the flask, and remove the denture and sprues (Fig. 10-17).

18. Place the lower part of the flask, that is, the cast side, in a humidor or under a wet towel.

19. Dry the tooth indentations in the alginate carefully. Use a gentle stream of air or a strip of cleansing tissue to remove water from the tooth imprints (Fig. 10-18).

20. Add autopolymerizing tooth-colored resin of the proper shade to the tooth indentations by the sprinkle-on or paint-on method (Fig. 10-19).

21. Carefully add the tooth-colored resin in increments, and fill the indentations to the cervical line (Fig. 10-20). Exercise care to improve materially the resultant

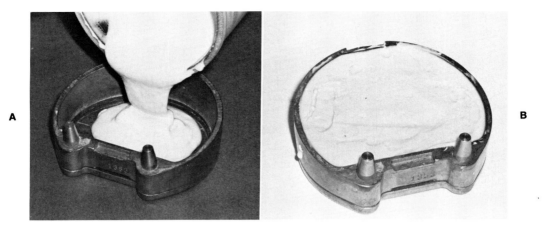

Fig. 10-10. A, Remaining alginate is placed in flask. **B,** Flask half filled with alginate.

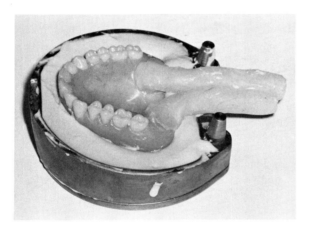

Fig. 10-11. Filled denture is settled into alginate-filled flask.

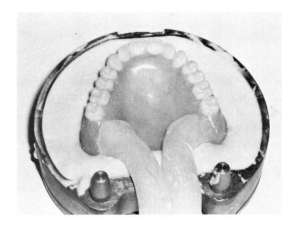

Fig. 10-12. Wax sprues are pressed into back side of flask to support denture and prevent sinking.

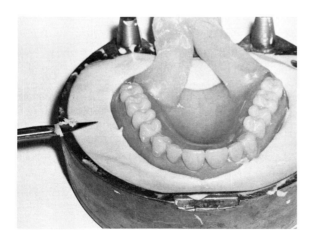

Fig. 10-13. Any alginate extending onto edges of flask is removed.

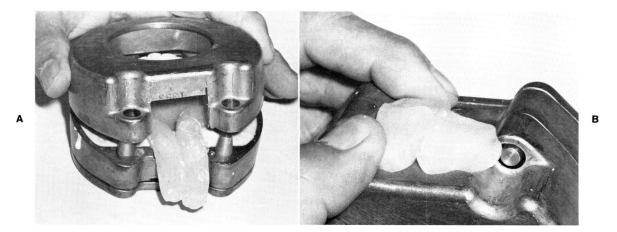

Fig. 10-14. **A,** Flask halves assembled. **B,** Fingers are used to mold wax sprues to make watertight seal. Here lower flask is being used.

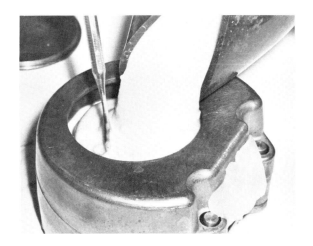

Fig. 10-15. Teeth are coated with alginate using brush, finger, or spatula. Lower flask is shown here. Hence alginate is poured through round plate opening.

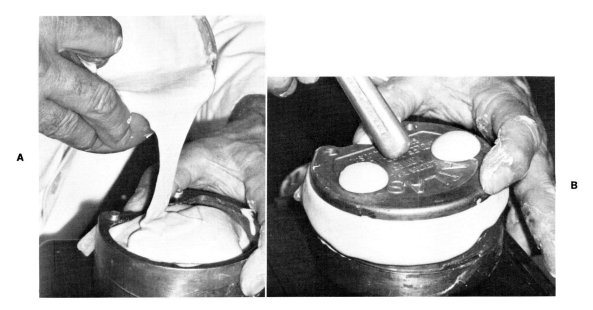

Fig. 10-16. **A,** Upper flask is filled completely with alginate, and lid is replaced. **B,** Lid is tapped to assure complete seating. If upper flask is used, pour through open top.

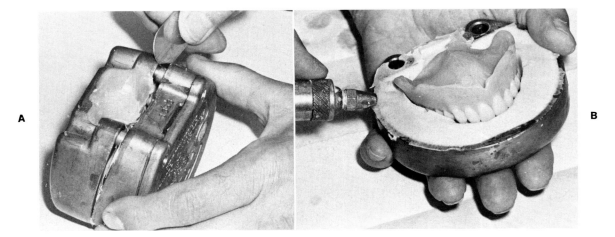

Fig. 10-17. A, Spatula is used to separate flask halves. **B,** Denture and wax sprues are removed from investing alginate. Gentle stream of air will often lift denture from alginate.

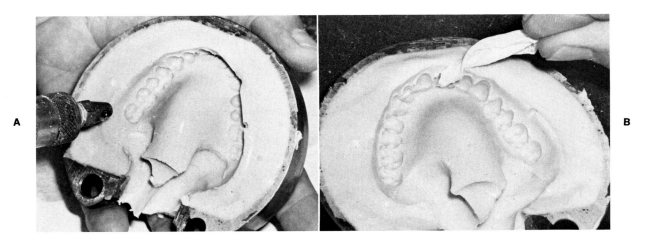

Fig. 10-18. A, Moisture is removed with gentle stream of air. **B,** Strip of absorbent tissue also can be used to remove moisture from tooth indentations.

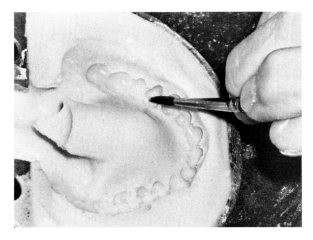

Fig. 10-19. Tooth shade–autopolymerizing resin is sprinkled or painted into indentations.

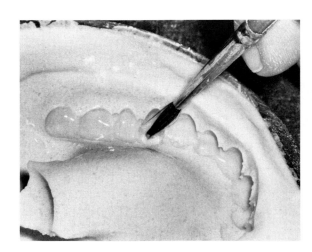

Fig. 10-20. Resin is painted or sifted to conform to cervical line. Do not overfill.

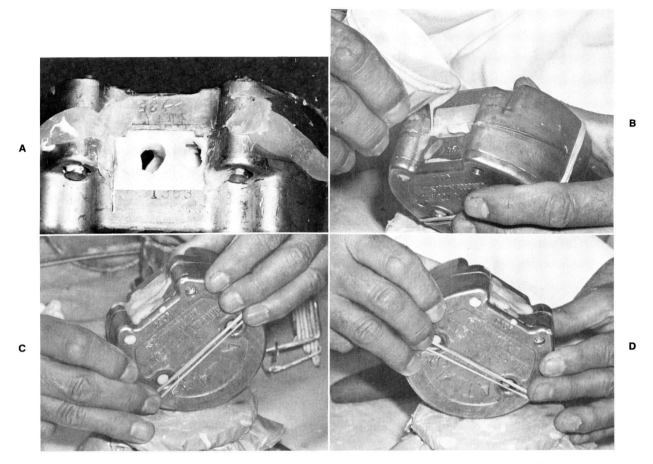

Fig. 10-21. A, Sprue hole. **B,** Resin is poured into one sprue hole only. **C** and **D,** Gently rock flask to left and right to minimize voids.

duplicate denture. It is possible to add incisal, body, and gingival shading, but it requires considerable skill to achieve good results.

22. Allow the tooth-shade resin to set for a few minutes before assembling the flask.

23. Carefully dry the alginate in the lower flask; then assemble the flask halves, and clamp or secure them with rubber bands.

24. Mix a pour-type resin* according to the manufacturer's recommendations, and pour it into one sprue hole (Fig. 10-21, *A* and *B*).

25. Rock the flask gently while pouring to minimize the entrapment of air (Fig. 10-21, *C* and *D*).

26. Fill one sprue until the resin fills the other sprue, thereby indicating that the mold is full.

27. Attach modeling clay to the filled flask, place it

sprues upward in warm water in a pressure container, and cure the denture at 20 psi for 30 minutes (Fig. 10-22).

28. Remove the cured denture, and examine it for nodules and voids (Fig. 10-23).

29. Cut off the sprues, and finish and polish the denture (Fig. 10-24), as described previously.

PROBLEM AREAS

The principal problems associated with this method are the inability to obtain a bubble-free voidless mold, failure to achieve an accurate duplication of denture teeth without rounded incisal angles, and difficulty in producing an accurate alginate mold and resultant duplicate denture (Table 10-1). Mixing the alginate in a mechanical spatulator under reduced atmospheric pressure helps to minimize voids. Painting the alginate into the denture with a finger or brush also results in fewer voids. Making acceptable autopolymerizing resin teeth in the denture requires skill and patience. Make certain

*Pronto II, Vernon-Benshoff Co., Inc., Albany, N.Y.; Pour-N-Cure, Coe Laboratories Inc., Chicago, Ill.; TruPour Fluid Resin System, Dentsply International, Inc., York, Pa.

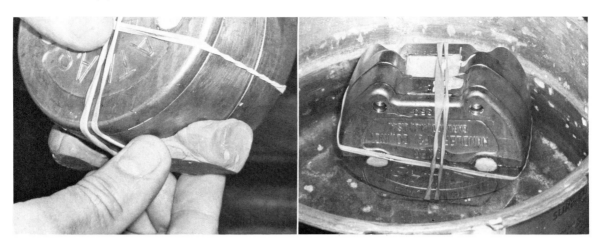

Fig. 10-22. Small pellets of modeling clay attached to flask permit it to remain with sprues upright in pressure container.

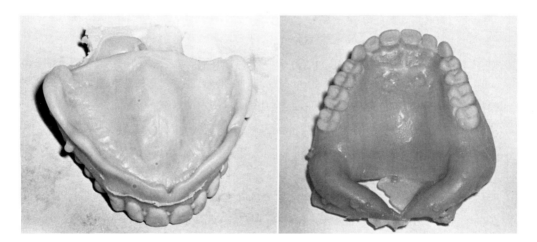

Fig. 10-23. Denture is examined carefully for voids or nodules.

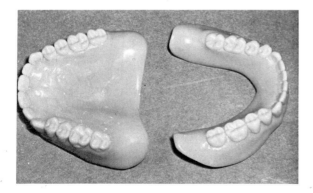

Fig. 10-24. Sprues are removed, and denture is polished.

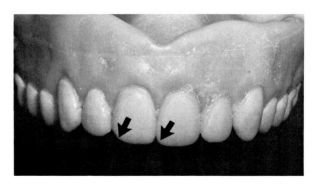

Fig. 10-25. Excess moisture is removed to reduce rounding of incisal angles (arrows).

Table 10-1. Modified–double flask method

Problem	Probable cause	Solution
Many bubbles and voids in alginate mold	Alginate not painted on denture with finger or brush	Minimize voids by painting alginate onto denture
	Alginate not mixed in mechanical spatulator contains excess air	Use mechanical spatulator to mix alginate under reduced atmospheric pressure
Duplicate denture incomplete because of voids	Thin areas in original denture	Thicken thin areas of original denture with wax to improve castability
	Sprues improperly attached	Attach sprues correctly to preclude entrapment of air
	Resin poured down both sprue holes	Pour resin into one sprue hole; use other as vent
	Flask not rocked while pouring resin	Rock flask gently during pouring to reduce possibility of entrapment of air and resultant voids in duplicate denture
Rounded incisal edges on teeth in duplicate dentures	Tooth indentations in alginate mold not dried before pouring resin	Dry tooth indentations in alginate mold with gentle stream of air or strip of absorbent tissue to remove moisture
	Moisture trapped in indentation, preventing sharp reproduction	
Teeth on duplicate denture pink in gingival third	Tooth indentations in alginate mold not completely filled with tooth resin	Fill mold indentations completely to gingival margin with tooth resin
Tooth-shaded resin on gingival papillae of denture base	Tooth resin applied improperly, permitting tooth-shaded resin to extend into papillae	Take care to confine resin to tooth indentation by using brush if necessary
Duplicate denture porous	Wrong type of resin used	Use pour-type autopolymerizing resin
	Mixing instructions of manufacturer not followed	Follow mixing instructions of manufacturer

that the tooth indentations in the alginate are dry to minimize the possibility of rounded incisal angles in the resin teeth (Fig. 10-25). Add the resin in increments, and tilt the flask while pouring. This procedure results in a controlled flow of resin. If tooth-shade resin does not fill the indentations completely, pink resin will fill the remaining portion and produce an unsatisfactory result. Adding too much tooth-colored resin may cause part of the gingival portion of the denture base to be tooth shade rather than pink and therefore undesirable. A small brush is helpful in adding resin to specific areas of the indentation, and practice assures more uniform and acceptable results.

It appears, at least clinically, that the duplicate denture made by the alginate mold–pour resin system does not exhibit the same adaptation to the tissues as the original denture. Therefore the duplicate may require more adjustment by the dentist. It is best to consider the duplicate denture a spare one for emergency use only.

Pour-resin–flask method

It is possible to make satisfactory duplicate dentures by using autopolymerizing pour-type resin, a special flask for these resins (Fig. 10-26), and reversible hydrocolloid. Boos and Carpenter (1974) have described an excellent method, and the following technique is an adaptation of theirs.

PROCEDURE

1. Mount the denture to be duplicated on the lower plate of a pour-resin flask, using heat-stable clay. Adapt the clay to form a base approximately 6 mm thick, and develop a land area around the denture border 4 to 5 mm wide and perpendicular to the denture flanges (Fig. 10-27).

2. Assemble the pour-resin flask,* and fill it with reversible hydrocolloid† (Fig. 10-28).

---

*Pour-N-Cure Flask, Coe Laboratories Inc., Chicago, Ill.
†Reversible hydrocolloid.

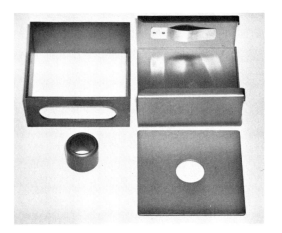

Fig. 10-26. Several types of pour resin flasks are available. Flask shown here is manufactured by Coe Laboratories Inc., Chicago, Ill.

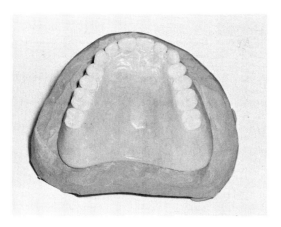

Fig. 10-27. Clay base simulating cast is formed around denture. Borders made 4 to 5 mm wide and 2 to 3 mm above denture borders.

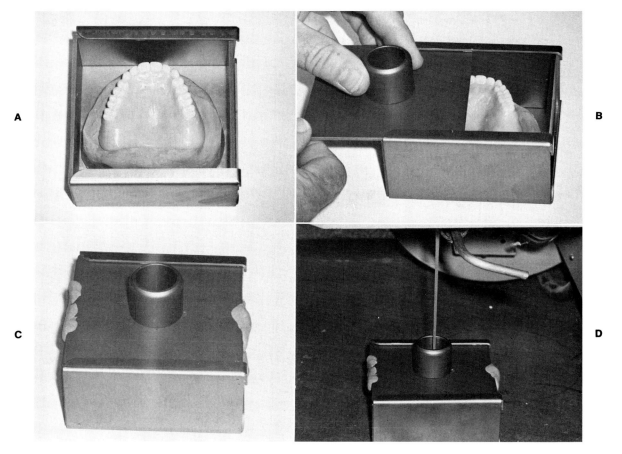

Fig. 10-28. A, Flask is assembled. **B** and **C,** Plates are slipped into position. **D,** Flask is filled with reversible hydrocolloid.

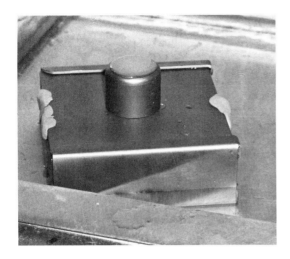

Fig. 10-29. Flask is placed in water to cool hydrocolloid.

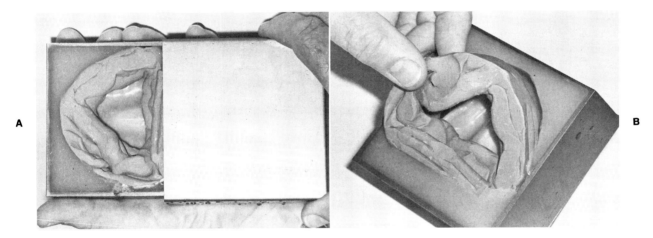

A   B

Fig. 10-30. A, Opened flask. **B,** Clay is removed.

3. Cool the filled flask in water (Fig. 10-29).

4. After the reversible hydrocolloid has gelled, disassemble the flask, and remove the denture and clay (Fig. 10-30).

5. Cleanse the denture, and reposition it in the mold (Fig. 10-31).

6. Switch the bottom plate of the flask to pour the tissue side of the denture (Fig. 10-32).

7. Fill the flask with the hydrocolloid, and cool it in the same manner as before (Fig. 10-33).

8. After the hydrocolloid has gelled, remove it from the cooling bath, and place it in water at 115° F (46° C) for 5 minutes prior to removing the denture.

9. Open the mold, and use a gentle stream of air to facilitate separation of the hydrocolloid pours (Fig. 10-34).

10. Dry the tooth indentations in the mold with a gentle stream of air, or use a thin slip of absorbent tissue to blot the moisture (Fig. 10-35).

11. Place the cast portion of the hydrocolloid mold in a humidor or cover it with a damp towel to minimize dehydration (Fig. 10-36).

12. Paint tooth shade–autopolymerizing resin into the tooth indentations with a brush, and exercise care to avoid the entrapment of air (Fig. 10-37).

13. Fill the tooth indentations with the resin carefully, and pay special attention to maintain the gingival outline. Do not remove the resin teeth from the mold.

14. Using a cork borer, cut sprue holes through the hydrocolloid resin (Fig. 10-38).

15. Assemble the mold, mix and pour the resin into one sprue only (Fig. 10-39), and gently rock the flask to minimize the entrapment of air within the mold.

16. Place the mold with the sprue holes upright in a

Text continued on p. 327.

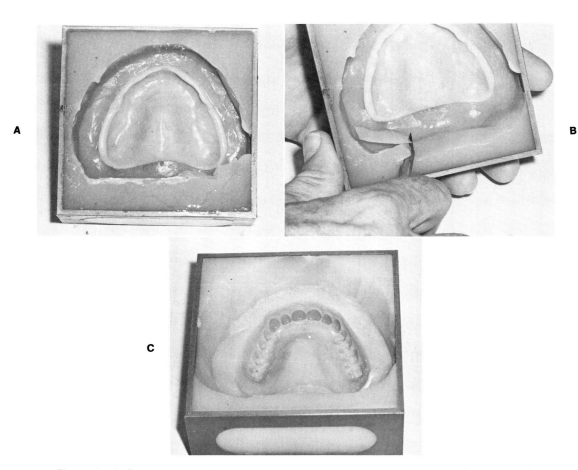

Fig. 10-31. A, Clay is removed from denture, and denture is replaced in mold. **B** and **C,** Undercuts in hydrocolloid are trimmed with knife to facilitate separation later.

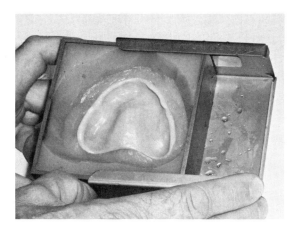

Fig. 10-32. Bottom plate of flask is switched.

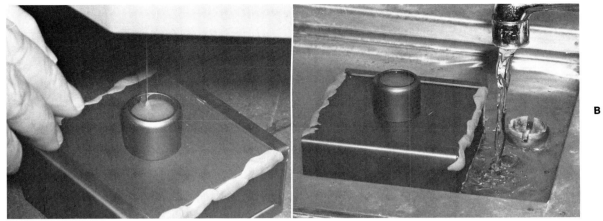

Fig. 10-33. A, Reversible hydrocolloid is poured in flask. Flask should be filled completely. **B,** Flask is cooled in water.

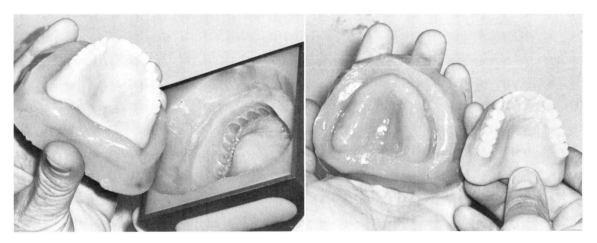

Fig. 10-34. Flask halves are separated with stream of air.

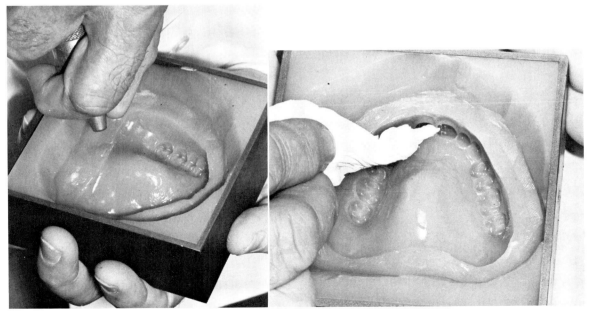

Fig. 10-35. Tooth indentations are dried with air (**A**) or absorbent tissue (**B**) to minimize rounding of incisal angles.

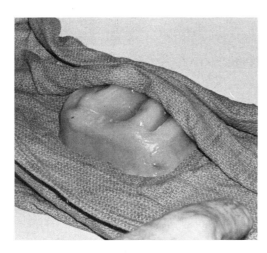

Fig. 10-36. Hydrocolloid mold is covered with damp towel to prevent drying and resultant shrinkage of mold.

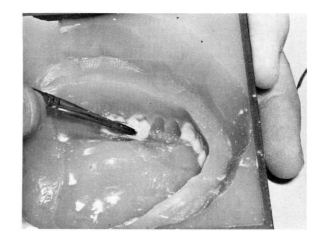

Fig. 10-37. Tooth-shade resin is placed in indentations. Gingival outline is maintained while adding tooth resin.

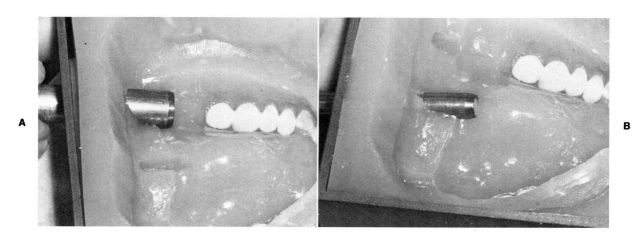

Fig. 10-38. A, Small cork borer is used first to achieve proper approach to denture, then larger cork borer is used to trace path of small borer. **B,** Small cork borer can be used to create vent in midline of posterior border of upper denture.

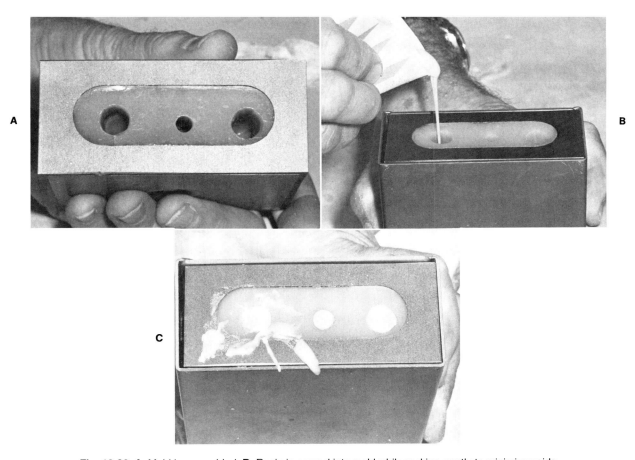

Fig. 10-39. A, Mold is assembled. **B,** Resin is poured into mold while rocking gently to minimize voids. **C,** Resin is added until sprue holes are filled.

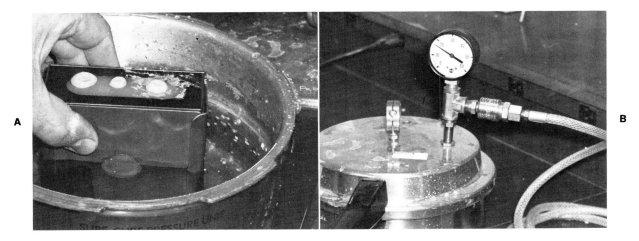

Fig. 10-40. A, Resin-filled flask is placed upright in warm water in pressure container. **B,** Flask is cured at 15 to 20 psi for 30 minutes.

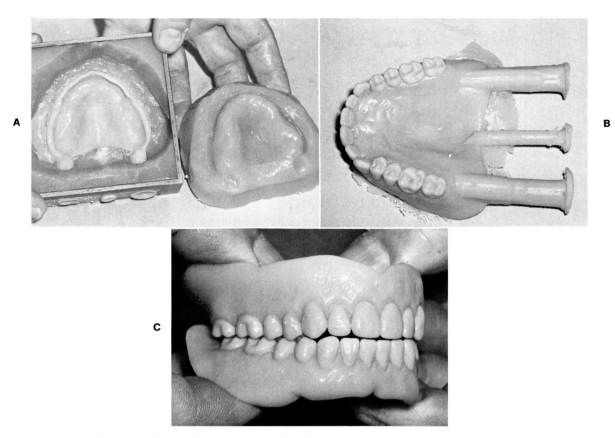

Fig. 10-41. A and **B,** Cured denture removed from flask. **C,** Sprues are cut from dentures and duplicate dentures are polished.

Table 10-2. Pour resin—flask method

Problem	Probable cause	Solution
Voids along posterior borders of duplicate denture	Sprues improperly attached	Attach sprues to denture so that denture does not extend above sprue feed
	Resin poured into both sprue holes, entrapping air	Pour resin into one sprue only
	Flask not rocked during pouring	Rock flask gently from side to side while pouring
Incisal edges of teeth on duplicate denture rounded	Water not removed from mold	Blot moisture from tooth indentations with absorbent tissue
	Mold not warmed in water at 115° F (46° C) for 5 minutes to reduce sweating	Minimize sweating by placing mold in water at 115° F (46° C) for 5 minutes prior to pouring
Teeth on duplicate denture pink in gingival third	Mold indentations not completely filled with tooth-shade resin	Fill tooth indentations carefully to level of gingival margin
Gingival papillae on duplicate denture blanched	Tooth indentations overfilled with tooth-shade resin, resulting in blanching of papillae	Do not overfill tooth indentations with tooth-shade resin

pressure container of water at 120° F (45.5° C), and cure at 20 psi for 30 minutes (Fig. 10-40).

17. Remove the cured duplicate, and trim it, and polish it (Fig. 10-41).

PROBLEM AREAS

Obtaining a duplicate denture free of voids is the principal problem of the pour-resin–flask method (Table 10-2). Correct spruing procedures and careful pouring techniques will minimize voids. In addition, a special flask and the equipment for liquefying reversible hydrocolloids are essential.

Cup-flask method

Wagner (1970) has described a method of duplicating complete dentures by using reversible or irreversible

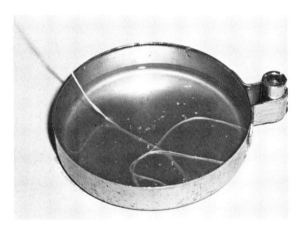

Fig. 10-42. Orthodontic tray wax is melted and dental floss pulled through it to make the floss tacky. Dental floss also can be made tacky by rubbing it with orthodontic tray wax.

hydrocolloid and a cup as a flask. Singer (1975) has modified the method by introducing a particularly convenient zipper technique that uses dental floss to section an alginate irreversible hydrocolloid mold poured in a 12-ounce ceramic cup. This zipper method is equally effective for reversible and irreversible hydrocolloid molds.

The methods described are adapted from those of Wagner and Singer. Although reversible hydrocolloid or irreversible hydrocolloid is usable for making molds, we prefer reversible hydrocolloid because of the resultant smoother resin surfaces.

PROCEDURE

1. Slowly pull 16-inch (40-cm) lengths of dental floss through liquefied orthodontic tray wax (Fig. 10-42). This soft wax will enable the floss to adhere to the denture flanges readily.

2. Tie the floss into a loop, and adapt it to the denture flanges 2 to 3 mm from the borders and across the posterior border of the maxillary denture (Fig. 10-43).

3. Use two loops for the mandibular denture. Adapt one loop to the lingual flange approximately 4 mm from the border (Fig. 10-44), and adapt the other loop to the buccal flanges of the denture.

4. Make soft utility wax or caulking compound sprues approximately 75 mm long and 12 mm thick, and adapt them to the maxillary and mandibular dentures as described previously (Fig. 10-45). An optional vent sprue that extends from the center of the maxillary denture is useful, but it is unnecessary if care is exercised when pouring.

5. For the maxillary denture, press the remainder of the loop into the inner and outer surfaces of one sprue.

6. Press the floss loop from the lingual flange of the

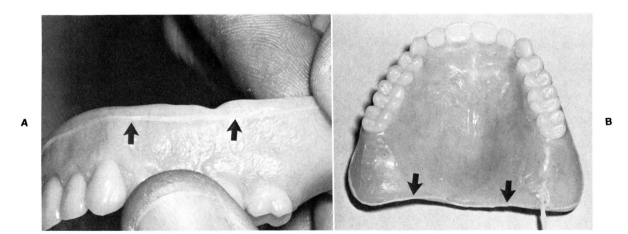

Fig. 10-43. A, Floss is adapted to flanges approximately 2 to 3 mm below borders (arrows). **B,** Floss is attached to posterior border also (arrows).

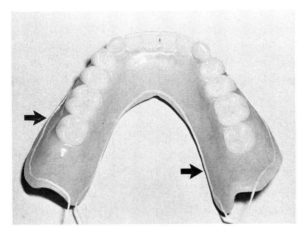

Fig. 10-44. One length of floss is adapted to lingual flanges of denture and another to outer or buccal flanges (arrows).

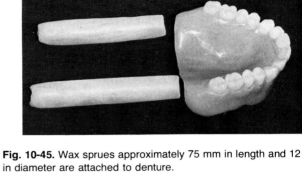

Fig. 10-45. Wax sprues approximately 75 mm in length and 12 mm in diameter are attached to denture.

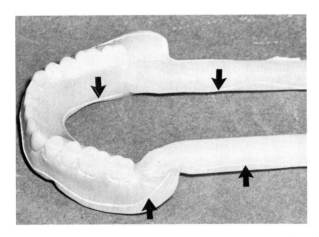

Fig. 10-46. Floss loop from lingual flanges is attached to inside of one sprue (upper arrows), and floss loop from buccal flanges is attached to outside of sprue (lower arrows).

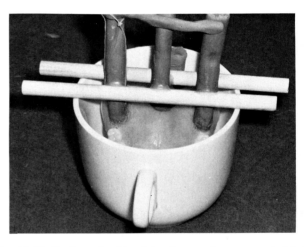

Fig. 10-47. Denture should not touch cup when suspended in it.

lower into the inner surface of the wax sprue and the floss from the buccal surfaces into the outer surface of the wax sprue (Fig. 10-46).

7. Attach the wax sprues between two ¼-inch (6 mm) wood dowel rods approximately 6 inches (15.2 cm) long to suspend the denture in a 12-ounce ceramic cup without contacting the bottom of the cup (Fig. 10-47).

8. Place a modeling clay wedge in the cup opposite the handle to facilitate removal of the mold after pouring (Fig. 10-48).

9. Suspend the sprued denture in the cup (Fig. 10-49)

10. Fill the mold with a pourable mix of alginate (Fig. 10-50) or reversible hydrocolloid (Fig. 10-51). Alginate mixed with approximately three times the recommended volume of water makes a pourable mix. A mix of six scoops of alginate and three times the recommended

amount of water will fill the 12-ounce cup approximately. A smoother bubble-free mix results from mixing in a mechanical spatulator under reduced atmospheric pressure.* An 800-gm mixing bowl is recommended. An optional pouring technique involves filling the cup first, then settling the denture into the mix, though there is greater risk of touching the cup with the denture.

11. Allow the irreversible hydrocolloid to set on the bench (Fig. 10-52, *A*). Place the reversible hydrocolloid in cool water until gelation occurs (Fig. 10-52, *B*).

12. Remove the dowel rods from the mold and the clay wedge from the hydrocolloid (Fig. 10-53).

13. Remove the mold containing the upper denture

---

*Combination Vac-U-Vester Power Mixer, Whip-Mix Corp., Louisville, Ky.

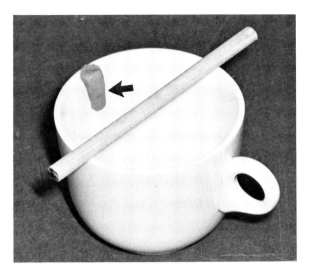

Fig. 10-48. Wedge of modeling clay is attached to inner surface of cup opposite handle (arrow).

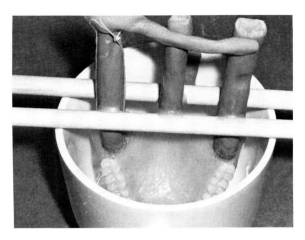

Fig. 10-49. Sprued denture is suspended in cup. Two dowel rods make it possible to stabilize denture without rocking.

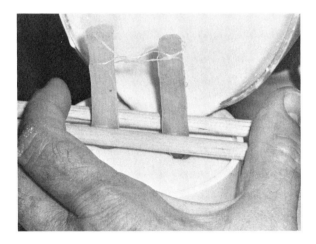

Fig. 10-50. Cup is filled with alginate irreversible hydrocolloid.

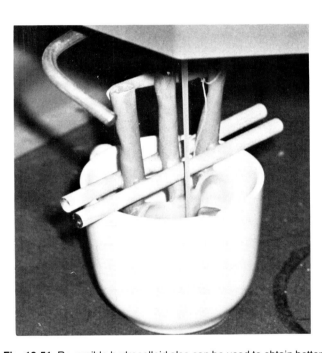

Fig. 10-51. Reversible hydrocolloid also can be used to obtain better denture surface.

from the cup. A gentle stream of air directed at the key-way will aid removal (Fig. 10-54).

14. Pull the dental floss across the posterior border and around the flanges of the upper denture (Fig. 10-55).

15. Open the mold, and retrieve the denture (Fig. 10-56).

16. Dry the tooth indentations with a stream of air and with absorbent tissue (Fig. 10-57).

17. Paint autopolymerizing resin of the proper shade into the tooth indentations as described previously (Fig. 10-58).

18. Assemble the mold in the cup in the original posi-

Text continued on p. 334.

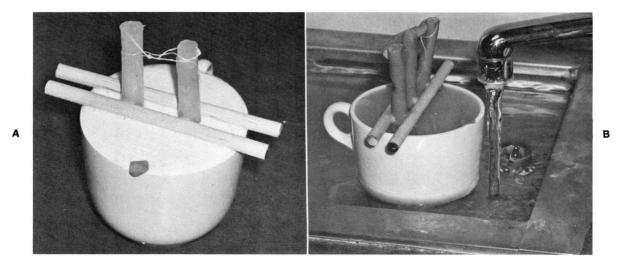

Fig. 10-52. **A,** Alginate is allowed to set on bench. **B,** Reversible hydrocolloid is placed in cool water to gel.

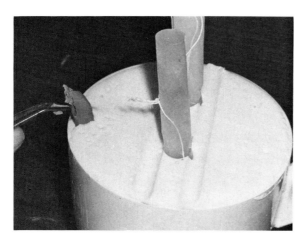

Fig. 10-53. Dowel rods are removed from mold. Clay wedge is removed from hydrocolloid.

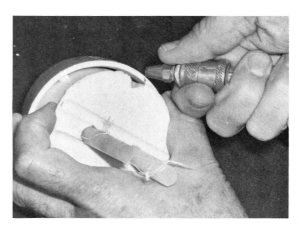

Fig. 10-54. Air is blown into keyway formed by clay wedge to remove mold from cup.

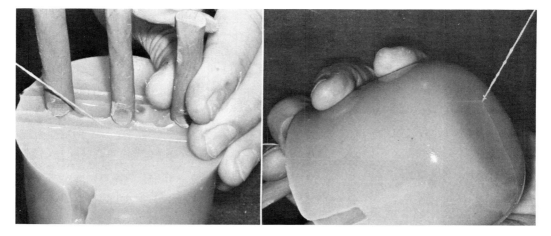

Fig. 10-55. Zipper floss is pulled across posterior border and around flanges.

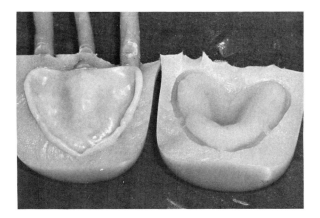

Fig. 10-56. Zippered mold is opened, and denture and sprues removed. Sprues can be removed earlier if desired.

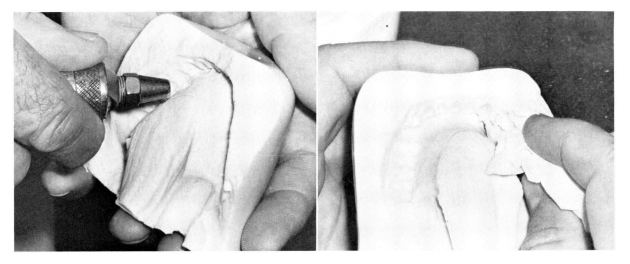

Fig. 10-57. Mold is dried with air or absorbent tissue.

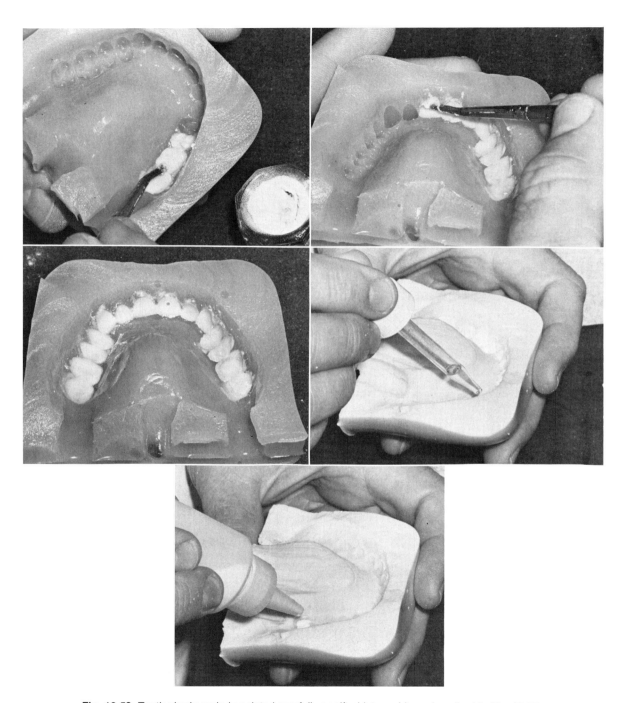

Fig. 10-58. Tooth-shade resin is painted carefully or sifted into mold, as described in Fig. 10-37.

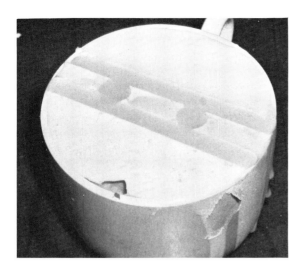

Fig. 10-59. Resin is poured into one sprue hole only. Mold is completely filled.

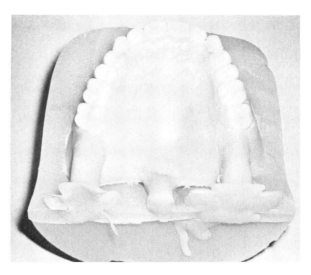

Fig. 10-60. Cured denture is checked for voids or nodules.

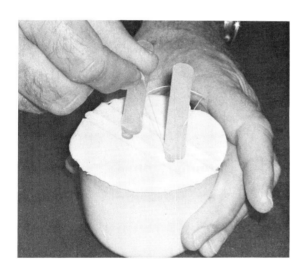

Fig. 10-61. Lingual flange zipper is pulled first.

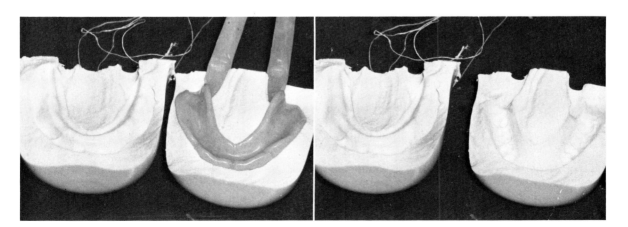

Fig. 10-62. Zipper floss is pulled around labial and buccal flanges.

tion. Mix pour-type resin, and pour it into one sprue, as described earlier (Fig. 10-59).

19. Cure the duplicate denture in warm water in a pressure container for 30 minutes at 20 psi.

20. Retrieve the denture, and examine it for voids or nodules (Fig. 10-60).

21. Polish the duplicate denture.

The mandibular denture is handled in much the same way; the main difference is in the placement of the waxed dental floss loops.

PROCEDURE

1. Cross the inner (lingual flange) dental floss loop, and pull it through the alginate or the reversible hydrocolloid before removing the mold from the cup (Fig. 10-61).

2. Remove the mold from the cup, and pull the floss around the labial and buccal flanges (Fig. 10-62).

3. Complete the mandibular denture in the manner described for the maxillary denture.

PROBLEM AREAS

The problems associated with the cup-flask method for duplicating dentures are the difficulty in obtaining a bubble-free mold, particularly with alginate, the rounding of incisal angles caused by improper drying of the tooth indentations in the hydrocolloid, and the difficulty of painting in the tooth-shade resin to make an esthetic duplicate (Table 10-3).

Mixing alginate materials in a mechanical spatulator under reduced atmospheric pressure minimizes bubbles in the mold. Drying the mold with a stream of air and absorbent tissue reduces rounding of the incisal angles. Practice and experience contribute to the improved skill that is required to apply the tooth-shade resin to the mold and significantly improve the quality of the duplicate denture.

SUMMARY

This chapter has presented three methods of constructing duplicate dentures. All of the methods use reversible or irreversible hydrocolloid for the mold and a pour-type resin for the duplicate denture. Reversible hydrocolloid molds produce a far better surface on the denture and are preferable to alginate. Reversible hydrocolloid is not as easy to use as alginate, since it must be liquefied first. However, we believe that the results with reversible hydrocolloid are clearly superior. Duplicate dentures constructed by these methods can be esthetically acceptable with proper attention to the individual steps.

Painting tooth shade resin in the mold is particularly important, and it requires extreme care for the best esthetic results. Duplicate dentures can be useful substitutes for the original dentures during necessary repair or modification. However, they should serve only as spare or backup prostheses.

REFERENCES

Adam, C. E.: Technique for duplicating an acrylic resin denture, J. Prosthet. Dent. 8:406-410, 1958.
Azarmehr, P., and Azarmehr, H. Y.: Duplicate dentures, J. Prosthet. Dent. 24:339-345, 1970.

Table 10-3. Cup-flask method

Problem	Probable cause	Solution
Bubbles in mold, producing nodules on denture	Alginate not mixed with mechanical spatulator	Mix alginate in mechanical spatulator under reduced atmospheric pressure
Voids in posterior border region of denture	Sprues improperly attached	Attach sprues so that denture does not extend above attachment
	Mold not rocked during pouring of resin	Rock mold gently during pouring of resin to preclude entrapment of air
	Resin poured down both sprues, resulting in entrapment of air	Pour resin into only one sprue
Rounded incisal angles on denture teeth	Mold not dry before resin added	Dry mold with air or absorbent tissue before adding resin
Denture teeth pink in gingival third	Tooth indentation not filled completely with tooth resin	Fill tooth indentation completely when adding tooth resin

Boss, R. H., and Carpenter, H. O., Jr.: Technique for duplicating a denture, J. Prosthet. Dent. **31:**329-334, 1974.

Boucher, C. O.: Clinical dental terminology: a glossary of accepted terms in all disciplines of dentistry, St. Louis, 1974, The C. V. Mosby Co.

Brewer, A. A., and Morrow, R. M.: Overdentures, St. Louis, 1975, The C. V. Mosby Co., pp. 209-213.

Gieger, E. C. K.: Duplication of the esthetics of an existing immediate denture, J. Prosthet. Dent. **5:**179-185, 1955.

Manoli, S. G., and Griffin, T. P.: Duplicate denture technique, J. Prosthet. Dent. **21:**104-107, 1969.

Shaw, D. R.: Duplicate immediate dentures, J. Prosthet. Dent. **12:** 47-57, 1962.

Singer, I. L.: The "zipper" technique for duplicating dentures; final impressions, replica dentures, and a complete denture splint, J. Prosthet. Dent. **33:**582-590, 1975.

Wagner, A. G.: Making duplicate dentures for use as final impression trays, J. Prosthet. Dent. **24:**111-113, 1970.

Zoeller, G. N., and Beetar, R. F.: Duplicating dentures, J. Prosthet. Dent. **23:**346-353, 1970.

CHAPTER 11

RELINING AND REBASING

KENNETH D. RUDD, ROBERT M. MORROW, R. NEAL EDWARDS,
and AMBROCIO V. ESPINOZA

reline To resurface the tissue side (basal surface) of a denture with new base material to provide a more accurate fit.

rebase A process of refitting a denture by replacing the denture base material without changing the occlusal relations of the teeth.

Relining a complete denture to improve its fit is a frequently used procedure in dental practice and has been referred to as one of the most difficult procedures in dentistry. This is reflected in the relining procedures advocated, which vary from relatively simple to complex. The clinical phase of relining involves making an impression in the denture to improve fit without incorporating errors in the occlusion. Thus the laboratory phase begins with the denture readapted to the denture-supporting tissues with a suitable impression material and correctly related to the opposing teeth.

ARTICULATOR METHOD

PROCEDURE

1. Box the denture with impression material before pouring a cast in artificial stone (Fig. 11-1).

2. Pour artificial stone into the boxed denture impression to form a cast (Fig. 11-2).

3. After the stone has set, remove the cast with the denture in place, and index the base. Paint the base with a separating medium (Fig. 11-3).

4. Fill the palatal section of maxillary dentures and the lingual region of mandibular dentures with clay. Adapt clay to the facial surfaces of the teeth and denture, exposing the occlusal third of the denture teeth (Fig. 11-4). This blockout of clay will prevent the in-

dex stone from engaging undercuts on the denture teeth.

5. Mix artificial stone, and place a patty of stone on the lower member of the articulator (Fig. 11-5).

6. Smooth the stone with a spatula, and seat the denture into the stone (Fig. 11-6). The clay will prevent the denture from being placed too deep into the stone (Fig. 11-7).

7. After the stone on the lower member has set, close the articulator to estimate the volume of stone needed to attach the cast (Fig. 11-8).

8. Mix the artificial stone, and place it on the cast, taking care to fill the index grooves (Fig. 11-9).

9. Place additional stone on the upper member of the articulator, and close the articulator (Fig. 11-10). Tap the articulator to determine that it is fully closed (Fig. 11-11).

10. Allow the stone to set, and remove the modeling clay from the denture (Fig. 11-12).

11. Separate the denture from the cast, and remove all traces of impression material from the denture (Fig. 11-13).

12. With an acrylic bur in a handpiece, remove a thin layer of resin from the interior of the denture to freshen the surface (Fig. 11-14).

13. Reduce the borders 2 to 3 mm with a bur (Fig. 11-15).

14. Deepen frena notches with a handpiece-mounted tapered fissure bur (Fig. 11-16).

15. Blow off acrylic-resin grindings with a stream of air (Fig. 11-17). Be sure the compressed air does not contain an aerosol of oil, which could compromise the bond

Text continued on p. 342.

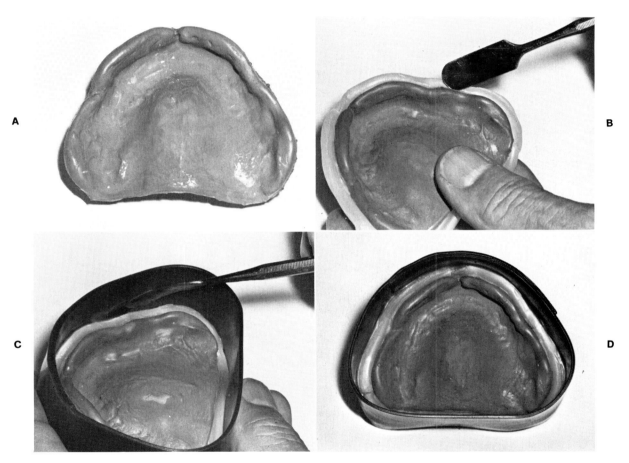

Fig. 11-1. A, Impression is made in complete denture that is to be relined. **B,** Beading wax placed and sealed to impression, keeping wax 2 to 3 mm below denture border. **C,** Boxing wax is adapted around beaded impression and sealed to beading wax with hot spatula. **D,** Boxed denture impression ready for pouring.

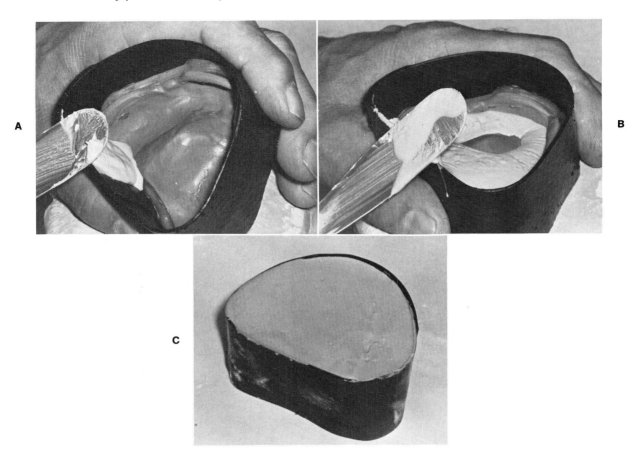

Fig. 11-2. A, Artificial stone is mixed and poured into boxed denture impression. **B,** Stone is added, taking care to avoid air inclusions or voids. **C,** Poured denture impression placed aside to set.

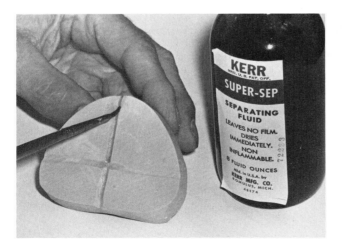

Fig. 11-3. Separating medium is painted on base of cast, using care to coat index grooves.

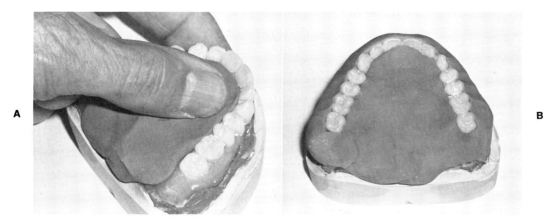

Fig. 11-4. A, Modeling clay is adapted to denture, blocking out all denture surfaces, except occlusal surfaces of teeth. **B,** Clay prevents stone extensions into undercuts on denture base and teeth, which would make separation difficult.

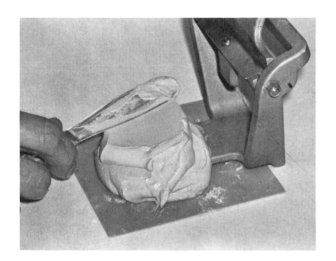

Fig. 11-5. Artificial stone is mixed and placed on lower member of articulator. Simple but sturdy hinge-type articulator is adequate.

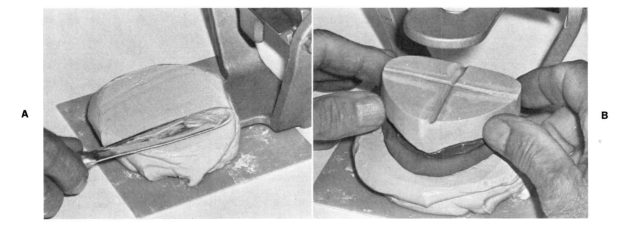

Fig. 11-6. A, Stone surface is smoothed with spatula. **B,** Denture is settled in stone mix. Stone can be placed on occlusal surfaces of denture teeth with finger before seating in stone. Position denture in stone so that occlusal surfaces are approximately parallel to bench top.

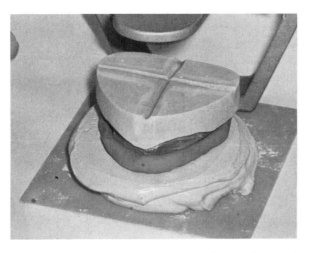

Fig. 11-7. Modeling clay will prevent denture from settling too deep in stone.

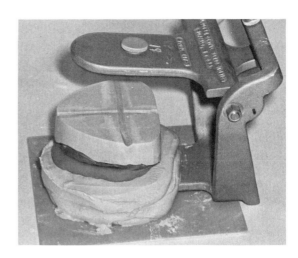

Fig. 11-8. Articulator is closed to estimate volume of stone required to attach cast.

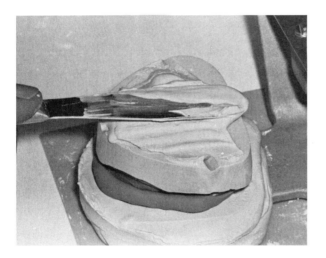

Fig. 11-9. Stone is placed on cast base, using care to fill index grooves.

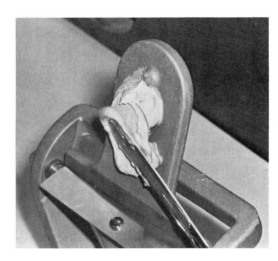

Fig. 11-10. Additional stone is placed on upper member of articulator.

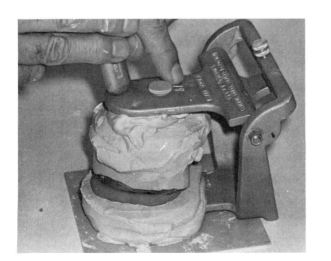

Fig. 11-11. Articulator is closed, and upper member tapped, making certain that articulator is closed to its stop.

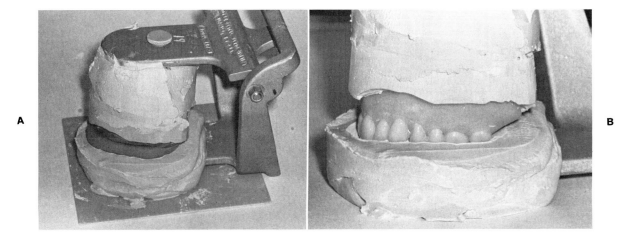

Fig. 11-12. A, Mounting stone is allowed to set. **B,** Modeling clay has been removed from denture surface. Note depth of index was controlled by clay.

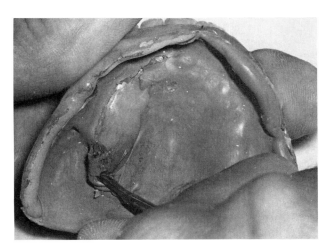

Fig. 11-13. All impression material must be removed from denture. Scraper or bur can be used to remove impression materials.

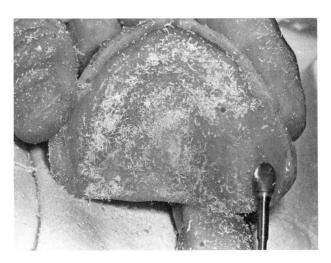

Fig. 11-14. Handpiece or lathe-mounted acrylic bur is used to remove thin layer of resin from interior of denture.

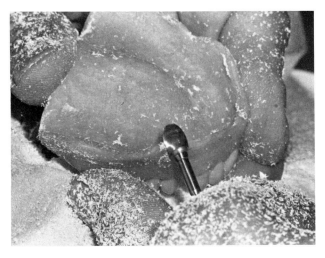

Fig. 11-15. Borders are reduced 2 to 3 mm with bur.

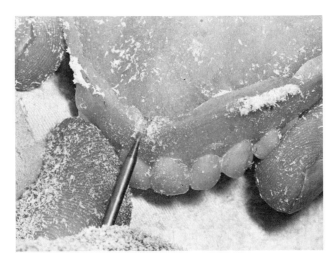

Fig. 11-16. Frena notches are deepened with No. 557 cross-cut fissure bur.

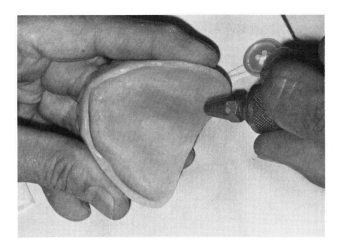

Fig. 11-17. Resin grindings are removed with stream of air. Air must not be contaminated with compressor oil or water, or bonding may be compromised.

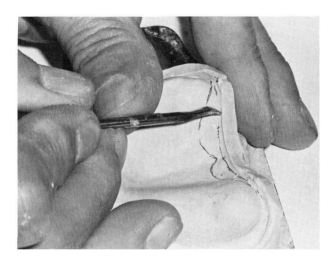

Fig. 11-18. Posterior palatal seal is placed in cast, unless provided for in impression.

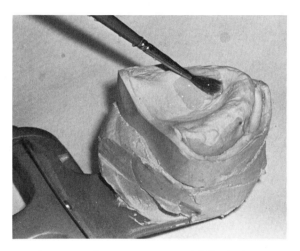

Fig. 11-19. Cast is coated with tinfoil substitute.

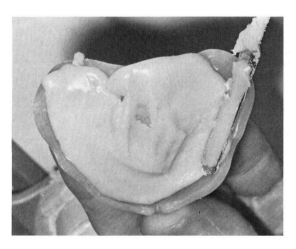

Fig. 11-20. Autopolymerizing resin is mixed according to manufacturer's recommendations and placed in denture, taking care to avoid air entrapment.

between old denture resin and the autopolymerizing resin to be added.

16. Place the posterior palatal seal in the maxillary casts (Fig. 11-18).

17. Paint the cast with tinfoil substitute (Fig. 11-19).

18. Mix autopolymerizing resin in accordance with the manufacturer's recommendations, and add resin to the interior of the denture with a spatula (Fig. 11-20).

19. Place additional resin on the cast, taking care to fill the borders of the cast (Fig. 11-21).

20. Seat the denture into the indentations, and close the articulator, expressing the excess resin (Fig. 11-22).

21. Cure the relined denture in a pressure container to minimize porosity (Fig. 11-23).

22. After curing the relined denture, remove from the cast, and finish and polish it (Fig. 11-24).

PROBLEM AREAS

The principal problem associated with this relining method is related to failure to eliminate voids when adding the autopolymerizing resin to the denture and cast. The resultant voids in the relined denture must be repaired. If the relined denture is not cured in a pressure container, the resin may develop porosity (Table 11-1). Carefully adding the resin with a spatula to preclude air inclusions and curing the relined denture in a pressure container will contribute to a relined denture of acceptable quality.

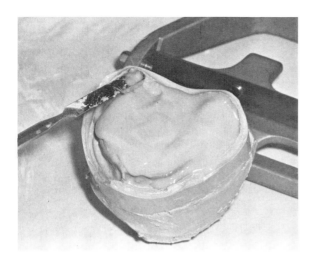

Fig. 11-21. Resin is placed on cast and in border reflections.

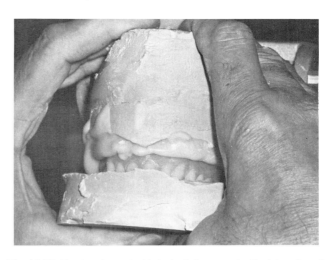

Fig. 11-22. Denture is seated in indentations, and articulator closed. Resin can be added to deficient areas if needed.

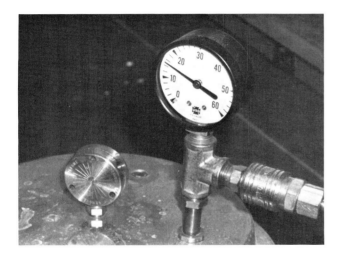

Fig. 11-23. Relined denture is cured in pressure container at 15 to 20 psi for 30 minutes. (Method and time of curing will vary with resin used.)

A

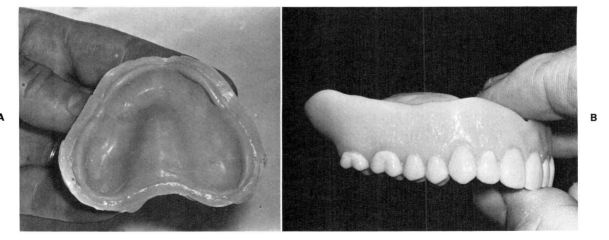

B

Fig. 11-24. A, Relined denture is removed and examined for voids and nodules of resin. **B,** Denture is finished, polished, and stored in water until needed.

Table 11-1. Relining procedures

Problem	Probable cause	Solution
Voids in resin of relined denture	Autopolymerizing resin not placed throughout the interior of denture or into border reflections of cast	Place resin over entire tissue surface of denture and cast; take care to minimize voids, using adequate volume of material
Completed reline shows line between denture base and added resin	Denture resin not freshened or thoroughly cleaned prior to adding autopolymerizing resin Aerosol of oil in compressed air; coated denture resin Autopolymerizing resin mix too dry when placed in denture	Grind surface of denture to receive new resin; thoroughly remove all traces of impression material; wet denture with a brush and monomer prior to adding resin Do not use air blasts to remove resin grindings if air source contaminated with oil or water Pack resin at proper stage before it begins to set
Relined denture is porous	Relined denture not cured in pressure pot	Cure relined denture in pressure pot for 30 minutes at 15 to 20 psi
Relined denture not retentive	Posterior palatal seal not placed in cast Initial impression not adequate	Scrape posterior palatal seal in cast prior to adding resin Examine reline impression carefully for damage in transit

RELINING JIG METHOD
PROCEDURE

1. Box the denture and impression, and pour a cast as described for the articulator method (Fig. 11-25).

2. Use modeling clay to block out the denture, and seat the denture in a stone patty on the lower member of the reline jig* (Fig. 11-26).

3. After the stone index has set, paint the indexed cast with a separating medium, and mount the cast to the upper member of the reline jig (Fig. 11-27).

4. After the stone has set, remove the modeling clay, open the jig, and separate the denture from the index (Fig. 11-28).

5. Carefully lift the denture off the cast (Fig. 11-29). A stream of air can sometimes be used to remove the denture (Fig. 11-30).

6. Remove all impression material from the denture, and prepare the surface as described for the articulator method (Fig. 11-31).

7. Seat the denture in the stone index (Fig. 11-32).

8. Paint the cast with tinfoil substitute (Fig. 11-33).

9. Moisten the resin surface of the denture with an autopolymerizing monomer (Fig. 11-34).

Text continued on p. 349.

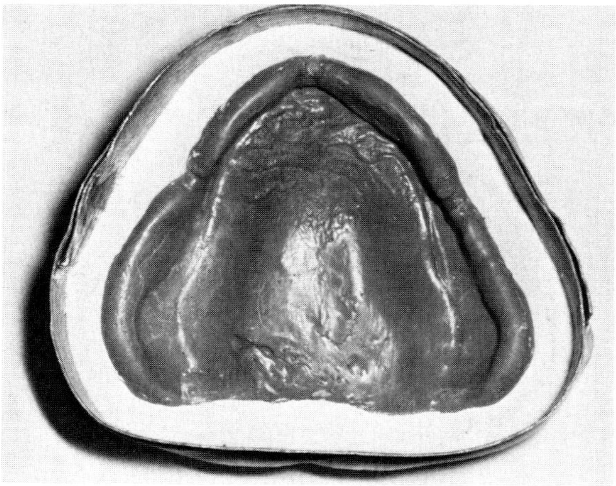

Fig. 11-25. Denture and impression are boxed prior to pouring cast. Caulking compound was used to bead impression in this case.

---

*Reline Jig, Howmedica, Inc., Chicago, Ill.; Hooper Duplicator, Teledyne Dental Products Co., Hanau Division, Buffalo, N.Y.; or equivalent.

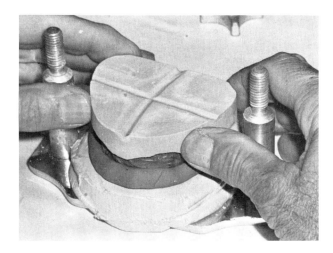

Fig. 11-26. Blocked out denture is seated in stone on lower member of relining jig.

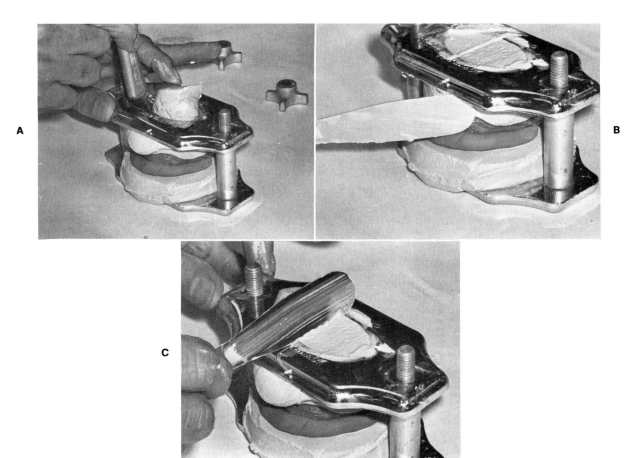

Fig. 11-27. A, Stone is placed on cast base and relining jig assembled. Tap jig with spatula handle to make certain that it is seated. **B,** Mounting stone is smoothed with spatula. **C,** Excess stone extruding through top of jig is removed. Locknuts are screwed down to secure upper member while stone sets.

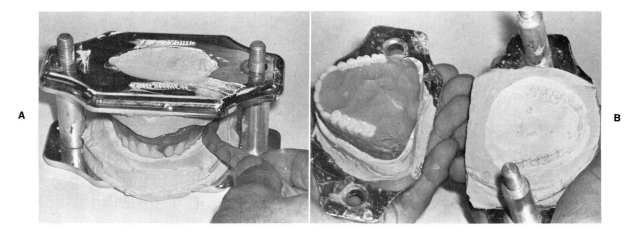

Fig. 11-28. **A,** Locknuts and modeling clay are removed. **B,** Jig is opened exposing occlusal indentations.

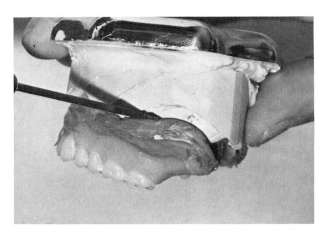

Fig. 11-29. Denture is carefully lifted off cast by prying gently at borders.

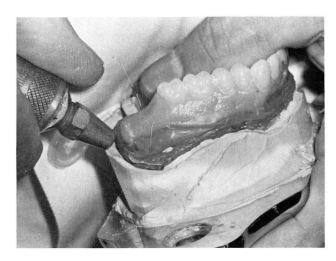

Fig. 11-30. Blowing air under denture will often lift it from cast.

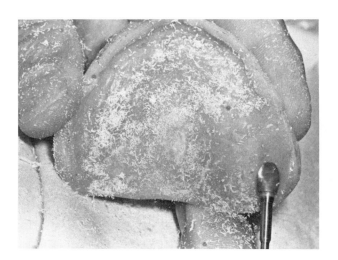

Fig. 11-31. Denture basal surface is prepared.

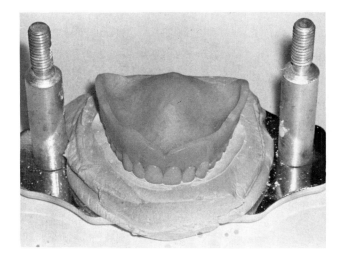

Fig. 11-32. Clean prepared denture is seated in stone index, making certain that it is completely seated.

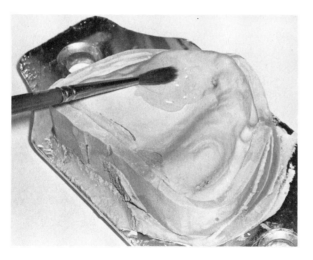

Fig. 11-33. Cast is painted with tinfoil substitute.

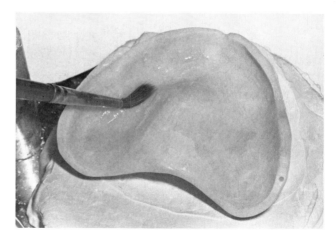

Fig. 11-34. Resin surface is moistened with autopolymerizing monomer.

A 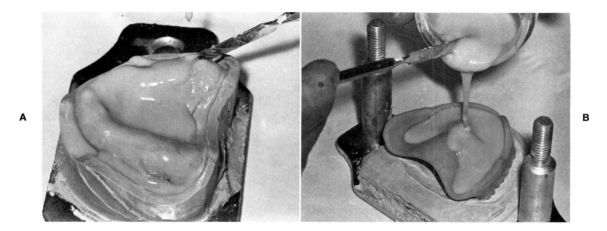 B

Fig. 11-35. A, Resin is mixed and placed on cast, using care to minimize voids. **B,** Resin is placed in denture.

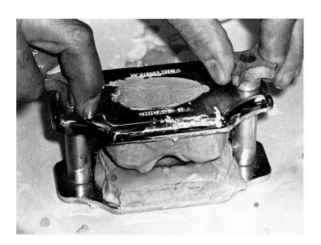

Fig. 11-36. Jig is assembled and locknuts tightened.

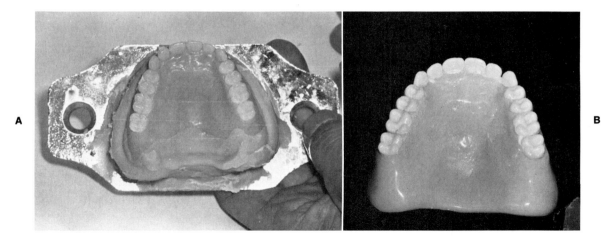

Fig. 11-37. A, Relining jig is separated and relined denture examined for voids. **B,** Relined denture is polished.

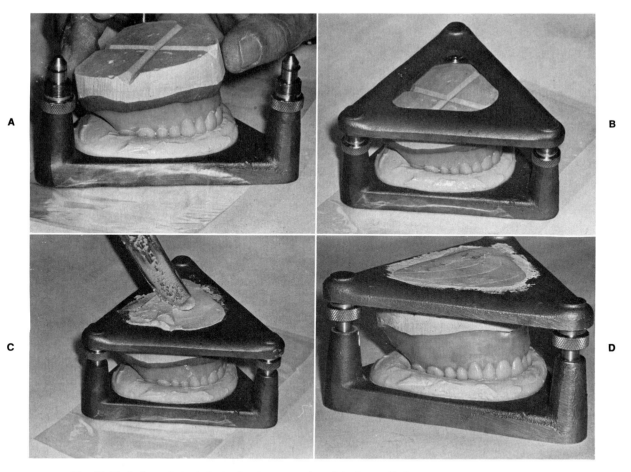

Fig. 11-38. A, Stone index is formed on lower member of duplicator. **B,** Denture to be rebased is seated in index in Hooper Duplicator. **C,** Cast is attached to upper member with stone and locknuts secured. **D,** Stone is allowed to set.

10. Mix the autopolymerizing resin, and place it on the cast and in the denture (Fig. 11-35).

11. Assemble the reline jig and secure it with locknuts (Fig. 11-36).

12. Cure the relined denture in a pressure container of warm water at 15 psi for 30 minutes.

13. Separate the jig, remove the relined denture, and finish and polish it as described for the articulator method (Fig. 11-37).

PROBLEM AREAS

Problems associated with the relining jig method are similar to those for the articulator method (Table 11-1).

REBASING

Rebasing may be necessary when the existing denture base is discolored or if the denture base resin is too light or dark in color for the patient. Rebasing may also be required in the laboratory if a newly processed denture exhibits porosity. Denture rebasing in which all of the denture base is replaced can be accomplished using a reline jig, articulator, or denture flask.

Jig method
PROCEDURE

1. Mount the denture on its cast in a reline jig* or articulator as described for the articulator method and relining jig method (Fig. 11-38).

2. Open the jig, or articulator, and carefully remove the denture from the cast.

3. If the teeth are porcelain, heat each tooth with a hot spatula, and remove it from the denture base (Fig. 11-39).

4. Place each denture tooth in its corresponding indentation (Fig. 11-40).

5. If the denture teeth are resin, cut them from the denture base in units with a bur, and seat them in their indentations.

---

*Hooper Duplicator, Teledyne Dental Products Co., Hanau Division, Buffalo, N.Y.

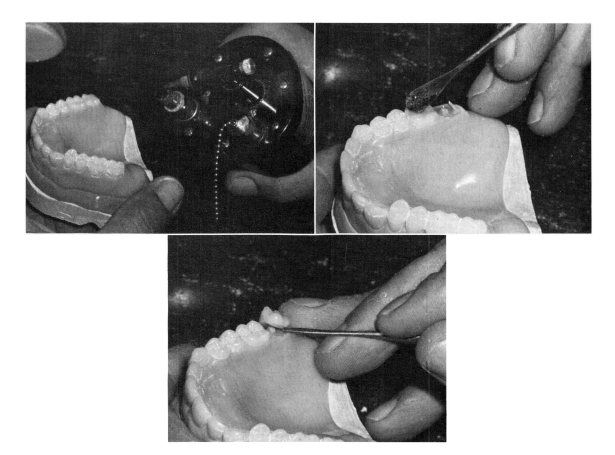

Fig. 11-39. Porcelain denture teeth can be removed from denture by heating carefully with alcohol torch or with hot spatula.

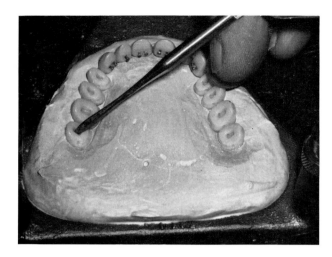

Fig. 11-40. Each porcelain tooth is replaced in its indentation in stone index.

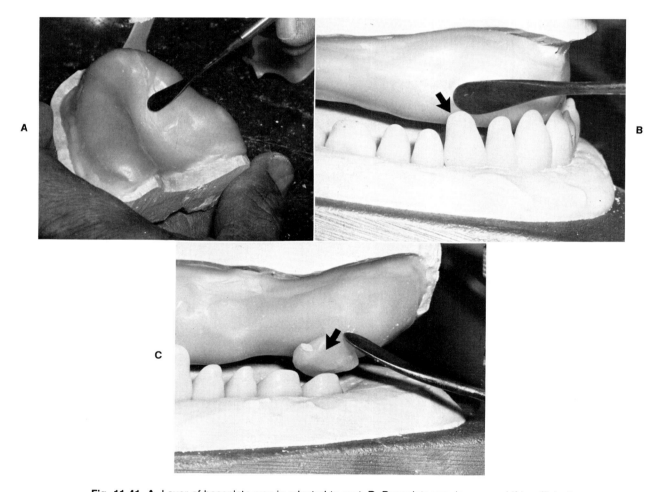

Fig. 11-41. A, Layer of baseplate wax is adapted to cast. **B,** Baseplate wax is removed if insufficient space exists between ridge lap of tooth and cast (arrow). **C,** Add additional thicknesses, or pieces, of baseplate wax where space is large (arrow) to help prevent occlusal changes as result of wax shrinkage.

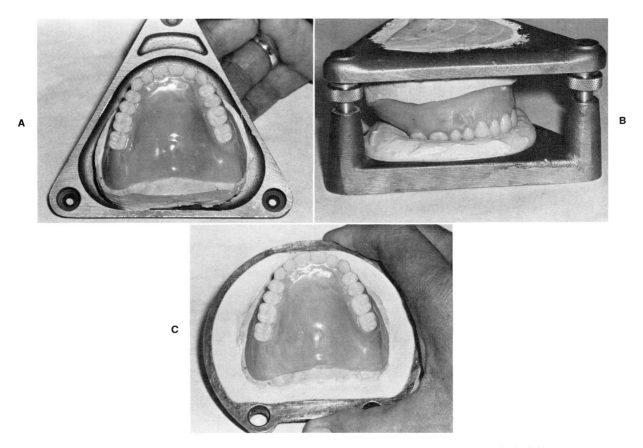

Fig. 11-42. A and **B,** Wax-up is completed on jig. **C,** Waxed denture is removed and flasked. Heat-curing denture base resin will be used for rebasing procedure.

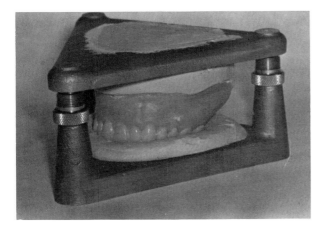

Fig. 11-43. Rebased denture is replaced on jig.

6. Adapt a layer of baseplate wax to the cast, assemble the jig or close the articulator, and wax the denture teeth to the wax (Fig. 11-41).

7. Complete the wax-up on the jig, or articulator, remove the cast, and flask and process it (Fig. 11-42).

8. Replace the cured denture on the jig, or articulator; check and correct the occlusion; then finish and polish the denture (Fig. 11-43).

PROBLEM AREAS

Principal problems associated with this procedure are related to separating the denture from the cast without breaking either the cast or denture; shrinkage of wax when the denture teeth are waxed to the cast, producing errors in occlusion; and the usual problems associated with waxing, flasking, packing, and curing a complete denture (Table 11-2). Undercuts must be removed from the interior of the denture before the rebase impression is made. Failure to remove undercuts will make removal of the denture from the cast difficult and can damage both the denture and cast. If considerable space exists between the denture teeth and the baseplate wax on the

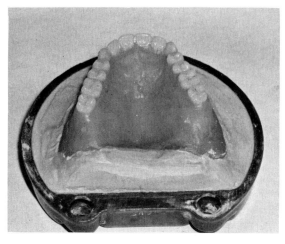

Fig. 11-44. Denture is half-flasked using standard procedure.

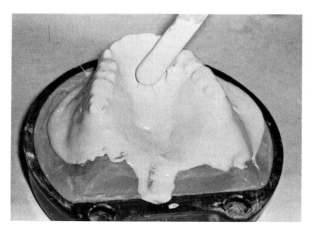

Fig. 11-45. Silicone mold material is painted on denture and teeth. Making coat too thin would not provide sufficient flexibility to remove denture.

Table 11-2. Jig or articulator rebasing method

Problem	Probable cause	Solution
Denture cannot be separated from cast without breaking cast or denture	Undercuts in denture not removed before making impression	Remove undercuts from denture with bur prior to making rebase impression
Rebased denture occlusion is in error	Denture teeth not seated properly in indentations	Seat denture teeth firmly in indentations
	Wax shrinkage withdrew teeth from indentations, resulting in lack of occlusal contact	Add chips of cooled wax to space between tooth ridge laps and cast to minimize wax shrinkage
	Occlusion not properly related by rebase impression	Make rebase impression at proper occlusal relationship
	Flask halves fit together poorly	Use flasks that fit together accurately without rocking

cast, add chips of cooled wax to minimize wax contraction. The use of melted wax alone can produce significant occlusal changes as a result of shrinkage. Careful attention during waxing and processing procedures will contribute to a better restoration.

Flask method
PROCEDURE

1. Pour a cast in the denture as described earlier.
2. Half-flask the denture in an accurate denture flask (Fig. 11-44).
3. Paint silicone mold material* over the denture as described in Chapter 9 (Fig. 11-45).
4. Complete flasking the denture.
5. Open the flask after the flasking stone has set. The

---

*Vescote, Dentsply International, Inc., York, Pa.

resilient silicone will allow the denture to be withdrawn without damage (Fig. 11-46).

6. Remove the porcelain or resin teeth from the denture as described for the jig method.
7. Replace the teeth in the silicone mold (Fig. 11-47).
8. Place a posterior palatal seal in the maxillary cast.
9. Paint the cast and investing stone with tinfoil substitute (Fig. 11-48).
10. Pack denture resin in the mold, and cure, finish, and polish the denture (Fig. 11-49).
11. Correct processing errors after the remounting procedure.

PROBLEM AREAS

Principal problems associated with this method are incorporating air inclusions in the silicone material, producing resin nodules on the rebased denture; the pos-

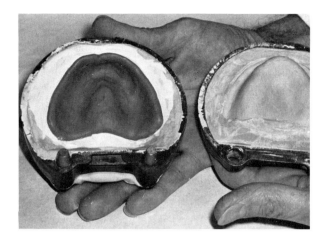

Fig. 11-46. Flask is opened. Here denture remained in upper half of flask.

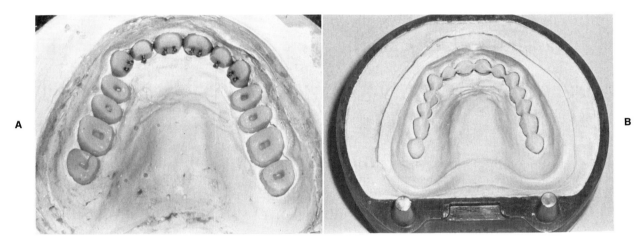

A   B

Fig. 11-47. A, Porcelain denture teeth are removed and placed in silicone mold. **B,** Resin teeth are cut from denture base and placed in mold.

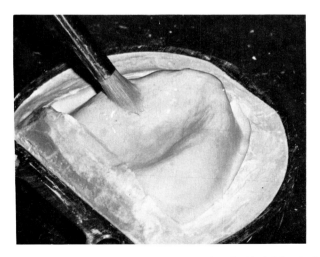

Fig. 11-48. Cast and investing stone are painted with tinfoil substitute.

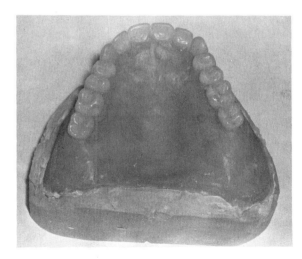

Fig. 11-49. Cured denture is ready for finishing and polishing.

Table 11-3. Flask rebasing method

Problem	Probable cause	Solution
Rebased denture has nodules of resin that require additional finishing time	Air incorporated in silicone mold material during mixing	Mix material carefully; do not whip air into mix
	Silicone material not painted on denture with stiff brush or spatula	Painting silicone over denture to preclude voids
Rebased denture occlusion is incorrect	Flasks do not fit properly	Use accurately fitting flasks that do not rock
	Resin not trial packed adequately	Trial pack resin until flash is eliminated
	Initial impression not related to proper jaw position	Make certain that impression is related to proper occlusal position (clinical); examine impression for damage that may have occured in transit to laboratory

sibility of occlusal errors if the flasks do not fit together accurately; and the potential for dislodging a denture tooth from the flexible silicone mold when packing the resin (Table 11-3).

SUMMARY

Methods for relining and rebasing complete dentures were discussed in this chapter. Each of the described methods can produce a satisfactory result. The relining procedures involved the use of autopolymerizing resin, which is cured in a pressure container. The rebasing procedure described used conventional heat-curing resin to rebase the denture. Whereas the laboratory phases of relining and rebasing methods are critical to success, the completed restoration will not be successful unless the prerequisite clinical procedures were completed properly.

BIBLIOGRAPHY

Body, L. H.: Relining immediate dentures utilizing cephalometries, J. Prosthet. Dent. 11:864-872, 1961.

Boucher, C. O.: The relining of complete dentures, J. Prosthet. Dent. 30:521-526, 1973.

Braver, F. M., White, E. E., Burns, C. L., and Woelfel, J. B.: Denture reliners—direct, hard, self-curing resin, J. Am. Dent. Assoc. 59:270-283, 1959.

Buchman, J.: Relining full upper and lower dentures, J. Prosthet. Dent. 2:703-710, 1952.

Christensen, F. T.: The wing relining technique, J. Prosthet. Dent. 22:268-270, 1969.

Christensen, F. T.: Relining techniques for complete dentures, J. Prosthet. Dent. 26:373-381, 1971.

Christie, D. R.: Relining acrylic dentures without distortion, J. Can. Dent. Assoc. 17:374-377, 1951.

Feldmann, E. E., Morrow, R. M., and Jamison, W. S.: Relining complete dentures with an oral cure silicone elastomer and a duplicate denture, J. Prosthet. Dent. 23:387-393, 1970.

Friedman, S.: Rebasing the complete maxillary denture, NY State Dent. J. 40:19-22, Jan., 1974.

Gillis, R. R.: A relining technique for mandibular dentures, J. Prosthet. Dent. 10:405-410, 1960.

Hardy, I. R.: Rebasing the maxillary denture, Dent. Digest 55: 23-27, 1949.

Hooper, B. B.: Rebasing or duplicating dentures: a method of restoring facial contour and correct faulty retention, Dent. Digest 38: 206-213, 1932.

Jordan, L. G.: Relining the complete maxillary denture, J. Prosthet. Dent. 28:637-641, 1972.

Ostrem, C. T.: Relining complete dentures, J. Prosthet. Dent. 11: 204-213, 1961.

Payne, S. H.: Denture base materials and the refitting of dentures, J. Am. Dent. Assoc. 49:562-566, 1954.

Sears, V. H.: Functional impressions for rebasing full dentures, J. Am. Dent. Assoc. 23:1031-1035, 1936.

Shaffer, F. W.: Relining complete dentures with a minimum of error, J. Prosthet. Dent. 25:366-370, 1971.

Smith, D. E., Lord, J. L., and Bolender, C. L.: Complete denture relines with autopolymerizing acrylic resin processed in H_2O under air pressure, J. Prosthet. Dent. 18:103-115, 1967.

Smith, R. V.: Rebasing technique for full dentures, Iowa Dent. Bull. 39:240, 1953.

Stout, C. J.: Rebasing complete dentures using infrared heat, J. Prosthet. Dent. 11:665-667, 1961.

Terrell, W. H.: Relines, rebases, or transfers and repairs, J. Prosthet. Dent. 1:244-253, 1951.

Tucker, K. M.: Relining complete dentures with the use of a functional impression, J. Prosthet. Dent. 16:1054-1057, 1966.

Wolfe, H. E.: Denture relining or rebasing with a fluid resin, J. Prosthet. Dent. 31:460-465, 1974.

CHAPTER 12

REPAIRS

KENNETH D. RUDD, ROBERT M. MORROW, and ALEXANDER R. HALPERIN

Unfortunately, complete dentures occasionally break when in function or when dropped onto a hard surface. Often the fractured denture can be repaired; several repair methods will be described in this chapter.

REPAIRING DENTURE WITH FRACTURED TEETH

Fracturing or chipping a denture tooth is not an uncommon problem. Although porcelain teeth are more prone to breakage, particularly when dropped onto a hard surface, either porcelain or plastic denture teeth may be fractured. The method used to replace these teeth depends on the tooth material.

Plastic anterior tooth replacement

Replacement of plastic teeth requires the fractured tooth to first be removed by grinding. Occasionally a lack of bonding between the denture base resin and tooth allows a plastic tooth to be dislodged from the denture. This can occur if wax elimination is not thorough or if tinfoil substitute inadvertently placed on the ridge laps of the teeth is not removed prior to packing.

PROCEDURE

1. Remove the fractured tooth by grinding it with a No. 8 round bur (Fig. 12-1).
2. Do not grind the labial gingival margin (Fig. 12-2).

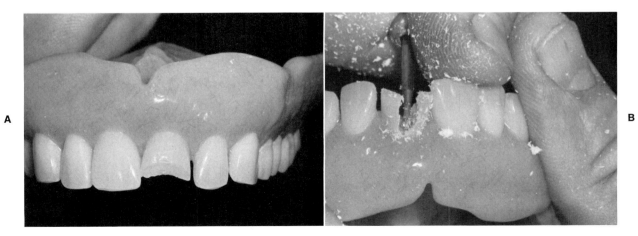

Fig. 12-1. Fractured plastic tooth to be replaced **(A)** is removed by grinding **(B).** Care must be taken to not perforate denture base.

355

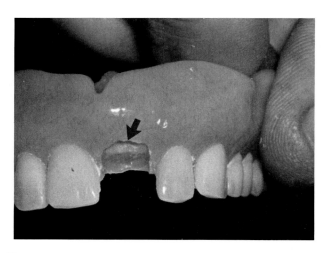

Fig. 12-2. Labial margin (arrow) is left intact to preserve esthetics.

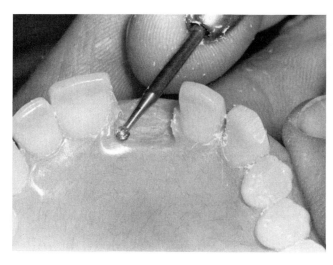

Fig. 12-3. Resin is removed from lingual aspect to provide for addition of repair resin.

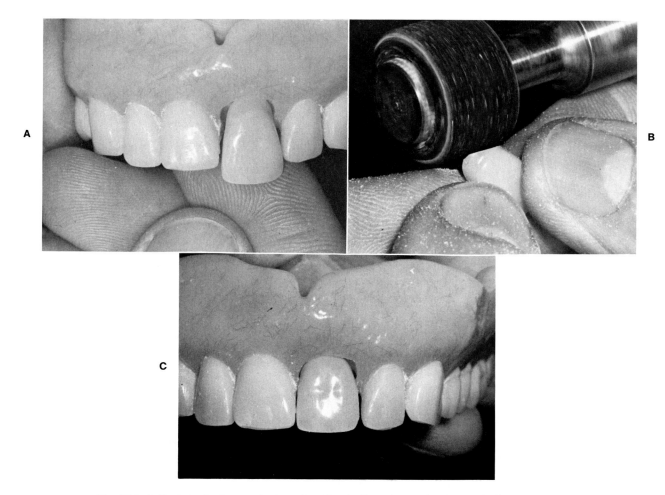

Fig. 12-4. A, Resin tooth of same shade and mold as tooth on denture is selected. **B,** Ridge lap of tooth is ground so that it can be placed on denture in same position as original. Small indentation can be placed in ridge lap at this time to improve attachment strength. **C,** Modified tooth is positioned.

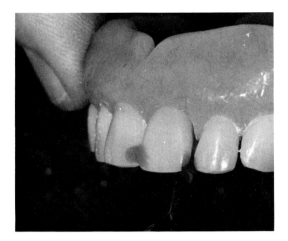

Fig. 12-5. After tooth position has been verified, it is sticky waxed into position.

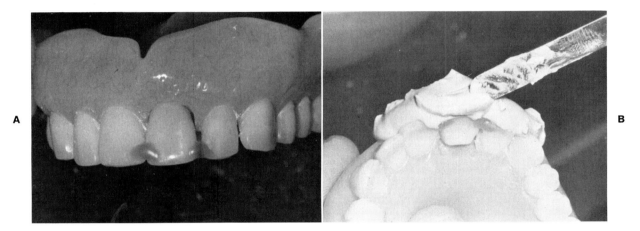

A

B

Fig. 12-6. Tooth position is checked again **(A)** and if acceptable, plaster index is poured **(B)**.

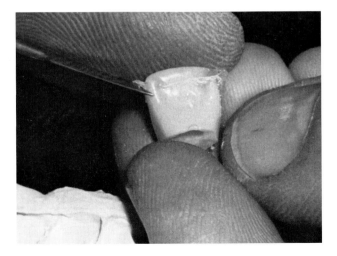

Fig. 12-7. Index is separated, and sticky wax removed.

3. Remove denture base resin from the denture lingual surface adjacent to the tooth to be replaced. Do not perforate the base (Fig. 12-3).

4. Select a plastic tooth of the appropriate size and shade, and custom grind its ridge lap to facilitate correct positioning on the denture (Fig. 12-4).

5. Check the replacement-tooth position from front and above views. Sticky wax may be used to secure it in position (Fig. 12-5).

6. When the tooth position is acceptable, pour a plaster index onto the labial surface of the tooth to be replaced and on the labial surfaces of adjoining teeth on each side (Fig. 12-6).

7. After the plaster sets, separate the index and tooth from the denture, and remove all traces of sticky wax (Fig. 12-7).

8. With a No. 6 bur, place shallow indentations in the denture-tooth ridge lap to provide an additional bonding area (Fig. 12-8).

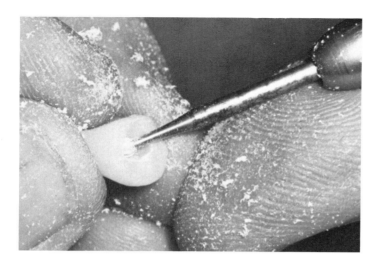

Fig. 12-8. If not done earlier, shallow indentations should now be placed in ridge laps of tooth to ensure stronger repair.

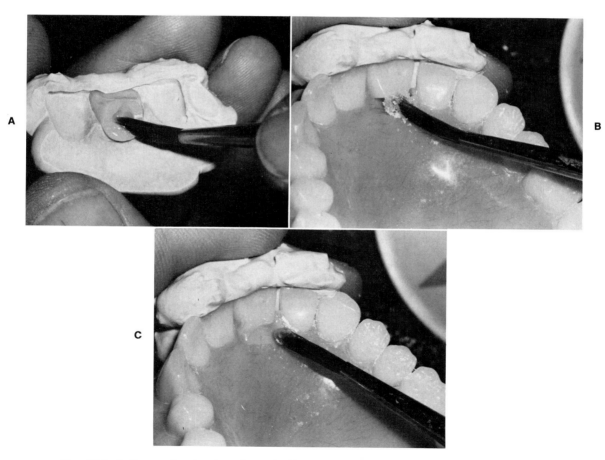

Fig. 12-9. A, Prepared region is moistened with monomer, and autopolymerizing resin is painted carefully into lingual prepared area, allowing resin to flow between ridge lap and denture base. **B,** Care must be taken to not entrap air, thus producing voids. **C,** Palatal surface is built up to desired contour.

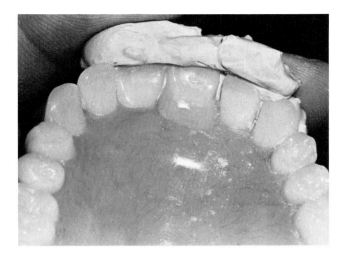

Fig. 12-10. Resin is added to build up slight excess, which will be finished to original contour after polymerizing.

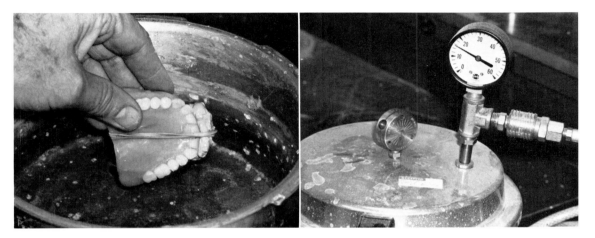

Fig. 12-11. Denture cured in pressure pot.

9. Replace the index and tooth on the denture, and carefully paint in autopolymerizing resin from the lingual or palatal side (Fig. 12-9).

10. Continue to add resin, taking care to minimize voids. Build it up to the desired contour (Fig. 12-10).

11. Place the repaired denture in a pressure pot of warm water, and cure it at 20 psi for 30 minutes (Fig. 12-11).

12. Remove the denture, and polish the autopolymerizing resin with flour of pumice and either a rag wheel (Fig. 12-12) or rubber prophy cup on a standard handpiece that reduces the likelihood of overreducing the denture surfaces (Fig. 12-13).

PROBLEM AREAS

Principal problems that occur with replacing anterior denture teeth are related to failure to duplicate the position of the original denture tooth; failure to control the flow of autopolymerizing resin when painting it on the denture; and permitting the autopolymerizing resin surface to dry, thus producing porosity in the cured resin (Table 12-1).

Porcelain anterior tooth replacement

The procedure for replacing porcelain denture teeth differs from that for plastic teeth in the manner of removing the fractured tooth from the denture base.

PROCEDURE

1. Heat the end of a roach carver or wax spatula in a flame, and press it against the fractured porcelain tooth (Fig. 12-14). Several applications may be necessary to heat the tooth sufficiently.

2. Gently pry the porcelain tooth from the denture base (Fig. 12-15). The tooth should separate cleanly from the base.

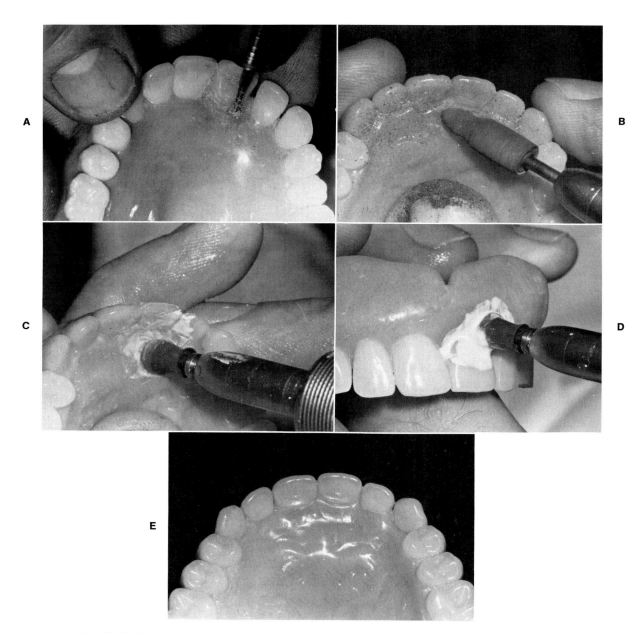

Fig. 12-12. A, Excess bulk is reduced with handpiece-mounted No. 8 bur. **B,** Resin is smoothed with mounted rubber point. **C,** Repair is polished with slurry of flour of pumice and handpiece-mounted prophy cup. **D,** High polish is achieved with prophy cup and prepared chalk. **E,** Repaired denture is polished, using care to not overpolish, thus obliterating contours of plastic replacement tooth.

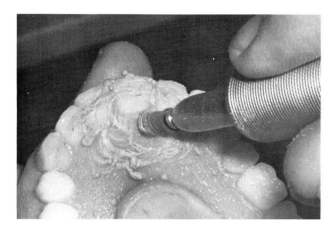

Fig. 12-13. Rubber prophy cup mounted in laboratory handpiece will reduce likelihood of overpolishing.

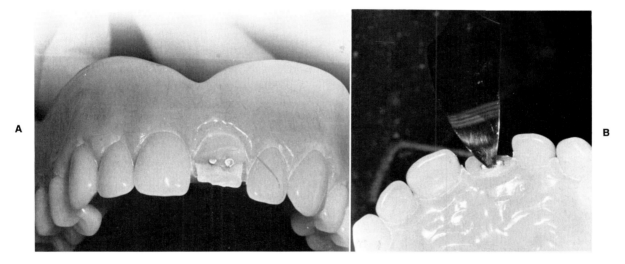

A

B

Fig. 12-14. A, Fractured tooth. **B,** Heated instrument is held against fractured tooth to soften adjacent denture base resin. Do not overheat, and check softening repeatedly by prying on tooth.

Fig. 12-15. Porcelain tooth is pried from denture base resin.

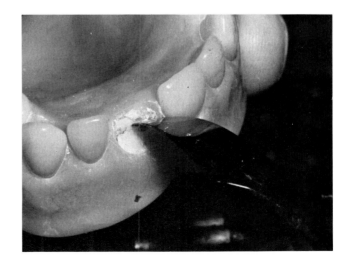

Table 12-1. Replacing anterior denture teeth

Problem	Probable cause	Solution
Replacement tooth too long, too short, or incorrectly positioned buccolingually	Tooth not modified to permit correct placement	Grind replacement tooth ridge lap to facilitate proper placement Check position carefully prior to pouring index
Replacement tooth wrong shade	Shade selection in error	Check shade under variety of lighting conditions to assure proper shade
Repair resin on polished denture surface	Too much resin added during paint-on procedure Too much monomer resulted in fluid resin mix	Paint resin on in increments to avoid overfilling Use only enough monomer to assure proper wetting
Porous repair resin	Repair-resin surface monomer evaporated	Keep surface of repair resin moistened with monomer; do not permit monomer to flow onto polished surface of denture Place repaired denture in pressure container for curing Use good-quality repair resin

3. Examine the ridge lap of the tooth for mold identification marks (Fig. 12-16). See Chapter 6 on artificial teeth.

4. Select a replacement tooth of correct mold and shade.

5. To provide space for repair resin to be added later, remove the denture base resin from the lingual or pin, area. Do not remove resin from the labial margin of the socket or perforate the base (Fig. 12-17).

6. Try the tooth in position, and adjust it if required (Fig. 12-18). A fine-cut wheel* is good for reducing porcelain.

7. Wax the tooth in position with two droplets of sticky wax on the incisal edge, and check its position carefully (Fig. 12-19).

8. Pour a plaster index as described previously for plastic teeth (steps 6 to 8).

9. After removing the wax and preparing the tooth, paint repair resin between the ridge lap and denture base. Take care to avoid air entrapment (Fig. 12-20).

10. Cure the repaired denture in a pressure container at 20 psi for 30 minutes.

11. Polish the repaired denture with flour of pumice and a rag wheel or a rubber prophy cup (Fig. 12-21).

PROBLEM AREAS

Principal problems are similar to those for plastic teeth. (See Table 12-1).

---

*Fine-cut wheel No. 328, ⅞ × ⅛ inch (2.2 × 0.32 cm), Dental Development and Manufacturing Co., Brooklyn, N.Y.

Plastic posterior tooth replacement

The method for replacing fractured plastic and porcelain posterior teeth is similar to that for anterior teeth, but with a significant difference. Since occlusion is usually a factor when replacing posterior teeth, the denture will need to be remounted for occlusal correction. This is particularly important for plastic teeth, since their occlusal surfaces are often worn, and a new tooth of the same mold will differ considerably in occlusal contour. A possible exception would occur if the plastic posterior tooth was fractured during deflasking or while the denture was being constructed. In this situation the new tooth would be added, and the occlusion adjusted in the articulator when the processing error was corrected.

PROCEDURE

1. Mount the denture in an articulator to facilitate correcting the occlusion (Fig. 12-22).

2. Remove the fractured resin posterior tooth by grinding it with a No. 8 round bur (Fig. 12-23), taking care to not perforate the denture base. Preserve the facial gingival margin of the denture base resin.

3. Select a resin posterior replacement tooth.

4. Grind the ridge lap of the replacement tooth to allow correct placement on the denture (Fig. 12-24). The tooth can be occluded and sealed to the opposing denture tooth during this procedure (Fig. 12-25).

5. Paint autopolymerizing resin into the ridge lap area to seal the tooth to the denture base (Fig. 12-26).

6. Place the denture in a pressure container of warm water, and cure it for 30 minutes at 20 psi.

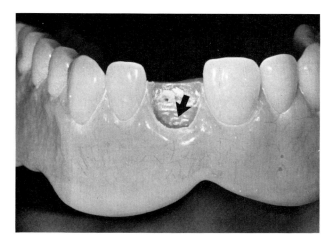

Fig. 12-16. Depending on type of tooth used, it may be possible to see mold number impressed in denture resin socket (arrow) if ridge lap of original tooth was not ground.

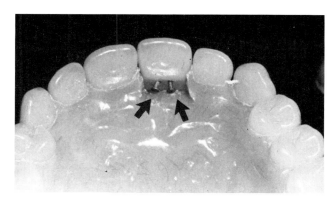

Fig. 12-17. Resin is removed from lingual surface (arrows) to accommodate retention pins on replacement tooth.

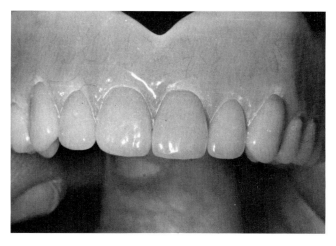

Fig. 12-18. Ridge lap of replacement tooth is shaped to permit replacement in same position as original.

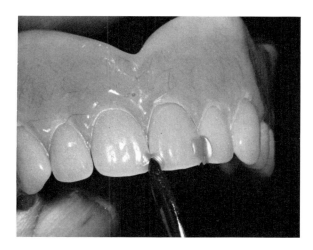

Fig. 12-19. Tooth sticky waxed into position, and position verified.

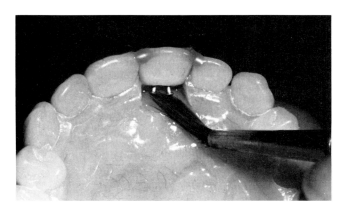

Fig. 12-20. Prepared resin is moistened with monomer. Plaster index is replaced, if used, and autopolymerizing resin is painted. No voids should remain around retention pins.

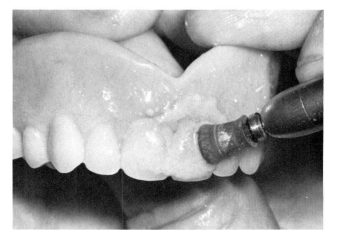

Fig. 12-21. Repaired denture is polished with flour of pumice and handpiece-mounted rubber prophy cup.

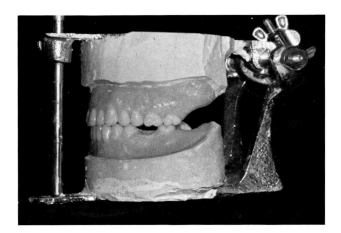

Fig. 12-22. Denture mounted in simple articulator.

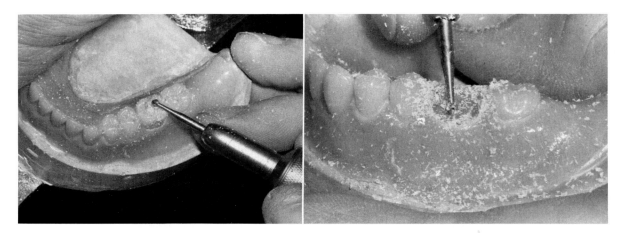

Fig. 12-23. Fractured plastic tooth is ground away with No. 8 round bur, preserving facial margin, and using care to not perforate base.

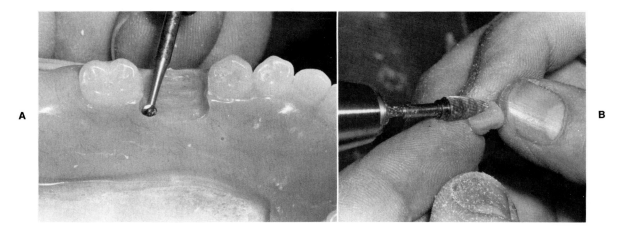

Fig. 12-24. A, Ridge-lap area of denture is hollow ground to permit placement of replacement tooth. B, Ridge lap of replacement tooth is modified as needed.

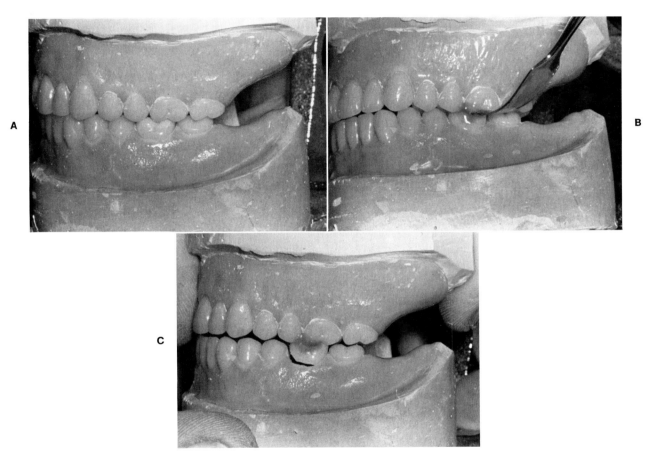

Fig. 12-25. A, Articulator is closed, and occlusion checked. **B** and **C,** If correct, replacement tooth is sealed to opposing tooth or index with sticky wax.

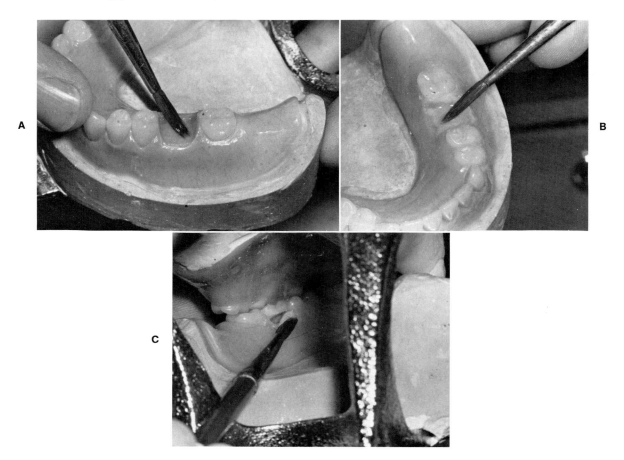

Fig. 12-26. A, Denture indentation and ridge lap of tooth are moistened with monomer. **B** and **C,** While tooth is secured with sticky wax, autopolymerizing resin is first painted into indentation on denture base and then between tooth and denture base, using care to avoid air entrapment.

7. Polish the repair, and adjust the occlusion (Fig. 12-27).

Porcelain posterior tooth replacement
PROCEDURE

1. Mount the denture on an articulator.

2. Heat the broken porcelain tooth with a hot wax spatula to remove it from the denture base (Fig. 12-28). Grind away the denture base resin extending into the retentive recess of the denture tooth.

3. Check the indentation in the denture base to determine if the mold number is discernible (Fig. 12-29). An impression of the indentation can be made in inlay wax: then the impressed mold number can be read in the wax (Fig. 12-30).

4. Select a replacement tooth, and grind the ridge lap if necessary to achieve the correct position (Fig. 12-31).

5. Occlude the replacement tooth, and seal it with sticky wax to the opposing tooth or index (Fig. 12-32).

6. With the tooth secured in this position, paint autopolymerizing resin into its retention recess and into the denture base indentation (Fig. 12-33). Close the articulator.

7. Place the denture in a pressure container of warm water at 20 psi for 30 minutes.

8. Remove the denture, polish it, and adjust the occlusion (Fig. 12-34).

If the occlusal surface of a fractured tooth is not affected, an occlusal index can be made of plaster before the fractured tooth is removed. This eliminates the need to mount the denture in an articulator. For occlusion adjustment, use the index instead of the opposing occlusion.

PROBLEM AREAS

The principal problems with posterior tooth replacement are similar to those for anterior teeth (Tables 12-1 and 12-2). An additional problem exists, however, with the occlusion. The posterior replacement tooth must harmonize with the existing occlusion to avoid deflective

Text continued on p. 371.

A B C D

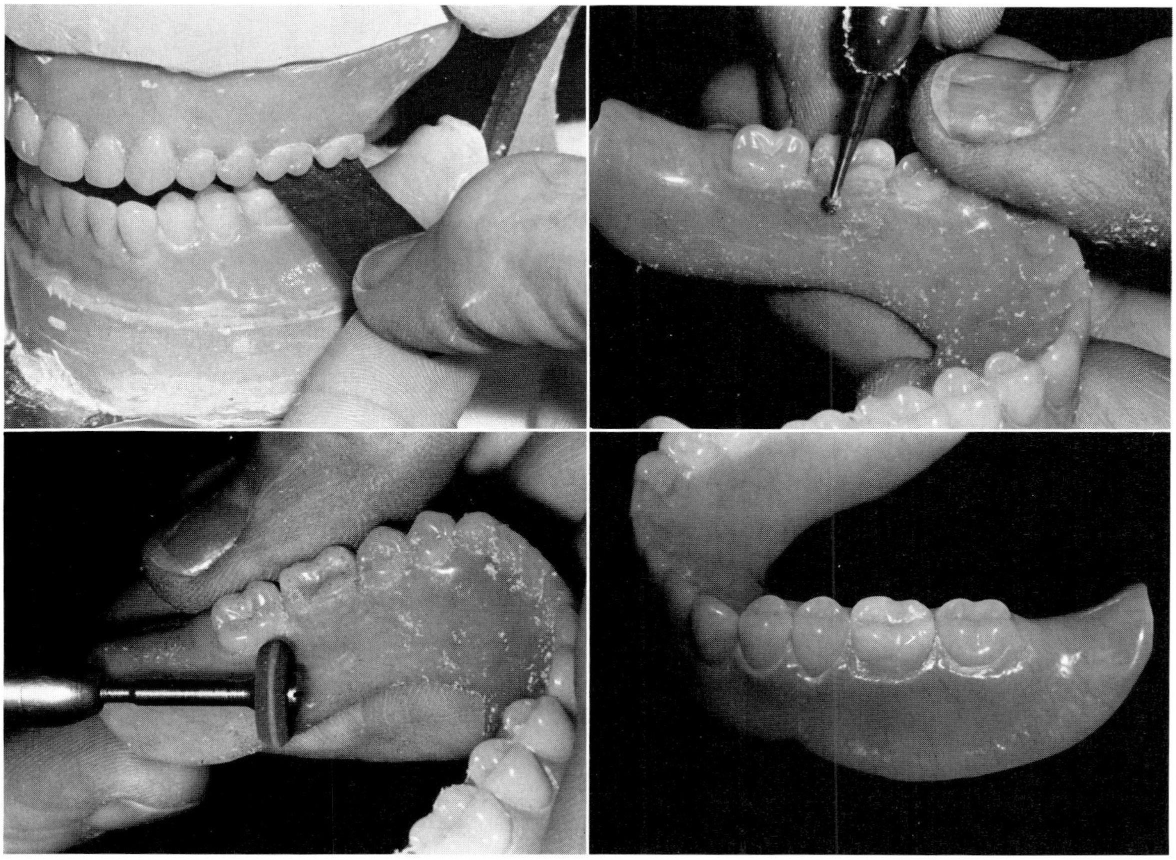

Fig. 12-27. Occlusion is checked and repair polished **(A)**. Bur **(B)** and pumice-impregnated rubber wheel **(C)** are used to smooth resin before pumicing. Polished repair **(D)**.

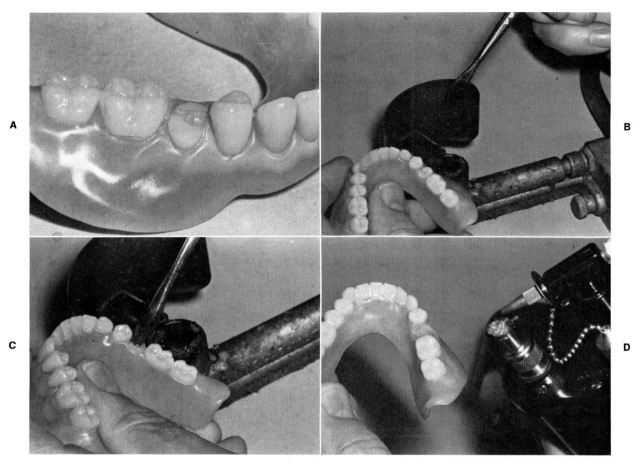

Fig. 12-28. **A,** Fractured porcelain tooth. **B,** Spatula is heated in flame. **C,** Hot spatula is held against fractured porcelain tooth. **D,** Broken tooth can often be removed after heating carefully with alcohol torch.

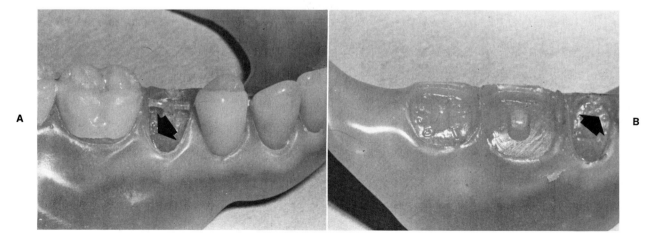

Fig. 12-29. **A,** Indentation in denture base (arrow) is checked to determine if mold number is readable. **B,** Dots (arrow) indicate that tooth is second bicuspid. Dots are on mesial ridge lap. (Teeth made by Dentsply International Inc., York, Pa.)

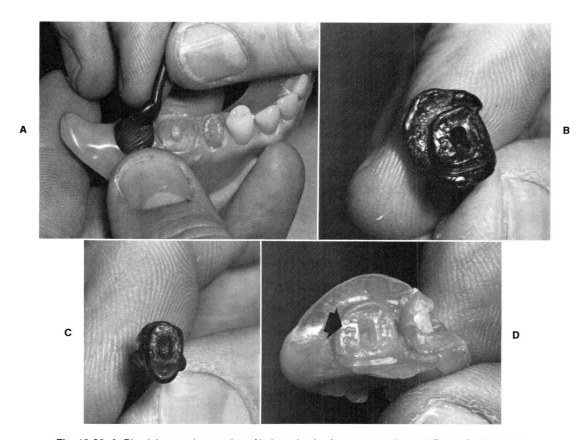

Fig. 12-30. A, Blue inlay wax impression of indentation is often more easily read. **B** and **C,** Wax impression may be readable, thus identifying original mold. All wax must be completely removed before adding resin. **D,** Baseplate wax can be used in same manner. Mold number is visible in wax (arrow).

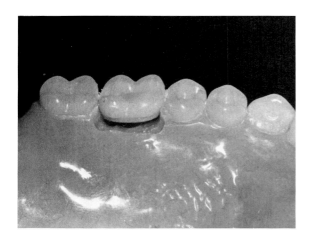

Fig. 12-31. Ridge lap is ground, if necessary, to place tooth correctly. Be sure to check occlusion.

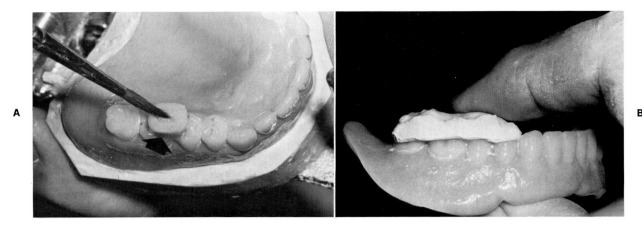

A **B**

Fig. 12-32. A, Replacement tooth is sealed to opposing tooth with sticky wax (arrow). Resin is painted into retention recess of tooth and indentation in denture base before closing articulator. In this instance, lower first molar is being replaced. **B,** Stone index can also be used to check occlusion if occlusal surface of fractured tooth was intact. Index would be made prior to removal of fractured tooth.

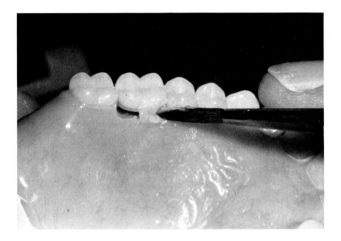

Fig. 12-33. Additional resin is painted into deficient areas as needed.

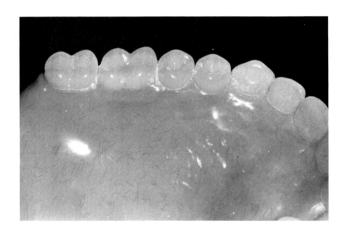

Fig. 12-34. Repair is polished, and occlusion adjusted to opposing teeth or index.

Table 12-2. Replacing posterior denture teeth

Problem	Probable cause	Solution
Posterior replacement is too high or too short, producing error in occlusion	Dentures not mounted prior to fractured-tooth replacement	Mount denture in articulator prior to repair or construct occlusal index
	Replacement-tooth ridge lap not modified properly	Prepare ridge lap to assure correct positioning
	Occlusion not adjusted after repair	With articulating paper, adjust denture occlusion after repairing
Replacement tooth wrong shade	Shade selection made in wrong light	Check shade under variety of lighting conditions
Repair resin on polished denture surface	Too much resin used during paint-on procedure	Use only enough resin to fill in between tooth and denture base resin
Porous repair resin	Repair not cured in pressure container	Cure denture in pressure container

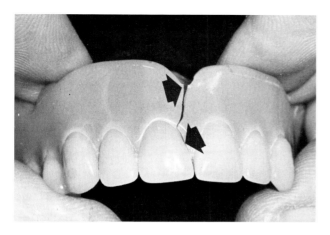

Fig. 12-35. Denture is examined to determine extent of fracture line. Gently flexing denture will aid this determination, but use care to prevent breakage. Fracture originating at labial notch and progressing alongside tooth is common (arrows).

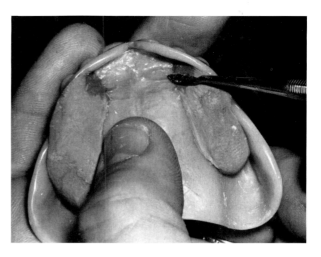

Fig. 12-36. If fractured denture self-approximates, undercuts are blocked out with clay, and repair cast poured. Stone cast poured in denture.

contacts. Careful placement of the tooth and correction of the occlusion after the repair resin has set will reduce occlusion problems.

REPAIRING FRACTURED DENTURE
Nonseparated fracture

This type of fracture often occurs in the midline of a maxillary denture, with the fracture line frequently originating at a deep labial frenum notch.

PROCEDURE

1. Carefully examine the denture to determine the extent of the fracture (Fig. 12-35). Gently flexing the denture, but taking care to prevent breakage, will aid this determination.

2. If the fractured denture is self-approximating, pour plaster into the denture to form a repair cast (Fig. 12-36). Depending on the size of the fracture, pouring the denture completely may not be necessary; instead, pour a cast incorporating the fracture and extending approximately 10 mm to either side of the fracture line (Fig. 12-37).

3. If the denture is undercut in the region of the repair, place a mix of silicone mold release into the undercut area to facilitate removing and replacing the denture after the cast has set (Fig. 12-38).

4. Remove the denture from the set cast, and use a No. 558 bur to grind out the fracture line from beginning to end (Fig. 12-39). Bevel the cut outward to increase the bonding surface (Fig. 12-40). In the palate of maxillary dentures, place dovetails to strengthen the repair joint (Fig. 12-41).

5. Paint the stone cast with tinfoil substitute, and al-

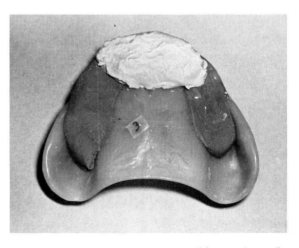

Fig. 12-37. Full cast is not necessary if fracture is small.

low it to dry (Fig. 12-42). Do not place the denture onto the cast before the tinfoil substitute is thoroughly dry; otherwise, coating of the resin may occur, which will severely reduce the repair strength.

6. Replace the denture carefully on the cast (Fig. 12-43).

7. Paint autopolymerizing resin into the groove, taking care to avoid air entrapment (Fig. 12-44).

8. Build up the repair resin slightly above the surface of the denture (Fig. 12-45).

9. Secure the denture to the cast with a rubber band, and cure it for 30 minutes in a pressure container (Fig. 12-46).

10. Remove the cured denture from the cast, then finish and polish it (Fig. 12-47).

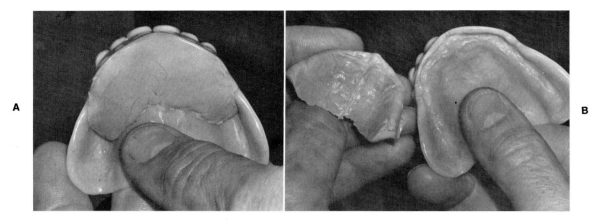

Fig. 12-38. A, Silicone mold material can be placed in undercut, resulting in flexible cast permitting removal of denture, yet maintaining tissue contours essential for repair. **B,** Repair cast of silicone mold release that can be withdrawn from undercuts.

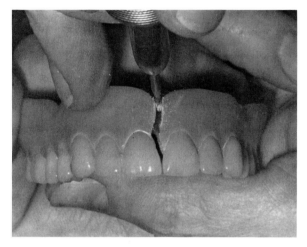

Fig. 12-39. Fracture line is widened from beginning to end with No. 558 bur.

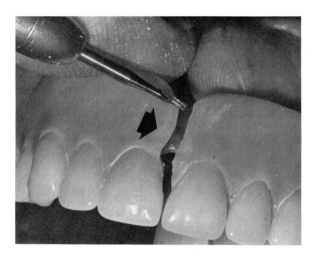

Fig. 12-40. Widened cut is beveled outward (arrow) to increase bonding area.

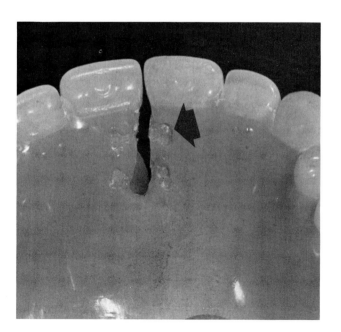

Fig. 12-41. Widened trough can be dovetailed (arrow) on palatal surface to further strengthen repair. Beveled margin is moistened with monomer before repair resin is added.

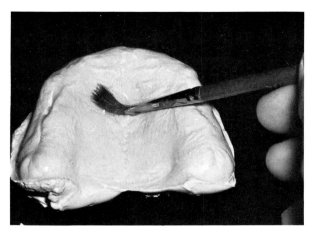

Fig. 12-42. Stone cast is painted with tinfoil substitute and allowed to dry. If denture is placed on cast before tinfoil substitute is thoroughly dry, resin may be coated, reducing repair strength.

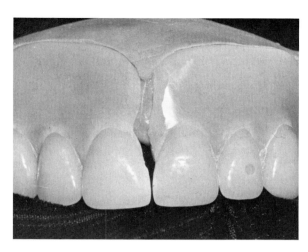

Fig. 12-43. Denture is replaced on cast. Moisten prepared surfaces with monomer before adding resin.

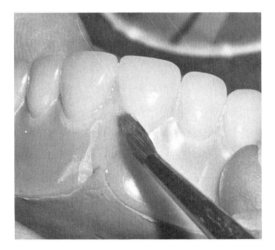

Fig. 12-44. Repair resin is painted in groove, using care to not create voids.

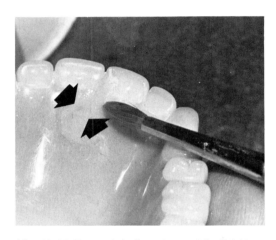

Fig. 12-45. Excess is built up (arrows) for finishing.

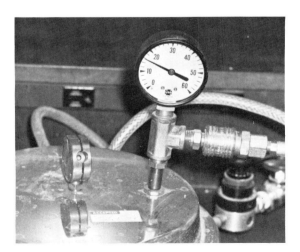

Fig. 12-46. Denture is cured in pressure container for 30 minutes.

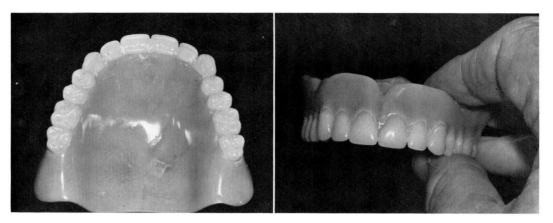

Fig. 12-47. Cured repair is removed, finished, and polished.

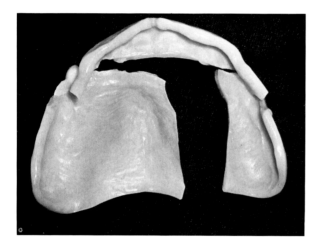

Fig. 12-48. Fragmented dentures require cast after assembly.

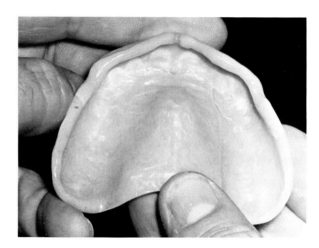

Fig. 12-49. Denture is assembled, noting whether all fragments are present.

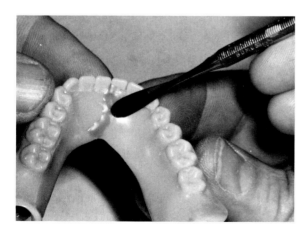

Fig. 12-50. Sticky wax can be used to lute sections together.

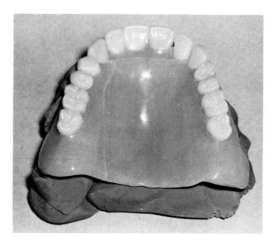

Fig. 12-51. Modeling clay used as scaffold can aid reassembly when assistance is not available.

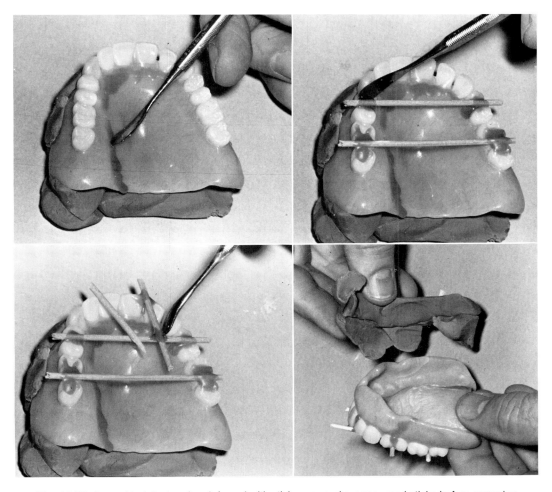

Fig. 12-52. Assembled denture is reinforced with sticky wax and orange wood sticks before removing from clay.

Denture fractured into two or more parts (components)

A denture fractured into two or more parts (components) often occurs when the denture is dropped on a hard surface. This type of breakage requires care to assure that the components are accurately oriented before a cast is poured (Fig. 12-48).

PROCEDURE

1. Examine the denture to determine that all pieces are present (Fig. 12-49).

2. Assemble the individual pieces carefully and lute them together with sticky wax (Fig. 12-50). An assistant may be needed to seal the wax while the denture is being held together. Modeling clay can often be used to hold the pieces in contact while the denture is being luted together (Figs. 12-51 and 12-52).

3. Pour a stone cast into the reassembled denture (Fig. 12-53). Undercut relief may not be required, de-

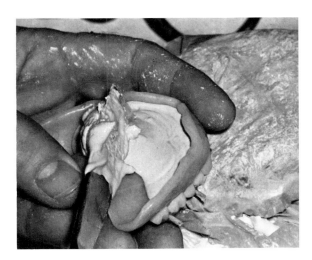

Fig. 12-53. Cast is poured in assembled denture. Undercut relief may not be required depending on degree of fragmentation. Mold release material or alginate can be used if needed.

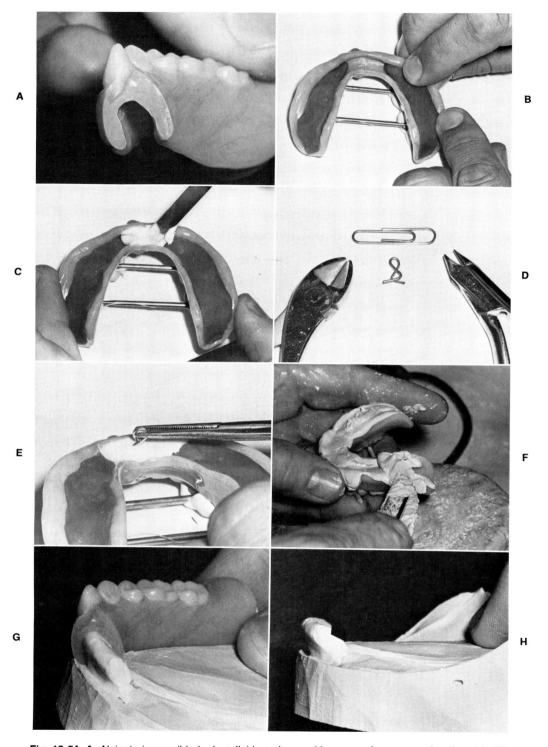

Fig. 12-54. A, Alginate irreversible hydrocolloid can be used because of pronounced undercut in this mandibular denture. **B,** Denture is blocked out with clay similar to method used for constructing mounting casts. Undercut midline fracture region is not blocked out. **C,** Alginate is mixed and painted into denture. **D,** Paper clip is bent to form figure eight retentive wire. **E,** Wire is placed in alginate and held in position until set. **F,** Stone cast is poured. **G,** Flexible alginate permits denture removal, yet preserves contour of undercut ridge. **H,** Cast is removed after denture. Note alginate ridge duplicates tissue surface.

pending on the degree of fragmentation. When needed, a silicone mold release or alginate irreversible hydrocolloid can be placed in denture undercuts to facilitate removal and replacement (Fig. 12-54).

4. After the cast has set, remove the denture, and groove and dovetail the various pieces as previously described; use wire reinforcement to strengthen the repair if desired (Fig. 12-55). Moisten the margin with monomer before painting the repair resin.

5. Paint tinfoil substitute on the cast, and allow it to dry. It is not necessary to paint the alginate with tinfoil substitute.

6. Replace the denture on the cast, and carefully paint autopolymerizing resin into each groove and dovetail (Fig. 12-56). Use antopolymerizing resin that is compatible in color and fiber content to the original denture. Build up the repair resin as previously described.

7. Secure the denture to the cast with plaster or rubber bands, and cure it in a pressure container of warm water for 30 minutes at 20 psi (Fig. 12-57).

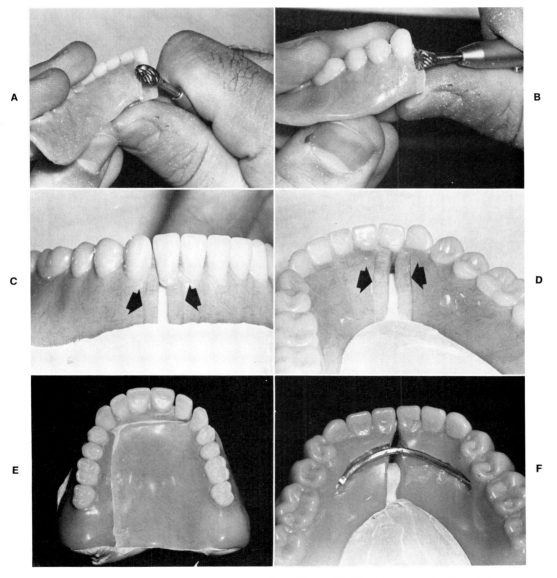

Fig. 12-55. A, Margin of each fragment is beveled with bur. **B,** Handpiece-mounted inverted cone acrylic bur can be used to place bevel. **C,** Mandibular denture labial bevel (arrows). **D,** Mandibular denture lingual bevel (arrows). **E,** Beveled maxillary denture on repair cast. **F,** Wire or screen mesh reinforcement can be incorporated in repair to gain additional strength.

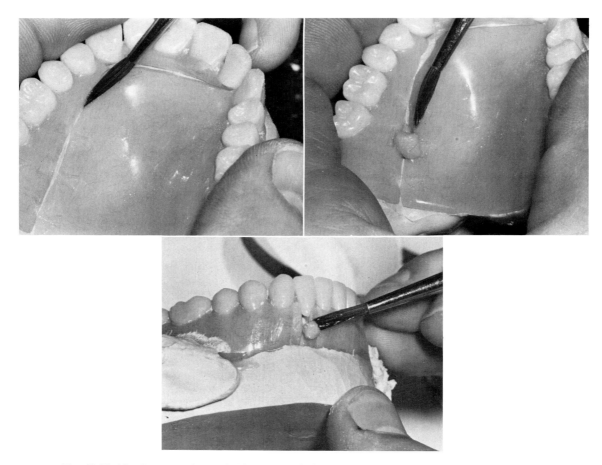

Fig. 12-56. Margins are moistened with monomer before painting repair resin. Autopolymerizing resin is painted in each groove and dovetail, building up excess.

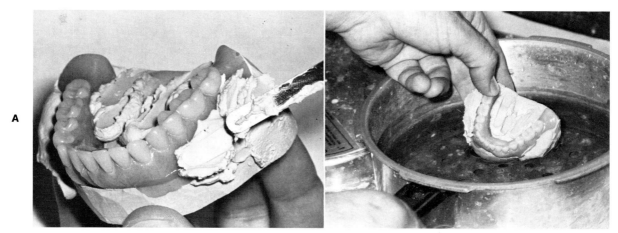

Fig. 12-57. A, Mix of quick-setting plaster can be used to hold denture and cast together. **B,** Repair is cured in pressure container for 30 minutes.

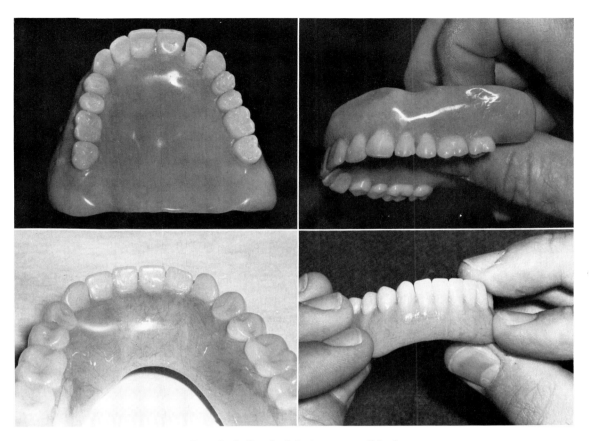

Fig. 12-58. Repaired dentures are polished.

8. Remove the repaired denture from the cast, and finish and polish it (Fig. 12-58).

Fractured denture with section(s) missing

A fractured denture with a section missing will usually require the dentist to make an impression with the denture in place to make a cast, particularly when a flange is broken, and the broken flange section has been lost. In addition, if the denture is broken into several sections, the denture may require a preliminary repair as previously described, prior to making the impression of the lost flange. Autopolymerizing resin is then painted onto the cast to replace the missing portion. The repair is very similar to constructing a resin baseplate.

PROBLEM AREAS

When repairing complete dentures, the principal problems are associated with correctly aligning the denture sections and achieving a strong break-resistant repair (Table 12-3). Alignment problems can be minimized if proper relationship of the various parts is assured as the broken denture is assembled. A high-quality denture repair resin and pressure-container curing will improve the physical properties of the repair.

ADDING A POSTERIOR PALATAL SEAL

Occasionally it may be necessary to add a posterior palatal seal to a maxillary denture after the denture has been constructed. The dentist should use wax or an impression compound to develop the desired thickness and extension of the seal. The laboratory converts this to autopolymerizing resin.

PROCEDURE

1. Pour an artificial stone cast into the denture. The cast must include all of the posterior palatal seal addition and extend 4 to 6 mm beyond it posteriorly (Fig. 12-59).

2. After the cast has set, remove the denture (Fig. 12-60). The denture may be placed in warm water for a few minutes to soften the wax or compound addition prior to removal.

3. Trim the cast, and remove all traces of wax and compound from the denture (Fig. 12-61).

4. Check the fit of the denture to the cast.

5. Paint the cast with tinfoil substitute (Fig. 12-62).

6. With autopolymerizing monomer, moisten the denture surface that is to receive the resin (Fig. 12-63).

7. Add autopolymerizing resin to the cast, and paint additional resin on the denture surface (Fig. 12-64).

Text continued on p. 384.

Table 12-3. Repairing complete denture

Problem	Probable cause	Solution
Repaired denture does not fit properly	Denture sections not aligned properly	Align parts accurately; lute together accurately
	Sticky-wax seal broken or distorted when pouring cast	Use adequate, good-quality sticky wax on dry surface
	Denture repair not allowed adequate setting time	Allow repaired denture to set at least 30 minutes in pressure container before polishing
	Denture did not fit well before breakage	Do not repair ill-fitting denture
Porous denture repair	Denture not cured in pressure container	Cure denture in warm water in pressure pot
	Denture repair-resin surface not kept moistened when painting on additional resin	Keep surface of repair resin moistened with monomer throughout adding resin procedure
Denture repair not rigid	Monomer contaminated	Use noncontaminated monomer; pour monomer from main container into small dappen dish; paint from that
	Wrong monomer (heat-curing) used	Do not substitute heat-curing monomer for autopolymerizing monomer
	Wire reinforcement not used	Use wire reinforcement to add rigidity to repair
Denture repair fails	Prepared edges of denture contaminated with tinfoil substitute	Avoid getting tinfoil substitute on denture edges adjacent to repair
	Wire reinforcement not used	Embed reinforcing wire in denture for additional strength
	Denture fits poorly; occlusion errors present	Refit denture by relining or remounting to adjust occlusion

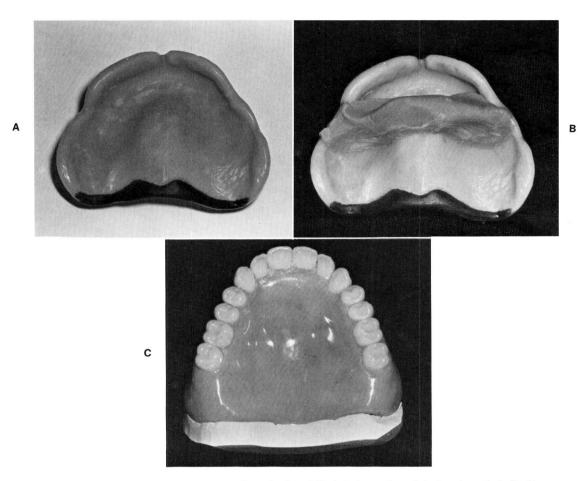

Fig. 12-59. A, Denture with wax posterior palatal seal. **B,** Anterior portion of denture is sealed off with clay. **C,** Cast is constructed to extend 4 to 6 mm beyond posterior border of denture. Denture can be blocked out, since complete cast is not required.

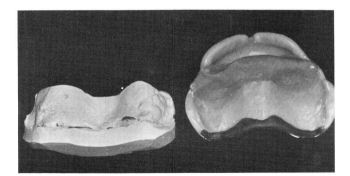

Fig. 12-60. Denture removed from cast.

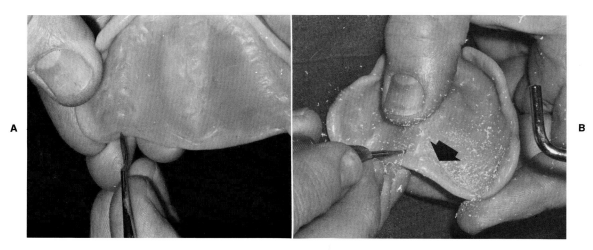

Fig. 12-61. A, All traces of impression compound or wax are removed from denture and cast. **B,** Anterior finish line (arrow) is made with No. 2 round bur.

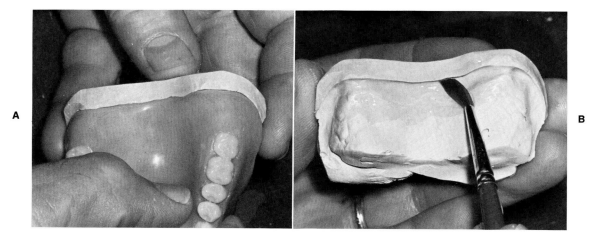

Fig. 12-62. A, Fit of denture is checked on cast. **B,** Cast is painted with tinfoil substitute and allowed to dry.

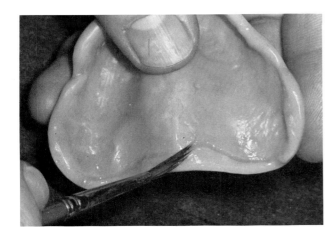

Fig. 12-63. Surface of denture to receive resin is moistened with monomer.

Fig. 12-64. Autopolymerizing resin is mixed and placed on cast, and additional resin is placed on denture.

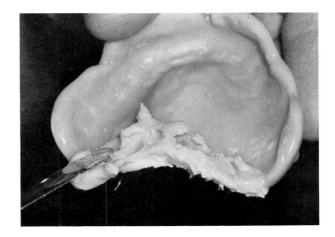

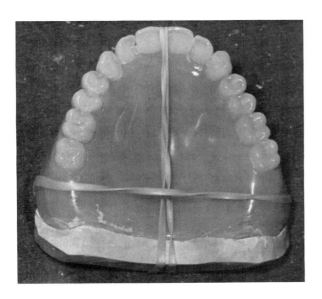

Fig. 12-65. Denture is placed on cast, and firm finger pressure is used to squeeze out excess resin posteriorly. Rubber bands are used to hold denture against cast during curing.

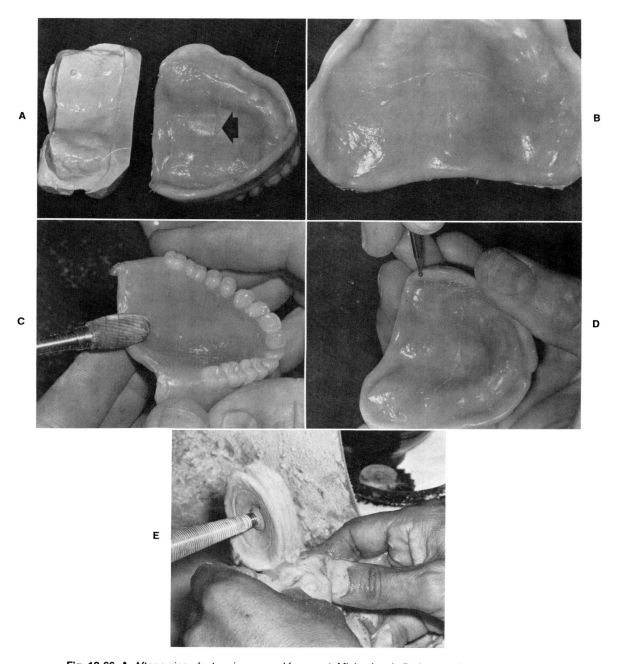

Fig. 12-66. **A,** After curing, denture is removed from cast. Minimal resin flash extending anteriorly must be removed (arrow). **B,** Surface of added resin is smooth, glossy, and devoid of porosity. **C,** Over-extensions are removed with lathe-mounted bur. **D,** Resin nodules or rough edges are smoothed with handpiece-mounted bur. **E,** Posterior border is lightly pumiced to produce smooth surface.

8. Assemble the denture and cast, and use firm finger pressure to squeeze out the excess resin.

9. Secure the cast and denture with a rubber band, and cure it in a pressure container (Fig. 12-65).

10. Remove the cast after curing, and finish and polish it (Fig. 12-66).

PROBLEM AREAS

Problems associated with adding a posterior palatal seal to an existing denture are related to controlling the amount of resin added and preventing voids in the completed addition (Table 12-4). The amount of resin added to the cast should approximate the volume of the wax

Table 12-4. Adding posterior palatal seal

Problem	Probable cause	Solution
Resin flash extends forward onto denture	Too much resin used Denture not seated firmly against cast to express excess resin posteriorly	Control amount of resin added Seat denture firmly with finger pressure to express excess resin posteriorly
Posterior palatal seal has voids	Inadequate resin used Denture not held firmly against cast	Use enough resin to assure complete fill Maintain pressure once denture is seated and resin expressed

or compound used to make the posterior palatal seal. Excessive resin will flow forward onto the tissue-contacting surface of the denture and will require removal. Too little resin will result in undesirable voids in the posterior palatal seal, which will have to be filled with resin.

SUMMARY

Several methods for repairing dentures with autopolymerizing resin have been described in this chapter, as well as a method for adding a posterior palatal seal to an existing denture. Successful denture repairs, providing adequate strength and minimal distortion, result only from painstaking attention to detail.

BIBLIOGRAPHY

Air Force Manual 160-29, Dental Laboratory Technician's Manual, Washington, D.C., 1959, The United States Air Force.

Boone, M. E.: Denture repairs involving midline fracture, J. Prosthet. Dent. **13:**676-678, 1963.

Boucher, C. O., Hickey, C., and Zarb, G. A.: Prosthodontic treatment of edentulous patients, ed. 7, St. Louis, 1975, The C. V. Mosby Co. pp. 556-559.

Martinelli, N.: Dental laboratory technology, ed. 2, St. Louis, 1975, The C. V. Mosby Co., pp. 159-160.

Molner, E. J., and Rice, W. S.: Bonding (repairing) acrylates with self-polymerizing acrylates—advantages and disadvantages, Int. Assoc. Dent. Res. **34:**87, 1956 (abstract).

Sharry, J. J.: Complete denture prosthodontics, ed. 3, New York, 1974, McGraw-Hill Book Co.

Sowter, J. B.: Dental laboratory technology, prosthodontic techniques, Chapel Hill, N.C., 1968, The University of North Carolina Press.

CHAPTER 13

IMMEDIATE DENTURES

KENNETH D. RUDD and ROBERT M. MORROW

immediate denture A removable dental prosthesis constructed for placement immediately after removal of the remaining natural teeth.

Many patients receive an immediate denture for their initial complete denture prosthesis. Immediate dentures offer several advantages. Since the patient receives the denture immediately after the last hopeless teeth are removed, the patient is spared the needless embarrassment of having to appear without teeth. The immediate denture can protect the surgical site, and its appearance is usually excellent, since the natural teeth served as guides for positioning the denture teeth.

CONSTRUCTING IMMEDIATE DENTURES

Laboratory procedures for constructing immediate dentures are similar to conventional complete dentures, except for the method of setting teeth. Preliminary immediate procedures, such as impression-tray and baseplate construction, were described in Chapters 2 and 4.

PROCEDURE

If casts are not received mounted in the articulator, they should be mounted in the laboratory using the centric jaw relation record furnished by the dentist (Fig. 13-1). The procedure for constructing a maxillary immediate denture is as follows:

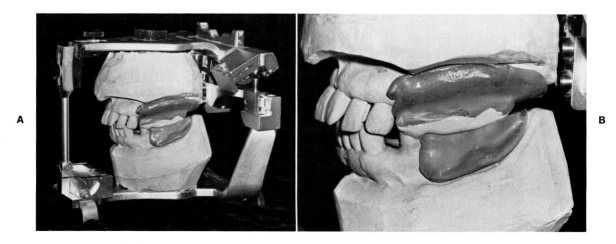

Fig. 13-1. **A,** Casts may be received mounted in articulator. **B,** Usually only anterior teeth remain on casts. This immediate maxillary denture will oppose interim removable partial denture in lower arch.

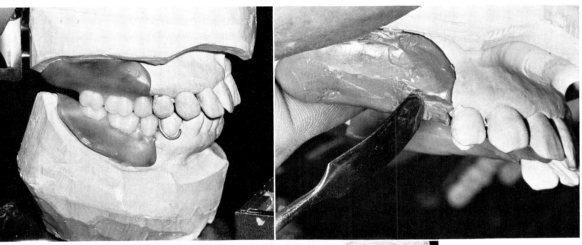

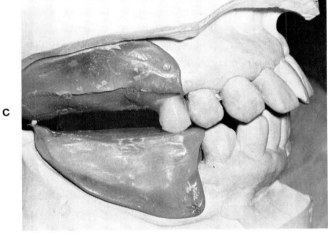

Fig. 13-2. A, Posterior denture teeth are positioned on baseplates for try-in if requested. In this situation, posterior teeth were set on lower cast to determine plane of occlusion and buccolingual tooth position. **B,** Commonly, it is necessary to reduce baseplate thickness prior to positioning tooth. **C,** Premolar in position on relieved baseplate.

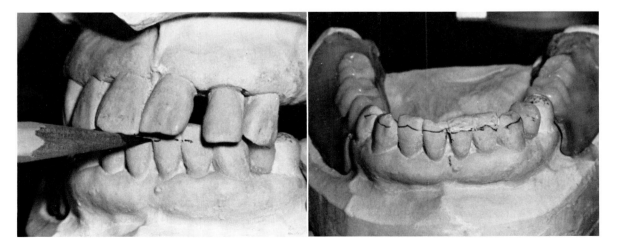

Fig. 13-3. Pencil line placed on labial surfaces of lower anterior teeth indicates vertical overlap in natural dentition and is guide for setting denture teeth.

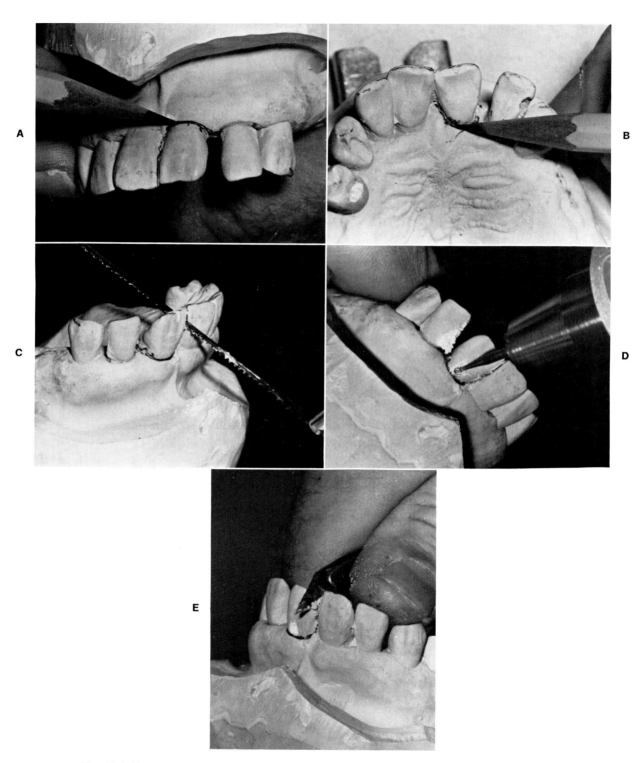

Fig. 13-4. Line indicates gingival margin of tooth to be removed **(A** and **B)**. Tooth is removed from the cast using a saw **(C)**, bur **(D)**, or knife **(E)**.

Immediate dentures   **389**

1. The dentist may wish to try in the posterior teeth to verify tooth shade, position, and accuracy of the jaw relation record. If this is desired, set the posterior teeth on the baseplate, and wax them for try-in (Fig. 13-2). After the try-in is completed, set the anterior teeth.

2. Draw a line on the lower anterior teeth at the level of the upper anterior teeth incisal edges (Fig. 13-3).

3. With a sharp pencil, indicate the gingival margin of the upper anterior teeth before removing one tooth from the cast with a knife or saw (Fig. 13-4).

4. Carve a small depression on the ridge portion of the cast to make a shallow socket (Fig. 13-5).

5. Select a denture tooth of the proper size, shape, and shade, and wax it in the position formerly occupied by the cast tooth (Fig. 13-6). It may be necessary to grind the denture tooth, or change its position, if the natural tooth was malpositioned (Fig. 13-7).

6. Remove alternating teeth on the cast, and set the

corresponding denture teeth (Fig. 13-8). In this manner the cast teeth serve as guides for the shape and position of the denture teeth (Fig. 13-9).

7. Complete the wax-up as previously described (Fig. 13-10).

8. Flask the immediate denture.

9. Eliminate the wax, and allow the flask to cool (Fig. 13-11).

10. Trim the cast according to the instructions of the dentist, or have the dentist trim the cast (Fig. 13-12).

11. Wet the cast in slurry water to prevent sticking, and make an impression of the cast in the flask (Fig. 13-13).

12. Separate the impression, and pour stone in the impression to form a cast (Fig. 13-14). This cast will be used to make a transparent resin surgical template (Fig. 13-15).

13. Paint the stone in the flask with tinfoil substitute

Text continued on p. 395.

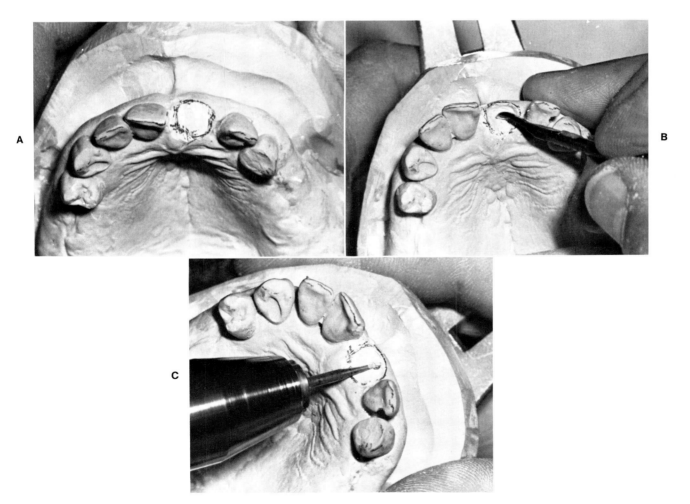

Fig. 13-5. A, Shallow socket is scraped in cast inside pencil mark, indicating gingival margin. **B,** Scraper can be used to taper depression from zero depth lingually to approximately 2 mm in depth facially. **C,** Handpiece-mounted No. 6 bur works well when creating facial depth.

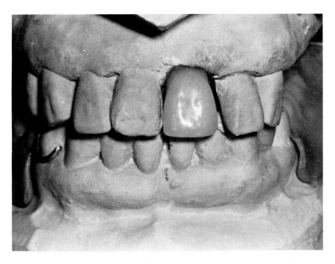

Fig. 13-6. Denture tooth positioned on cast and sealed with base-plate wax.

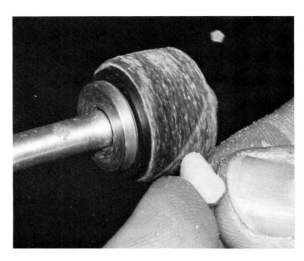

Fig. 13-7. It may be necessary to modify denture tooth by grinding to improve function or esthetics.

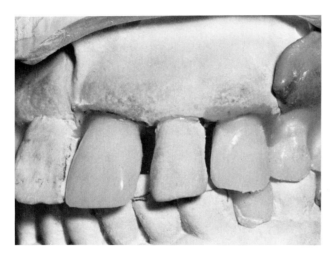

Fig. 13-8. Teeth set in alternating sequence to assure proper position.

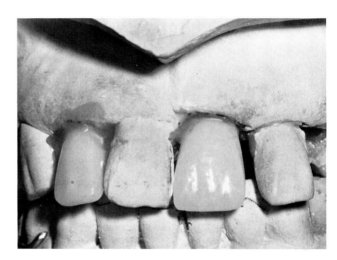

Fig. 13-9. Cast tooth adjacent to denture tooth is guide for proper positioning.

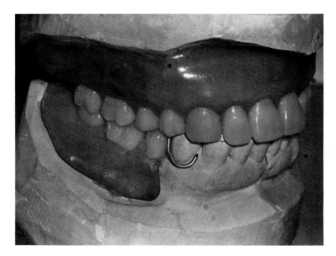

Fig. 13-10. Denture waxed in usual manner. Posterior palatal seal may be placed in cast prior to waxing palate, but *must* be placed before processing denture.

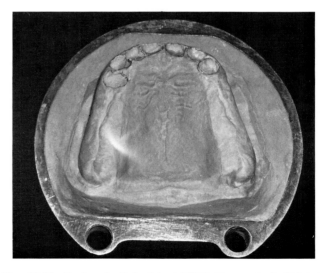

Fig. 13-11. Denture is flasked in artificial stone, wax boiled out, and flask cooled.

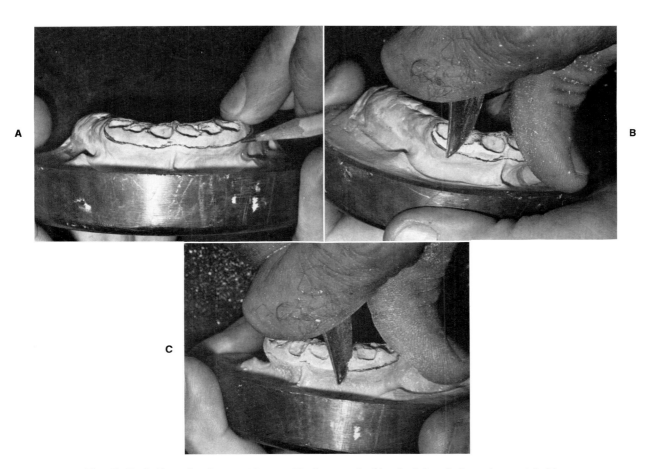

Fig. 13-12. A, Cast trimming must be specifically prescribed by dentist, or better yet, completed by dentist. **B** and **C,** Trim only as specified because overtrimming results in ill-fitting denture.

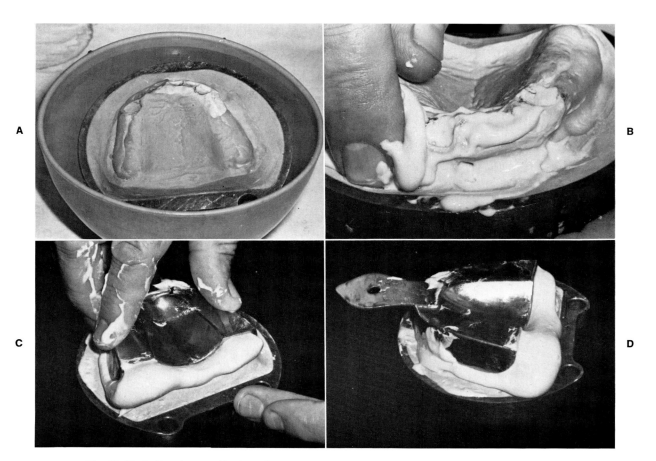

Fig. 13-13. A, Cast is wet with clear slurry water to prevent alginate from sticking. **B,** Alginate placed on cast with finger to minimize voids. **C,** Filled tray is placed in position, and impression made of flasked cast. **D,** Alginate is allowed to set.

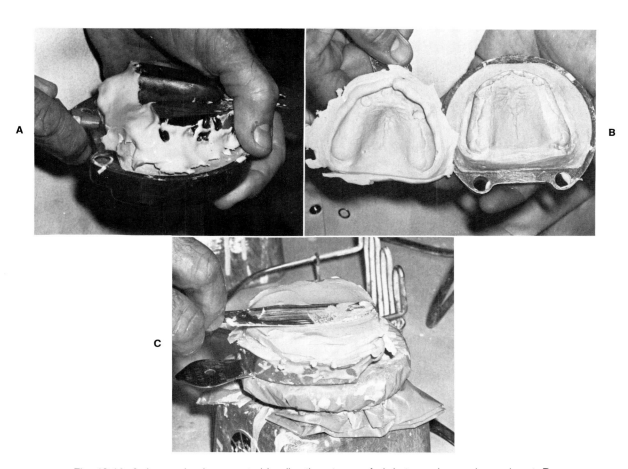

Fig. 13-14. A, Impression is separated by directing stream of air between impression and cast. **B,** Impression is examined to determine if it is acceptable. **C,** Stone is poured in impression to make cast. Cast will be used to construct transparent surgical template.

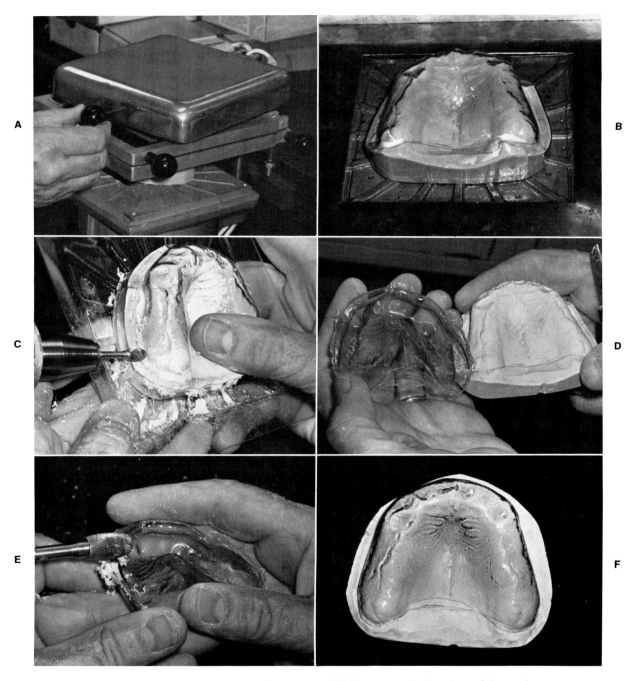

Fig. 13-15. A, Transparent surgical template made quickly by vacuum-forming sheet of clear resin over cast. Cast poured in alginate impression is one used for template. **B,** Heated resin sheet has been formed over cast. Careful finger molding at this stage can improve adaptation. **C,** After cooling, lathe-mounted laboratory bur is used to trim around borders of cast. **D,** Template is removed and examined. **E,** Borders are trimmed and smoothed with lathe-mounted laboratory bur. **F,** Template is stored on cast.

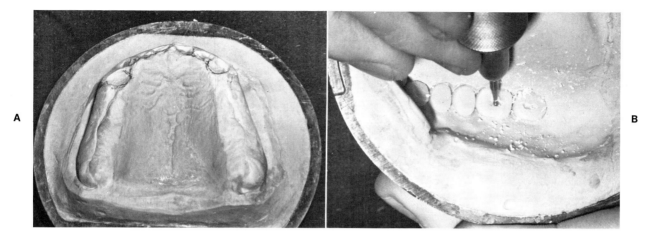

Fig. 13-16. A, Cast and stone are painted with tinfoil substitute, using care to not place tinfoil substitute on ridge laps of teeth. **B,** Indentations placed in ridge laps of resin teeth improve bonding to denture base.

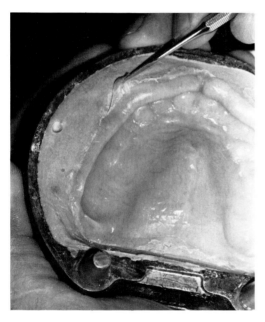

Fig. 13-17. Denture base resin is mixed according to manufacturer's recommendations, and denture is trial packed to assure minimum flash.

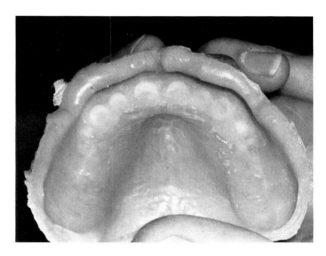

Fig. 13-18. After processing and recovering denture from mold, it is examined for resin nodules or sharp fins.

(Fig. 13-16, *A*). Indentations placed in ridge laps of resin denture teeth can improve the attachment of teeth to the denture base (Fig. 13-16, *B*).

14. Mix the denture base resin, and pack the immediate denture (Fig. 13-17).

15. Cure the immediate denture as recommended by the resin manufacturer.

16. After curing, cool it to room temperature, and recover the denture as described in Chapter 9.

17. Remount the denture in the articulator, and correct processing errors as previously described.

18. Construct a face-bow index to permit remounting of the maxillary denture later as described in Chapter 9.

19. Remove the denture from the cast, and examine it carefully (Fig. 13-18). Sharp fins, resin projections formed by the sockets, and nodules can be removed from the interior of the denture with a bur (Fig. 13-19).

20. Polish the immediate denture (Fig. 13-20).

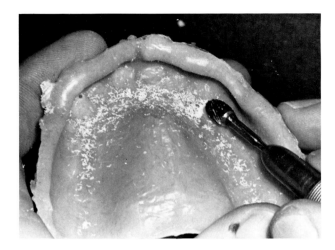

Fig. 13-19. Sharp projections on denture are smoothed with bur. Remove resin projections that were formed by sockets carved into cast.

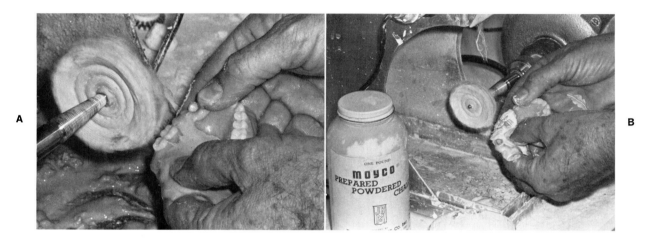

Fig. 13-20. A, Carefully pumice denture, paying particular attention to borders. **B,** High shine achieved with soft rag wheel and slurry of prepared powdered chalk.

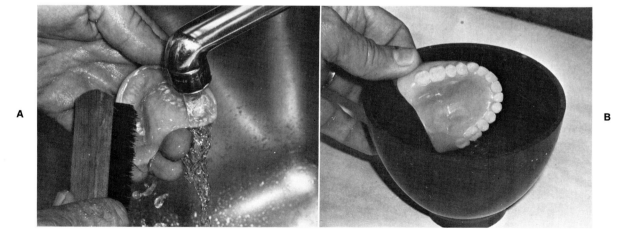

Fig. 13-21. A, Denture is scrubbed to remove polishing agent. **B,** Store denture in water or 1:10 dilution of 5% to 6% sodium hypochlorite and water. Dentures with teeth that have metal occlusal surfaces should not be stored in sodium hypochlorite solution.

Table 13-1. Constructing immediate dentures

Problem	Probable cause	Solution
Esthetics of immediate denture not acceptable because of drastic change in appearance of patient	Denture teeth not placed in position of natural teeth Position of denture teeth differs significantly from position of natural teeth because of overcorrection	Place denture teeth in same position as natural teeth where acceptable Avoid drastic correction, which may produce poor esthetic results, when compensating for malpositioned natural teeth
Immediate denture and surgical template do not demonstrate good adaptation on insertion	Cast overtrimmed prior to packing immediate denture	Trim cast only as prescribed by dentist or dentist can trim cast

21. Scrub the denture thoroughly with soap and water and store it in water or diluted sodium hypochlorite (Fig. 13-21).

PROBLEM AREAS

Principal problems associated with construction of immediate dentures are similar to those for conventional complete dentures (Chapters 8 and 9). Problems unique to immediate dentures are related to failure to duplicate the position of natural teeth (Table 13-1). This can occur when attempting to correct the positions of natural teeth with the denture teeth and overtrimming the cast prior to packing.

Denture teeth can be positioned on the cast to improve the esthetics of the completed denture. This is particularly true when the natural teeth are malpositioned with unslightly diastemas and overlap. The cast should not be overtrimmed prior to packing the denture, and this procedure should be prescribed or accomplished by the dentist.

SUMMARY

This chapter described procedures used during the construction of an immediate denture that differ from comparable procedures for conventional complete dentures.

CHAPTER 14

FLUID RESIN COMPLETE DENTURES

PART ONE

Denture base processing with a hydrocolloid investment

WALTER L. SHEPARD

festooning Carving of the denture base material to simulate the contours of the natural tissues that are to be replaced by the denture.

fluid resin (pour resin) An autopolymerizing or lower temperature–curing resin that can be introduced into a mold in a liquid state.

Traditionally, methods of denture base formation consisted of carving, casting, or forming the base under varying degrees of pressure. Dentists hand carved early dentures from various organic materials, such as ivory, wood, or animal horn, and usually fitted them directly to the oral tissues. After the advent of techniques for making impressions of the mouth, they devised methods of making denture bases of swaged gold, tin, aluminum, and porcelain. Vulcanization probably brought to dentistry the first relatively inexpensive method of producing a denture base that was accurate and durable. Although in the late 1930s vulcanite lost its popularity as a primary means of processing denture bases, dentists continue to find the occasional patient who still wears vulcanite dentures.

The methyl methacrylate denture, which possessed superior esthetic characteristics and offered other advantages over denture bases of vulcanite and other materials, primarily condensites, first appeared in 1937. The inherent properties of methyl methacrylate cause it to remain the denture base material of choice today. No other denture base materials have proved equal to methyl methacrylate denture base materials, in spite of other claims of superiority.

Mirza (1961) described a method of producing a denture base that used a pourable methyl methacrylate resin and a hydrocolloid investing medium. Thereafter, numerous reports about this type of denture base processing appeared, and several manufacturers produced resins that dentists could introduce into a mold in a liquid state. Winkler (1967) described a technique, and Shepard (1968) reported the results of producing more than 14,000 dentures in a 2-year period, using a hydrocolloid investment and a liquid resin.

The substitution of hydrocolloid for gypsum as an investing medium offered several advantages. It considerably reduced the working time required for flasking and deflasking. Tooth breakage was less likely to occur during deflasking, hydrocolloid material was both cleaner to handle and reusable, curing was faster, and it was possible for the dentist to receive the finished denture sooner. Axinn et al. (1975) reported that the results obtained with this method compared favorably with conventional packing techniques.

As in almost all procedures in dentistry, disadvantages offset some advantages. Usually, a slight loss in the vertical dimension of the occlusion occurred, but it was possible to compensate for it when making jaw records or setting teeth. Increasing the interocclusal distance 0.5 mm in the incisal guide-pin area of the articulator offset curing shrinkage. Occasionally, individual tooth movement occurred, particularly if it was necessary to reduce excessively the length of the denture tooth to accommodate the lack of interocclusal space. The denture base contouring phase of the waxing procedures required more attention to detail.

398

REQUIREMENTS FOR DENTAL RESIN

Phillips (1973) stated the properties of an ideal resin as follows:

1. The material should exhibit a translucency or transparency that would make it possible to duplicate esthetically the oral tissues that it was to replace.

2. No change should occur in the color or appearance of the material after fabrication, whether accomplished inside or outside of the mouth.

3. It should not expand, contract, or warp during processing or subsequent use by the patient.

4. It should possess adequate strength, resilience, and abrasion resistance to withstand all normal use.

5. It should be sufficiently impermeable to oral fluids so that it would remain sanitary and not acquire a disagreeable taste or odor.

6. It should be completely insoluble in the oral fluids or any substances taken into the mouth, show no evidence of corrosive attack, and not absorb these fluids.

7. It should be tasteless, odorless, nontoxic, and nonirritating to the oral tissues.

8. It should have a low specific gravity.

9. Its softening temperature should be well above the temperature of any hot foods or liquids taken into the mouth.

10. In case of unavoidable breakage, it should be possible to repair easily and efficiently.

11. It should be easy to make the material into a dental appliance with only simple equipment.

Although no known dental resin would satisfy all of these requirements, acrylic resins, such as methyl methacrylate, as well as the resins described in this technique, have essentially all of these properties.

SYNOPSIS OF METHOD

1. Place the waxed denture in a modified duplicating flask,* and surround it with a hydrocolloid.

2. Chill the hydrocolloid.

3. Remove the waxed denture from the mold, and sprue the mold.

4. Remove the teeth and wax from the cast, clean them, and replace them in the mold.

5. Reassemble the flask.

6. Mix the resin, and pour it into the mold.

7. Cure the denture.

8. Deflask the denture, and finish and polish it by the conventional method.

MATERIALS AND EQUIPMENT REQUIRED

1. Pourable methyl methacrylate resin
2. Suitable flask (Fig. 14-1)
3. Reversible hydrocolloid
4. Hydrocolloid conditioner
5. No. 4 and No. 5 cork borers
6. Tinfoil substitute
7. Wax detergent
8. Compartmentalized strainer for cleaning teeth†
9. Pneumatic curing unit

---

*V-102 Flask, Vernon-Benshoff Co., Inc., Albany, N.Y.
†Howmedica, Inc., Chicago, Ill.

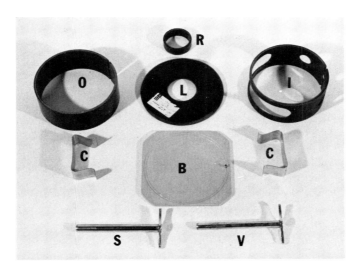

Fig. 14-1. Flask disassembled. Inner ring *(I)* has large opening to permit cutting of sprues and vents. Split outer ring *(O)* confines hydrocolloid within flask. Reservoir *(R)* is tapered to fit snugly into lid *(L)*. Metal base *(B)* is held securely in position by flexible metal retaining clips *(C)*. No. 5 cork borer *(S)* is used for spruing. No. 4 cork borer *(V)* is used for venting.

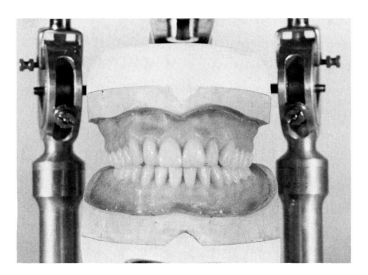

Fig. 14-2. Cast should be tapered so that it will have adequate land area.

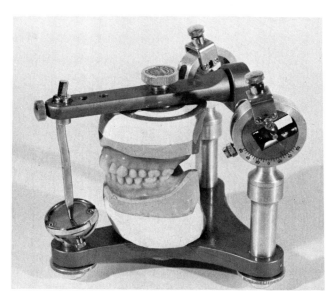

Fig. 14-3. Waxed denture should be made to conform to desired finished contours and be well sealed to cast. Teeth should be free of wax residue.

PREPARATION OF CAST AND WAX PATTERN
PROCEDURE

1. Make the cast so that it has an adequate shelf or land area, 3 to 5 mm, to support the cast in the mold after dewaxing.

2. Taper the sides of the cast so that they will converge slightly toward the occlusal aspect, thereby facilitating removal from the chilled hydrocolloid (Fig. 14-2). The base should be flat, and the cast should be free of contaminants.

3. Contour the wax in exactly the same manner as desired in the finished denture (Fig. 14-3). The ability of the hydrocolloid to duplicate minute details makes it worthwhile to spend additional time on festooning. Exercising care with this procedure will espedite finishing and polishing.

4. It is extremely important to have no wax residue left on the artificial teeth prior to investing. Carelessness at this point not only increases finishing time, but it also can result in dislodging the teeth during pouring procedures. It is essential to remember that the hydrocolloid will duplicate accurately any wax remaining on the teeth as well as the waxed denture. Any wax left on the tooth surface will result in a void between the tooth and hydrocolloid after dewaxing and repositioning the tooth in the mold. In this instance, a resin flash will occur on the tooth surface during the pouring of the denture.

5. It is necessary to take advantage of existing undercuts on the teeth by trimming the wax down to the collar. This gives the teeth better retention in the mold

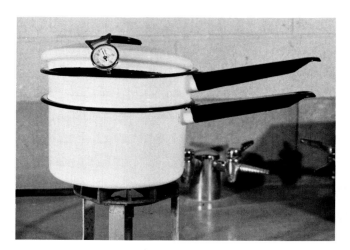

Fig. 14-4. Double boiler may be used to break down hydrocolloid. Use of aluminum utensils should be avoided because of adverse effect on hydrocolloid.

and reduces the likelihood of tooth movement during pouring.

6. When using a preformed palatal pattern, it is essential to seal the cast with a thin coating of wax before adapting it. Firm adaptation of the pattern in position is necessary to prevent any lifting away from the cast when pouring the hydrocolloid.

PREPARATION OF HYDROCOLLOID
PROCEDURE

1. Break down the hydrocolloid in a simple double boiler or conditioning machine (Fig. 14-4). Bring it to

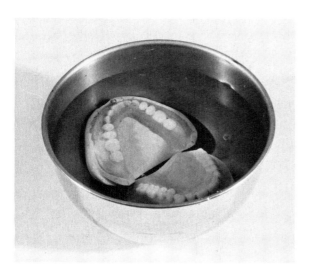 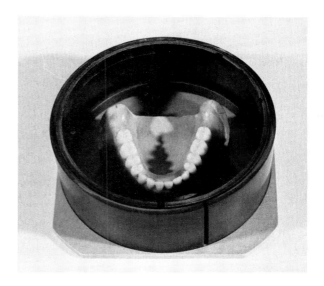

Fig. 14-5. Waxed dentures are soaked in slurry water to displace air in casts. Note bubbles being released.

Fig. 14-6. Waxed denture is centered in ring with distal aspect toward large opening of inner ring.

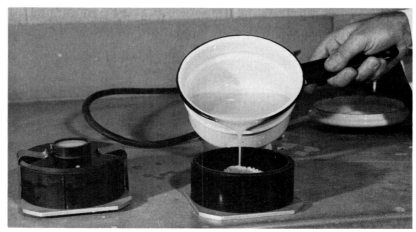

Fig. 14-7. Hydrocolloid is poured so that flask is filled from base upward.

a temperature that produces a fluid without lumps, and then cool it to a temperature between 120° and 125° F 50° to 53° C). Hydrocolloids that contain glycerin or those that are water thinned are satisfactory investment media. The glycerin-type hydrocolloid appears to be tougher and have a longer life as well as a desirable tacky surface. However, it is impossible to use it in duplicating casts because it adversely affects the setting of gypsum products. Reuse of either material is satisfactory until it no longer cuts sharply with a sprue former.

2. Wash the hydrocolloid free of all debris after use, and store it in a moist atmosphere.

INVESTMENT
PROCEDURE

1. Soak the cast with the waxed denture in slurry water at room temperature for 10 minutes prior to in-

vesting (Fig. 14-5) to displace any air within the cast and prevent bubble formation in the hydrocolloid investment.

2. Assemble the flask without the top, and center the waxed denture in the flask. It is important to center the waxed denture so that an equal amount of hydrocolloid surrounds it and thereby prevent distortion. The distal aspect of the denture should face the large opening of the inner ring (Fig. 14-6) to allow access to areas of the denture base through which sprues and vents can be cut.

3. Pour the hydrocolloid into the side of the ring to fill it from the base upward (Fig. 14-7). After covering the teeth, assemble the top of the flask, position the retaining clips, and add the reservoir. Continue pouring through the reservoir until it is full.

4. Place the flask in cool circulating water no deeper than half the height of the flask (Fig. 14-8). The metal base will conduct the heat from the mold so that the

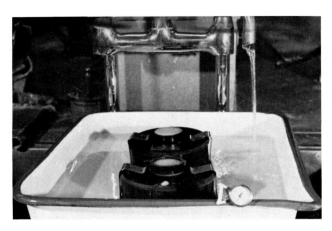

Fig. 14-8. Flasks should remain in cool circulating water until hydrocolloid has gelled.

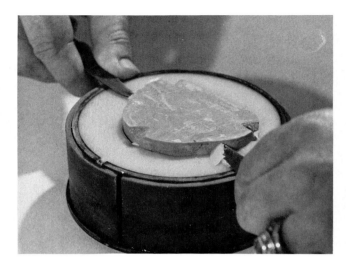

Fig. 14-9. Hydrocolloid is removed from areas in which cast has been keyed and beveled to gain access to base. All torn fragments of hydrocolloid must be cleared away carefully after removal of cast and waxed denture.

hydrocolloid will gel and shrink toward the base, resulting in a more accurate mold. Allow the flask to remain in the water for 45 minutes to assure complete gelation.

DEWAXING
PROCEDURE

1. Remove the retaining clips and reservoir after gelation, and trim the hydrocolloid reservoir flush with the lid of the flask.

2. Remove the base of the flask and any hydrocolloid from the areas used in keying the cast.

3. Bevel the hydrocolloid around the base of the cast slightly to permit access with a knife blade on each side of the cast to facilitate removal of the cast and waxed denture.

4. Grip the knive blades firmly at each side of the base of the cast, and apply downward leverage with the knife handles to remove the waxed denture from the mold (Fig. 14-9).

5. Remove any torn fragments of hydrocolloid carefully from the beveled surface to keep them from falling into the mold (Fig. 14-10).

6. Dislodge the denture teeth from the wax, and place them in the compartmentalized strainer in proper sequence (Fig. 14-11).

7. Clean the teeth with detergent to remove all wax residue, and rinse them in clear, hot water (Fig. 14-12).

8. Remove the waxed denture base, clean the cast with detergent, and rinse it with hot water.

9. Apply a thin coat of separating medium (tinfoil substitute) evenly over the impression surface of the cast

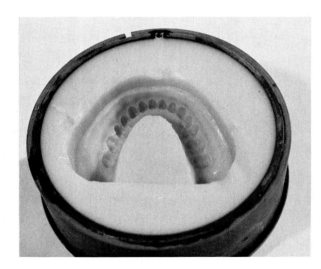

Fig. 14-10. Mold should be inspected carefully for any loose pieces of hydrocolloid.

while it is still hot (Fig. 14-13). Set the cast aside, and permit it to cool.

10. Exercise care to avoid pooling the separating medium on any part of the cast. Since the resin is fluid, it does not require any packing pressure and will not displace thick areas of separating medium during processing. Therefore voids can occur on the impression surface and border areas of the finished denture. The paintbrush can carry small stone particles back into the separating medium, contaminate it, and cause it to thicken. Pour a small amount of fresh separating me-

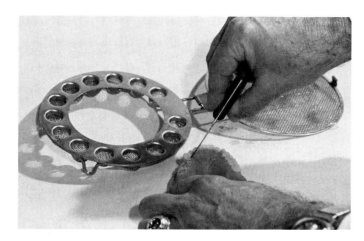

Fig. 14-11. Denture teeth are removed and placed in proper compartments of strainer.

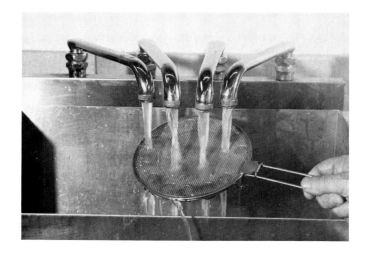

Fig. 14-12. Teeth must be cleaned thoroughly of all wax residue.

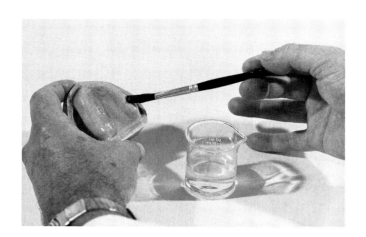

Fig. 14-13. Thin coating of uncontaminated separating medium is applied to clean cast. Care is taken to prevent pooling of medium.

dium into a clean container, and discard any unused portion at the end of the working period.

SPRUING AND VENTING
PROCEDURE

1. Remove the outer ring of the flask to expose the area designated for the vents and sprues.

2. Position the No. 4 cork borer so that it will cut through the hydrocolloid to the most distal area of the mold to provide a vent. Usually these areas are the distolingual flange area of the lower denture and the hamular notch area of the upper denture. After cutting the vents and removing the hydrocolloid plugs, make the main pouring sprue.

3. Make the slightly larger pouring sprue with a No. 5 cork borer. Position it so that it will make contact with the denture base in the distal midline area of the upper

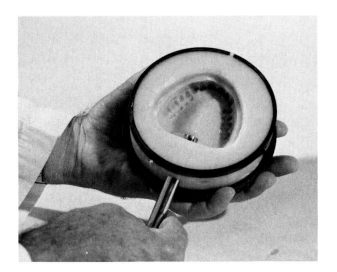

Fig. 14-14. Main pouring sprue is cut after vents are made. Vents and pouring sprue should be as close to parallel as possible.

denture and distolingual midline area of the lower denture (Fig. 14-14).

4. The principal consideration when spruing is having the fluid resin reach the most central anterior area of the denture as quickly as possible and permitting it to travel up the lateral aspects of the denture and force air out ahead of it.

5. Some assistance with a sharp blade may be necessary to release the hydrocolloid plug from the mold after the cork borer has cut into the denture base portion.

6. Scrutinize the mold carefully for any loose fragments of hydrocolloid, and remove them to prevent their incorporation in the resin.

REPLACING TEETH IN MOLD
PROCEDURE

1. Remove the thoroughly cleaned teeth from the strainer with cotton pliers, and replace them in their respective positions in the mold (Fig. 14-15). When using resin teeth, grind the ridge-lap area lightly prior to replacing the teeth in the mold. Civjan et al. (1972) reported that removal of the glaze will result in a stronger bond at the denture base and tooth interface. It is more expedient to grind resin teeth lightly during setup procedures. When using porcelain teeth, remove any water remaining in the diatoric portion of the tooth with a blast of air.

2. After repositioning the teeth in the mold, invert the flask, and shake it gently to make certain that the teeth remain in position.

3. If any tooth becomes dislodged at this point, use a small amount of petroleum jelly on the occlusal or incisal surface to hold it in place. Eastman 910 adhesive* also works well for this purpose. Exercise care to prevent contact between either of these materials and the

---

*Buffalo Dental Manufacturing Co., Inc., Brooklyn, N.Y.

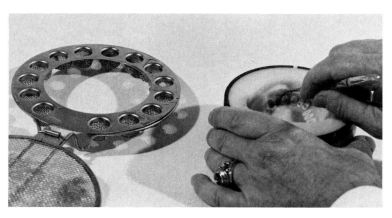

Fig. 14-15. Teeth are replaced in their respective positions in mold.

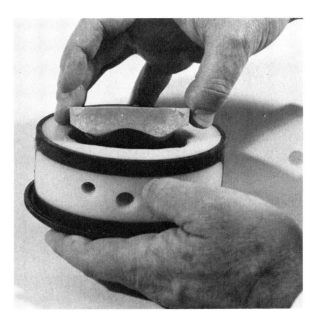

Fig. 14-16. Cool cast is replaced carefully in mold.

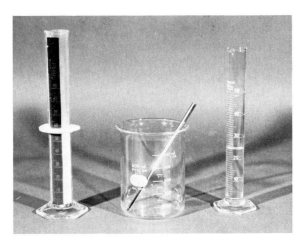

Fig. 14-17. Proportions must be accurate, and mixing utensils must be clean.

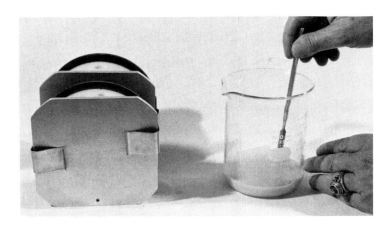

Fig. 14-18. Mixing is done slowly for 15 to 30 seconds.

ridge-lap area of the teeth because the result will be a poor bond between the tooth and resin.

MIXING AND POURING RESIN
PROCEDURE

1. Replace the cast in the mold (Fig. 14-16), and reposition the base of the flask and retaining clips. Make certain that the cast is not warm at this point.

2. Measure the powder and liquid accurately to assure proper color, dimensional stability, and curing and pouring of the resin. Follow the manufacturer's directions accurately because mixing procedures vary between manufacturers.

3. Use resins with a higher percentage of polymer in relation to monomer to produce the best results because less curing shrinkage is likely to occur. Winkler (1972) states some resins use two volumes of polymer to one volume of monomer, and at least one resin uses three volumes of polymer to one volume of monomer. Though more viscous in its pouring state, the latter* produces excellent results, similar to resins using a 2.5:1† or an 8:3‡ ratio. Therefore, the higher polymer ratio resins are preferable.

4. All of the currently available fluid resins allow sufficient working time for pouring two dentures from the same mix. Clean the mixing equipment thoroughly (Fig. 14-17).

5. Add the polymer to the monomer, and stir slowly for 15 to 30 seconds until the mixutre has a uniform consistency (Fig. 14-18). A glass or polyethylene mixing beaker is suitable for the purpose. Overspatulation can cause the undesirable incorporation of air in the resin.

6. Rotate the beaker slowly for 10 to 15 seconds to assure homogeneity before pouring.

7. Handle the flask carefully to avoid dropping or

---

*Flow, Cosmos Dental Products, Mt. Vernon, N.Y.
†Pronto II, Vernon-Benshoff Co., Inc., Albany, N.Y.
‡Myerson's Porit, Myerson Tooth Corp., Cambridge, Mass.

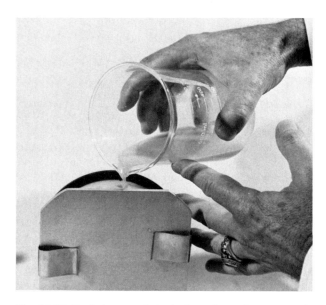

Fig. 14-19. Resin is poured slowly through pouring sprue only.

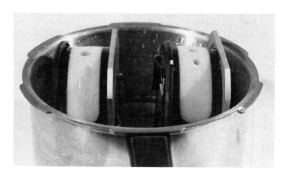

Fig. 14-20. Flasks are placed in curing unit carefully to prevent initial air input from disturbing resin.

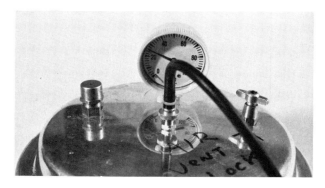

Fig. 14-21. Air pressure at 20 to 30 psi is maintained for 30 minutes. Pressure must be monitored.

jarring it. If either occurs, discard the mix, and disassemble the flask to make certain that there has been no tooth movement.

8. Pour the resin slowly through the main pouring sprue only (Fig. 14-19). Do not add any resin in the vents. Adding resin through the vents could produce voids. Continue pouring until the resin overflows through the vents.

9. Rock the flask gently from side to side for 10 to 15 seconds to displace any air bubbles that may have become trapped during pouring. It is possible to add more material if the sprue level drops as a result of overflow through the vents, but add it only to the main pouring sprue. Then the dentures are ready for curing.

CURING DENTURES
PROCEDURE

1. The curing procedure varies slightly from one resin to another. Some are autopolymerizing, whereas others require low curing temperatures. A temperature-controlled pneumatic curing unit is helpful, but not absolutely necessary. Follow the manufacturer's directions as to the temperature and depth of the water in the curing unit. The temperatures vary from 100° to 125° F (38° to 51.5° C). One resin requires a starting temperature of 120° F (49° C) in a curing unit.

2. Position the flasks carefully in the curing unit so that the sprues or vents are not directly beneath the air inlet (Fig. 14-20). This precaution will prevent an initial intake of air in the curing unit from disturbing the fluid resin.

3. Position the top of the curing unit securely, and add 20 to 30 psi air pressure (Fig. 14-21).

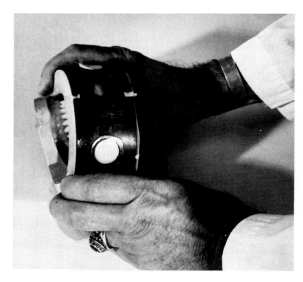

Fig. 14-22. Cured denture is ejected from mold with finger pressure.

4. Monitor the pressure gauge to make certain that the unit does not lose pressure.

5. After 30 minutes in the curing unit at 20 to 30 psi, release the pressure, and remove the flasks. The dentures are cured.

DEFLASKING
PROCEDURE

1. A major advantage of this method of processing is the ease with which it is possible to recover the dentures after curing. To recover the dentures after curing disassemble the flask, and eject the dentures with finger pressure (Fig. 14-22).

2. Wash the hydrocolloid clean of any debris, and store it for further use.

FINISHING AND POLISHING
PROCEDURE

1. If the sprues or vents interfere with remounting, remove them with a separating disk at this time (Fig. 14-23). If it is possible to remount the dentures without interference, remove the sprues and vents later (Fig. 14-24).

2. Equilibrate the occlusion, remove the casts, and finish and polish the dentures in the conventional manner (Fig. 14-25).

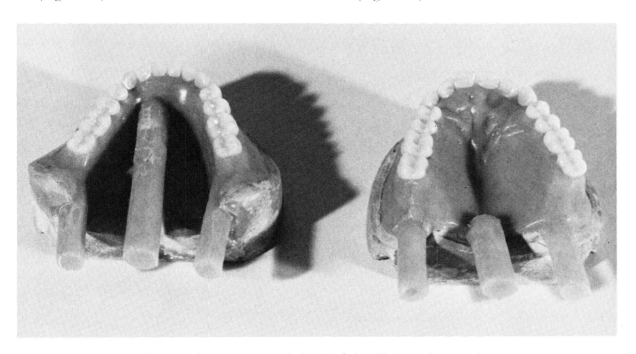

Fig. 14-23. Sprues are removed when interfering with remounting procedures.

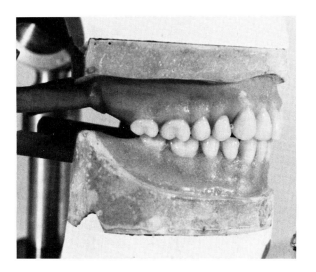

Fig. 14-24. Dentures are remounted prior to equilibration. Note slight loss in vertical dimension, indicated by opening between maxillary cast and mounting.

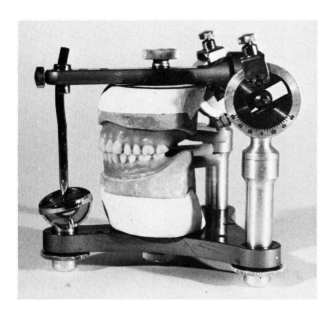

Fig. 14-25. Dentures after occlusal equilibration.

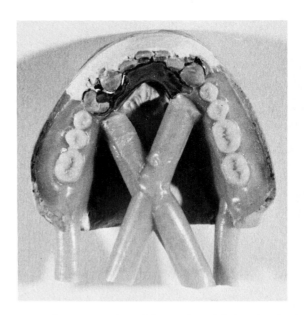

Fig. 14-26. Processed bilateral free-end partial denture showing sprue and vent positions. Area beneath lingual bar has been blocked out with quick-setting plaster of Paris.

REMOVABLE PARTIAL DENTURES

PROCEDURE

1. Spruing procedures vary when processing partial dentures, according to the type and position of the denture base areas. The principle is the same as for complete dentures, that is, having the sprue connect the most anterior accessible denture base area and making the vents at the most distal aspect of the denture base.

2. Block out gross undercuts of the cast with quick-setting plaster of Paris to prevent tearing of the hydrocolloid when removing the cast from the mold. Do not use modeling clay in this procedure because it can change shape during handling in the dewaxing procedures and prevent proper reseating of the cast back in the mold. The areas requiring blockout are generally the labial aspect of the anterior teeth and beneath the lingual major connector of the lower partial dentures (Fig. 14-26). Block out any other severe undercut areas, but do not extend the plaster over the clasp arms as the framework is removed from the cast during dewaxing procedures (Fig. 14-27).

3. Bilateral and unilateral free-end partial dentures require no modifications prior to investing other than plaster blockout. In instances when a distal abutment tooth prevents access for a vent, attach a roll of wax of approximately the size of the vent to the most distal aspect of the denture base, and bring it back to an accessible area of the cast. Cut the vent to the space in the mold formed by the roll of wax (Fig. 14-28).

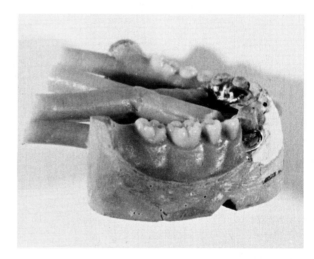

Fig. 14-27. Anterior undercut area also is blocked out with plaster of Paris. Plaster should not cover clasp arms.

4. For partial dentures containing only an anterior denture base, attach a roll of wax to the labial aspect of the denture base in the buccal fold area, and continue it posteriorly to an accessible venting area.

5. Cut the pouring sprue through to the denture base at the lingual aspect of the anterior teeth, and vent it where the roll of wax ended (Fig. 14-29).

6. When there are both an anterior denture base and a unilateral posterior denture base, attach one roll of wax to the buccal fold area from the anterior base to the

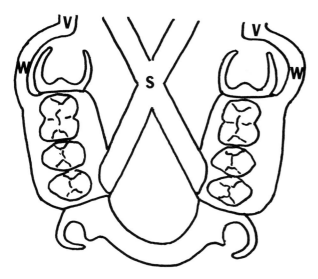

Fig. 14-28. Bilateral partial denture with distal abutments. Sprues *(S)* are cut to most anterior lingual segment. Rolls of wax *(W)* were connected to denture base and brought distally to accessible vent *(V)* area prior to investment.

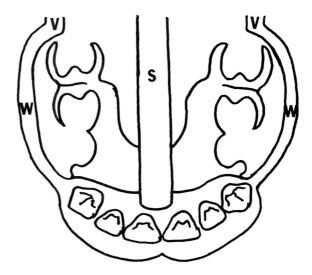

Fig. 14-29. Partial denture with only anterior edentulous area. Sprue *(S)* is cut to lingual area. Rolls of wax *(W)* were connected to most distal area of denture base and continued to accessible vent *(V)* area prior to investment.

posterior base on one side; also attach another roll to the other side, and bring it back to the most distal accessible area of the cast. Cut the pouring sprue to the most anterior area of the denture base and the vents to the most posterior areas.

7. When there are bilateral posterior edentulous areas and an anterior area, treat each side as in the unilateral situation (Fig. 14-30).

8. Remove the framework from the cast during dewaxing.

9. Clean the cast and framework of all wax, and coat the cast with a separating medium.

10. Sprue, vent, and clean the teeth, and replace them in the mold.

11. Replace the framework on the cast, and replace the cast in the mold.

12. Accomplish the remaining steps in the same manner as for complete dentures.

13. Pouring generally takes longer with partial dentures because the retentive meshwork impedes the resin flow to some extent. Less restrictive meshwork patterns are best to use when making the metal framework. The screen-type retentive meshwork pattern is not satisfactory because it impedes the flow of resin too much and can cause voids in the denture base.

14. A major advantage of a fluid resin method of processing, in the instance where the denture base has a free-end extension, is the absence of packing pressure on the retentive meshwork of the partial denture. Packing pressures frequently cause warping of the meshwork during processing. The release of stresses after removal

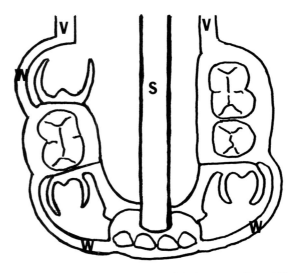

Fig. 14-30. Unilateral free-end partial denture with additional anterior and posterior denture base area. Sprue *(S)* is cut to lingual aspect of anterior teeth. Rolls of wax *(W)* were connected to posterior denture base areas prior to investment. Vent *(V)* on left side is cut into denture base area. Vent *(V)* on right side is cut into what was extension of roll of wax *(W)*.

of the partial denture from the cast causes the meshwork to resume its original position. When the pressure-packed free-end extension partial denture is inserted in the mouth of the patient, the dentist often finds that the denture has an anteroposterior displacement. It becomes evident when finger pressure is applied to the occlusal surface of the posterior denture teeth and metallic portions of the partial denture anterior to the most distal rest move upward out of proper position. The fluid resin processing method eliminates the warping effect because it requires no application of pressure.

15. Another advantage is the ability to recover the partial denture from the mold without damage to the cast. This situation greatly facilitates remounting procedures for occlusal correction after processing.

REBASING
PROCEDURE

1. It is impossible to reline dentures properly by this method of processing. It is essential to rebase instead of reline dentures.

2. All undercuts should have been removed from the basal surface of the denture prior to making the impression to permit removal of the denture from the cast without damage.

3. After the impression has been made, box the denture, and make a cast of improved stone.

4. Taper the cast on the sides, and make the base flat.

5. Remove carefully any impression material from the polished surface of the denture up to the peripheral roll without removing the denture from the cast.

6. Do the investment, cooling, removal, spruing, cast cleaning, and painting with a separating medium in the same manner as when the denture is an original.

7. If the denture has porcelain teeth, remove them from the denture base, clean them, and replace them in the hydrocolloid mold individually. If the denture has resin teeth, cut the denture base away up to the teeth, clean the entire arch, and replace it in the mold as a unit.

8. The remaining procedures for processing are the same as those for original dentures.

REPAIRING
PROCEDURE

1. Make repairs with autopolymerizing or low-heat resin, using the pneumatic curing unit to avoid porosity. Any fluid resins can be used for repair if they are autopolymerizing or low-temperature polymerizing.

2. Repair any denture made originally of fluid resin with the same resin if possible. Then the repaired area is undetectible.

PROBLEM AREAS

Some problems can arise in this method of processing, but generally they result from carelessness or lack of attention to detail (Table 14-1).

It is essential to handle the cast with care. Contamination with silicone or acrylic spray, talcum, and oils; failure to clean the cast properly before pouring; or per-

mitting the separating medium to form pools will affect the impression surface of the denture adversely. These resins are autopolymerizing, and some contaminants will prevent proper curing. Exercising care when using impression materials that contain eugenol is essential. When it is necessary to soften a zinc-oxide–eugenol wash impression that has been border molded with modeling plastic before separating the cast from the impression tray, heat it quickly and moderately. It is necessary to avoid placing the impression in an oven or under an infrared lamp to soften it, since either type of heat tends to make the stone cast take up the eugenol. An adequate land area, proper tapering, and a flat base are essential for the cast.

Festooning should conform exactly to what is desired in the denture after minimal finishing. The teeth must be entirely free of wax prior to investing. If one is unable or unwilling to remove all of the wax, it is preferable to use some other method of processing.

Spruing and venting correctly and understanding the basic concepts of the technique are essential for success. Some partial dentures require rather complicated spruing and venting procedures, but pouring works well when the resin reaches the most anterior area first and is able to escape through the most distal area without interruption. Voids result when air is trapped anywhere along the route. The mold must be free of loose pieces of hydrocolloid because they become incorporated in the denture base.

Only precise mixing of the resin according to the proportions specified by the manufacturer assures the best results. Higher polymer-ratio resins are recommended. Cleanliness of mixing utensils is critical for consistent results. It is impractical to use the monomer of one manufacturer with the polymer of another because this combination can result in unpredictable polymerization of the resin. Inverting the measuring graduate containing the monomer after use is essential for complete drainage, or the polymerized monomer can build up gradually in the bottom of the graduate and render it inaccurate. Since the monomer is relatively clear, and all of it does not drain out during decanting for mixing, it may be impossible to detect a buildup. If ambient temperatures are high, refrigeration of the monomer will increase the working time.

Pouring slowly and only through the pouring sprue is essential because pouring through the vents will result in voids. Pouring too rapidly can cause entrapment of air. Careful handling of the flask will avoid tooth dislodgment. If the resin is too viscous as a result of some delay after mixing it, there should be no attempt to pour it.

For good results, it is necessary to do the curing with

Table 14-1. Denture base processing with a hydrocolloid investment

Problem	Probable cause	Solution
Voids in denture base	Air trapped within mold as result of improper spruing and venting	Follow spruing and venting procedures properly
	Air trapped within mold as result of improper pouring	Pour slowly through pouring sprue only; gently rock flask from side to side to displace bubbles
	Air trapped within mold because of too viscous mixture	Follow manufacturer's recommendations exactly as to proportioning monomer and polymer; pour within prescribed time limitations
Hydrocolloid particles in denture base	Loose pieces of hydrocolloid left in mold	Inspect mold carefully before reassembling; remove any loose hydrocolloid particles
Palatal form of improper contour or excessively thick	Preformed palatal pattern lifted away from cast during investing	Seal palatal area of cast with wax; firmly adapt pattern
Blebs on denture surface	Bubble formation in hydrocolloid mold	Soak cast in slurry water prior to investing to displace air contained in cast; exercise care in pouring hydrocolloid
Tooth movement	Tooth not held in position properly by hydrocolloid during pouring	Trim wax down to collar of tooth surface during festooning; use adhesive to hold tooth in position when ridge lap ground excessively
	Tooth out of position prior to pouring	Exercise care in handling flask after reassembly; place correct tooth in proper position in mold
Porous denture base	Inadequate air pressure	Monitor pneumatic curing unit to make certain that pressure is maintained at 20 to 30 psi during curing cycle
	Denture placed in curing unit after polymerization begun	Avoid excessive delay in placing flask in unit after pouring
	Accelerated polymerization	Make certain that water temperature in curing unit is not too high and that cast is cool before placing it in mold
Irregularities on impression surface of denture	Improper treatment of cast prior to pouring resin	Avoid contamination of cast with oils, sprays, talcum; do not permit separating medium to pool or use contaminated separating medium; clean cast properly prior to coating, reassembly, pouring
Tooth detachment from denture base during finishing or after delivery to patient	Inadequate treatment of resin tooth at denture interface	Clean teeth properly to remove wax residue; grind ridge-lap area to assure proper bond
Denture base acrylic on tooth surface	Wax left on tooth surface prior to investing	Clean teeth of wax meticulously during festooning

adequate air pressure, and at a specific temperature if advocated. Otherwise, porosity of the denture base or improper polymerization will result.

SUMMARY

This section of the chapter described a method for producing dentures from resins that do not require a gypsum investment. Considerable processing time can be saved when this method is used. Consistent results depend on attention to detail. Attempts to circumvent certain procedures will result in less than satisfactory results.

PART TWO
A fluid resin system for processing dentures in a rigid mold

RICHARD A. SMITH, HUGH E. WOLFE, FRANK F. KOBLITZ, and LAURENCE T. OLIVER

Various fluid resin techniques use reversible hydrocolloid as the mold for processing denture bases. These have been described by Mirza (1961), Fairchild (1967), Winkler (1967), Shepard (1968), Weaver et al. (1969), and Stanford (1972-1973). This method is said to simplify flasking and deflasking, reduce the time required for finishing, and permit the use of relatively inexpensive equipment. However, these fluid resin methods have presented some problems, such as movement of the teeth, tilting of the cast, decrease in the vertical dimension, and seepage of resin onto the teeth as described by Shepard (1968), Dutton et al. (1968), Civjan et al. (1968), Weaver et al. (1969), Inge et al. (1970), Goodkind et al. (1970), Winkler et al. (1971), Kraut (1971), Grant et al. (1971), Winkler (1972), and Stanford (1972-1973).

In an approach to the problems associated with fluid resin processing, a system* has been designed that combines elements of the conventional investment technique with those of the pour technique. A modified gypsum investment poured into expendable plastic accessories replaces the hydrocolloid investment. This chapter will describe the technique for processing complete dentures, removable partial dentures, immediate complete dentures, and for relining or rebasing. These methods are described previously by Koblitz et al. (1973), Wolfe et al. (1974), and Oliver et al. (1975).

This processing requires the use of a unique rigid

---

*TRUPOUR Fluid Resin System, Dentsply International Inc., York, Pa.

mold. Since the investing material is firm enough to serve as its own flask, there is no need for another metallic container to enclose it. At the same time, the investment is friable enough to permit easy removal from the completed denture with a laboratory knife after polymerization of the fluid resin.

METHOD FOR COMPLETE DENTURES

All generally accepted practices for tooth arrangement (setup) and wax denture contouring (wax-up), are completed prior to processing with a fluid resin.

PROCEDURE

1. Remove excess wax from the surfaces of the teeth, and seal the waxed-up denture to the cast in the usual manner. Make the cast taper from the base approximately 5 degrees occlusally toward the land area, which is approximately ⅛ inch (0.32 cm) wide.

2. Attach the stone cast to the surface of the plastic base with wax (Fig. 14-31).

3. Attach soft wax sprues to appropriate areas of the denture wax-up. For a maxillary denture, use three sprues approximately parallel to the occlusal plane and extending horizontally: one from the most distal portion of each tuberosity area and one from the midline of the palate (Fig. 14-32). For a mandibular denture, use two sprues: one at the most distal point of each side of the denture (Fig. 14-33). Extend these sprues until they are approximately even with the inner step of the plastic base.

4. Wrap a plastic strip from the kit around the first step of the base, and staple the ends together (Fig. 14-34).

5. Measure 12 ounces (340 gm) by volume of the investment powder supplied and 6 ounces (180 ml) by volume of water. Mix the powder and water in a plaster bowl with 15 to 30 seconds of hand spatulation. Mechanical or vacuum spatulation is preferable if available.

6. Pour the investment into one side of the plastic flask while holding it on a vibrator (Fig. 14-35). Cover the teeth and/or cast with at least ¼ inch (0.64 cm) of investment, and continue vibrating for a few seconds to promote the escape of air bubbles.

7. After the investment has set, remove the staples, plastic strip, and plastic base from the hardened investment (Fig. 14-36).

8. Trim enough of the investment material from the base of the cast in a **V** groove to expose the cast base to a depth of ⅛ inch (0.32 cm) (Fig. 14-37).

9. Trim the investment away from the sprue holes (Fig. 14-38). If the investment has covered the ends of the wax sprues, the distinctive shadowy appearance of the investment makes it easy to locate them.

10. Cut a flat surface on the side of the investment

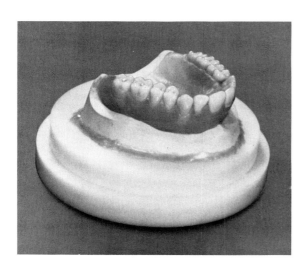

Fig. 14-31. Cast with denture wax-up has been attached to surface of plastic base supplied by manufacturer.

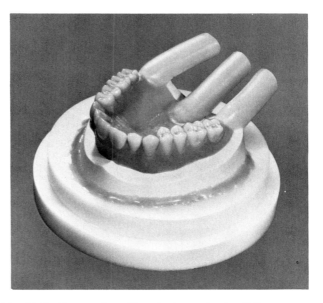

Fig. 14-32. Sprues of maxillary denture extend until they are even with inner step of plastic base.

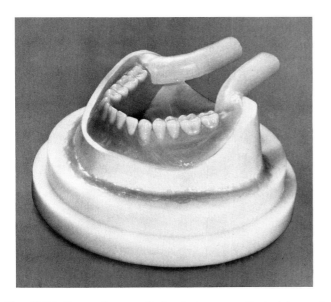

Fig. 14-33. Sprues for mandibular denture are attached to most distal point of each heel area. Note taper of base of each cast.

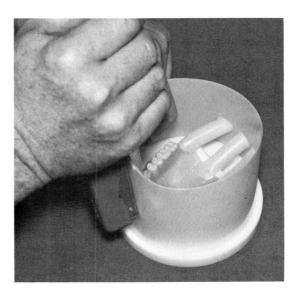

Fig. 14-34. Plastic strip provided by manufacturer is wrapped around inside rim of plastic base and stapled.

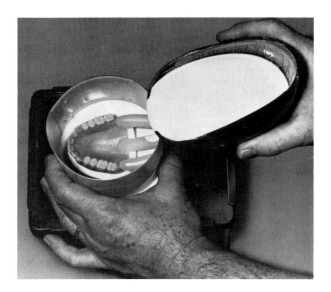

Fig. 14-35. Investment is poured into plastic flask while it is held on vibrator.

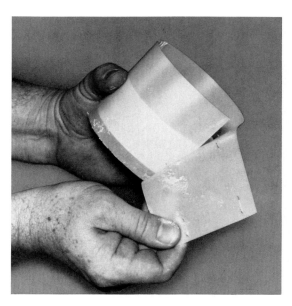

Fig. 14-36. Staples, plastic strip, and plastic base are removed from hardened investment.

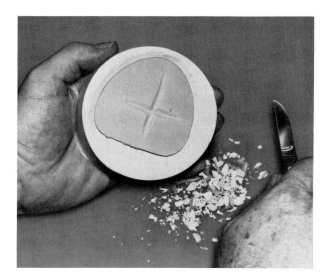

Fig. 14-37. Investment is trimmed away from base of cast in V groove approximately ⅛ inch (0.3 cm) deep to expose edges of base. This method of trimming leaves gripping area used in removing cast after boiling it out.

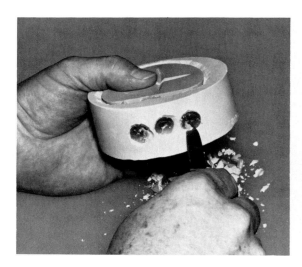

Fig. 14-38. Investment is trimmed away from sprue holes.

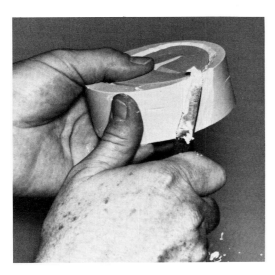

Fig. 14-39. Flat surface cut with knife on side opposite sprues permits invested denture to stand upright by itself in later procedures.

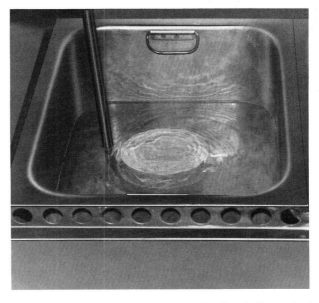

Fig. 14-40. Invested denture is submerged in clean boiling water for 8 minutes or until wax is softened.

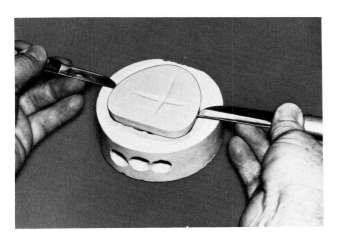

Fig. 14-41. Cast is teased gently from investment mold.

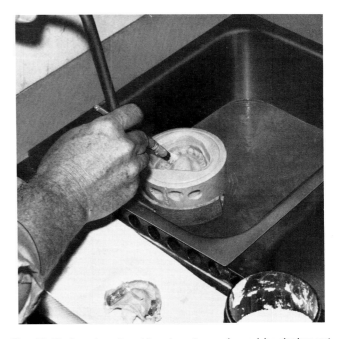

Fig. 14-42. Investment mold and cast are cleaned by rinsing out residual wax with boiling water and scrubbing them gently with powdered detergent. They are rinsed again with clear, clean boiling water.

opposite the sprue holes. This flat area of the side of the investment permits the invested denture to stand upright with the sprue openings up (Fig. 14-39).

11. Immerse the invested denture in boiling water for 8 minutes (Fig. 14-40) or until the wax is soft.

12. Remove it from the water, and gently tease the cast from the investing material (Fig. 14-41).

13. Remove the softened wax from the mold, and rinse away any wax remaining from both the cast and investment with clean boiling water.

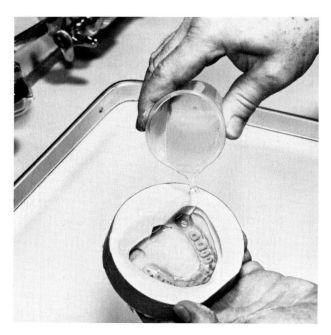

Fig. 14-43. As soon as surface moisture has drained and evaporated from investment, approximately 30 seconds, separating medium provided by manufacturer is flooded or brushed liberally over mold cavity and cast.

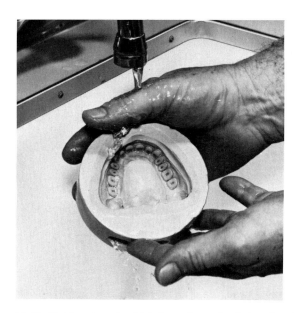

Fig. 14-44. Mold and cast, which have been flooded or brushed liberally with separating medium, are rinsed under gentle stream of water.

14. Gently scrub the cast and investment with a soft brush and powdered household detergent (Fig. 14-42), and then rinse with clear, clean boiling water. Attention to thorough cleanliness and neatness is essential for the best results.

15. Pour approximately 1 ounce (30 ml) of the separator supplied into a small glass or paper cup.

16. Flood or brush the separator liberally onto the hot cast. Rinse it immediately with a gently running stream of water. Then apply the separator liberally throughout the hot denture mold. This may be done as soon as the surface moisture left from the boiling-water rinse has drained and evaporated (Fig. 14-43).

17. Then rinse immediately with a gently running stream of cool, 65° F (18.5° C), water (Fig. 14-44) to prevent excessive buildup of separator thickness. NOTE: Both the mold and cast should be rinsed immediately after application of the separator.

18. Stand both the investment and the cast vertically to drain and dry for approximately 10 minutes.

19. Submerge both the cast and the flask in cool 65° F (18.5° C), water for approximately 10 minutes.

20. Remove and stand both the cast and the flask upright to drain until they are free of water (Fig. 14-45). Carefully blot any excess water from the pins and diatoric areas of the porcelain teeth (Fig. 14-46).

21. Apply the bonding agent supplied by the manufac-

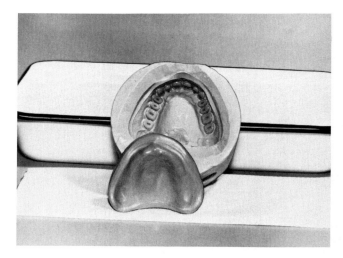

Fig. 14-45. After they have drained and dried for 10 minutes, both cast and mold are submerged in cool water, about 65° F (18.5° C), for 10 minutes. Then they are removed and stood upright to drain until free of surface water.

turer to the plastic teeth, but use it sparingly (Fig. 14-47).

22. Reseat the cast in position (Fig. 14-48). Secure it in place with a rubber band and a small jar lid or a retaining cap (Fig. 14-49).

23. Stand the mold with the reseated cast on the

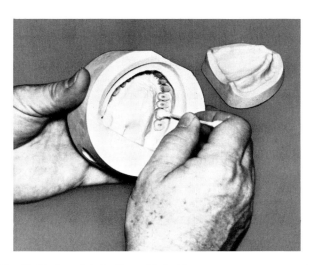

Fig. 14-46. Porcelain teeth are blotted to remove any excess moisture trapped in diatoric and vent holes.

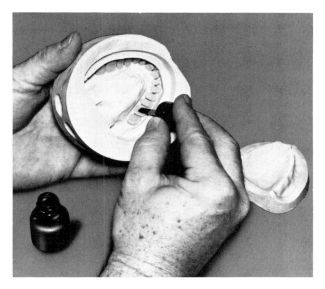

Fig. 14-47. Bonding agent supplied by manufacturer is applied to ridge lap of plastic teeth.

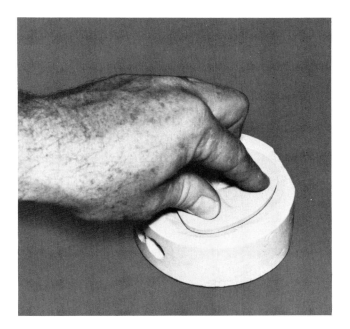

Fig. 14-48. Cast is reseated snugly in position.

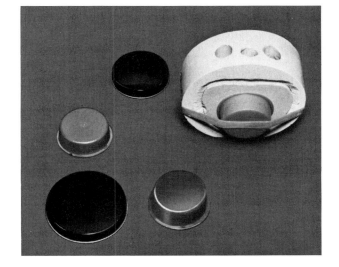

Fig. 14-49. Cast, which has been reseated into its keyway in investment, is held securely with retaining cap and rubber band.

bench top with the sprues up and the base of the cast facing away from the operator.

Processing acrylic resin
PROCEDURE

1. Mix 28 ml of denture base powder and 13 ml of liquid in the receptacles provided, and stir gently for 15 seconds. The mixture can stand 15 seconds longer to release any entrapped air.

2. Holding the flask assemblage in one hand, tilt it at approximately a 45-degree angle toward yourself, and pour the mixed fluid denture base material down a side sprue until the flask is half full (Fig. 14-50).

3. Elevate the flask to as near a horizontal position as possible with the cast up, and rock the flask gently from side to side two or three times to promote release of entrapped air bubbles between the teeth, and any entrained air in the resin mixture. Then pour the re-

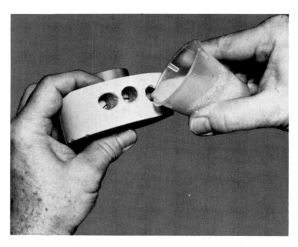

Fig. 14-50. Fluid resin is poured carefully into side sprue hole.

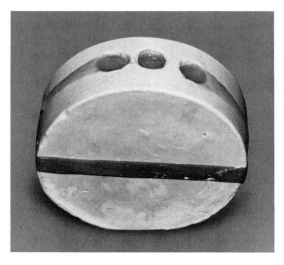

Fig. 14-51. Fluid resin has filled cavity of mold. Mold is allowed to stand on bench top for 3 to 5 minutes to permit escape of air bubbles.

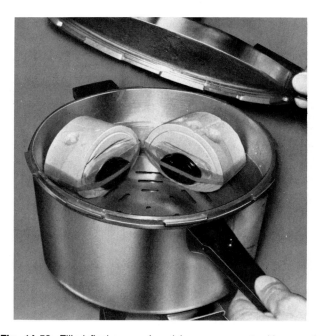

Fig. 14-52. Filled flasks are placed in pressure pot with enough water at 140° F (60° C) to immerse them to within 1 inch (2.5 cm) of sprue openings.

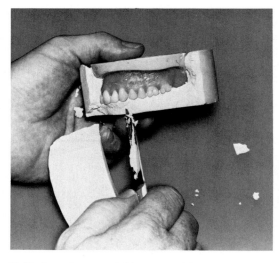

Fig. 14-53. Investing material is removed from processed denture readily with plaster knife.

mainder of the mixture in the same hole until it fills every sprue.

4. Stand this assemblage on its flattened edge on the bench top for 3 to 5 minutes (Fig. 14-51).

5. Place it in a pressure pot with sufficient water (140° F [60° C] to immerse the flask to within 1 inch (2.54 cm) of the sprue openings (Fig. 14-52).

6. Process the denture for 30 minutes at a pressure of 20 psi. A thermostatically controlled pressure pot is preferable for maintaining water at a constant temperature.

FINISHING DENTURES
PROCEDURE

1. Remove the processed denture in its flask, and immerse it in cool water for 15 minutes.

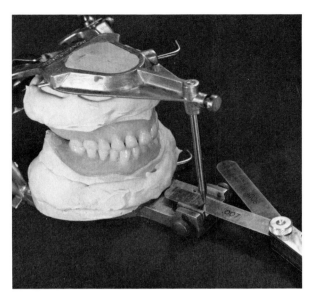

Fig. 14-54. Dentures have been repositioned on articulating instrument for occlusal correction. In this instance, incisal pin opening was 0.07 inch or approximately 0.2 mm.

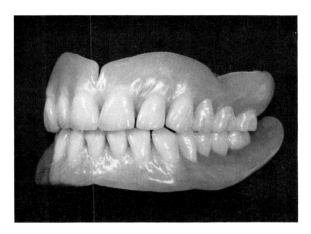

Fig. 14-55. Dentures have been removed from cast, trimmed, and polished.

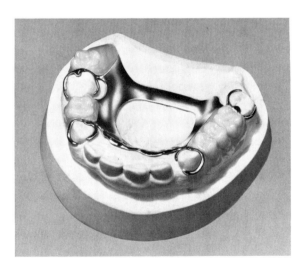

Fig. 14-56. Typical maxillary removable partial denture with metallic palatal connectors is shown with completed setup.

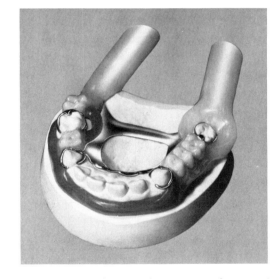

Fig. 14-57. Wax is used for secondary or connecting sprue to allow free flow of resin between right and left posterior areas.

2. Remove the investing material with a plaster knife (Fig. 14-53).

3. Remove the acrylic resin sprues from the denture with an appropriate instrument.

4. Position the denture on the articulating instrument for occlusal corrections before removing the cast from the inner aspect of the denture (Fig. 14-54).

5. Finish and polish the denture in a routine manner (Fig. 14-55).

METHOD FOR REMOVABLE PARTIAL DENTURES
PROCEDURE

The technique for processing removable partial dentures is almost the same as that for complete dentures. The main difference is the need for blocking out undercuts on the cast. This may be done with either a combination of plaster and wax or wax alone (Figs. 14-56 to 14-70). Three typical partial denture configurations are shown with both types of blockout.

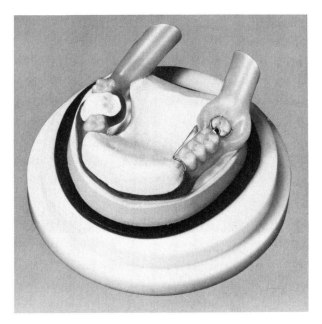

Fig. 14-58. Plaster completes blockout of remaining undercut areas and holds partial denture frame on cast. Denture is ready for investing.

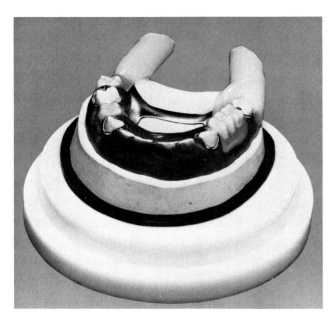

Fig. 14-59. Same type of denture as in Figs. 14-56 to 14-58 is shown with only wax used to block out undercuts.

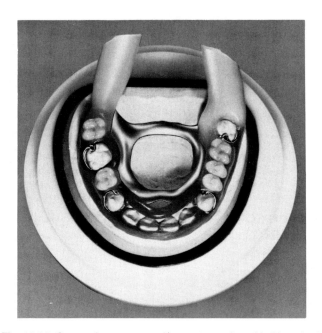

Fig. 14-60. Connecting sprues and/or vents can be added in palatal areas to promote flow of resin and prevent entrapment of air.

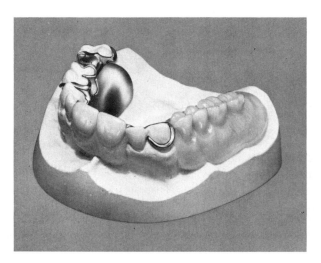

Fig. 14-61. Another maxillary removable partial denture is shown with completed setup.

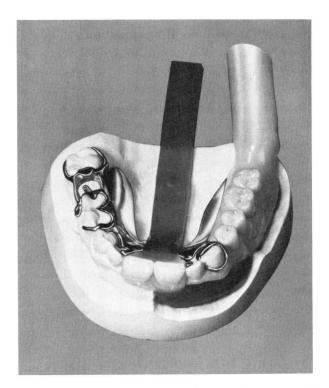

Fig. 14-62. Wax is used on labial aspect for secondary or connecting sprue between posterior and anterior areas. It partially fills undercut area. Note palatal sprue or vent to promote escape of air from anterior area.

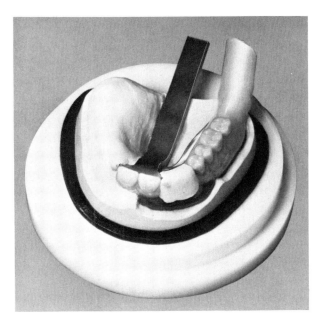

Fig. 14-63. Plaster completes blockout of remaining undercut areas and holds partial denture frame on cast. Denture is ready for investing.

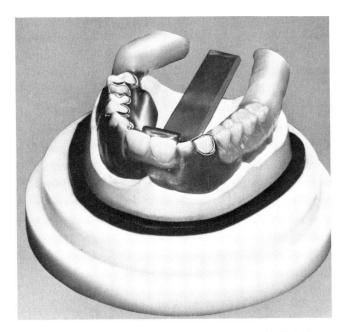

Fig. 14-64. Same type of denture as in Figs. 14-61 to 14-63 is shown with only wax used to block out undercuts.

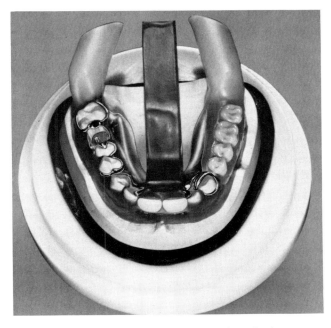

Fig. 14-65. Additional sprues and/or vents in palatal areas can promote flow of resin, facilitate escape of air, and block out undercuts. Denture is ready for investing.

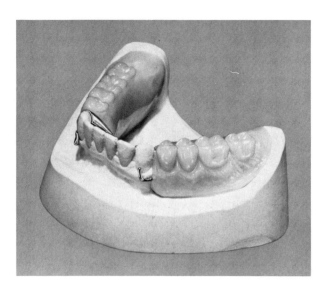

Fig. 14-66. Typical bilateral distal extension mandibular removable partial denture is shown with completed setup.

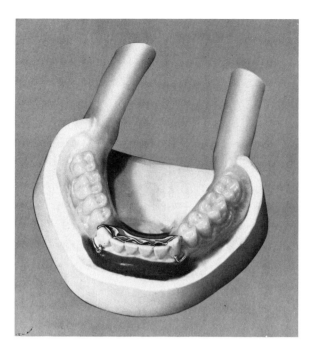

Fig. 14-67. Wax, which is used on labial aspect for secondary or connecting sprue between posterior areas, partially fills labial undercut area. Note addition of lingual secondary sprue.

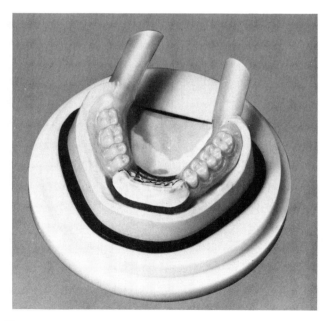

Fig. 14-68. Plaster completes blockout of remaining undercut areas and holds partial denture frame on cast. Denture is ready for investing.

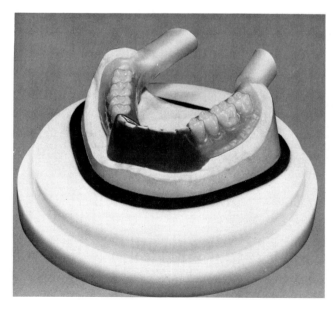

Fig. 14-69. Same type of denture as in Figs. 14-66 to 14-68 is shown with only wax used to block out undercuts.

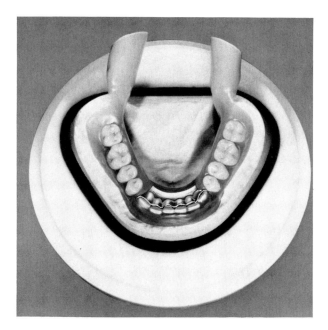

Fig. 14-70. Connecting sprues and/or vents can be added to lingual areas to promote flow of resin, prevent entrapment of air, and block out additional lingual undercut areas. Denture is ready for investing.

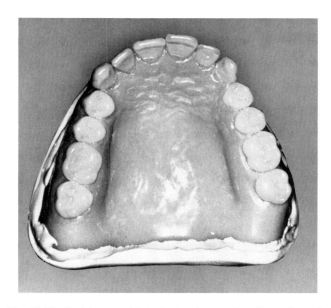

Fig. 14-71. Cast is poured into denture impression. Base of cast is tapered approximately 5 degrees toward land areas.

Blockout with a combination of plaster and wax holds the frame on the cast. Use of wax alone for blockout permits both removal of the framework from the cast for easier cleaning and thorough flooding of the entire cast with the separator. In each method, the resin replaces the boiled out wax blockout material. A few quick cuts with a separating disk or a bur readily remove the resin.

Some suggestions for methods of determining the configuration of the sprues for removable partial dentures processing are as follows:

1. Attach primary sprues at the most distal and/or highest points of the wax-up.

2. Attach secondary sprues or connectors facially, lingually, or both facially and lingually, depending on the design of the denture, and make them thick enough to permit the resin to flow freely between the resin body areas.

3. Select the attachment areas for sprues and vents visually by holding the wax-up in the pouring position.

4. Use additional venting in isolated areas to promote the escape of all entrapped air, if required. Eliminate any area that might act as a trap for an air bubble by attaching more secondary or connecting sprues to promote the flow of the fluid resin.

5. Instead of spruing exceedingly small or remote areas, which may necessitate the use of several long sprues and vents, hold the artificial teeth involved with a matrix, and pour each area individually as when making a simple repair.

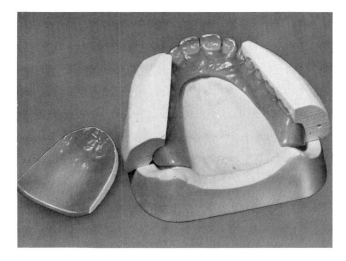

Fig. 14-72. Denture is removed from cast after occlusal indices have been made. Peripheral area is reduced, and palatal section is cut out. Impression material can be cleaned from denture at this time.

METHOD FOR RELINING OR REBASING
PROCEDURE

1. Relieve the inner aspect of the denture to eliminate undercuts in the acrylic resin, and make an impression by an accepted clinical method.

2. Pour the cast with mechanically spatulated stone, and taper the base approximately 5 degrees toward land areas (Fig. 14-71).

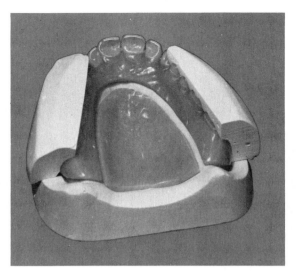

Fig. 14-73. Denture is repositioned on cast with indices. Palatal section is replaced.

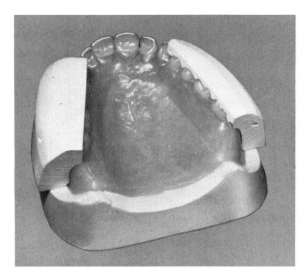

Fig. 14-74. Wax-up is completed. Denture is ready for investing.

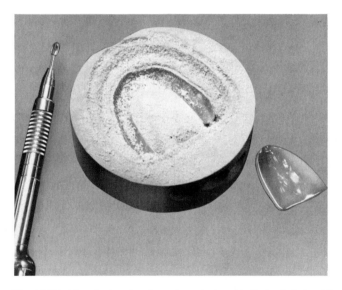

Fig. 14-75. After denture has been invested and boiled out, it should be further reduced to ensure surface cleanliness and to increase available flow space.

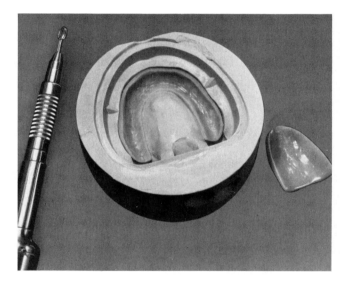

Fig. 14-76. Denture is ready for pouring. Palatal section is discarded.

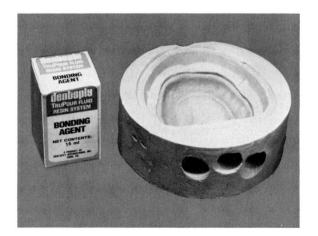

Fig. 14-77. Bonding agent furnished by manufacturer can be applied to original denture base material if desired.

3. Construct the occlusal indices, remove the denture from the cast, reduce the periphery, and cut out the palatal section (Fig. 14-72).

4. Reposition the denture on the cast with the indices, and replace the palatal section (Fig. 14-73).

5. Wax the palate to the main portion (Fig. 14-74), and complete any peripheral waxing required.

6. Sprue and invest according to the manufacturer's directions.

7. Follow the recommended procedures for separating the cast from the investment and eliminating the wax; discard the palatal portion.

8. Further reduce the tissue surface of the denture to ensure surface cleanliness and to increase the available flow space (Figs. 14-75 and 14-76).

9. Apply the bonding agent to the original denture base material (Fig. 14-77).

10. Follow the recommended procedures for mixing, pouring, and processing.

11. Recover the denture from the mold, and finish it (Fig. 14-78).

ALTERNATE PROCEDURE

1. After pouring the cast and tapering its base, mount the cast with the denture attached on an articulating

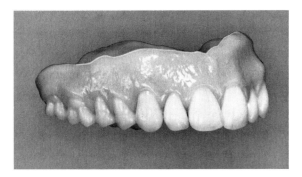

Fig. 14-78. Normal finishing and polishing procedures complete relining or rebasing.

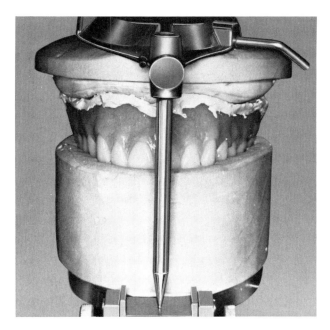

Fig. 14-79. After cast is poured and mounted on articulating instrument, occlusal index is made to maintain vertical dimension.

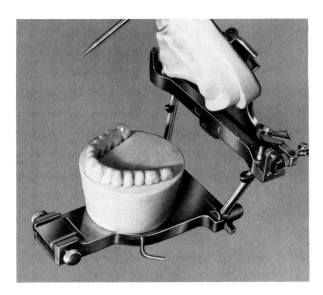

Fig. 14-80. Most of old denture base material has been removed, other than narrow arch in ridge-lap area, to aid in maintaining original tooth position.

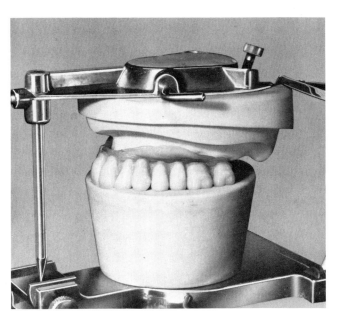

Fig. 14-81. Teeth are attached to cast with wax.

instrument, and make an occlusal index to maintain the vertical dimension (Fig. 14-79).

2. Remove most of the old denture base material, leaving a narrow arch in the ridge-lap area (Fig. 14-80), and reposition the teeth in the occlusal index.

3. Attach the teeth to the cast with wax (Fig. 14-81).

4. Complete the wax-up (Fig. 14-82); then flask the denture, and eliminate the wax in a manner similar to that described previously (Fig. 14-83).

5. Apply the bonding agent ot the original denture base material and the ridge-lap areas of the teeth (Fig. 14-84).

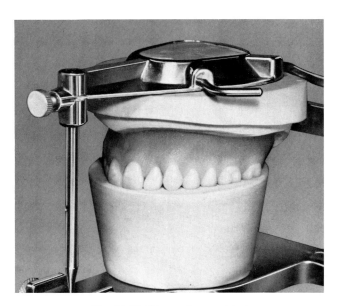

Fig. 14-82. Wax-up is completed.

6. After pouring and processing the resin, reposition the denture on the articulating instrument for any needed occlusal corrections (Fig. 14-85).

7. Use the normal finishing and polishing procedures to complete the rebasing (Fig. 14-86).

METHOD FOR IMMEDIATE COMPLETE DENTURES

One problem in processing immediate complete dentures by conventional compression-molding methods is the recovery of the processed denture from the cast. Removal of the processed denture from the cast can be time consuming and difficult because of the thin flanges and the presence of undercuts, particularly in the anterior region. Additionally, the denture base may fracture and therefore require various repair procedures.

The purpose of this section is to describe a method of processing an immediate complete denture with this fluid resin system in a rigid, but readily friable mold. Significantly, the cast used while processing the denture *also* is made of the unique investment material provided with the system. Use of the same material facilitates recovery of the denture from both the mold and the cast.

The basic fluid resin technique, as described previously, is used for processing.

PROCEDURE

1. Complete the tooth arrangement and wax contouring for the immediate denture in the usual manner on a conventional artificial stone working cast (Fig. 14-87). Note that the base of the cast is slightly tapered occlusally.

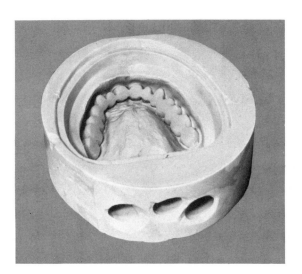

Fig. 14-83. Wax elimination procedures have been completed, and mold is prepared for processing.

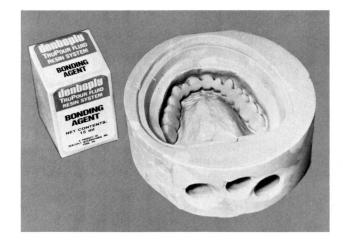

Fig. 14-84. Bonding agent furnished by manufacturer is applied to arch of original denture base material and to ridge-lap areas of teeth if desired.

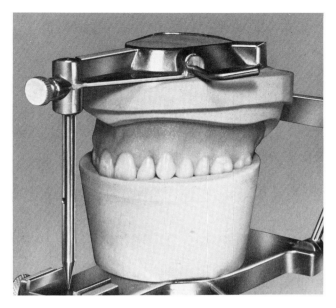

Fig. 14-85. Completed denture is repositioned in occlusal index.

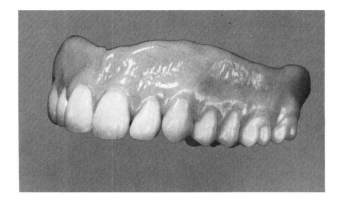

Fig. 14-86. Denture is finished.

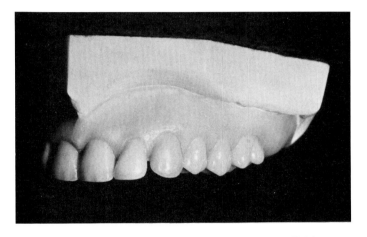

Fig. 14-87. Immediate denture has been waxed on artificial stone cast with its base tapered slightly toward occlusal surface.

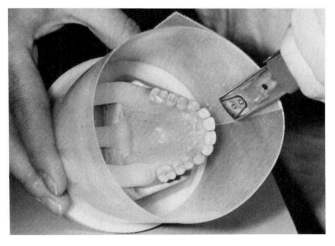

Fig. 14-88. After wax sprues are attached, denture is flasked, as described in Figs. 14-34 and 14-41.

2. Seal the cast to a plastic base, and attach sprues to the wax denture. Surround the assemblage with a plastic strip from the kit supplied by the manufacturer for the fluid resin system (Fig. 14-88).

3. Mix and vibrate the investing medium over the wax denture in its flask, according to the manufacturer's directions (Fig. 14-89). After the investment has hardened, immerse it in boiling water for 8 minutes or until the wax is soft.

4. Carefully lift the artificial stone cast from the investment mold (Fig. 14-90), and complete the wax-elimination procedures.

5. Apply the separating agent provided in the kit to the mold, rinse the mold immediately with a gentle stream of water, and permit the mold to drain.

6. Seal the investment mold in a plastic bag that also contains a damp sponge (Fig. 14-91). This container serves as a humidifier and prevents dehydration of the mold.

7. Duplicate the working cast by means of an irreversible hydrocolloid (alginate) impression.* Pour the duplicate cast with the blue investment material provided in the kit.

8. When the blue investment has hardened, remove

---

*JELTRATE (regular), The L. D. Caulk Co., Milford, Del.

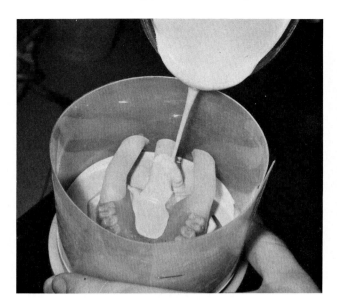

Fig. 14-89. Investment is poured.

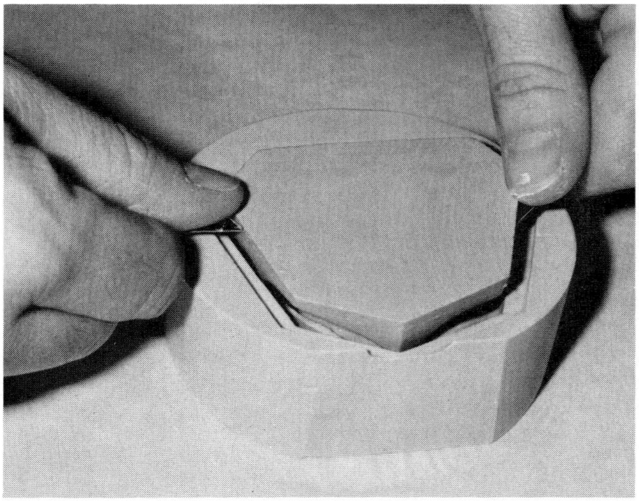

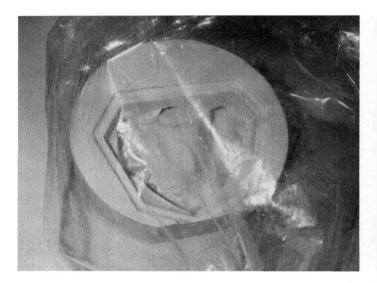

Fig. 14-90. Cast is teased from mold.

the duplicate cast from the irreversible hydrocolloid (alginate) impression (Fig. 14-92). Note that the investment cast should not be allowed to become dehydrated.

9. Dip the duplicate cast in clean boiling water for 1 minute. Remove the cast, and apply a separating medium to the hot cast in the same manner as for the investment mold. Allow the cast to drain and dry for approximately 10 minutes.

10. Submerge the blue investment cast in cool, 65° F (18.5° C), water for approximately 10 minutes.

11. Remove the cast from the water bath, and permit it to drain.

12. Remove the rigid mold from the plastic-bag humidifier, and blot any excess moisture off the teeth. Position the duplicate cast in the mold, and hold it securely with a plastic cap and rubber band (Fig. 14-93).

13. Mix and pour the fluid resin according to the manufacturer's directions (Fig. 14-94). Process the denture in a pressure pot for 30 minutes at 140° F (60° C) and 20 psi.

14. While the denture is processing, form a clear surgical template on the original working cast by using a molding apparatus* (Fig. 14-95).

15. Cool the mold in water at room temperature for 10 to 15 minutes before removing the processed denture from the investment mold (Fig. 14-96).

16. Remove the processing cast from the denture with a laboratory knife (Fig. 14-97).

17. Finish the denture by cutting off the sprues and polishing the borders (Fig. 14-98).

18. The denture and the template are ready to be

---

*VACU-PRESS, Dentsply International Inc., York, Pa.

placed in the mouth after removal of the patient's teeth (Fig. 14-99).

The minimal degree of tooth movement associated with this method of processing will not normally be of clinical significance.

PROBLEM AREAS

If the recommended procedures of the manufacturer are closely followed, the user should experience few, if any, problems in denture fabrication. A lapse in technique may result in problems (Table 14-2).

Fig. 14-91. Blue investment mold is sealed in plastic bag with damp sponge to act as humidifier.

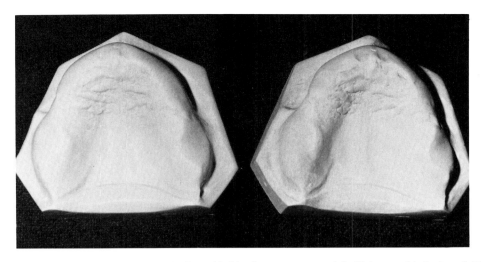

Fig. 14-92. Working cast has been duplicated in blue investment material with irreversible hydrocolloid (alginate) impression.

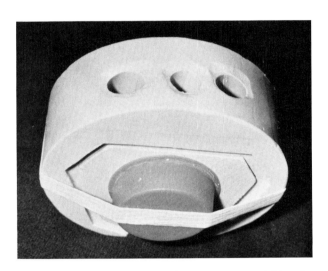

Fig. 14-93. Duplicate cast made of investment material has been placed in rigid mold and is held in position with plastic cap and rubber band.

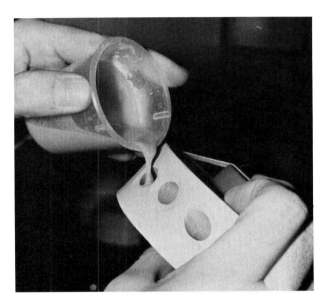

Fig. 14-94. Denture is poured, as described in Figs. 14-49 to 14-51.

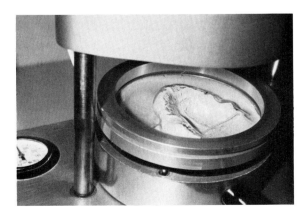

Fig. 14-95. During processing of denture, surgical template is formed on original stone working cast.

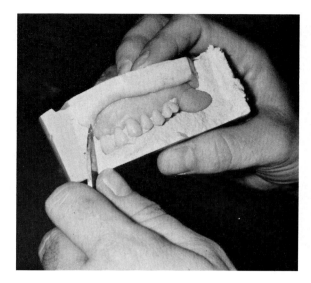

Fig. 14-96. Processed denture is removed from mold with ease.

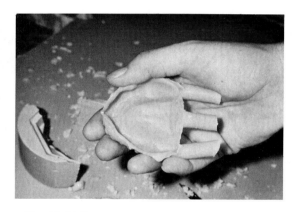

Fig. 14-97. Processing cast also is removed easily.

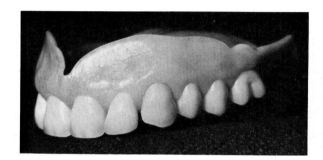

Fig. 14-98. Denture is finished.

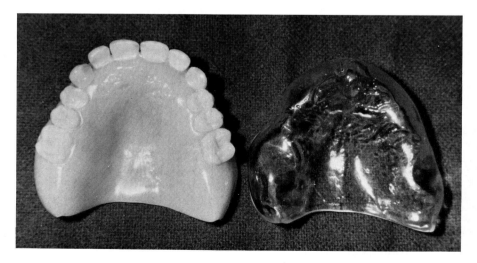

Fig. 14-99. Denture and surgical template are ready for placement in mouth.

Table 14-2. Processing dentures in a rigid mold with a fluid resin

Problem	Probable cause	Solution
Separation of teeth from denture	Wax film on teeth	Use proper wax elimination procedures, including clean rinse water
	Detergent film on teeth	Use powdered household detergent and proper rinsing procedures
	Separator buildup on teeth	Carefully apply separator; carefully remove any separator remaining on surfaces of teeth
Bubbles, voids, porosity of denture base	Too much delay before pouring resin	Avoid undue delay in mixing and pouring procedures
	Improper rocking of mold during pouring procedure	Follow recommended pouring procedures
	Too much delay before application of air pressure to processing apparatus	Apply air pressure as soon as practicable after pouring
	Improper temperature for processing	Process at recommended temperature
Undue shrinkage of denture base	Improperly proportioned powder and/or liquid	Proportion materials carefully
	Use of incorrect size sprues, too short and/or too small in diameter	Use sprue size of sufficient length and diameter

SUMMARY

The second part of this chapter has described a system for processing complete dentures, removable partial dentures, immediate complete dentures, and for relining or rebasing. The method requires no specialized equipment, such as metal flasks or a hydrocolloid conditioning apparatus, and eliminates the time-consuming step of sorting and replacing artificial teeth in a hydrocolloid mold. As with all denture processing techniques, attention to detail is the prime requirement for continuing excellent results.

REFERENCES

Axinn, S., Kopp, E. N., and Hansen, J. G.: Trouble-shooting the pour resins, J. Prosthet. Dent. **33**:689-601, 1975.

Civjan, S., Gardner, T. V., Worthen, D. F., and de Simon, L. B.: Evaluation of a "fluid" denture base resin, Int. Assoc. Dent. Res. Abst. No. 233, March, 1968.

Civjan, S., Huget, E. F., and de Simon, L. B.: Modifications of the fluid resin technique, J. Am. Dent. Assoc. **85**:109-112, 1972.

Dutton, D. A., Swoope, C. C., and Moffa, J. P.: A comparison of vertical changes in dentures processed by two methods, Int. Assoc. Dent. Res. Abst. No. 236, March, 1968.

Fairchild, J. M.: The fluid resin technique of denture base formation, J. Calif. Dent. Assoc. **43**:127-138, 1967.

Goodkind, R. J., and Schulte, R. C.: Dimensional accuracy of pour acrylic resin and conventional processing of cold-curing acrylic resin bases, J. Prosthet. Dent. **24**:662-668, 1970.

Grant, A. A., and Atkinson, H. F.: Comparison between dimensional accuracy of dentures produced with pour-type resin and with heat-processed materials, J. Prosthet. Dent. **26**:296-301, 1971.

Inge, W. A., Jr., and Taylor, D. F.: Dimensional changes in dentures processed by the fluid resin technique, Int. Assoc. Dent. Res. Abst. No. 273, March, 1970.

Koblitz, F. F., Smith, R. A., and Wolfe, H. E.: Fluid denture resin processing in a rigid mold, J. Prosthet. Dent. **30**:339-346, 1973.

Kraut, R. A.: A comparison of denture base accuracy, J. Am. Dent. Assoc. **83**:352-357, 1971.

Mirza, F. D.: Dimensional stability of acrylic resin dentures, J. Prosthet. Dent. **11**:848-857, 1961.

Oliver, L. T., Smith, R. A., Wolfe, H. E., and Koblitz, F. F.: Immediate denture processing with a fluid resin, J. Prosthet. Dent. **34**:216-220, 1975.

Phillips, R. W.: Skinner's science of dental materials, ed. 7, Philadelphia, 1973, W. B. Saunders Co., pp. 158-159.

Shepard, W. L.: Denture bases processed from a fluid resin, J. Prosthet. Dent. **19**:561-572, 1968.

Stanford, J. W., editor: Guide to dental materials and devices, ed. 6, Chicago, 1972-1973, American Dental Association, pp. 98-99.

Weaver, R. G., and Ryge, G.: Advancements in processing techniques, J. Ala. Dent. Assoc. **53**:22-27, 1969.

Winkler, S.: Pour technique for denture base processing, Dent. Digest **73**:200-203, 1967.

Winkler, S.: The current status of pour resins, J. Prosthet. Dent. **28**:580-584, 1972.

Winkler, S., Morris, H. F., Thongthammachat, S., and Shorr, J. H.: Investing mediums for pour resins, J. Am. Dent. Assoc. **83**:848-851, 1971.

Winkler, S., Ortman, H. R., Morris, H. F., and Plezia, R. A.: Processing changes in complete dentures constructed from pour resins, J. Am. Dent. Assoc. **82**:349-353, 1971.

Wolfe, H. E., Smith, R. A., and Koblitz, F. F.: Denture relining or rebasing with a fluid resin, J. Prosthet. Dent. **31**:460-465, 1974.

CHAPTER 15

SOFT LINERS

MICHAEL J. MAGINNIS and GERALD T. GAUBERT

resilient denture base liner A layer of compressible material that separates the hard denture base material from the oral mucosa of the residual ridge.

The indications for use of a resilient liner are existence of thin, nonresilient mucosal coverage of the residual ridge, poor ridge morphology, persistent denture-sore mouth, and acquired or congenital oral defects.

Storer (1962) states that the rationale for using a soft lining material is that part of the energy transferred from it to the denture aids in deforming the denture elastically and consequently reduces the direct load of mastication on the atrophied area. In addition, the soft lining produces an equal amount of pressure over the bone of the ridge and thereby avoids resistance from the prominent spicules to a larger amount of applied force.

Ortman and Ortman (1975) have described the ideal properties of a resilient liner and recommended that these liners serve merely as aids in solving the problem and not as the total solution.

REQUIREMENTS OF RESILIENT DENTURE BASE LINERS

The requirements of soft liners are as follows:

1. They should be of a biologically inert material that is compatible with the oral tissues and does not support bacterial or fungal growth.

2. They should be resilient and capable of maintaining this characteristic. Dentists agree that the average period of satisfactory service for a denture is 7 years; however, patients that need this resilient lining have special problems that often require more frequent ser-

vice. For them, a reasonable period of service expected from such a material may be 2 years.

3. After curing, they should be dimensionally stable and insoluble in oral fluids to maintain proper tissue contact.

4. They should be color stable throughout their useful life, resistant to staining, and impervious to odors.

5. Even though flexible, they should resist abrasion and thereby allow the practice of proper hygiene of the surface.

6. On curing, they should maintain their bond to the denture base without damaging it.

7. It should be relatively easy to work with them, including during fabrication of the lining and its subsequent adjustment; however, it is not essential for the liner to be a chairside material.

RESILIENT LINER MATERIALS

Materials available for use as resilient liners are natural rubber, soft acrylic materials, vinyls, and silicone rubbers (Table 15-1). Natural rubber has only a limited service period because of deterioration, fouling, and poor dimensional stability.

Soft resin materials are the largest group of resilient liners; they are either cold-cure or heat-cure systems, and frequently they depend on the addition of plasticizer for their resilience. A plasticizer eventually leaches out, leaving the material hard and often fissured, thereby promoting staining. Vinyls have shortcomings similar to those of resins because they may harden in service gradually. Lower resistance to abrasion also is a problem and may contribute to the poor fit of dentures (Ortman and Ortman, 1975).

Table 15-1. Materials and manufacturers

Material	Manufacturer
Silicone rubber materials	
Flexibase	Flexico Developments Ltd., London, England
Simpa	A. Kettenback, West Germany
Cardex-Stabon	Cardex, Austria
Molloplast-B	Kostner and Co., Germany
Primasoft	Buffalo Dental Manufacturing Co., Inc., Brooklyn, New York
Soft acrylic materials	
Coe-soft	Coe Laboratories, Inc., Chicago, Illinois
Soft Oryl	Teledyne Dental Products Co., Getz/Opotow Division, Elk Grove Village, Illinois
Coe-Super soft	Coe Laboratories, Inc., Chicago, Illinois
Palasiv 62	Kulzer and Co., Germany
Soft Nobiltone	Nobilium, Chicago, Illinois
Virina	Virina Dental Products, Ltd., Canada
Verno Soft	Vernon-Benshoff Co., Inc., Albany, New York
Other materials	
Hydrocryl Soft Liner	Hydro Dent, Los Angeles, California
Cole Polymers	R. H. Cole and Co., Ltd., London, England
Natural rubber	The Malaysian Rubber Producer's Research Association, Malaysia

Silicone rubbers probably are closest to being the ideal material. Achieving a satisfactory bond strength between the silicone lining and denture base resin for a reasonable service life has been a problem. Use of newer bonding agents seems to have increased the service life. Although silicone rubber is a suitable medium for the growth of fungus, proper denture hygiene minimizes this problem.

Silicone rubber materials

Having no natural adhesion to polymethyl methacrylate, silicone rubbers depend on an adhesive or a bonding agent, such as a silicone polymer in a volatile solvent, for adherence of the lining to the denture base. The molecules of the polymer penetrate the acrylic of the denture base and anchor in it after evaporation of the solvent. As the resilient lining material cures, it adheres to the denture base by cross-linkage with the silicone polymer (Wright, 1976).

Bates and Smith (1965) have suggested that the rate of diffusion and total water absorption of ideal resilient lining materials should be similar to that of polymethyl methacrylate, approximately 2.2%. Presumably, this rate is sufficient to reduce the likelihood of a breakdown of the bond to the denture base.

Wright (1976) has investigated fifteen resilient liner materials and analyzed them for water absorption, water solubility, viscoelastic properties, and the effect of bonding these materials to polymethyl methacrylate. He notes that silicone rubbers are well established resilient lining materials. They have 10% to 35% inorganic silicates that determine their water absorption characteristics. The results of his study indicate that Molloplast-B* has a lasting softness and an especially low water absorption rate similar to that of the acrylic of the denture base.

Suchatlampong et al. (1976) have determined that silicone rubber materials are most satisfactory with regard to compressibility. They produce a stress-relieving action that is adequate if they are at least 2 mm thick. The study indicates that a 2 to 3 mm thick section of Molloplast-B has superior compressibility. Wright (1976) has found that silicone rubber 3 mm thick is eight times as soft as one that is 1 mm thick.

Lining denture bases
PROCEDURE

1. To control the thickness of the silicone rubber, process the liner in the same manner as when relining a previously fabricated appliance rather than including it in the initial construction of the appliance. Complete the denture to be lined with the resilient liner in the conventional manner using a high-impact denture base resin,† return it to the patient, remount it, and adjust the occlusion. Remove approximately 2 mm of the denture base material from the tissue side and borders of the denture, and replace it with a tissue conditioner.‡ During a 1-week period, adjust the tissue surface and borders to relieve overextensions and impingements, as well as to make the final thickness of the tissue conditioner 2 to 3 mm immediately prior to processing (Fig. 15-1).

2. Place the denture with the tissue conditioner liner in the lower half of a conventional denture flask in such a manner that the impression surface is upright. Also make certain to embed the teeth in a vacuum spatulated mix of one-half dental stone and one-half dental plaster.

---

*Molloplast-B, Kostner and Co., Germany. Marketed by Buffalo Dental Manufacturing Co., Inc., Brooklyn, N.Y.
†Lucitone 199, L. D. Caulk Co., Milford, Del., or equivalent.
‡Coe-soft, Coe Laboratories, Inc., Chicago, Ill., or equivalent.

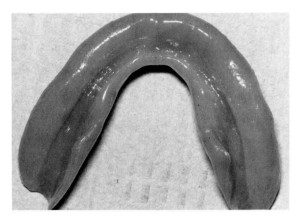

Fig. 15-1. Denture with soft tissue–conditioner preparatory to flasking and processing with Molloplast-B.

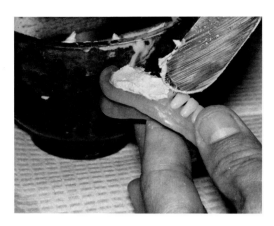

Fig. 15-2. Stone-plaster mix is spatulated onto outer surface of denture so as to avoid trapping air and to assure filling interproximal spaces.

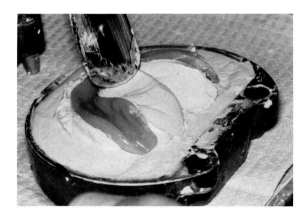

Fig. 15-3. Denture is inverted into lower half of denture flask filled with stone-plaster mix. Position denture above rim of flask to contain border rolls in upper half of flask.

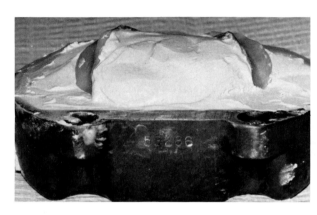

Fig. 15-4. Stone-plaster surface should slant down and away from border rolls to avoid creating undercut in lower half of flask.

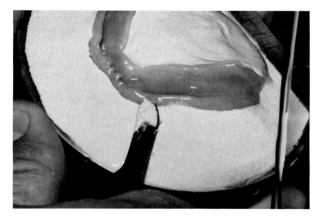

Fig. 15-5. Entire denture border rolls are exposed with plaster knife while stone-plaster mix is still soft. Care is exercised to avoid touching border roll of tissue conditioner.

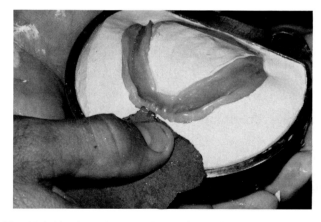

Fig. 15-6. No. 320 grit wet or dry sandpaper is used to put smooth finish on stone-plaster surface and to facilitate separation of halves of flask prior to removal of tissue conditioner. Also care is exercised to avoid touching or distorting soft material.

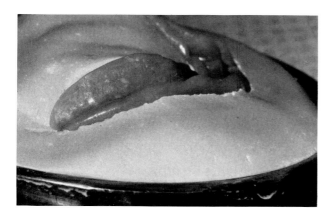

Fig. 15-7. Fully exposed denture border roll will be contained in top half of flask when second pour is made to assure accurate replication and prevent any change in shape of border contours during subsequent removal of tissue conditioner.

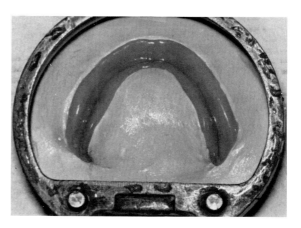

Fig. 15-8. When stone-plaster mix has reached its final set, thin coat of petroleum jelly is painted on surface to act as separator. Second half of flask has been placed in position.

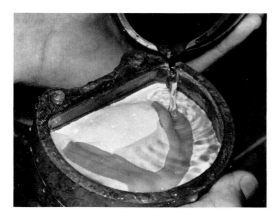

Fig. 15-9. Upper half of flask is positioned, and flask is filled with water at room temperature to wet surface of tissue conditioner and to prevent air bubbles from clinging to material during second pour. Water remaining in flask while mix of dental stone is made for second pour is emptied immediately prior to addition of stone.

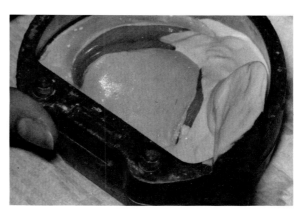

Fig. 15-10. Vacuum-spatulated mix of dental stone is vibrated carefully into upper half of flask to complete flasking. After flask is filled, lid is positioned.

Have the border rolls of the denture above the rim of the flask and the stone-plaster surface slope down and away from the denture borders (Figs. 15-2 to 15-4).

3. Before the stone-plaster mix reaches its final set, remove the excess with a plaster knife to expose fully the tissue rolls of the denture borders (Fig. 15-5). This action assures inclusion of all of the border rolls in the upper half of the flask and prevents damage during removal of the impression material. Contour the remainder of the stone-plaster mix with a wet finger, and sand it smooth with No. 320 grit wet or dry sandpaper; exercise care to avoid touching or distorting the impression material (Figs. 15-6 and 15-7).

4. After the stone-plaster mix has reached its final set, coat the surface with a thin layer of petroleum jelly,

and place the upper half of the flask in position (Fig. 15-8). Fill the flask with water that is at room temperature, and allow it to stand while mixing dental stone for the second pour (Fig. 15-9). The water wets the surface of the impression material and prevents air bubbles from clinging to it during the second pour.

5. Pour the water out of the flask, vibrate the vacuum-spatulated mix of dental stone into the top half of the flask, and make certain to avoid trapping any air bubbles (Fig. 15-10). Fill the flask to the top with the second pour, and position the flask lid.

6. After the stone has reached its final set, immerse the flask in hot, 130° F (54° C), tap water for approximately 5 minutes (Fig. 15-11). Gently pry the flask apart, and separate the halves of the flask carefully to

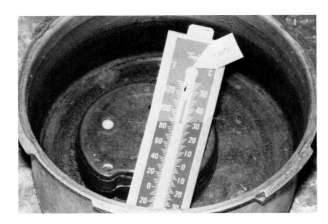

Fig. 15-11. After stone of second pour of denture flask has reached its final set, flask is immersed in hot water, 130° F (54° C), for approximately 5 minutes to soften tissue conditioner and facilitate separation of halves of flask. Boiling out is unnecessary. Halves of flask are pried apart gently to avoid fracturing stone investing medium.

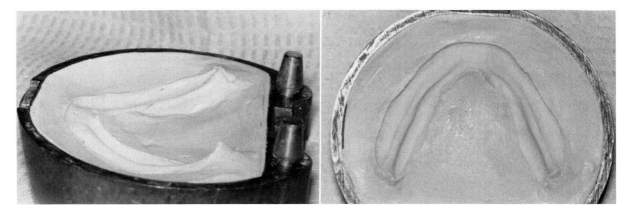

Fig. 15-12. Full rolls of denture border are reproduced accurately in stone investing medium of second half of denture flask. Rolls are unaffected during removal of impression material from lower half of flask and preparation of denture base prior to addition of soft liner. Any manipulation of stone surface or denture base is done in lower half of flask.

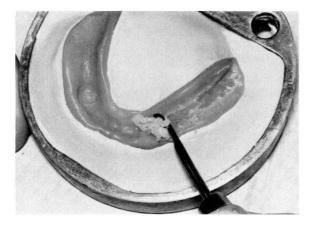

Fig. 15-13. Bulk of tissue conditioner can be removed quickly and easily with sharp vulcanite scraper.

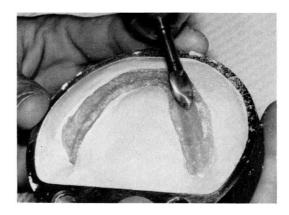

Fig. 15-14. After bulk of tissue conditioner has been removed with vulcanite scraper, remainder of material can be removed with carbide bur mounted in bench lathe.

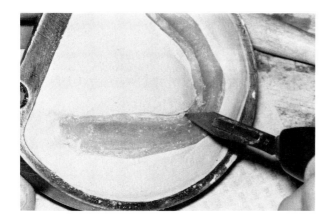

Fig. 15-15. Portion of tissue conditioner that forms sides of border molds can be removed from between denture base and stone investing medium with sharp blade. Small pieces of stone flash that might be included in Molloplast-B during trial packing later also can be removed.

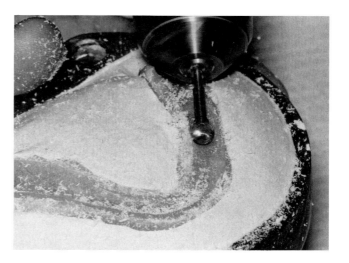

Fig. 15-16. Resin of denture base is roughened with carbide bur and, if necessary, part of it is removed to provide 2 to 3 mm thickness of Molloplast-B in all areas of denture base. Denture base material should be maintained at thickness of at least 3 mm over crest of ridge to reduce possibility of producing fracture site.

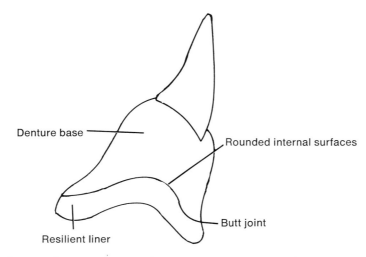

Fig. 15-17. Borders of denture base are flattened to provide butt joint for finishing Molloplast-B on external surface of denture. All surfaces of inner aspect of denture base are rounded to remove sharp angles.

avoid fracturing the stone. The top half of the flask should contain an accurate replication of the impression surface of the denture, including the full rolls of the denture borders (Fig. 15-12).

7. Remove the bulk of the tissue conditioner with a sharp vulcanite scraper (Fig. 15-13), and use a large carbide bur mounted in a bench lathe to remove the remainder of this material (Fig. 15-14). With a sharp blade (Fig. 15-15), remove the tissue conditioner from

the sides of the denture below the stone surface. Also take out small pieces of stone flash to prevent their inclusion in the Molloplast-B during the trial packing.

8. Prepare the denture base with a carbide bur to roughen the acrylic surface (Fig. 15-16). If necessary, remove additional acrylic to make the Molloplast-B 2 to 3 mm thick in all areas of the denture base. At the same time, maintain at least a 3 mm thickness of acrylic base material over the crest of the ridge to reduce the pos-

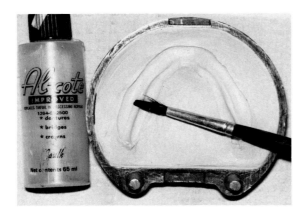

Fig. 15-18. Tinfoil substitute is applied to all gypsum surfaces of both halves of flask to facilitate separation after processing. After approximately 5 minutes material is thoroughly dry and ready for trial packing of Molloplast-B.

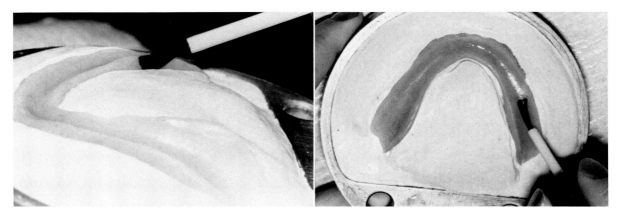

Fig. 15-19. Bonding agent is applied to all exposed surfaces of resin denture base. Bonding agent is applied immediately prior to trial packing, and 1- to 5-minute wait before trial packing is recommended by some manufacturers.

sibility of producing a fracture site. Flatten the denture borders to make a butt joint and to remove any sharp angles in the denture base material (Fig. 15-17).

9. Apply a tinfoil substitute* to all gypsum surfaces of both halves of the flask (Fig. 15-18), and allow them to dry thoroughly (approximately 5 minutes).

10. Coat all exposed resin surfaces thoroughly with a bonding agent (Fig. 15-19) immediately prior to trial packing with Molloplast-B. It is essential to use a bonding agent to assure adhesion of the Molloplast-B to the denture base. Primo† and Primabond‡ are silicone polymer bonding agents in a volatile solvent. After application to the resin surfaces and evaporation of the solvent, the silicone polymer becomes anchored to the denture base and serves as sites for attaching the Molloplast-B by cross-linkage.

11. The pregelled Molloplast-B is ready to use directly from the container because it requires no extra catalyst or mixing (Fig. 15-20). Roll the puttylike Molloplast-B into the shape of a hot dog, place it on the denture base (Fig. 15-21), and cover it with a thin plastic sheet.* Position the top half of the flask, and trial pack it with minimal packing pressure to produce an even distribution of material (Fig. 15-22).

12. Open the flask, and remove the flash with a sharp blade. Trial pack at least twice more until only a minimal amount of flash is produced (Fig. 15-23). Generally, the addition of more material after the first trial pack is unnecessary unless there is no flash.

13. Remove the plastic sheet prior to final closure, and achieve metal-to-metal contact between the halves of the flask before placing them in the flask press for processing. The manufacturer stresses the importance of maintaining sufficient pressure at all times to prevent

---

*Al-cote, L. D. Caulk, Co., Milford, Del., or equivalent.
†Primo, Guthapfel and Co., Switzerland.
‡Primabond, Buffalo Dental Manufacturing Co., Inc., Brooklyn, N.Y.

---

*Plastipac, Yates Dental Products, Chicago, Ill., or equivalent.

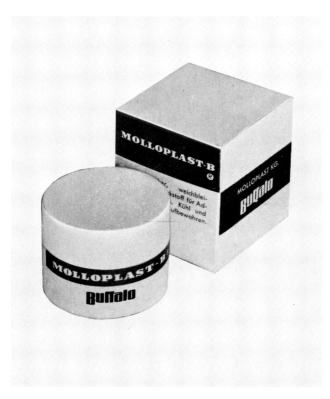

Fig. 15-20. Pregelled Molloplast-B is ready to use directly from its container and requires no additional catalyst.

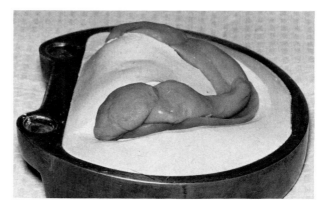

Fig. 15-21. Putty-like Molloplast-B is formed into roll and placed on denture base. If excessive amount is used at this stage, no more material will be required during trial packing.

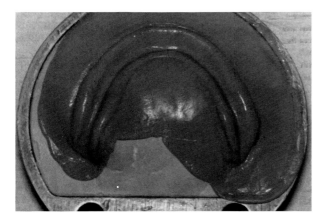

Fig. 15-22. Trial packing with minimal packing pressure should produce even distribution of material. Flash can be removed with sharp blade.

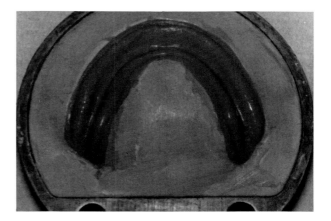

Fig. 15-23. Minimum of three trial packs usually is required to produce minimal amount of flash prior to final closure of flask.

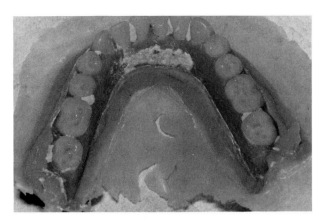

Fig. 15-24. Processed denture is deflasked. Stone of investing medium that clings to surface of denture can be removed ultrasonically in plaster and stone remover solution.

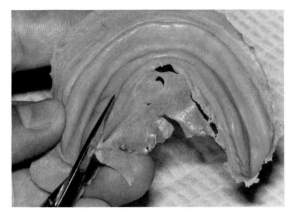

Fig. 15-25. Molloplast-B flash is trimmed with sharp scissors.

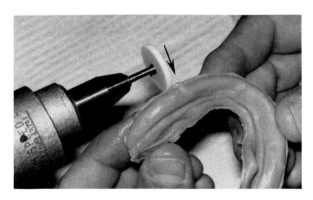

Fig. 15-26. Bulk of excess Molloplast-B can be removed with No. 60 LG grinding wheel. This wheel also can be used to reduce and contour excess material. Direction of rotation of wheel (arrow) should be from soft material to hard denture base.

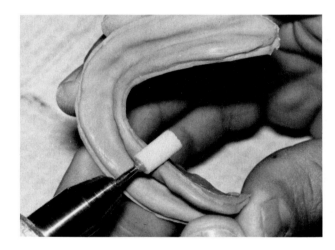

Fig. 15-27. No. 228 barrel-shaped LG mounted point can be used for final finishing and smoothing of Molloplast-B resilient liner.

the escape of the oxygen catalyst from the Molloplast-B; otherwise, bubbles can form, and subsequently the acrylic and silicone rubber liner can separate.

14. Insert the flask in cold water in a Hanau curing unit,* bring the temperature of the water to 160° F (71° C) within 30 minutes, and maintain this temperature for 30 minutes. During the next 30 minutes bring the water to a boil, and then boil it for 2 hours. The total curing time is 3½ hours.

15. Bench cool and deflask the denture (Fig. 15-24). Clean it ultrasonically in a plaster- and stone-remover solution.

16. Trim the bulk of the flash from the denture borders with a sharp scissors (Fig. 15-25). Reduce and contour the remainder of the flash with a No. 60 LG grinding wheel.* Make certain that the direction of the rotation of the stone is from the soft material to the hard denture base (Fig. 15-26). Silicone rubber resilient liners are always difficult to trim and polish. The manufacturer recommends trimming them at slow speeds with disks and rubber wheels. However, experience has shown that fine stones revolving at high speeds produce the best finish.

17. Do the final finishing and smoothing with a No. 228 barrel-shaped or a No. 230 tapered LG mounted point* (Fig. 15-27). Mount the wheels and points in a high-speed lathe or handpiece that will reach speeds of at least 25,000 revolutions per minute (rpm). No

---

*Hanau curing unit, Teledyne Dental Products, Hanau Division, Buffalo, N.Y.

*J. F. Jelenko & Co., LG Division, Chicago, Ill.

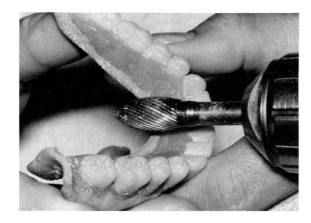

Fig. 15-28. Any areas of denture base that were nicked or scarred during processing and finishing should be smoothed and contoured with carbide bur.

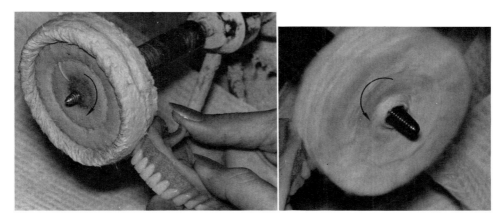

Fig. 15-29. Denture base material is pumiced and then brought to high shine with mounted rag wheels that rotate in direction from soft liner to hard denture base (arrows). Care is exercised to avoid separating resilient liner from denture base.

further finishing or polishing of the Molloplast-B is necessary.

18. Use a carbide bur to smooth any areas on the denture base that are nicked or scarred during processing and finishing (Fig. 15-28).

19. Pumice and polish the acrylic, but exercise care to avoid separating the resilient liner from the denture base (Fig. 15-29).

20. Clean the denture ultrasonically in an all-purpose solution. Then the completed denture with the resilient liner is ready for delivery to the patient (Fig. 15-30).

PROBLEM AREAS

In the past, the major problems associated with the use of resilient liners have been inadequate bonding of the liner to the denture base, color instability, loss of resiliency, and support of bacterial growth.

Use of the newer silicone rubber liners has overcome the problem of loss of resiliency. Although the material may become lighter in color with age, it should have no effect on the performance of the material. Bacterial growth is only an infrequent problem, controllable with proper denture hygiene and use of an antibacterial agent.* Use of the newer bonding agents appears to have improved the bond strength between silicone rubber liners and the denture base. A discussion of the other problems encountered with processing resilient denture base liners, their causes, and solutions follows (Table 15-2).

1. Large subsurface voids that occur during the initial stages of flasking fill with Molloplast-B later and become a problem during finishing (Fig. 15-31). Failure to apply the stone-plaster mix carefully to the external surface of the denture before inserting it in the bottom half of the flask causes voids. Therefore spread the vacuum-spatulated stone-plaster mix on the external surface of the

*Mersene, Colgate-Palmolive Co., New York, N.Y.

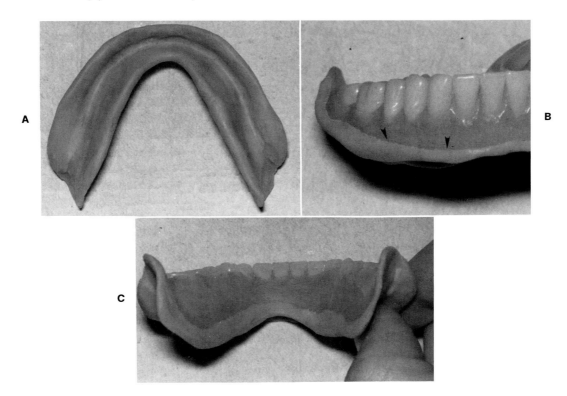

Fig. 15-30. A, Completed denture with resilient Molloplast-B liner. Tissue rolls have been reproduced and carried onto external surface of denture. **B,** Butt joint placed in denture base (arrows) makes smooth finishing line. **C,** LG wheels and points mounted in high-speed lathe produce excellent finish.

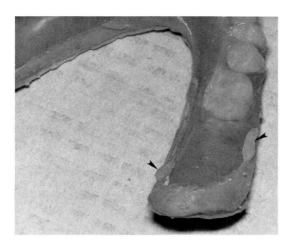

Fig. 15-31. During first half of flasking procedure, care is taken to avoid trapping any air bubbles on surface of denture and creating voids that will fill with Molloplast-B (arrows) later during trial packing. Generally, it is easy to remove these bubbles of resilient liner during finishing, but they can make border roll inaccurate.

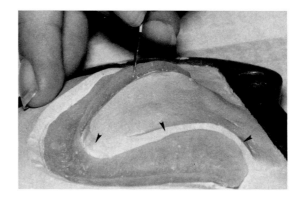

Fig. 15-32. Stone from around denture base in lower half of flask can be removed (arrows) to provide access to denture base without affecting shape and accuracy of denture border roll. Resultant thickness of Molloplast-B above border roll can be removed during finishing.

Table 15-2. Resilient denture base liners

Problem	Probable cause	Solution
Subsurface voids during initial flasking stages	Improper application of stone-plaster mix to surface of denture	Carefully apply stone-plaster mix to assure filling interproximal areas and avoid trapping air Vacuum spatulate stone-plaster mix in mechanical spatulator
Inadequate duplication of denture border rolls	Improper flasking	Flask so as to assure inclusion of border rolls of impression in top half of the flask Fully expose border rolls prior to final set of stone-plaster mix
Adherence of tissue conditioner to stone surface	Too much free liquid remaining in tissue conditioner	Alter powder-liquid ratio Prolong wearing time of tissue conditioner until flasking
Chalky, rough, pitted stone surface	See above	See above
Voids in top half of flask	Dry surface of tissue conditioner Improper flasking	Wet surface of tissue conditioner with water before pouring second half of flask Use mechanical vibration to avoid entrapment of air bubbles Use vacuum-mixed dental stone
Denture base visible through resilient liner on adjustment	Resilient liner too thin Inadequate removal of denture base material	Remove adequate amount of denture base material to assure resilient liner 2 to 3 mm thick prior to packing and processing
Fracture of denture base during usage	Weak denture base material Denture base material too thin	Use high-impact resin Leave minimum of 3 mm of denture base material over crest of ridge
Separation of resilient liner from denture base material	No bonding agent used All surfaces not coated with bonding agent	Use bonding agent recommended by manufacturer Apply bonding agent thoroughly to all surfaces to be covered with resilient liner

denture, and exercise care to fill the interproximal embrasures of the teeth, and cover their occlusal surfaces without trapping air bubbles (Fig. 15-2).

2. Improper flasking can result in inadequate duplication of the denture border rolls, overfinished borders, and loss of accuracy in the rolls of soft-tissue conditioner. To assure accurate replication of the denture borders, it is essential to trim the stone-plaster mix prior to its final set (Fig. 15-5). This trimming makes it possible to contain the border rolls of tissue conditioner in the top half of the flask. Later, during removal of the tissue conditioner and preparation of the denture base, it is possible to remove stone from around the denture base in the lower half of the flask for access to the acrylic base without affecting either the shape or accuracy of the denture borders (Fig. 15-32). The resultant thickness of Molloplast-B is produced above the border rolls (Fig. 15-33) and permits removal druing finishing.

3. The tissue conditioner adheres to the cast, resists easy removal, and produces a chalky and pitted stone surface (Figs. 15-34 and 15-35). This problem results from the presence of too much free liquid in the tissue conditioner. The dentist can rectify the problem most effectively by altering the powder-liquid ratio or by increasing the amount of time that the patient wears the appliance with the soft-tissue conditioner prior to removal from the mouth and flasking.

4. Voids in the top half of the flask (Fig. 15-36) that later fill with Molloplast-B produce inaccuracies in the borders of the finished denture. Pouring the second half of the flask without first wetting the surface of the tissue conditioner traps air bubbles, which produces voids. It is necessary to fill the flask with water at room temperature, allow it to stand while mixing dental stone for the second pour, and then pour the water out of the flask immediately prior to filling it with the vacuum-spatulated mix of dental stone.

5. The denture base shows through the resilient liner

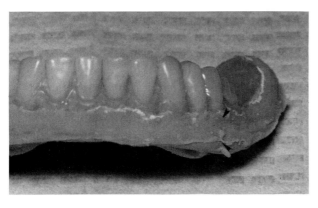

Fig. 15-33. Removal of stone from bottom half of flask to provide access to denture base during removal of tissue conditioner often produces excessive amount of Molloplast-B above denture border roll (arrows). Excess can be removed easily during finishing without affecting shape or accuracy of denture border roll.

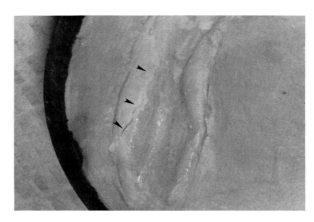

Fig. 15-34. Chalky and pitted stone surface (arrows) in top half of flask results when tissue conditioner adheres to cast and resists easy removal. This problem is caused by presence of too much free liquid in tissue conditioner.

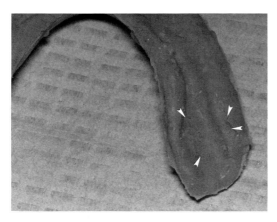

Fig. 15-35. Too much free liquid in tissue conditioner will produce chalky and pitted stone surface in top half of flask (arrows) and result in roughened surface on resilient liner.

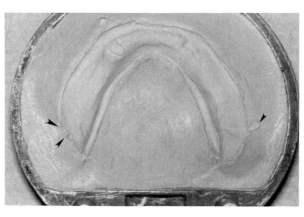

Fig. 15-36. Voids in top half of denture flask will produce inaccuracy in border roll of resilient liner (arrows). Voids result from clinging of air bubbles to surface of tissue conditioner during second pour of denture flasking procedure and can be eliminated by filling flask with water and wetting surface of tissue conditioner prior to making second pour.

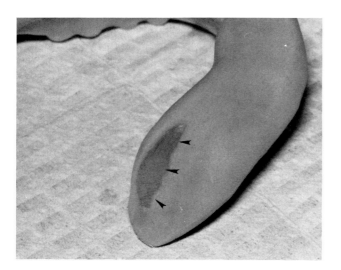

Fig. 15-37. Inadequate removal of denture base material during application of tissue conditioner or during preparation of denture base prior to trial packing will result in thin section of resilient liner (arrows) that can be removed during adjustment of denture base to provide tissue relief. This problem is avoided by removing adequate amount of denture base to provide 2 to 3 mm thickness of resilient liner. Area like this can reduce effectiveness of resilient liner and weaken bond between liner and denture base.

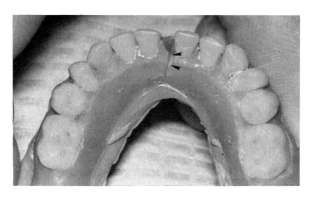

Fig. 15-38. Fracture in denture base (arrows) during use generally results from inadequate amount of denture base material over crest of ridge. If resilient liner is still intact, repair can be attempted. Use of high-impact resin and leaving thickness of at least 3 mm over crest of ridge can prevent problems of this type.

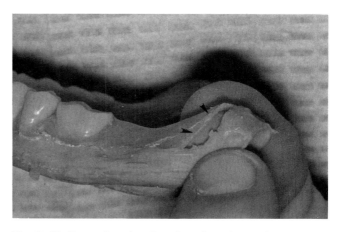

Fig. 15-39. Separation of resilient liner from denture base material (arrows) is caused by improper or inadequate use of bonding agent. All surfaces of denture base to be covered by resilient liner must be coated with bonding agent.

on adjustment to provide tissue relief (Fig. 15-37). The cause is the inadequate removal of the denture base material during the initial stages of applying the tissue conditioner or during preparation of the denture base prior to packing the Molloplast-B. It is necessary to remove 2 to 3 mm of resin from all areas of the tissue surface of the denture to provide for adequate thickness of the resilient liner. Although an area of resin like that shown in Fig. 15-37 does not produce a poor result necessarily, it can reduce the effectiveness of the resilient liner and weaken the bond between the liner and denture base.

6. The resilient-lined denture base fractures during usage (Fig. 15-38). The primary cause is use of an inadequate amount of denture base material over the crest of the ridge in the fracture site or failure to use a high-impact resin for the base material. Preparation of the denture base for a resilient liner more than 3 mm thick can leave an inadequate amount of base material (less than 3 mm) and produce a possible fracture site. When it is necessary to reduce the thickness of the denture base to less than 3 mm to allow for a 2 to 3 mm thickness of the resilient liner, use of such a liner is questionable; probably the height and thickness of the residual ridge permits use of a conventional denture base. If the resilient liner is still intact, it is possible to repair the denture base. However, this denture base is not dependable, inasmuch as the initial cause of the fracture still exists, and the denture base is even weaker after repair. If the liner tears, no repair is feasible, and it is necessary to reline the denture base.

7. The resilient liner separates from the denture base material (Fig. 15-39). Improper use of the bonding agent results in an inadequate bond between the resilient liner and denture base. It is essential to apply a coat of bonding agent to all surfaces to be covered by the resilient liner and to follow the manufacturer's instructions as to when to apply the agent and how long to wait before packing the resilient liner.

SUMMARY

Silicone rubber is an ideal resilient denture liner because its properties afford relief from the problems associated with badly resorbed ridges covered by thin, nonresilient mucosa. However, its use is not without limits as stated by Ortman and Ortman (1975):

Too often linings are used by dentists out of frustration. The basis for this frustration is, unfortunately, poor diagnosis of the original problem. No soft lining ever relieved chronic soreness due to an open vertical dimension of occlusion. Nor did it ever relieve an unstable thrusting type of occlusion. It cannot eliminate tissue trauma caused by inadequate tissue coverage. No soft denture lining will replace sound prosthodontic principles.

REFERENCES

Barnhart, G. W.: Silicone materials for lining dentures, Dent. Progress 3:246-252, 1963.

Bascom, P. W.: Resilient denture base materials, J. Prosthet. Dent. 16:646-649, 1966.

Bates, J. F., and Smith, D. C.: Evaluation of indirect resilient liners for dentures: laboratory and clinical test, J. Am. Dent. Assoc. 70: 344-353, 1965.

Boone, M. E.: Three R's—resilient, resistance, research, J. Am. Soc. Ger. Dent. 4:2-4, Jan., 1969.

Braden, M., and Clarke, R. L.: Viscoelastic properties of soft lining materials, J. Dent. Res. 81:1525-1528, 1972.

Cawson, R. A.: Symposium on denture sore mouth, II, the role of Candida, Dent. Pract. (Bristol) 16:138-142, Dec., 1965.

Craig, R. G., and Gibbons, P.: Properties of resilient denture liners, J. Am. Dent. Assoc. 63:382-390, 1961.

Gibbons, P.: Clinical and bacteriological findings in patients wearing Silastic 390 soft liner, J. Mich. Dent. Assoc. **47:**65-67, March, 1967.

Gonzales, J. B., and Laney, W. R.: Resilient materials for denture prostheses, J. Prosthet. Dent. **16:**438-444, 1966.

Griem, M. L., Robinson, J. E., and Barnhart, G. W.: The use of a soft denture base material in the management of post radiation denture problem, Radiology **82:**320-321, 1964.

Gruber, R. G., Lucatorto, F. M., and Molnar, E. J.: Fungus growth on tissue conditioners and soft denture liners, J. Am. Dent. Assoc. **73:**641-643, 1966.

Guide to dental materials and devices, ed. 6, Chicago, 1972-1973, American Dental Association, p. 106.

Harris, E.: Plea for more research on denture-base materials, J. Prosthet. Dent. **11:**673-676, 1961.

Lammie, G. A., and Storer, R.: A preliminary report on resilient denture plastics, J. Prosthet. Dent. **8:**411-424, 1958.

Laney, W. R.: Processed resilient denture liners, Dent. Clin. North Am. **14:**531-551, 1970.

Larsen, H. D., McDonald, G. T., and Purcell, J. P.: Resilient denture linings, J. La. Dent. Assoc. **35**(2):9-11, 1977.

Lytle, R. B.: Management of abused oral tissues in complete denture construction, J. Prosthet. Dent. **7:**27-42, Jan., 1957.

Mason, H. J.: Extreme warpage of resin dentures in routine grinding and polishing, North-West Dent. **43:**97-99, March-April, 1964.

Morrow, R. M., Reiner, P. R., Feldman, E. E. et al.: Metal reinforced silicone-lined dentures, J. Prosthet. Dent. **19:**219-229, 1968.

Mowrey, W. E., Burns, C. L., Dickson, G., and Sweeney, W. T.: Dimensional stability of denture base resins, J. Am. Dent. Assoc. **57:**345-353, 1958.

Ohashi, M., Woelfel, J. B., and Paffenbarger, G. C.: Pressures exerted on complete dentures during swallowing. J. Am. Dent. Assoc. **73:**625-630, 1966.

Ortman, H. R.: Factors of bone resorption of residual ridge, J. Prosthet. Dent. **12:**429-440, 1962.

Ortman, H. R.: Discussion of impact reduction in complete and partial dentures, J. Prosthet. Dent. **16:**246-250, 1966.

Ortman, H. R., and Ortman, L. F.: Denture refitting with today's concepts and materials, Dent. Clin. North Am. **19:**269-290, 1975.

Robinson, J. E.: Clinical experiments and experiences with silicone rubber in dental prosthetics, J. Prosthet. Dent. **13:**669-675, 1963.

Robinson, J. E., and Barnhart, G. W.: Silicone rubber soft denture base material: technique and clinical applications, Dent. Digest **70:**362-369, 1964.

Rudd, K. D.: Processing complete dentures without tooth movement, Dent. Clin. North Am. pp. 675-691, 1964.

Sauer, J. L., Jr.: Relining dentures with silicone rubber, J. Mich. Dent. Assoc. **46:**101-106, April, 1964.

Sauer, J. L., Jr.: A clinical evaluation of Silastic 390 as a lining material for dentures, J. Prosthet. Dent. **16:**650-660, 1966.

Storer, R.: Resilient denture base materials. Part I. Introduction and laboratory evaluation, Br. Dent. J. **113:**195-203, Sept., 1962.

Storer, R.: Resilient denture base materials. Part II. Clinical trial, Br. Dent. J. **113:**231-238, Oct., 1962.

Suchatlampong, C., Davies, E. H., and von Fraunhofer, J. A.: Some physical properties of four resilient lining materials, J. Dent. **4**(1): 19-27, 1976.

Sweeney, W. T.: Acrylic resins in prosthetic dentistry, Dent. Clin. North Am. pp. 593-601, 1958.

Travaglini, E. A., Gibbons, P., and Craig, R. G.: Resilient liners for dentures, J. Prosthet. Dent. **10:**664-672, 1960.

West, W. H.: RTV silicone rubbers in prosthetic dentistry, Dent. Progress **3:**125-126, Jan., 1963.

Woelfel, J. B., and Paffenbarger, G. C.: Evaluation of complete dentures lined with resilient silicone rubber, J. Am. Dent. Assoc. **76:**582-590, 1968.

Woelfel, J. B., and Paffenbarger, G. C.: Method of evaluating the clinical effect of warping a denture: a report of a case, J. Am. Dent. Assoc. **59:**250-260, 1959.

Woelfel, J. B., Paffenbarger, G. C., and Sweeney, W. T.: Clinical evaluation of complete dentures made of 11 different types of denture base materials, J. Am. Dent. Assoc. **70:**1170-1188, 1965.

Wright, P. S.: Soft lining materials: their status and prospects, J. Dent. **4:**247-256, 1976.

Young, G., Resca, H. G., and Sullivan, M. T.: Yeasts of the normal mouth and their relation to salivary acidity, J. Dent. Res. **30:**426-430, June, 1951.

CHAPTER 16

METAL BASES

JAMES S. BRUDVIK

metal base The metallic portion of a denture base, forming a part or all of the basal surface of the denture. It serves as a base for the attachment of the plastic (resin) part of the denture and teeth.

References to metal bases for complete dentures can be found in antiquity. Certainly their use was well understood by the time dentistry entered its modern era.

In 1867, Bean received a patent on a device for casting aluminum bases. Descriptions of swaged aluminum bases appeared in the dental literature of the late 1800s. More recently, Campbell (1923) described aluminum casting techniques that are still applicable in part.

Cast gold alloys, and later cast chrome base alloys, completed the armamentarium for complete denture metal bases. Grunewald's classic article (1964) defined the advantages of gold alloy bases, whereas Bell et al. (1977) discussed chrome alloy bases and Lundquist (1963), aluminum alloy bases.

The three alloys mentioned here have a place in the current practice of prosthodontics. Faber (1957) has given the following advantages of metal bases: (1) prevention of acrylic warpage, (2) more strength, (3) increased accuracy, (4) less tissue change under the base, (5) less porosity and therefore easier to clean and keep clean, (6) thermal conductivity, and (7) less deformation in function. He also has given the following disadvantages: (1) cost, (2) difficulty of refitting (relining), and (3) time-consuming construction.

REQUIREMENTS FOR CAST METAL BASES

The requirements for acceptable cast metal bases mirror the advantages. The bases should be (1) as thin as possible, and at the same time rigid, depending on the alloy used; (2) dense; (3) accurate, that is, having a positive fit on the master cast without rocking; and (4) of a biologically acceptable alloy.

DESIGN PRINCIPLES

Although some aspects of construction of cast metal bases depend entirely on the alloy chosen, the principles of design remain essentially the same. The design of the cast metal base always must be a clinical decision. A prescription or pencil drawing on the master cast must determine the amount of coverage, placement of finishing lines, and type of resin retention used.

Maxillary bases

The maxillary base can cover (1) only the palate, (2) the palate and the ridge crest, or (3) the entire denture-bearing area (Figs. 16-1 to 16-3). The most satisfactory design covers the complete palate and ridge crest, but leaves the denture borders in resin. An acceptable variation of this design also places the posterior palatal seal area in metal and begins the resin periphery at the pterygomaxillary notch area (Fig. 16-4).

If the posterior palatal seal is to be in metal, it is essential that the dentist establish this critical area accurately. Scraping of the cast by the technician to establish the seal area is inadvisable.

Mandibular bases

The mandibular cast base is of only two types: (1) with crest of the ridge coverage and (2) with complete coverage of the mandibular denture space (Figs. 16-5 and 16-6). Since exact determination and registration of the mandibular denture space is difficult clinically, the crest

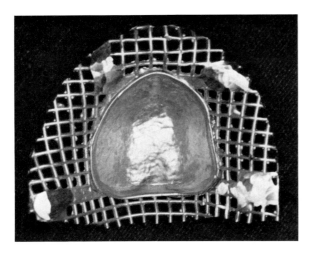

Fig. 16-1. Maxillary base covering only center palate area with relieved retention mesh. This design has been used to aid patient with history of repeated midline fractures of maxillary denture. It is inferior design because it places thin, porous resin over ridge crest.

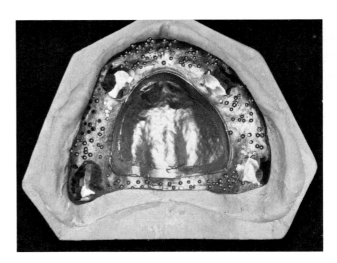

Fig. 16-2. Maxillary coverage of palate and ridge crest. Posterior palatal seal area will be in resin to facilitate adjustments.

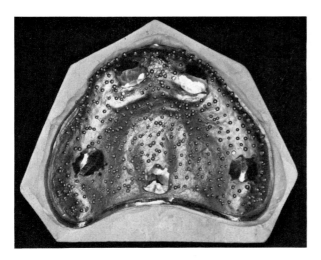

Fig. 16-3. Entire denture-bearing area is covered with metal. This design is seldom used because weight of metal is excessive.

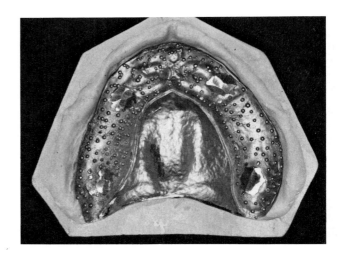

Fig. 16-4. When posterior palatal seal area is well defined on master cast, posterior border can be placed in metal. This design reduces bulk of denture base in posterior area.

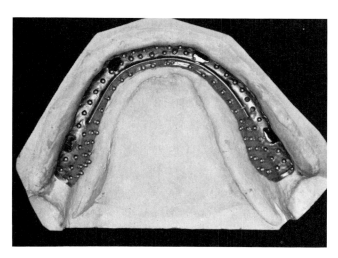

Fig. 16-5. Mandibular cast bases that are short of peripheries are simple to make and adjust. Base outline is drawn to follow heights of contour without entering any prominent undercuts.

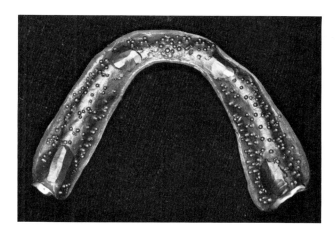

Fig. 16-6. If considerable weight is desired in mandibular casting, it can be cast of gold alloy to outline covering complete denture space. Careful determination of peripheries during final impression is essential with this type of base.

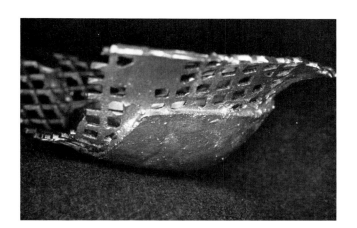

Fig. 16-7. Relieved retention mesh should allow at least 1 mm for resin beneath it.

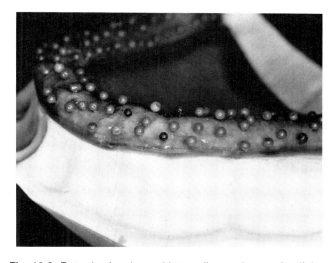

Fig. 16-8. Retentive beads provide excellent resin retention if they are No. 14 or larger and space between them is twice their diameter.

of the ridge coverage with resin peripheries is preferable, especially when using chrome base alloys because adjustment and subsequent repolishing are much more difficult than when using resin peripheries.

Resin retention

Resin retention for maxillary or mandibular bases is of four types: (1) raised (relieved) retention mesh, (2) nonrelieved retention of beads, (3) "nailheads," and (4) loops (Figs. 16-7 to 16-10). Since relieved retention places thin resin adjacent to denture-bearing tissues, it is inferior to nonrelieved types, which permit a butt joint of thicker resin. In addition, nonrelieved retention

uses less interridge space and thereby facilitates positioning of the denture teeth.

Blockout and relief

Aspects of concern in both maxillary and mandibular bases are the blockout of soft-tissue undercuts under the bases and placement of arbitrary relief areas. These two steps require clinical observation and judgment and normally are completed by the dentist. Placement of relief chambers cannot be arbitrary. However, it is possible to block out extremely sharp soft-tissue folds and crevices as well as pronounced rugae contours arbitrarily to eliminate problems in seating the cast-

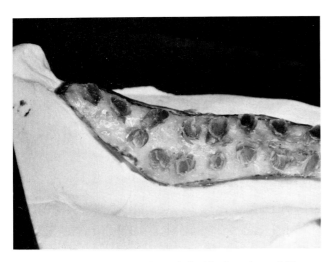

Fig. 16-9. Nailhead retention is made by blunting piece of 18-gauge wax and attaching it to stipple sheet with tacky liquid.

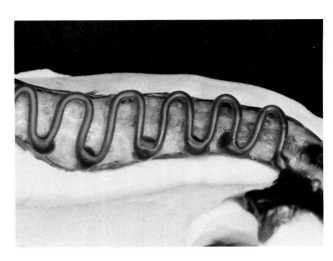

Fig. 16-10. Retentive loops made of 18- or 20-gauge round wax can be adapted to base wax-up for effective retention. They have disadvantage of intruding into denture space more than bead or nailhead retention.

ing back on the master cast (Fig. 16-11). This blockout also reduces the number of sharp metal projections on the tissue surface to be removed during finishing.

Materials for cast metal bases

Three groups of alloys are used to construct cast metal bases for complete dentures. They have had clinical evaluation, and many references to their use appear in the literature.

Gold alloys

Gold alloys of Types III and IV are sufficiently rigid for use as cast metal bases. Casting in gypsum-bound investments with a uniform thickness as thin as 28 gauge is easy. The gold alloys are most frequently cast in 20 to 24 gauge. They contain copper, silver, palladium, platinum, and some trace elements, and differ slightly in content with the various manufacturers, but all that satisfy the American Dental Association specifications will be acceptable.

Chrome base alloys

All of the commonly used removable partial denture alloys are equally acceptable for cast metal bases for complete dentures. Casting at a 26-gauge thickness is dependable, but chrome base alloys generally are at 22 to 24 gauge to be sufficiently rigid. The low-heat chrome alloy offers only one advantage: casting in gypsum-bound investments with a 1300° F (704.5° C) burnout.

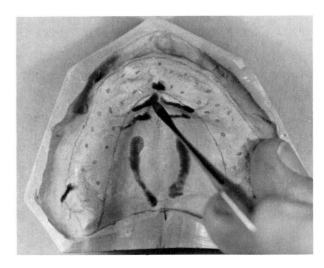

Fig. 16-11. Blockout of soft tissue undercuts should be guided by clinical judgment, as indicated on prescription form. If casting is to enter undercuts without blockout, adjustments *must* be made on master cast to allow seating of cast base.

Aluminum alloys

Unlike the gold and chrome base alloys, aluminum is usable in its pure state. However, its use as an alloy with 2% to 4% magnesium and slight amounts of silicon is more common. The casting temperature of aluminum in gypsum-bound investment alloys is between 1300° F (704.5° C) and 1500° F (815.5° C). It is possible to anodize aluminum, although this practice is not essential. Aluminum oxidizes easily and can become pitted. There-

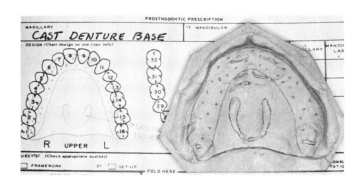

Fig. 16-12. Design as seen on two-dimensional prescription must be transferred to master cast before blockout procedures are begun.

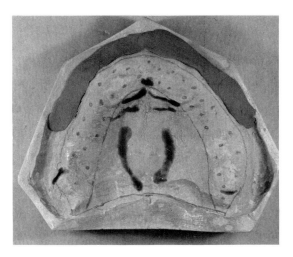

Fig. 16-13. Clay or mortite (window caulking) is used to block out undercuts on peripheries of master cast.

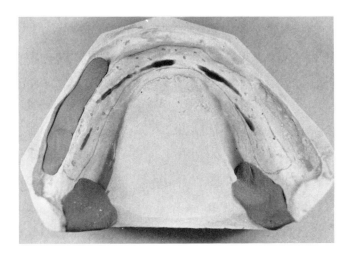

Fig. 16-14. Mandibular cast, properly blocked out, is ready for duplication.

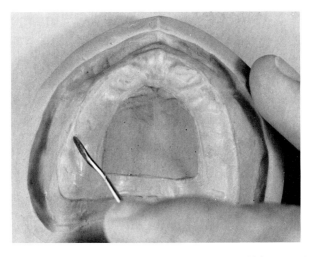

Fig. 16-15. Relief pad wax is sealed to master cast with hot spatula. In addition to periphery, wax is sealed by crosshatching entire pad area to prevent pad from becoming displaced during duplication.

fore no commercial denture base cleansers should be used when soaking it overnight. Warm water and soap used after each meal are adequate for maintaining a clean surface.

Gold alloy cast base
PROCEDURE

1. Ideally, the master cast arrives at the laboratory with the base outlined in pencil. When this is impossible, the technician transfers the design to the master cast from the information obtained from the prescription (Fig. 16-12).

2. The technician holds the designed master cast in front of a suction outlet, and sprays it lightly with a model spray.* This prevents the design from being washed away in subsequent procedures. It also fills minute pores in the cast and strengthens chalky areas against abrasion.

3. Blockout of the master casts consists of two separate stages. First, with any standard blockout wax, block out the areas within the outline of the cast base requiring relief or recontouring, as indicated by the prescription. Next, the undercut areas outside of the outline are blocked out with clay or caulking compound (Fig. 16-13).

---

*Jelenko Model Spray, J. F. Jelenko & Co., New Rochelle, N.Y., or equivalent.

The standard outline of a maxillary cast base extends barely over the crest of the ridge; therefore place this material along the buccal and facial ridge surfaces and into any other cast undercuts or discrepancies that may distort the duplicating material and make the refractory cast inaccurate (Table 16-1). The mandibular cast usually requires blockout in the retromolar area as well as the sharp, soft-tissue folds (Fig. 16-14). If raised retention mesh is desired, relief pads must be placed at this point. The minimum acceptable thickness is equal to approximately that of one sheet of standard baseplate wax. Seal this wax completely at the periphery to prevent it from raising up and becoming distorted during the duplicating process (Fig. 16-15).

4. Place the master cast in slurry water preheated to 100° F (38° C) for 20 minutes. This procedure prepares the cast for accurate duplication by warming it to the approximate temperature of the duplicating material. Slurry water is essential to prevent leaching action on the master cast.

5. Use any duplicating colloid, but follow the manufacturer's directions as to time and temperature because of slight differences in the materials. For example, it is essential to boil and spatulate Nobilloid* to break it down, to pour it at 125° to 130° F (51.5° to 54° C), and to let it set at 65° to 75° F (18.5° to 24° C) for at least 30 minutes. A variety of duplicating flasks are available, and they consist of a base and a cover. Usually, the base is of metal, so that cooling in cold water will pull the solidifying material toward the base and down onto the master cast. Center the cast in the flask and,

after the duplicating material reaches the recommended temperature, direct it in a small finger-size stream to the highest portion of the cast (Fig. 16-16, *A*). The material flows down the sides of the cast and fills it without entrapping air. Bench set the filled flask for 5 minutes, and then place it in the cooling tank from 30 minutes to an hour (Fig. 16-16, *B*). Have the water no deeper than the depth of the flask base to "pull" the colloid toward the cast.

6. After the colloid has set, remove the base. Cut away excess material around the cast base, and remove the master cast by forcing a blast of air gently along the walls of the cast, or by snapping out the cast with two knives (Figs. 16-17 to 16-19). Carefully inspect the mold under magnification for tears and distortions in the colloid.

7. Although the manufacturer recommends pouring the refractory material immediately, frequently it is impractical when doing a series of units at the same time. In the event of any delay, place the colloid mold in a humidor or at least cover it with a damp towel. Use any gypsum-bound refractory material for gold castings, but follow the manufacturer's directions. Investic,* the investment for Ticonium,* is a good example of a general-purpose gypsum-bound refractory material. Mix 100 gm of investment with 29 ml of distilled water. As with any gypsum-bound refractory material, more water decreases the expansion, and less water increases the expansion. It may be necessary to use 30 ml of distilled water for extra-large castings. When mixing these investments in small amounts, such as for a single cast, use

---

*Nobillium Products, Chicago, Ill.

*Ticonium, Albany, N.Y.

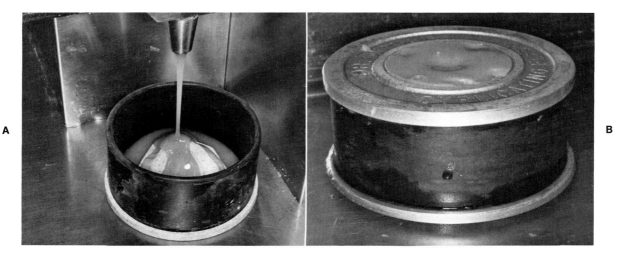

Fig. 16-16. A, Duplicating colloid is directed to highest point on master cast. **B,** Filled flask is put into cooling tank with water covering only base.

Table 16-1. Metal bases

Problem	Probable cause	Solution
Incomplete casting	Inadequate amount of metal cast	Reevaluate amount of metal to be used in casting (Table 16-2)
	Stipple sheet possibly stretched during application, causing wax-up to be too thin	Add flash of wax (0.5 mm) to refractory cast before applying stipple sheet in prominent areas or sharp contours where distortion of plastic sheet is liable to occur
	Mold too cold at casting	Check burnout furnace temperature control; do not bring mold from furnace until metal is ready to cast (30-second interval, maximum allowed); recalibrate induction casting machines; follow instructions of manufacturer exactly; preferably have manufacturer's representative demonstrate calibration procedure first time
		Practice hot and cold casting of metal bases with torch to train eye (practice castings can be made to simulate dimensions of desired metal bases by using stipple sheets)
Porosity in casting	Metal too hot at casting	Same as when metal too cold
Pits and inclusions in casting	Investment particles incorporated in molten mass	Round all angles in wax-up and spruing stage to avoid having sharp areas of refractory cast liable to be broken off by force of molten metal
Metal blebs on completed casting	Voids (air pockets) during paint-on stage	Apply paint-on layer in smaller increments
Failure to fit master cast	Inadequate blockout of undercuts	Identify interferences with disclosing medium (spray powder, Liqua-Mark,* or similar product); relieve metal with fine-cut stones; return casting for clinical try-in and if acceptable, relieve master cast under casting for soft-tissue undercuts when necessary for complete seat
	Distortion during duplication	Check time and temperature for entire duplication process
	Breakdown of refractory	Verify manufacturer's expiration date on investment
	Change in powder-water ratio	Verify powder-water ratio; check measuring devices (scales and graduates)
	Plastic pattern (stipple sheet) pulled from refractory cast	Apply tacky liquid carefully; apply small amounts of hot wax at stipple-sheet margin to seal patterns to cast

*The Wilkinson Co., Westlake Village, Calif.

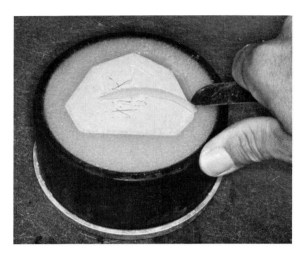

Fig. 16-17. Dull laboratory knife is used to trim colloid around base of cast.

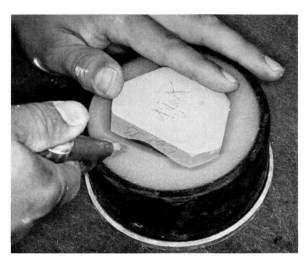

Fig. 16-18. Blast of compressed air directed along base of cast will free it from duplicating material.

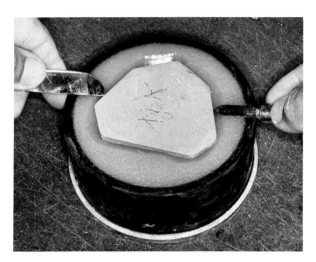

Fig. 16-19. Master cast also can be removed by prying on base of cast with two knives.

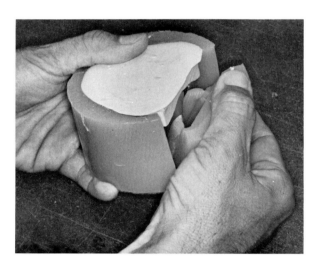

Fig. 16-20. Duplicating material is broken off from refractory cast and must be rinsed to remove stone particles before breaking it down for reuse.

of a syringe in measuring the water is essential. The possible error in reading the meniscus of a standard graduate is too great to risk. When mixing larger amounts, such as for many casts in large commercial laboratories, the meniscus error has less effect on the overall powder-water ratio.

The manufacturer states that Investic should be spatulated not more than 30 seconds mechanically, or 1 minute by hand. Remove any excess moisture from the mold with a gentle blast of air, and vibrate the refractory investment directly into the mold. Do not vibrate longer than is necessary to cover the surface of the mold.

8. Allow 1 hour to complete the set before removing the cast from the colloid. Leaving the cast in the mold

longer is detrimental because the water-based colloids can dry up and affect the refractory surface. Glycerin-based colloids, used with some chrome base alloys, do not exhibit this desiccation.

After breaking the colloid from the set refractory material, rinse it to remove the stone debris (Fig. 16-20). Then cut or break it into small pieces, and reboil it for future use, or store it in 100% humidity. Do not store it immersed in water because the material will absorb water and lose both strength and accuracy.

9. Trim the refractory cast with a model trimmer to within ½ inch (1.3 cm) of the desired base coverage. Then reduce it in height until the cast is ¼ inch (0.64 cm) thick at its thinnest vertical dimension (Fig. 16-21).

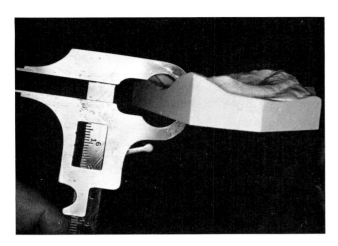

Fig. 16-21. Cast base must be trimmed to thickness of ¼ inch (0.64 cm) in thinnest portion to assure having pattern close to outside of investment mold.

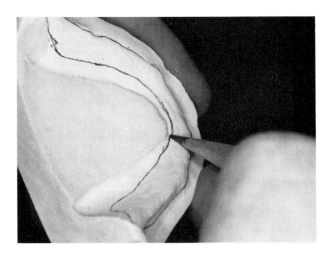

Fig. 16-22. Black pencil is used to indicate critical areas of design. Since plastic stipple sheet patterns are translucent, it is possible to trim exactly to line by using black pencil marks visible through sheet.

Table 16-2. Alloy, pattern gauge, and amount used for cast metal bases

Alloy	Pattern gauge	Average amount by type of cast
Gold Type IV	20 to 24	24 dwt, mandibular 30 dwt, maxillary
Chrome base alloys Ticonium, Vitallium, Nobillium, etc.	24	16 dwt, mandibular 19.5 dwt, maxillary
Aluminum Alcoa D214	22	25 ingots, mandibular 30 ingots, maxillary

Uniformity in thickness of the refractory cast is essential to position the wax pattern properly in the flask ring during the investing. Make it no more than ½ inch (1.3 cm) thick from the pattern to the outside of the refractory mold, and standardize this procedure for all castings.

Rinse the trimmed refractory casts quickly under running water to remove all slurry from the trimming. Any slurry allowed to remain on the refractory cast will set and distort it. Dry the cast with a blast of air, and place it in a drying oven at 200° F (93.5° C) for 1 hour.*

10. Close or fill all the pores in the refractory cast before waxing the base. Use a model spray,† or dip the hot cast in beeswax.‡ Usually, commercial deep fat

fryers are used to heat the beeswax to 300° F (149° C). Remove the refractory cast from the drying oven and submerge it in the hot beeswax. Soon it begins to bubble and foam; keep the cast in the wax for 15 seconds more before removing it and placing it on a paper towel to absorb the excess wax. When the cast is cool, it is ready for transfer of the design and waxing.

11. Transfer the outline showing the extent of the base coverage and the position of the finishing lines from the master cast to the refractory cast. It is unnecessary to draw the complete outline on the refractory cast, which is much softer than dental stone (Fig. 16-22). Any damage caused by excessive drawing will be reproduced in the metal.

12. Selection of the size of the plastic pattern is a clinical decision. In general, mandibular gold bases are strong enough if they are 1 mm thick (18 gauge). It is possible to make them from 0.75-mm (21-gauge) pattern sheets by reinforcing the peripheries. Maxillary bases

---

*Model 105-SS, Modern Laboratory Equipment Co., New York, N.Y., or equivalent.
†Jelenko Model Spray, J. F. Jelenko and Co., New Rochelle, N.Y., or equivalent.
‡Modern Material Manufacturing Co., St. Louis, Mo., or equivalent.

are strong enough in their thinner dimensions because their geometric form makes them more rigid than mandibular bases. The average thickness of a maxillary cast base is 0.61 mm (22 gauge) (Table 16-2).

13. For a maxillary cast gold base, make a "tacky liquid" by mixing 18 ml of acetone and enough plastic pattern material to raise the volume to 20 ml. This ratio makes it have the consistency of a thin syrup. Occasionally, it will be necessary to add more acetone to maintain this consistency. Paint this liquid on the refractory cast within the confines of the proposed base. Take one

thickness of a stipple sheet that is half the final thickness desired, and lay it down to the outlined base extension. A stipple sheet is a plastic pattern form available from any of the major manufacturers of removable partial denture alloys. It is available in 21 to 30 gauge and in both a stippled surface and a smooth one. Using a moistened finger or a pattern adapter,* adapt the stipple sheet to the refractory cast (Fig. 16-23). Begin the adaptation in the center of the palate, and work the

---

*Howmedica, Inc., Chicago, Ill.

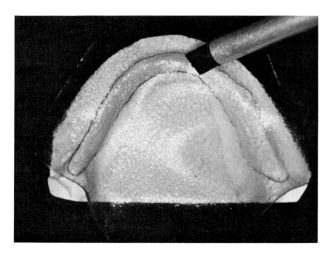

Fig. 16-23. Pattern adapter facilitates adaptation of plastic stipple sheets to refractory and minimizes risk of tearing or excessive thinning.

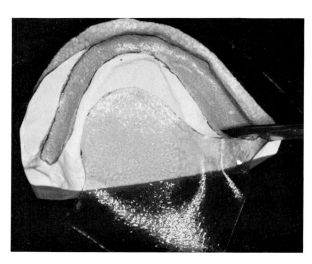

Fig. 16-24. If blade has been heated, pattern can be cut without distortion.

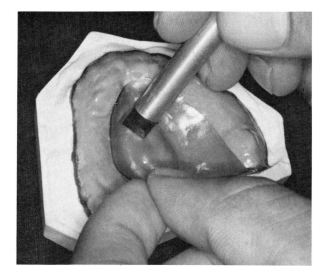

Fig. 16-25. Finishing line for junction of resin and metal is established when second sheet of plastic pattern is laid to cover first sheet partially.

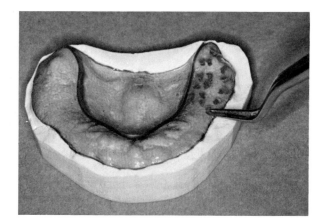

Fig. 16-26. Retentive beads can be placed on tacky liquid with cotton forceps. Fine brush also can be used to pick up and deposit beads if tip is moistened.

material out to the peripheries to prevent the sheet from folding over on itself. After making certain that the sheet is in place and well adapted, cut off the excess back exactly to the line with a No. 11 blade warmed over a Bunsen burner (Fig. 16-24).

14. Adapt a second sheet of stipple, also half the thickness of the final casting, to the first sheet with the aid of the tacky liquid. Trim this second sheet quite short of the first so that its border forms the external finishing line on the palate and allows a smooth transition from the metal to the resin lingual to the denture teeth (Fig. 16-25). Cut the second sheet at a 90-degree angle to the palatal surface so that the resin can have a butt joint with the metal.

15. Add retention beads for the resin to the ridge crest area. The beads should be 14 gauge or larger to retain the resin adequately. Form nailheads from 18-gauge round wax and retention loops from 18- or 21-gauge round wax. Place tacky liquid on the ridge crest area, and use cotton forceps to apply the beads or nailheads (Fig. 16-26). Place them in a regular pattern, and make the distance between them two and a half times their diameter. Exercise care to avoid setting the beads too deep in the tacky liquid because the retentive effect relies on having the maxium surface below the height of the contour.

16. Make a final inspection of the entire periphery at this point to make certain that the borders are sealed *completely* to the refractory cast (Fig. 16-27). Failure to seal any portions may allow it to rise slightly before investing and result in inaccuracies in the adaptation of the base.

17. Except for using a different gauge of stipple sheet and almost always making the base short of all borders, the techniques for waxing the mandibular cast are the same as for the maxillary cast. Since ridge loss often causes constriction of the labiolingual dimension of the mandibular base area, the mandibular cast base must be thicker than the maxillary. In some severe situations, the base requires more structural support in the form of an I-beam addition to the stipple sheet (Fig. 16-28). Generally, form a mandibular cast gold base from a 22-gauge plastic pattern sheet. Cut it at a 90-degree angle to the refractory cast surface to allow for a butt joint of resin. The outlined base should allow for a 3 to 5 mm extension of resin at all peripheries.

18. Sprue gold alloy cast bases from above by placing 8-gauge sprues in the cuspid and first molar areas. Join the sprues with a wax-cone sprue form centered above the base (Fig. 16-29). It is possible to construct the wax cone by cutting a circle of regular baseplate wax that has a diameter of 2½ inches (6.4 cm). Cut this circle of wax into two pieces, and roll each one to form an ideal sprue cone (Fig. 16-30). Round the tip of the cone by adding more wax by hand, and place the cone so that the sprue leads join it 3 to 5 mm up from the tip. Place the tip of the cone approximately 30 mm from the deepest portion of the palate or the center portion of the mandibular refractory cast (Fig. 16-31). This distance varies with the height of the ridge and palatal contour. It is essential that the sprue leads be inclined until they form an angle of approximately 135 degrees with the long axis of the sprue cone. Sometimes it is necessary to curve the sprues slightly to eliminate severely acute

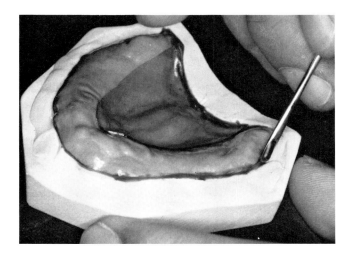

Fig. 16-27. Addition of small amount of blue wax to periphery with extremely hot spatula will assure having sheet in contact with cast throughout investing procedure.

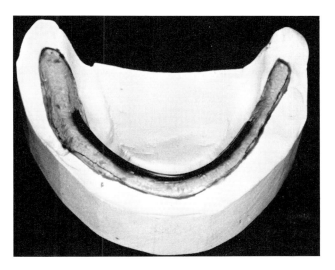

Fig. 16-28. Addition of half round strip of wax slightly to lingual area of ridge crest greatly strengthens thin mandibular casting without interfering with placement of denture teeth.

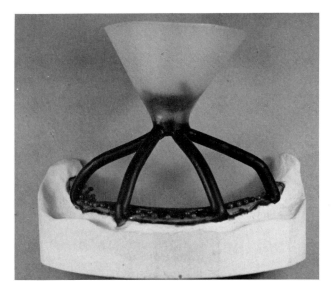

Fig. 16-29. Gold bases require four 8-gauge sprues curved slightly to reach ridge at almost 90-degree angle. This approach eliminates thin angle of investment that would result from acute angle and possible breakoff during casting.

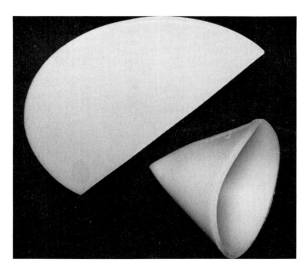

Fig. 16-30. Sprue cone formed from half circle of wax 2½ inch (6.4 cm) in diameter.

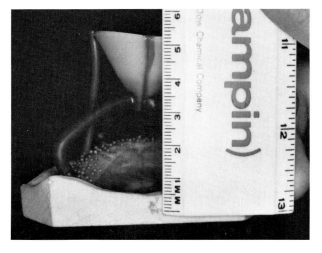

Fig. 16-31. Sprue cone tip needs to be approximately 30 mm from deepest portion of wax-up to allow space for curving sprue leads to approach cast at 90-degree angle and to maintain approximately 135-degree angle with long axis of sprue cone.

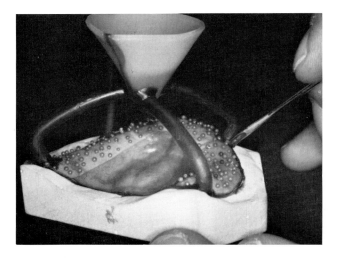

Fig. 16-32. More blue wax must be added to eliminate sharp edges in junction of sprue lead and wax-up.

angles where sprues join the appliances. The sprue leads join the waxed appliance in the resin retention area. Add wax at this junction to make a smooth transition into the stipple sheet (Fig. 16-32). Establish a similar smooth joint where the leads join the wax cone. Elimination of sharp angles in the wax in these areas is essential to preclude sharp edges in the refractory mold; they may break off during casting and become entrapped in the molten mass.

19. After properly spruing the completed wax-up, prepare it for investing by dipping it in a surface tension–reducing agent* and carefully blowing off the excess. Prepare the paint-on layer according to the powder-water ratio of the manufacturer (Investic, 100 gm : 30 ml). A 50-gm mixture is sufficient for the paint-on

*Debubblizer, Kerr Manufacturing Co., Romulus, Mich., or equivalent.

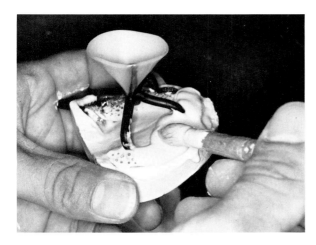

Fig. 16-33. Hand with brush is placed on vibrator table, and refractory is brought to brush tip. Paint-on layer is added in small amounts to prevent entrapment of air.

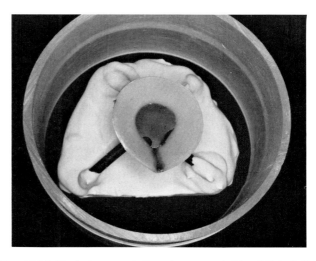

Fig. 16-34. Flask rings must allow clearance of at least ½ inch (1.3 cm) from paint-on layer to give adequate strength in final mold.

layer. Spatulate the material for 30 seconds mechanically or 1 minute by hand, and then vibrate it gently onto the waxed base (Fig. 16-33). Exercise care to avoid entrapping air bubbles or dislodging retentive beads or loops. The entire layer should be not more than ⅛ inch (0.32 cm) thick. This uniformly thin layer within the larger investment mold allows the gas to escape. It also increases the likelihood of complete castings by reducing the possibility of trapping air on the wax-up and by protecting the mold if the investment cracks during the burnout. When the paint-on layer has reached its initial set (in approximately 10 minutes), continue the investing. Select a flask ring that will allow a clearance of at least ½ inch (1.3 cm) around the refractory model and its paint-on layer (Fig. 16-34). Measure the rest of the refractory investment, and spatulate it in the same ratio and manner as the paint-on layer. Do not vacuum spatulate investment layers because the mold must be porous to eliminate gas. Place the flask ring on a flat bench surface and fill it three fourths full. Hold the cast by the sprue cone, and dip it in water to wet the paint-on layer and keep it from dehydrating the fresh mix of investment. Wiggle the cast into the investment flask ring until it touches the bottom, and then bring it ¼ inch (0.64 cm) back up toward the top (Fig. 16-35). The investment should be firm enough to support the cast in this position as the initial set begins. The final set requires approximately 15 minutes.

20. The investment flask rings can be of metal, Plexiglas, or polyvinyl chloride (PVC) pipe; a 4-inch (10.16-cm) diameter pipe split lengthwise with a 1½-inch (3.8-cm) cutoff disk makes an excellent homemade flask (Fig. 16-36). A larger diameter pipe is suitable for especially large castings. Split all rings to permit expansion and

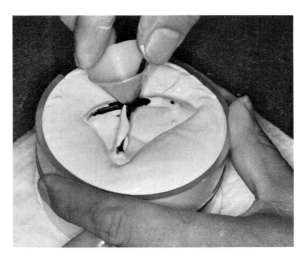

Fig. 16-35. Refractory is wiggled or twisted into partially filled ring. When cast touches bottom, it is twisted back up approximately ¼ inch (0.64 cm). Sprue cone must be positioned near center of ring to complete investing properly.

removal from the mold before placing it in the furnace. The flask ring chosen for the case must have enough vertical height for the sprue cone tip to be ½ to ¾ inch (1.3 to 1.9 cm) below the top of the ring (Fig. 16-37). This position will allow the recessed sprue lead to be at least ¼ inch (0.64 cm) in the completed mold.

21. Burnout cycles (time and temperature) vary with the refractory material used. Normally, a burnout time frame of 2 to 3 hours during which the furnace reaches 1300° to 1350° F (704.5° to 732° C) is used with a heat-soak period of 1 to 2 hours at the maximum temperature. Most large, modern burnout furnaces have electronic

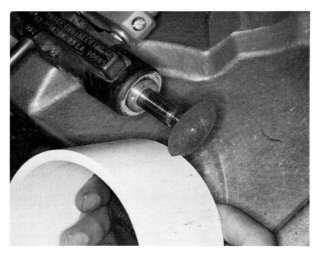

Fig. 16-36. Polyvinyl (PVC) pipe, available from plumbing supply store, makes durable investing ring when sectioned with cutoff disk.

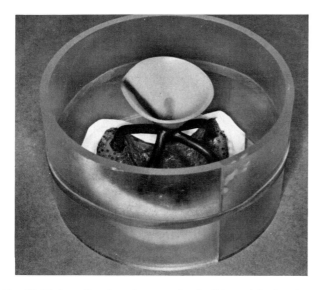

Fig. 16-37. Investing ring of proper size for this cast denture base.

timers to regulate the rate at which the temperature increases.

22. Always place the mold in the furnace with the sprue opening down and in such a position that·the mold touches neither the furnace walls nor other molds. Burnout eliminates the plastic and wax patterns, and allows the thermal expansion inherent in the particular refractory material to occur.

23. It is possible to cast the gold denture base in the conventional broken-arm machine with a gas-air or a gas-oxygen torch to melt the metal. However, use of an induction casting machine assures more repeatable results. Although every technician has a technique for torch castings, the essential aspects are: to use a crucible not contaminated from use with other alloys, to balance the casting arm for the weight of the mold, to clean and flux the metal properly, to bring the metal to the required temperature evenly and avoid overheating, to position the mold in the cradle as close as possible to the actual moment of casting to prevent excessive cooling of the mold, and to use a reducing flame on the torch.

24. Induction casting eliminates most of the human error from the process. Specific instructions accompany each induction casting machine. For example, with Jelenko's Thermotrol 2500, the casting temperature is set on the pyrometer, and the metal is placed in the crucible in the muffle at approximately 400° F (204.5° C) below the casting temperature. The arm is wound with two turns and locked into position. A buzzer sounds when the casting temperature is reached. It may be necessary to heat-soak the metal and visually verify that the mass of metal is truly molten. The ring is removed from the oven and placed in the cradle. With the metal at the desired temperature, the arm is unlocked by freeing it from the locking pin. At the drop of the pin, the arm can be released, and the casting completed. Howmedica's Electromatic Casting Machine is even more sophisticated. It releases the casting arm automatically when the radiation pyrometer indicates that the desired metal temperature has been reached. Since the arm is driven by a motor instead of a spring, the rpm of the arm can be set, and a constant rate established. Gold castings require a rate of 380 rpm. Other settings for the Electromatic are as follows: range switch, gold; temperature controller, approximately 150° F (13.1° C) above the midpoint of the alloy melting range; soak timer, 45 seconds; centrifuge, 380 rpm; centrifuge acceleration: large melts (more than 1 ounce [28 gm]), 40 to 50 and small melts (less than 1 ounce [28 gm]), 0 to 10; powder-selector switch: small melts, low and large melts, medium; and pyrometer angle, *forward.*

25. Remove the casting from the cradle, and allow it to bench cool. Tap the mold with a wood or hard rubber mallet to break away the refractory material easily down to the paint-on layer. Do not break away the remaining layer of investment with blows from a hammer. Since damage to the casting is too great a possibility, remove the final material with sand or walnut shell blasting.

26. Remove the sprue leads with a large cutoff disk mounted in a high-speed lathe. Do not attempt to cut the sprue right down to the casting, but remove it at a safe distance. Continue further reduction with a wheel or three disks mounted on the same mandrel. Stop the sprue reduction at the level of the middle of the retentive beads. Then remove the upper half of the retentive beads (Fig. 16-38). Square off the peripheries

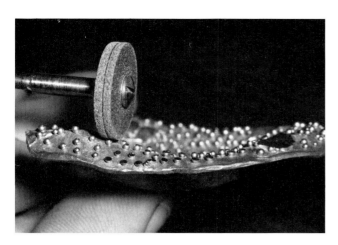

Fig. 16-38. Since upper halves of beads have no retentive value, they are removed with stone.

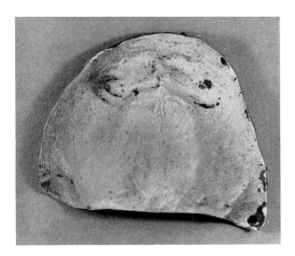

Fig. 16-39. Indicator spray identifies areas of initial contact.

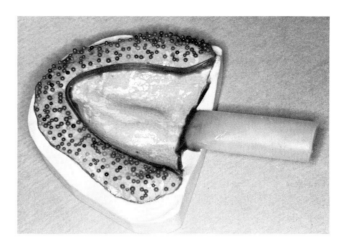

Fig. 16-40. Posterior sprue for Ticonium denture bases.

of the casting with a disk or wheel until they are at an angle of 90 degrees to the palatal surface, and no flash remains. The finished casting *must* fit the master cast without rocking. It is permissible to blunt sharp internal ridges with finishing stones before the first attempt at seating the casting. On the first indication of contact, use no more force. A powdered deodorant spray is an excellent disclosing material to demonstrate primary contact areas (Fig. 16-39). Continue to adjust the casting with finishing stones until the casting is fully seated. Finish those areas not to be covered by resin with fine stones, followed by rubber points and lathe polishing. At this time, a high shine on these areas offers little advantage. The casting will receive considerable handling before completion of the denture, and the final polishing will be done at that time.

Chrome alloy cast base
PROCEDURE

1. The techniques for chrome alloys differ from those for gold alloys, primarily in the investing and casting procedures. If Ticonium is the chrome alloy, the refractory material and investing and spruing techniques can be identical to those for the gold alloys. Only the casting temperature differs. With chrome alloys, a thinner cast base has enough rigidity, and often a 24-gauge stipple sheet is adequate. For high-heat chrome base alloys, such as Vitallium and Nobillium, it is essential to use a phosphate or silica-bound investment, different paint-on and investing techniques, and a much higher temperature burnout, 1800° to 2000° F (982° to 1093° C). Cast all chrome base alloys in automatic induction casting machines. Torch casting of alloys that melt above 2400° F (1315.5° C) is a demanding technique that requires considerable experience.

2. Master alternative techniques for spruing chrome alloy bases. These techniques are for specific alloys, and complete instructions are available from each manufacturer of an alloy. For example, it is possible to sprue and cast accurately Ticonium maxillary cast bases by using a single large sprue attached at the posterior border and parallel to the hard palate (Fig. 16-40). A mold for making these large sprues is available from the manufacturer.* On the other hand, it is best to sprue Vitallium from above by adding a fifth lead, or even a sixth, for exceptionally large casts (Fig. 16-41).

3. Sprue Ticonium mandibular cast bases through the base of the refractory cast like all Ticonium mandibular removable partial denture castings (Fig. 16-42). This type of spruing requires special preparation of the

---

*Ticonium, Albany, N.Y.

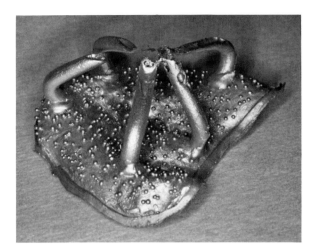

Fig. 16-41. Multiple sprue leads for Vitallium denture base castings. Insufficient metal was used in this casting.

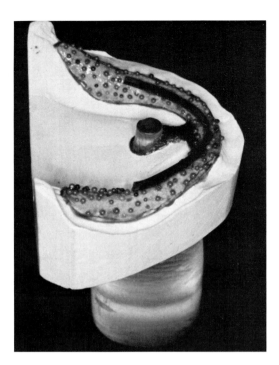

Fig. 16-42. Mandibular base sprued through refractory cast.

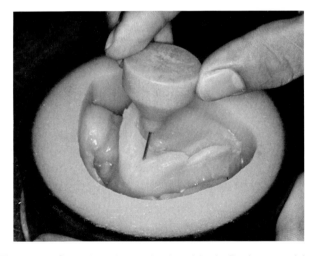

Fig. 16-43. Sprue hole former is placed in duplicating material to precisely locate sprue hole in relation to ridge.

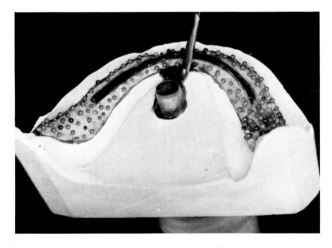

Fig. 16-44. Wax-up and sprue are connected by 8-gauge round wax lead that is flared where it is joined to wax-up.

mold during the pouring of the refractory cast (Fig. 16-43). During spruing, form a single wax lead from the sprue hole to the base of the casting at the lingual frenum area. Make this lead of 8-gauge round wax, and flare it at the junction point with additional wax to avoid forming sharp angles (Fig. 16-44). Wax the Ticonium sprue cone in place for the paint-on layer and final investing, and remove it before placing the ring in the furnace. Mark the mold to indicate the desired direction of metal flow during casting. Do this by aligning the single sprue lead toward the seam in the flask ring (Fig. 16-45).

Aluminum alloy cast base
PROCEDURE

1. Aluminum differs considerably from gold and chrome alloys. Being such a light metal, aluminum requires a modification of the spruing, burnout, and casting techniques to achieve repeatedly acceptable results. It is possible to cast Alcoa D214 aluminum alloy as thin

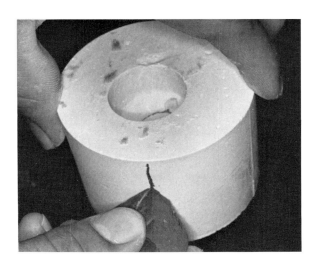

Fig. 16-45. Position of mold for casting mandibular base is marked on mold with jeweler's rouge.

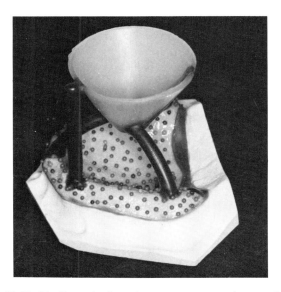

Fig. 16-46. Maxillary aluminum base wax-up properly sprued and ready for paint-on layer of investment.

as 26 gauge, but it is too fragile. A 22-gauge sheet is dependable for casting and rigidity in the maxillary cast base. Mandibular castings normally should have two thicknesses of 24-gauge aluminum alloy and additional reinforcement provided by hand waxing and an I-beam in the anterior area for special situations.

2. The remainder of the wax-up is identical to that for gold or chrome base castings. Sprue the cast bases with three 8-gauge round wax leads, one to the anterior midline and the other two to the second molar areas. Join these three leads over the center of the casting to the wax cone. Have the cone 1 inch (2.54 cm) above the ridge crests. Add another 8-gauge round wax lead to the crest of the ridge at the position of the right cuspid, and run it straight up to the side of the wax cone. Sprue the maxillary and mandibular bases in the same manner (Fig. 16-46).

3. The refractory material used for aluminum alloys is the same gypsum-bound investment used for gold or Ticonium. The powder-water ratios are identical; the refractory cast, paint-on layer, and final investing also are the same.

4. Place the mold in the burnout furnace at 1350° F (732° C). The burnout time is 1 hour at this temperature. At the end of this time, reduce the furnace control to 650° F (343.5° C). When the furnace reaches this temperature the mold is ready for casting.

5. Since D214 alloy melts at 1500° F (819° C) and solidifies at 650° F (343.5° C), keep the casting arm turning until the alloy has solidified. During this *vital* phase, an induction casting machine is essential for a casting technique to be dependable. The large induction machines used in routine chrome base alloy cast-

ings have belt-driven casting arms able to be set to deliver a specific rpm. Activated electrically, the arm runs until switched off. The following settings are applicable to the Howmedica Electromatic Casting Machine:* centrifugal accelerator, 30; melt, medium; multisoak, 0; and rpm of casting arm, 300. Other induction machines have similar settings, but it is essential to consult the manuals of each manufacturer for specific information. The lowest temperature setting for the Electromatic Casting Machine is 1600° F (871° C). The Ticomatic Machine† does not have a temperature-control reading in degrees F; it is necessary to cast the metal by visual reference.

6. With the mold in the furnace at 650° F (343.5° C), place the aluminum ingots in the induction crucible of the Electromatic Casting Machine. Use this crucible for *aluminum only.* Turn on the melt switch, and probe the ingots with a quartz rod as they melt. When it is possible to push the top ingots into the mass, turn off the melt switch, and allow the metal to cool until it turns gray.

7. Remove the mold from the furnace, and place it in the cradle. Turn on the melt switch, and watch the metal until it takes on the orange color of a harvest moon. At that point, throw the automatic cast switch, and complete the casting. Keep the arm rotating for a full 3 minutes.

8. Remove the cast and allow it to bench cool for 10 minutes before quenching it in running water. Re-

*Howmedica, Inc., Chicago, Ill.
†Ticonium, Albany, N.Y.

move the bulk of the refractory material with a wax spatula or a similar hand instrument under running water. Do the final cleansing of the refractory cast by blasting it carefully with walnut-shell abrasives. Do *not* use a sand blaster or a liquid hone under any conditions because either one will pit and dull the aluminum alloy.

9. Since the aluminum alloy is soft, exercise considerable care in fitting and finishing the casting. Cut off the sprue leads with a high-speed lathe. Do the rest of the finishing with a slow-speed lathe (Red Wing or a similar lathe), or with a laboratory handpiece, finishing stones, and burs. On a properly executed casting, the metal will have a clean, shiny surface and require no polishing.

Conversion of cast base to record base

1. The addition of autopolymerizing resin to the peripheries on the master cast is the most reliable method of converting the cast base to a record base. The resin need only engage the outer retention on the periphery of the casting (Fig. 16-47). This will facilitate removal of the resin during the boilout phase of packing and processing the completed denture. (See Chapter 4 for the technique used in adding this resin.)

2. Pack and process complete dentures with cast metal bases in the same manner as conventional complete dentures. There appears to be some advantage in a resin system that does not require trial packing because it is easy to displace the cast base when opening the flask. Myerson's Duraflow* or any fluid resin will

---

*Myerson Tooth Corp., Cambridge, Mass., or similar material.

serve this purpose. After boiling out the denture, remove the cast base, and burn off the peripheral resin by heating it with an alcohol torch until it softens, and remove it with cotton forceps, or a similar tool. Cleanse the metal carefully of all debris, and seat it back on the master cast immediately after painting it with tinfoil substitute. If the cast is warm and the separator is new, the casting will be fully seated and retained in place by the set separating medium.

3. If the casting fits the master cast accurately, no flash of cured resin should show on the tissue side. Any imperfection in this adaptation will result in a thin flash that is readily removable with a finishing bur or a stone run at slow speed (Fig. 16-48). An aluminum alloy base demands care in finishing to avoid cutting into the metal because it is much softer than a gold or chrome alloy base.

SUMMARY

Cast metal bases for complete dentures must be considered an adjunct to routine care for the dentulous patient. Fortunately, they are not complicated to construct, and when made of nonprecious alloys, they should not prove to be so costly as to eliminate them from consideration as an alternative to the conventional denture.

Cast metal bases are indicated as the treatment of choice under certain conditions: allergic reactions to dental resins, fracture-prone dentures, instances where additional weight is required in the mandibular denture, and similar special situations. For these reasons the master dental technician must be prepared to offer them as a treatment modality.

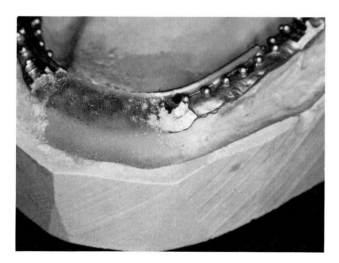

Fig. 16-47. Resin added to periphery of cast denture base.

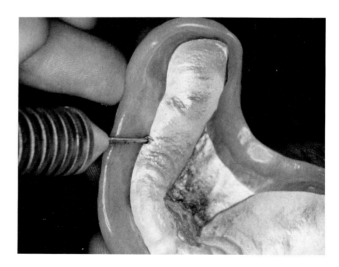

Fig. 16-48. Internal resin flash is removed with slow-speed round bur.

REFERENCES

Bell, D. H., Finnegan, F. J., and Ward, J. E.: Pros and cons of hard and resilient denture base materials, J. Am. Dent. Assoc. **94:**511, 1977.

DeFurio, A., and Gehl, D.: Clinical study of the retention of maxillary complete dentures with different base materials, J. Prosthet. Dent. **23:**374-380, 1970.

Faber, B. L.: Lower cast metal denture, J. Prosthet. Dent. **7:**51-54, 1957.

Grunewald, A. H.: Gold base lower dentures, J. Prosthet. Dent. **14:**432-441, 1964.

Hansen, C.: Phonetic considerations of chromium alloy palates for complete dentures, J. Prosthet. Dent. **34:**620-624, 1975.

Jha, M.: A study of tissue response to metallic (aluminum) denture base, J. Indian Dent. Assoc. **44:**122-126, 1972.

Landy, C.: Full dentures, St. Louis, 1958, The C. V. Mosby Co., p. 56.

Lang, B. R.: The use of gold in construction of mandibular denture bases, J. Prosthet. Dent. **32:**398-404, 1974.

Lundquist, D. O.: Aluminum alloy as a denture base material, J. Prosthet. Dent. **13:**102-110, 1963.

Moore, F. D.: Organic or metal bases for denture, J. Prosthet. Dent. **17:**227-231, 1967.

Regli, C. P., and Kydd, W. L.: Preliminary study of the lateral deformation of metal base dentures in relation to plastic base dentures, J. Prosthet. Dent. **3:**326-330, 1953.

Sizeland-Coe, J. W.: Superpurity aluminum in dental prosthesis, Br. Dent. J. **91:**263-268, 1951.

CHAPTER 17

MAXILLOFACIAL PROCEDURES

FREDRICK M. MATVIAS

obturator A prosthetic substitute that restores a defect by occupying a space created as the result of loss or absence of tissue, generally in the maxillary arch. An obturator should be light in weight, stable, nonirritating, comfortable, simple in design, readily removable, and capable of restoring both contour and physiologic function, such as speech and swallowing (Appleman, 1951). The total restoration of function, as well as anatomic contour, may be impossible.

immediate (surgical) obturator An obturator that is placed immediately after surgical removal of tissue, generally after tissue is taken from the hard or the soft palate.

In general terms, maxillofacial prosthetics is the art and science of anatomic, cosmetic, and/or functional reconstruction and rehabilitation of missing or defective body areas by means of prosthetic substitutes (Rahn and Boucher, 1970). The defects are acquired or congenital in nature.

All laboratory techniques should use proper and acceptable prosthodontic principles. Since success depends on the correct application of materials, it is essential to follow accurately all instructions of the manufacturer. A knowledge of basic head and neck anatomy is important. Training should include exposure to the many problems that challenge the imagination and lead to the development of many approaches that produce similar results. The purpose of this chapter is to present some of these approaches.

IMMEDIATE OBTURATORS
Requirements

Immediate obturators should restore the contours of the hard palate and, if possible, portions of the soft palate immediately after their loss, which has tremendous

psychologic benefit for the patient. Although it may be impossible to restore complete function at this time, food contamination and unfavorable scarring will be minimized.

Materials

Immediate obturators generally are of either chemically or thermally activated acrylic resin that is pink or clear. The use of metal is rarely feasible at this time. The impression can be of any material, but usually it is of irreversible hydrocolloid.

PROCEDURE

1. Pour the impression with artificial stone using the proper method designated by the clinician, and then trim it carefully to avoid loss of deliberate posterior and lateral extensions (Fig. 17-1).

2. Return the cast for outlining of the area to be removed surgically.

3. After completion of the outlining, duplicate the cast, cut off any teeth to be removed in a manner similar to that used in immediate denture fabrication, and prepare the cast to maintain or form a typical palatal contour.

4. Deepen the sulcus in the area of the defect, and round it to provide a smooth, round, slightly overextended peripheral roll, thereby avoiding trauma to the soft-tissue cut edges.

5. If the patient has any natural teeth left, block out unnecessary undercuts; however, if the patient is edentulous, block out severe undercuts minimally, and only if requested.

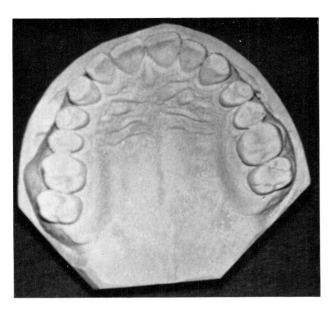

Fig. 17-1. Properly poured and trimmed cast used as pretreatment record.

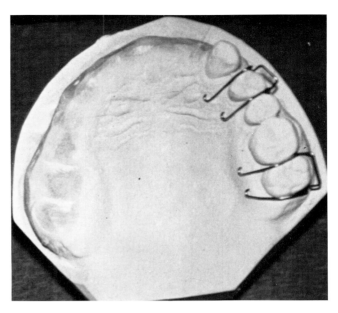

Fig. 17-2. Teeth are removed in area of surgery, cast is smoothed, clasps are adapted with tooth undercut blockout if needed, and peripheral vestibule is contoured to achieve smooth roll.

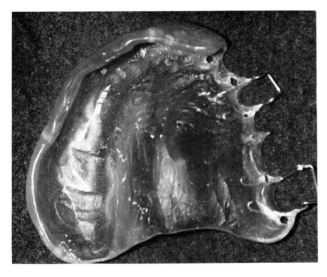

Fig. 17-3. Properly fabricated immediate obturator with smooth peripheral roll and interproximal holes for fixation.

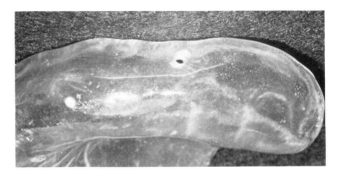

Fig. 17-4. Lateral hole placement for possible postoperative zygomatic wire fixation.

6. Duplicate this prepared cast, and adapt wire clasps at this time if desired (Fig. 17-2).

Chemically activated resin obturator
PROCEDURE

1. Make a chemically activated resin obturator in a manner quite similar to a record base. NOTE: soft resin from other methods of stabilization used in making record bases is not satisfactory for obturators initiated on properly prepared casts.

2. After completion of processing, chip away the working cast to avoid warping the resin.

3. Trim the acrylic resin, and polish it in a manner that does not result in loss of the desired form or contour.

4. Fit the obturator to the duplicate prepared cast to assure accuracy (Fig. 17-3).

5. If it is necessary to have retentive holes for wire or pin fixation, use a No. 6 round bur for the correct diameter. Place these holes approximately between the second premolar and first molar areas bilaterally and in the area lateral to the anterior frenum or in the middle of the palate where it is possible to use orthopedic screws (Fig. 17-4).

6. When natural teeth remain, use interproximal holes for wire fixation to the remaining teeth. The inclu-

sion of artificial teeth is rare; they must be anterior teeth only.

Thermally activated resin obturator
PROCEDURE

1. Allow the prepared cast to dry, and then adapt baseplate wax to a uniform thickness over the cast, usually approximately 2 mm.

2. Flame the wax smooth, and invest and separate the flask in the usual manner.

3. Mix and compression-mold the acrylic resin, and use a short or long cure.

4. Recover and polish the obturator.

5. Do not warp the obturator by trying to salvage the working cast.

6. Place the retentive holes as described previously.

INTERIM OBTURATORS

An interim obturator is a transitional obturator fabricated after the surgical removal of tissue but before complete healing. It may be the first obturator or a modification of the surgical obturator. Usually only anterior teeth are replaced, if any.

Requirements

Requirements of interim obturators include those of the immediate obturators. It is necessary to restore function, that is, speech and swallowing, to some extent at this point (Fig. 17-5).

Materials

Chemically activated or thermally activated acrylic resin or metal with either of the two resins are the materials of choice.

Chemically activated resin interim obturator
PROCEDURE

1. Pour the impression correctly with artificial stone. The impression can include the surgical obturator. Discard the obturator if it has served as a tray, but not if it is necessary to add an extension to the original obturator.

2. After obtaining the master cast, prepare it as when making a record base, but do not block out any undercuts.

3. If natural teeth are present, survey and block out the undercuts, adapt clasps, and use lug rests if not using a metal frame.

4. Apply resin by the method of choice.

5. Add teeth when a bite registration and an opposing cast are available.

6. Avoid warping the master cast during recovery.

7. If the defect is particularly large, make the bulb hollow to minimize the weight, as described later in this chapter.

8. Pumice and buff lightly the bulb portion of the obturator to preserve the surface detail.

9. Use tape to protect the teeth present from damage during polishing.

10. When adding a bulb to a previously fabricated

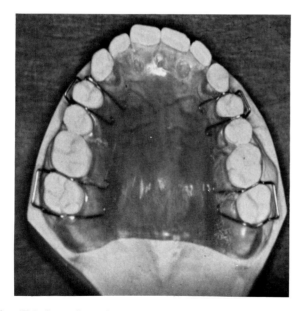

Fig. 17-5. Immediate obturator without loss of any teeth for hard palate resection only.

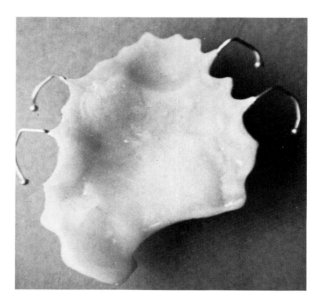

Fig. 17-6. Transitional obturator that provides some restoration of soft palate defect is made quickly from chemically activated resin.

surgical appliance, clean the old resin, free it of wax and other contaminants and, if needed, freshen it by roughening with a bur.

11. Provide mechanical retention if the previous appliance has been of thermally activated resin. The creation of dovetails is adequate, and a tapering or beveled finish is more acceptable than a butt-joint finish line (Fig. 17-6).

Thermally activated resin interim obturator
PROCEDURE

1. Dry the master cast, and trim it so that it will be conducive to flasking.

2. Reduce the severe undercuts by flowing wax into these areas.

3. Soften additional baseplate wax, and adapt it to form a base approximately 2 mm thick.

4. If the defect area is particularly large, use a hollow bulb to reduce the weight.

5. In setting artificial teeth on a cast mounted by means of an intermediate record base, arrange them for the best esthetic effect. Often a try-in aids in obtaining the best results.

6. Survey the natural teeth, and block them out with appropriate clasp adaptation.

7. Invest the waxed obturator with the clasps held in place by stone.

8. Process the case according to an established routine.

Metal framework with resin interim obturator
PROCEDURE

1. Survey and design a master cast to provide retentive areas that resist displacement forces. This retention consists of lingual retention with buccal reciprocation, alternate buccal and lingual retention, or possibly a well-designed latch or swing lock.

2. Follow the design accurately in blocking out, duplicating, and waxing.

3. Fill the defect with clay or wax, carve it to simulate normal palatal contour, and allow space for the resin to be retained by the metal (Figs. 17-7 and 17-8).

4. Place an internal finish line to allow the resin to flow in the area of the surgical cut on the hard palate, thereby facilitating relief in this area if needed.

5. The external finish line can simulate a median palatine fissure when appropriate, or it can be slightly lower in the defect, thereby resulting in a relatively smooth palatal contour (Fig. 17-9).

6. If the surgical excision involves the anterior labial frenum area, design the metal to allow ease of adjustment and to avoid metal impingement or overextension into the soft tissues.

7. Invest the cast as if it were a removable partial denture framework; cast, recover, and polish it (Fig. 17-10).

8. After try-in, return the framework for addition of resin to the defect using the original cast or a modified altered cast if needed to redefine the defect.

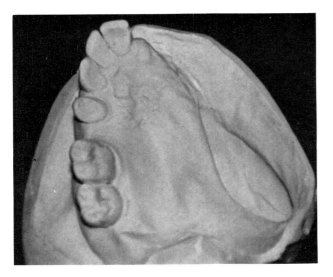

Fig. 17-7. Maxillary cast after pouring and proper trimming to preserve necessary structures, including defect area.

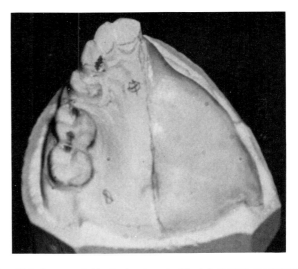

Fig. 17-8. Surveyed, blocked out cast with defect area recontoured prior to framework wax-up.

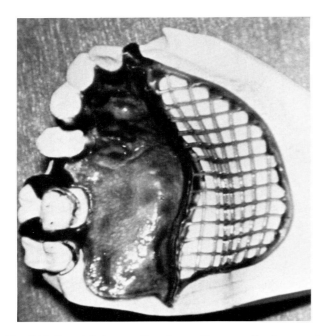

Fig. 17-9. Completed wax pattern for maxillary resection framework.

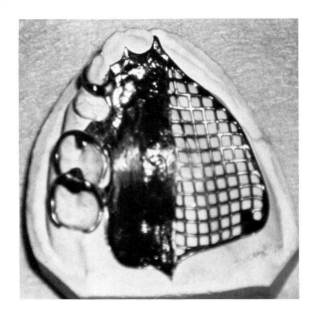

Fig. 17-10. Maxillary framework completed.

9. Add resin of either the chemically or thermally activated type (Fig. 17-11).

DEFINITIVE OBTURATORS

A definitive obturator is for patients whose healing after surgical management of a tumor or after trauma is complete. All healing changes have stabilized, and the patient has minimal discomfort. The patient can be totally edentulous, partially edentulous, or dentulous. The defect can involve the hard palate, the soft palate, or a combination of both.

Requirements

These obturators satisfy all requirements for surgical and interim obturators and provide a maximum seal during function to allow refinement of swallowing and speech. The addition of artificial teeth will restore esthetics and contours.

Materials

The prosthesis can be resin, metal, resin and metal, or resin and silicone. It is possible to attach the bulb of the defect portion of the obturator to the rest of the prosthesis or keep it separate.

Impressions can be of any type, but it is necessary to box them to make the stone of an adequate, uniform thickness throughout the defect area. Record bases or processed bases are used to obtain proper centric records. Set artificial teeth conventionally, according to the occlusal scheme selected by the clinician.

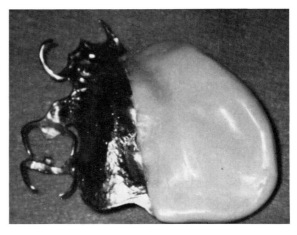

Fig. 17-11. Completed interim-type obturator with metal framework.

A hollow bulb reduces weight and increases the comfort of the patient. The bulb can be of silicone or acrylic resin, made in one piece or several pieces. The best approach is to simplify the design as much as possible.

Silicone bulb
PROCEDURE

1. Duplicate the master cast to form a working cast.
2. Outline the extension of the bulb. It usually follows the palatal contour (Fig. 17-12).
3. Adapt a uniformly thick wax shim.
4. Index or key the lip of the waxed bulb to pro-

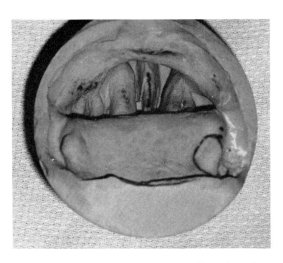

Fig. 17-12. Defect area prior to wax shim adaptation.

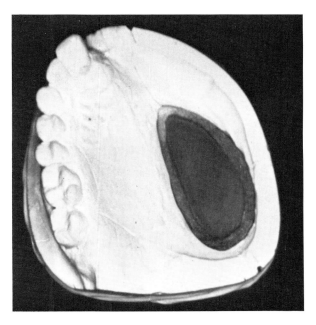

Fig. 17-13. Waxed obturator with blocked undercuts.

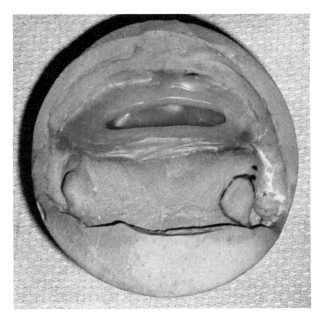

Fig. 17-14. Completed wax shim with lip and mechanical undercuts.

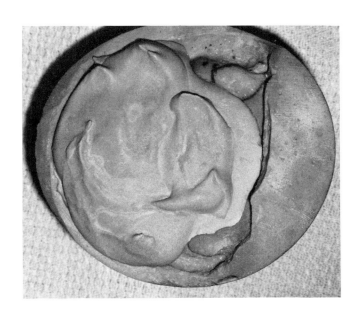

Fig. 17-15. Stone cap.

vide mechanical retention (Figs. 17-13 and 17-14).

5. Pour a stone cap into the wax bulb with stops after applying silicone release or foil (Fig. 17-15).

6. Boil out, separate, and dry the mold. It is critical to remove the foil at this time. Apply silicone release or liquid-soap separator to the cast and stone cap (Figs. 17-16 and 17-17).

7. Mix the Dow Corning MDX 4-4210* thoroughly (one part curing agent to each ten parts by weight of the base material) (Fig. 17-18). Entrapped air can be removed by exposure to a vacuum of 28 inches (71.1 cm) of mercury for 30 minutes. Allow the material to set for

---

*Dow Corning Corp., Midland, Mich.

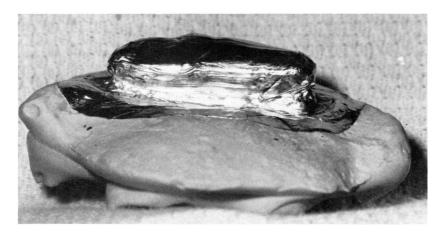

Fig. 17-16. Side view of cap showing mechanical retention bulb.

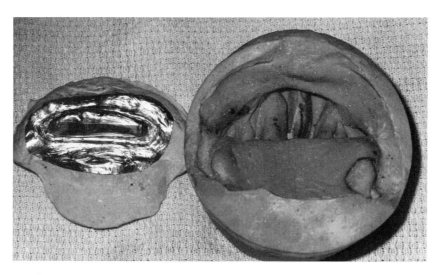

Fig. 17-17. Stone cap and defect areas devoid of wax. Foil is removed, and silicone release is applied.

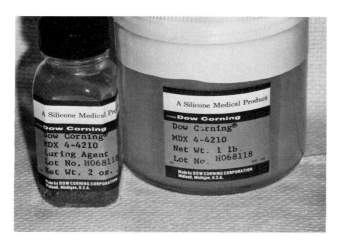

Fig. 17-18. Dow Corning MDX 4-4210 curing agent, *left,* and base silicone, *right.*

10 minutes to permit redissolving of trace gases into the polymer.

8. Pour the mixture into the defect area (Fig. 17-19). Place the stone core, and hold the halves to allow curing (Fig. 17-20). A cure of about 24 hours at 23° C is required. At 40° C, a 5-hour cure is noted. The material is cured in 5 minutes at 150° C, 15 minutes at 100° C, 30 minutes at 75° C, and 2 hours at 55° C.

9. Separate and save the key and cast (Fig. 17-21).

10. Duplicate the silicone bulb and cast with hydrocolloid to obtain a working stone cast (Fig. 17-22).

11. Remove the silicone bulb; it will be mechanically retained on the finished acrylic prosthesis (Fig. 17-23).

Hollow acrylic bulb
TWO-PIECE PROCEDURE

1. Use two flasks with interchangeable upper halves.
2. Invest the bulb in the bottom half (drag) of the

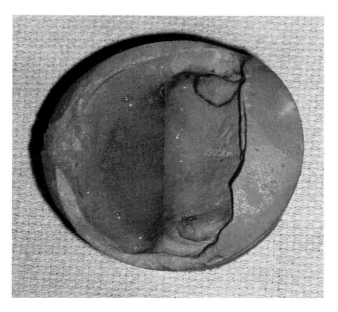

Fig. 17-19. Mixture poured into defect.

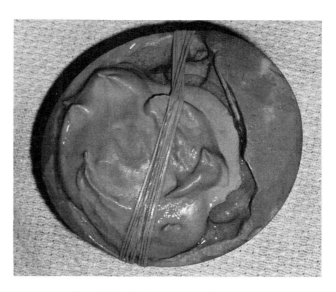

Fig. 17-20. Cap in place to allow curing.

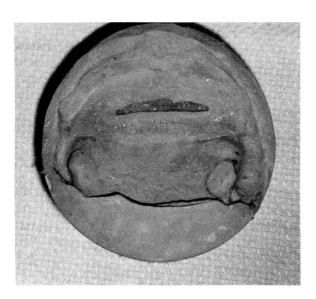

Fig. 17-21. Silicone bulb.

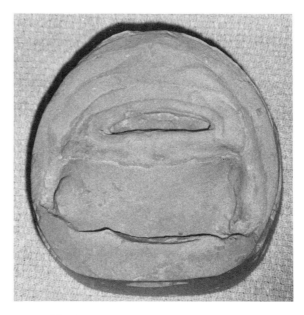

Fig. 17-22. Working (processing) cast.

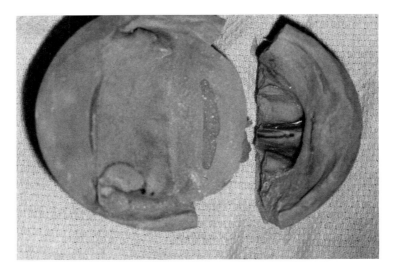

Fig. 17-23. Removal of silicone bulb.

flask, No. 1, and the remaining portion of the prosthesis in the top half (cope).

3. Separate, boil out, and allow it to dry.

4. Line the bulb form with a single thickness of baseplate wax after blocking out the undercuts. Avoid any mechanical lock, thereby preventing the stone core from drawing.

5. Press the top half of the first flask, and hold it in position relative to the bottom half of the flask to form a key or contact with the remaining prosthesis, or carve a key in the wax.

6. Remove the top half of flask No. 1.

7. Place the top of flask No. 2 with the bottom of flask No. 1, invest and complete the boilout procedure.

8. Compression-mold the bulb, and process it in a conventional manner.

9. Fill the bulb with stone up to the previously designed key, but do not interfere with the key. Place tinfoil substitute over the stone core and arcylic resin. Discard the upper half of flask No. 2.

10. Return the upper half of flask No. 1, pack and process.

11. Recover the obturator bulb, and trim the two pieces.

12. Use the previously established keys, and lute the two pieces together with chemically activated resin.

13. Verify the continuity of the seal by placing the bulb in a bowl of water, and check it for water seepage. If there is a leak, drain the bulb, and place a new seal.

14. Do not place the bulb in any pressurized container, such as a pressure pot, until after curing the seal to prevent perforation and seepage (Malson, 1955).

In a variation of the procedure, make the following changes:

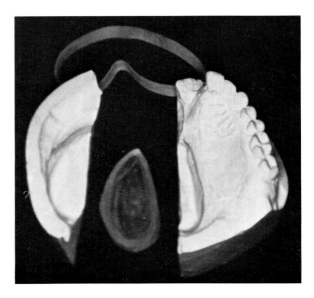

Fig. 17-24. Processed bulb with split master cast.

1. Pour the final impression with the appropriate artificial stone, and then duplicate the cast.

2. Wax the bulb portion, invest it, process it, and recover it from the investment.

3. Split the master cast by sawing through the stone partially, and then break the cast carefully. This procedure makes it possible to reorient the bulb to the remaining tissues (Figs. 17-24 and 17-25).

4. Hold the bulb in position with a rubber band, and then fill it with clay or blockout wax, but leave the key exposed.

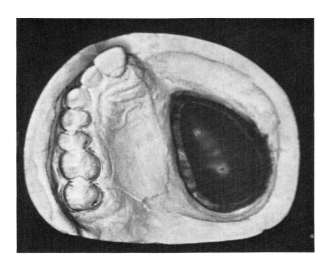

Fig. 17-25. Bulb repositioned in master cast.

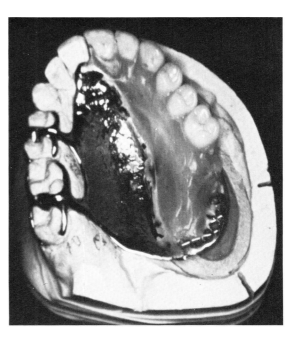

Fig. 17-26. Teeth can be set on master cast with previously processed bulb.

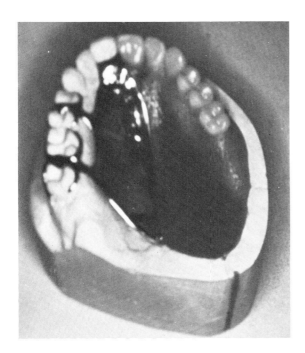

Fig. 17-27. Processed obturator.

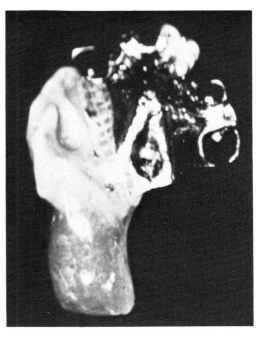

Fig. 17-28. Completed large acrylic resin hollow bulb obturator.

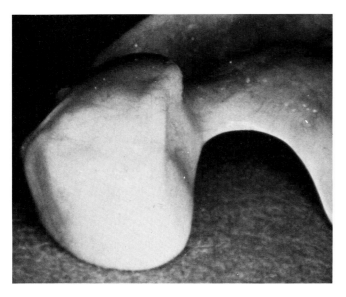

Fig. 17-29. Hollow bulb obturator was fabricated by grinding from superior surface and capping with chemically activated resin.

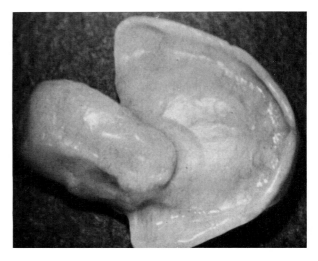

Fig. 17-30. Hollow bulb obturator from tissue side was fabricated in one-step procedure.

5. Duplicate the cast, and use it to fabricate record bases.

6. Set the teeth where indicated (Fig. 17-26).

7. Process the obturator against the keyed, duplicated cast (Fig. 17-27).

8. Process the halves separately, and lute them together with chemically activated resin (Fig. 17-28).

In another variation of the procedure, the following changes are made:

1. Make record bases on the master cast in the usual manner with the defect area blocked as needed.

2. Complete all final setups.

3. Wax, and prepare it for finishing.

4. Wax the bulb solid.

5. Complete the investing and processing procedures.

6. Recover, and hollow the bulb by grinding the resin with burs. Maintain approximately 2 mm for adjustments to the exterior surface of the bulb. Initiate the grinding from a noncritical area, and create a step or a key around the lip of the hole.

7. Use clay to fill the bulb, and form a proper contour for the external surface of the cap.

8. Adapt foil to the clay and the key, and make a chemically activated resin cover.

9. Seal the lid or cap to the bulb with chemically activated resin (Fig. 17-29) (Chalian and Drane, 1972).

ONE-PIECE PROCEDURE

1. Invest the waxed and festooned obturator in a denture flask in the usual manner.

2. Separate the obturator, clean it, and allow it to dry.

3. Block out severe undercuts, and adapt a wax shim

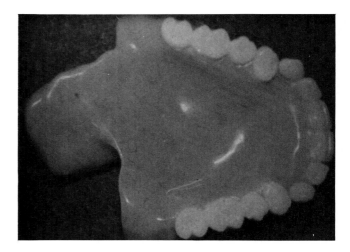

Fig. 17-31. Palatal view of obturator shown in Fig. 17-30.

in the defect areas in the upper and lower halves of the flask.

4. Press together the halves of the flasks to key the halves of the wax shim.

5. Cut a tripod system of stops to the stone in each half of the wax shim.

6. Mix chemically activated resin, and pour it in each half after placing tinfoil substitute in the stops.

7. Put the halves together, and rotate the cases during the curing cycle of the resin.

8. Separate the flask, thereby producing a hollow resin bulb core.

9. Mix the thermally activated resin, and compression-mold with the hollow core in place.

Table 17-1. Immediate obturators

Problem	Probable cause	Solution
Loss of lateral and posterior extension	Improper trimming and polishing	Refer to outlined cast after processing
Improper fit	Warpage during removal from working cast	Reduplicate prepared cast; review removal procedure
	Improper storage, polishing, processing	Review method for record base fabrication
Fracture of acrylic	Uneven placement of resin	Review method for record base fabrication

Table 17-2. Interim obturators

Problem	Probable cause	Solution
Loss of labial tooth form	Overpolishing	Cover teeth with tape prior to polishing; use rubber cup with pumice
Failure of new resin to bond to previous resin	Contamination	Use proper boilout with clear water
	Lack of mechanical retention	Provide mechanical retention, especially when adding chemical resin to thermally activated resin

10. Complete the processing, and recover the obturator (Figs. 17-30 and 17-31) (Chalian and Barnett, 1972).

PROBLEM AREAS FOR OBTURATORS

Some of the potential problems are noted in Tables 17-1 to 17-4. Most are caused by improper procedure sequence.

MANDIBULAR RESECTION DEVICES

A mandibular resection device is any appliance or device used to retrain the muscles so that the remaining mandibular segment functions in a more physiologic manner. It provides a degree of functional ability and restores esthetics by replacing teeth and improving facial profiles and contour in patients in whom a portion of the mandible has been removed to control cancer.

Mandibular resection devices are of two types, edentulous and dentulous. An edentulous patient uses a removable maxillary appliance with a guide ramp located in the palatal side of the maxillary teeth to guide the motion of the mandible to a relatively correct relationship. Maxillary and mandibular loops and guide bars of metal or acrylic resin attached to removable partial dentures also can provide a hingelike action.

Table 17-3. Definitive obturators

Problem	Probable cause	Solution
Loose record bases	Overrelief (blockout)	Minimize blockout
	Improper use of soft resin	Review technique
	Warpage during recovery	Review technique

Table 17-4. Hollow bulb obturators

Problem	Probable cause	Solution
Fluid leakage	Inadequate seal	Redesign keys; avoid rushing; do not use pressure pot; use adequate amount of chemically activated resin; use of adequate cementation (silicone bulb)
Perforation after adjustment	Improperly relating bulb to remainder of case	Wax patch with baseplate wax; form stone key; repair hole with chemically activated resin
	Inadequate thickness of bulb walls	Walls should be uniform in thickness

An edentulous patient requires a specifically designed occlusal scheme to provide function and possible correction of a mandibular deviation.

Requirements

The appliance should be comfortable and nonirritating, compatible with the oral environment, stable, and easy to clean. Restoration of function and esthetic contours may be secondary or obtainable only in part, but they are essential aspects to consider.

Materials

Mandibular resection devices can be of metal, acrylic, or acrylic and metal combined. Establishing a proper occlusal scheme is the major difficulty from the laboratory standpoint.

Edentulous mandibular resection device
PROCEDURE

1. Mount the maxillary and mandibular record bases, or key them in a position acceptable to the clinician.

2. Set the maxillary anterior teeth in a conventional manner.

3. Set the maxillary posterior teeth in an ideal position mediolaterally, but rotate them about their axes so that the lingual cusps are lower or more inferior to the buccal cusps on the nondefect side.

4. Place a piece of plastic or compound in the region of the second premolar to the second molar on the nondefect side, and lute it to the record base with hard wax or a compound such as modeling plastic. This ramp has its most medial margin (relative to the midline) inferior to the maxillary occlusal plane, and its lateral margin is continuous with the maxillary posterior rationale teeth.

5. Set the posterior teeth on the defect side conventionally if there are no opposing teeth or in a manner harmonious to the inclination of the ramp if there are teeth in the opposing arch.

6. Then position the mandibular anterior teeth with the midline corresponding to the maxillary anterior teeth and slightly anterior to the crest of the ridge.

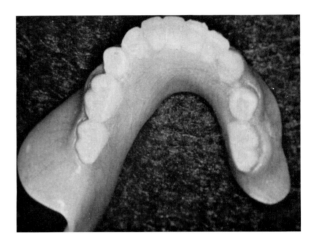

Fig. 17-32. Tentative placement of mandibular teeth.

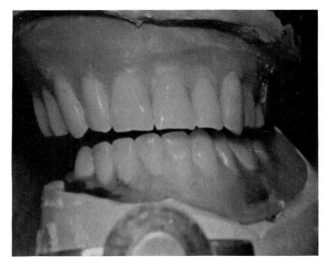

Fig. 17-33. Ridges are not parallel, and initial tooth placement should allow rotation of defect side superiorly.

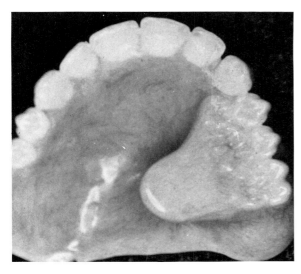

Fig. 17-34. Functionally generated occlusal surface of ramp.

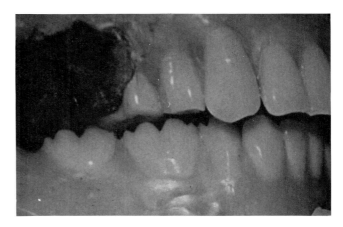

Fig. 17-35. Adjustment of ramp and posterior teeth with compound to allow mandibular movement.

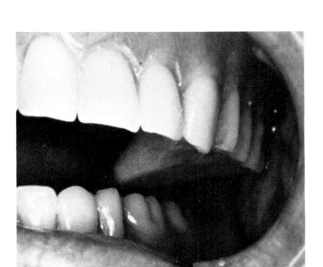

Fig. 17-36. Anteroposterior and mesiolateral positions are adjusted to provide proper initial contact and smooth sliding mechanism.

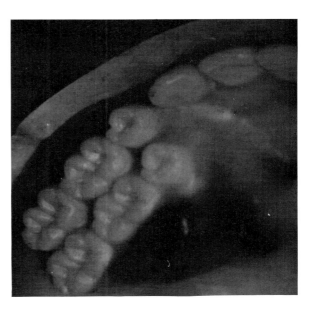

Fig. 17-37. Two rows of teeth have been set—one for appearance and one for function.

7. Position the mandibular posterior teeth mediolaterally with the cusp or the central groove over the crest of the ridge (Fig. 17-32).

8. Determine the height by the level of the maxillary teeth or halfway up the retromolar pad. The inclination of the posterior teeth harmonizes with the maxillary ramp. The interarch relationship may or may not appear conventional at this point. If the arches appear parallel anteroposteriorly, have the teeth on the defect side touch on complete closure. If the mandibular arch is not parallel, that is, usually open on the defect side, leave a space between the teeth (Fig. 17-33).

9. The patient returns for a try-in, and one of the following approaches is used: (a) wax of a functional nature is added to the ramp, and a functionally generated occlusion is established; (b) the ramp is adjusted in a mediolateral and an anteroposterior position and angle of inclination to guide the mandible smoothly to a more correct vertical and lateral relationship (Figs. 17-34 to 17-36). A new centric record is made at this time.

The resection appliance will be returned and remounted in the revised position. The teeth should be reset. If the mandibular position falls short of ideal, a

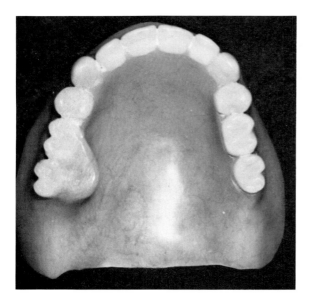

Fig. 17-38. Completed maxillary component of mandibular resection device.

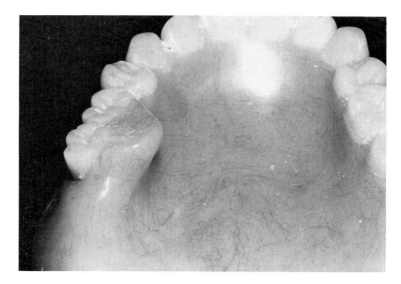

Fig. 17-39. Posterior view showing necessary angulation of ramp and teeth.

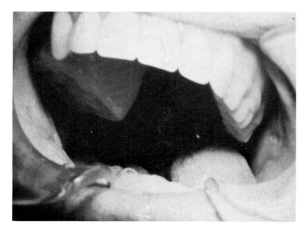

Fig. 17-40. Completed appliance inserted with patient's teeth in open position.

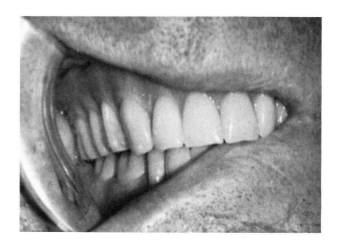

Fig. 17-41. Patient's teeth in closed position.

double row of teeth, one for esthetics and contour and one for function, may be set (Fig. 17-37). The functional row will establish an occlusal surface or table more satisfactory for mastication at the deviated position. The ramp should be smooth and continuous so that the mandibular teeth do not trip or catch during the closing cycle (Figs. 17-38 to 17-41).

10. Process in resin any functionally generated occlusal pattern developed on the ramp.

Dentulous mandibular resection device

Two approaches to use for patients with teeth are as follows: (1) make a maxillary removable appliance with a guide ramp or (2) make a mandibular guide prosthesis with or without the maxillary component. In both instances, the objective is to provide a method to correct the mandibular deviation on completion of closure.

PROCEDURE

1. Survey the cast to determine favorable undercuts.
2. Achieve appropriate blockout.

3. Duplicate the master cast.
4. Adapt clasps of choice, usually from orthodontic-type wire.
5. Add thermally or chemically activated resin to the palatal aspect of the maxillary cast.
6. Add a plastic ramp to the nondefect side with compound until the lingual cusps tips are flush with the surface of the ramp, so that the mandibular cusps will glide smoothly to the proper occlusal contact.
7. Return the appliance for ramp angulation and overall dimension determination.
8. Make a stone core.
9. Construct the ramp by adding more resin (Figs. 17-42 to 17-46).

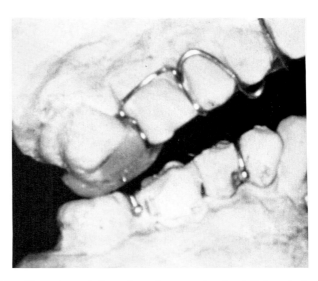

Fig. 17-43. Lateral view of acrylic ramp showing initial contact of mandibular teeth.

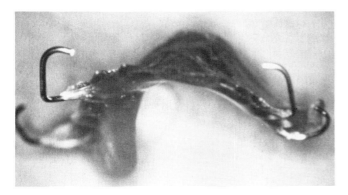

Fig. 17-42. Acrylic resin maxillary guide ramp.

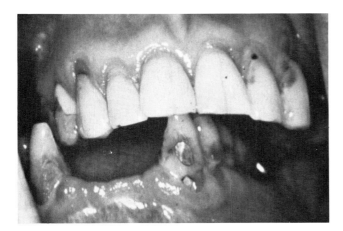

Fig. 17-44. Closure of patient's teeth without aid of guide ramp. Note deviation of mandible toward defect side.

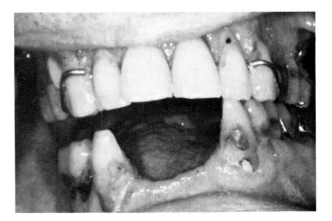

Fig. 17-45. Initial closure of patient's teeth with ramp placed on left. Note lack of closure on right.

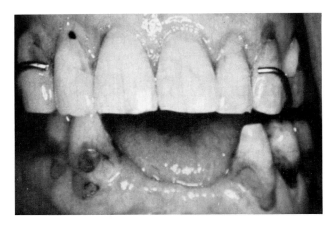

Fig. 17-46. Closure after adaptation to guide ramp.

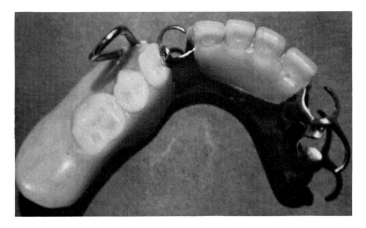

Fig. 17-47. Mandibular guide prosthesis with wire loop soldered to framework to guide mandible in hinge-like opening and closing.

Mandibular guide prosthesis
PROCEDURE

1. Design a removable partial denture framework that has lingual retention on the nondefect side and buccal retention on the defect side.
2. Cast a rigid metal loop. Design it for soldering to the buccal aspect of the mandibular framework.
3. Try in the partial denture, adjust it, and return it with a centric record for accurate mounting.
4. Position the loop so that it will contact the maxillary teeth during function. The vertical dimension is slightly less than the maximum opening to allow placement by the patient.
5. Solder the loop.
6. Set the artificial teeth (Fig. 17-47).

Following is an alternate approach to making a mandibular guide prosthesis:

1. Design a maxillary framework and cast with buccal retention on the nondefect side and lingual retention on the defect side.

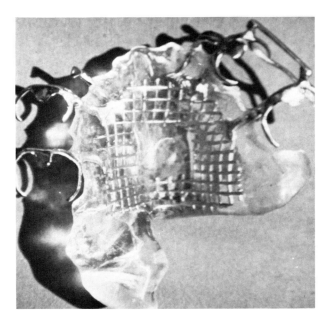

Fig. 17-48. Maxillary removable partial denture with guide bar soldered to clasps.

2. Solder a bar to the buccal clasps on the nondefect side of the buccal arms approximately the length of two teeth (Fig. 17-48).
3. Make the mandibular framework as described previously for mandibular guide prostheses, but have the loop glide over the maxillary bar rather than over the teeth.

Acrylic resin guide flange
PROCEDURE

1. Design the mandibular framework as described earlier.
2. Add an acrylic resin guide to the buccal aspect of the teeth on the nondefect side rather than on the metal loop (Ackerman, 1955).

PROBLEM AREAS FOR MANDIBULAR RESECTION DEVICES

The more common problem areas for mandibular resection devices are summarized in Table 17-5.

SPEECH AIDS

A speech aid is a prosthesis or an appliance used to help produce or improve the quality of speech in the patient for whom surgical correction of this problem is impossible, generally a patient with a congenital cleft palate. The aid can consist of an obturator-like bulb (Fig. 17-49) or a maxillary palatal midline extension known as a palatal lift (Fig. 17-50). A speech bulb compensates for a congenitally or surgically shortened soft palate. A lift raises the soft palate structures physically, and thereby promotes palatal function. It can serve as a

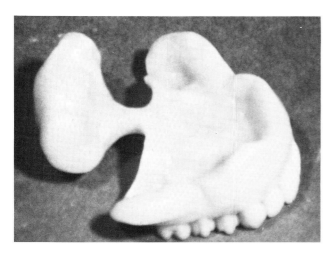

Fig. 17-49. Maxillary speech bulb for patients with edentulous cleft palates.

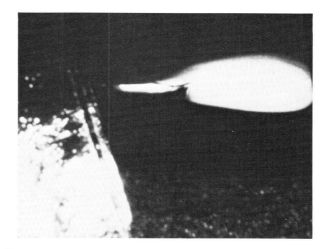

Fig. 17-50. Maxillary palatal lift with connector (i.e., partial denture framework).

Table 17-5. Mandibular resection device

Problem	Probable cause	Solution
Uneven ramp surface	Failure to fill spaces between rows of teeth	Give proper attention to waxing detail
Loss of posterior teeth during processing	Overmodification of esthetic row of teeth	Reduce excessive modification; cement teeth to stone prior to application of tinfoil substitute
Inadequate framework retention	Poor design	Review design principals
Inadequate loop height	Poor loop positioning	Obtain record of maximum opening

diagnostic tool to determine whether surgical repositioning of the palate would be beneficial.

Requirements

A speech aid should improve the quality of speech, and it must be easy to clean, lightweight, comfortable, and retained adequately.

Materials

Speech aids can be entirely acrylic or metal with an acrylic lift or bulb portion.

Acrylic resin palatal lift
PROCEDURE

1. Pour the impression with stone, and trim it, leaving the posterior extension intact.
2. Adapt wire clasps with distal undercuts. Adams clasps often are ideal.
3. Survey the teeth, and block them out.

4. Duplicate the cast.
5. Position the clasps.
6. Add acrylic resin, usually orthodontic type, with a midline posterior extension. Wherever indicated, initiate soft-palate relief.
7. As an alternative to chemically activated resin, process with thermally activated resin.
8. Polish the lift, and return it with wax or compound added to the tissue side when corrections are needed.
9. Use an altered cast technique or a stone core fabricated with the necessary corrections made of resin. Make the posterior extension thin, but not thin enough to fracture under stress.

Metal framework with reenforced acrylic posterior extension
PROCEDURE

1. Block out a master cast according to the designated design.

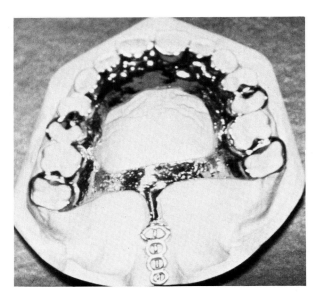

Fig. 17-51. Posterior extension is added to provide support for acrylic component of lift.

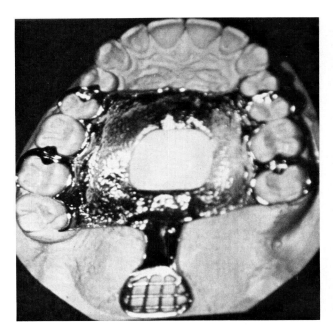

Fig. 17-52. Different design possibility for posterior extension.

2. Use distal retention generally.

3. Duplicate the cast in a refractory model, and complete the wax-up.

4. Make a metal extension posteriorly. Use a pattern for a mandibular lingual bar with retention placed in the posterior segment (Figs. 17-51 and 17-52).

5. Provide relief for the resin to encompass the distal extension retentive area.

6. Cast the distal extension separately, and solder it to the palatal major connector (Fig. 17-53).

7. Cast and finish the framework.

8. Return it for try-in.

9. Compound or wax is added for the appropriate amount of lift action.

10. Make an altered cast.

11. Section the tailpiece, and resolder it if necessary.

12. Add wax, and process the lift as if it were a partial denture.

Edentulous and dentulous maxillary speech bulb

A maxillary speech bulb uses many of the techniques associated with a maxillary obturator. Speech bulbs obturate, and thereby improve velopharyngeal valving and facilitate speech. They can be dentulous or edentulous.

PROCEDURE

1. Make and design the major connector or denture like any other complete denture or removable partial denture.

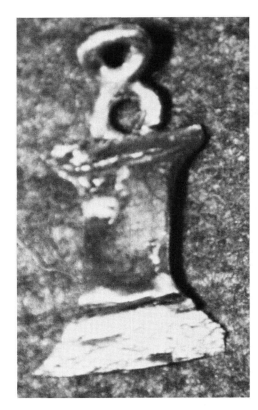

Fig. 17-53. Casting of separate tailpiece to be soldered later.

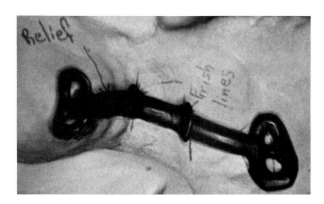

Fig. 17-54. Posterior connector or tailpiece should dip into defect. Finish lines and relief should be provided.

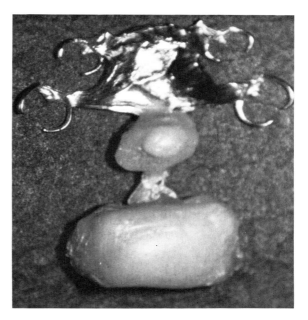

Fig. 17-55. Maxillary speech aid with distal retention, maxillary obturator for palatal defect, and hollow posterior speech bulb.

Table 17-6. Speech aids

Problem	Probable cause	Solution
Inadequate prostheses retention	Displacement forces not considered in design	Distal undercuts required
Soft-palate irritation	Inadequate tailpiece relief	Make sure resin or metal does not contact soft palate at rest
Fracture of posterior extension	Inadequate metal or resin thickness	Reenforce resin with metal or use mandibular lingual bar pattern for adequate thickness
Inferior placement of tailpiece	Failure to use altared cast	Cut and resolder metal; modify acrylic resin
Exposure of retention mesh	Failure to place retention mesh superiorly	Section and resolder tailpiece using new stone cast

2. Place the clasp retention to the distal side.

3. Make the connector between the bulb and base of the denture of metal or acrylic.

4. Indicate relief in the range of 30-gauge wax to prevent the connector from impinging on the soft palate. Incorporate a finish line in the design of the connector for both the bulb and the palatal portions.

5. Have the most posterior extension of the bulb connector dip into the defect, so that the acrylic bulb can begin at the soft palate and extend superiorly. Considerable inferior extension will result in impingement of the tongue during function (Fig. 17-54).

6. Return the frame with the bulb connector for an impression. Make an altered cast, that is, trim the posterior of the cast, seat the denture or metal base, and pour stone around the bulb impression.

7. Make the bulb hollow as for hollow maxillary bulb obturators (Fig. 17-55).

8. Process the denture and bulb portions simultaneously.

PROBLEM AREAS

Five problem areas in reference to speech aids are discussed in Table 17-6.

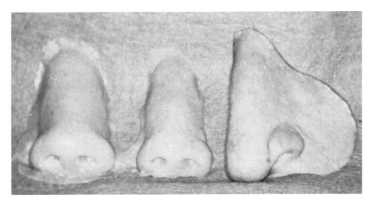

Fig. 17-56. Three nasal prostheses: polyurethane, *left;* silicone, *center;* and polyvinyl chloride, *right.*

FACIAL PROSTHESES

A facial prosthesis is an extraoral removable prosthesis used to restore a missing or defective area of the body. The restoration is usually anatomic, functional, and esthetic. It may be a nasal, orbital, ocular, or auricular (ear) prosthesis, or some other type.

Requirements

Facial prostheses should be comfortable, nontoxic, nonallergenic, reasonably esthetic, translucent, easy to clean, capable of accepting makeup and intrinsic and extrinsic coloration, flexible and natural to touch, easy to make, inexpensive, retentive of fine detail for a long time, mechanically retentive or receptive to adhesive with a fine line marginal contact, and easy to duplicate. Maximum esthetics depend on matching shades and reproducing details by sculpting (Fonseca, 1966).

Materials

The most popularly used materials are vinyl chloride polymers and copolymers; types of acrylic material, such as methyl methacrylate; and heat-vulcanizing and room temperature–vulcanizing silicones and polyurethanes. Each has favorable and unfavorable characteristics. The material of choice depends on the needs of the particular patient and the preference of the clinician. All materials require a mold, generally of metal, stone, or epoxy resins. The working characteristics of each brand of material may be different. Exact and close adherence to the manufacturer's suggestions is essential (Fig. 17-56).

Laboratory facility requirements

The following items are necessary for making facial prostheses: a heating unit for reversible hydrocolloid; large investment rings, usually of galvanized sheet metal; gray, or other high-heat, investment material;

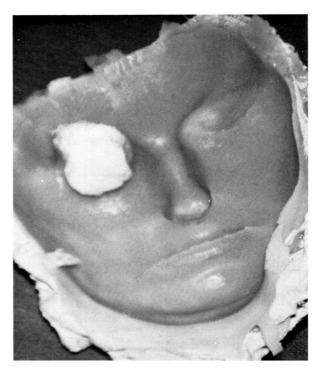

Fig. 17-57. Reversible hydrocolloid impression of face and defect area of patient.

a large dry-heat oven; and other routine laboratory supplies.

Metal mold fabrication
PROCEDURE

1. Pour an impression of the defect, and separate it (Figs. 17-57 to 17-59).
2. Prepare a sculptured, extremely detailed clay or wax prosthesis pattern on the cast. Return it for trial placement by the clinician. Then seal the margins of

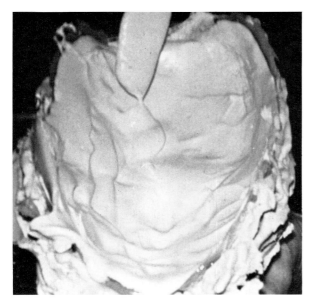

Fig. 17-58. Pouring the impression with artificial stone.

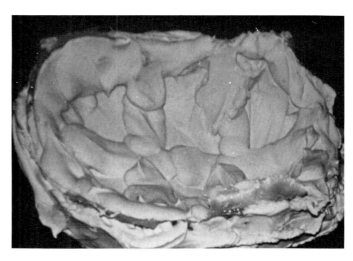

Fig. 17-59. Properly poured and reinforced impression of facial defect.

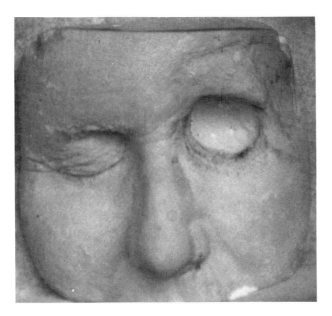

Fig. 17-60. Master cast separated and prepared for fabrication of clay pattern.

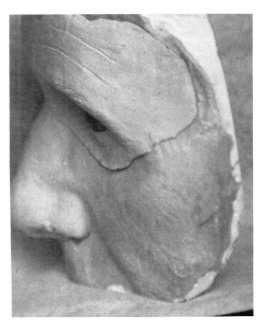

Fig. 17-61. Clay pattern positioned on cast.

the pattern to the cast, and place keys in the peripheral area (Figs. 17-60 and 17-61).

3. Box the pattern and keyed areas with wax, and pour alginate into the boxed area. Mix it with approximately twice as much water as required. Pour a stone or plaster core over the alginate for support after placing wire mechanical retention mesh.

4. Remove the impression, box it, and pour it with gray investment.

5. Block out the defect area not to be used for retention by drilling a hole through the back of the master cast and vibrating stone through the hole with the pattern in place. The effect is to minimize the thickness of the facial prosthesis. Thin the pattern as much as

possible prior to this blockout procedure. Avoid creating mechanical undercuts that prevent the molds from seating. In making an orbital prosthesis allow an undercut under the ocular area, and key the ocular prosthesis, that is, the artificial eye, to relate it to the master cast prior to making an impression for the tissue side of the mold and to form a retentive lip in the final prosthesis to maintain the eye.

6. Remove the clay pattern, replace the ocular prosthesis, and make a boxed impression in the manner described previously for the other half of the mold.

7. Box the impression, make another impression of the first impression, and back the latter with stone.

8. Discard the first impression. Use gentle compressed air to facilitate separation of the two impressions.

9. Box the second impression, and pour it with gray investment.

10. Check both patterns for detail. It is possible to make minor surface detail changes to the tissue side at this time.

11. Wax the patterns with approximately 3 mm of baseplate wax. Add a strip of beading wax to the periphery of the pattern to aid in later retention of the clasp.

12. Attach sprues to the patterns at the lowest points on the periphery of the mold.

13. Place several vents at the highest points on the pattern.

14. Invest the waxed patterns with more investment by using large rings screwed or clamped together at one point to permit removal prior to elimination of the wax. The main sprue is 1 inch (2.54 cm) from the wall of the ring.

15. Invest the pattern, and boil it out with hot water or burn it out in an oven.

16. Dry the molds thoroughly to prevent fracture from vaporization of retained moisture during the introduction of molten metal. Place them in a dry-heat oven at 70° C.

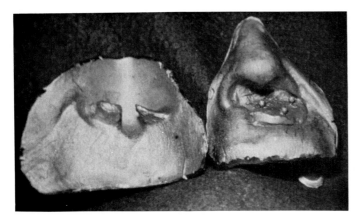

Fig. 17-62. Metal molds prior to fitting and adjustment by spot grinding.

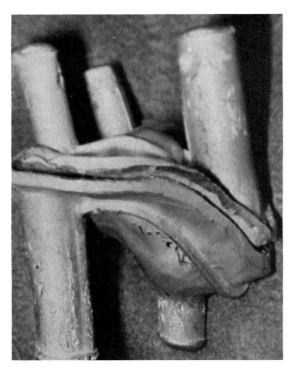

Fig. 17-63. Metal molds fitted properly with sprues and vents trimmed to form stand for molds.

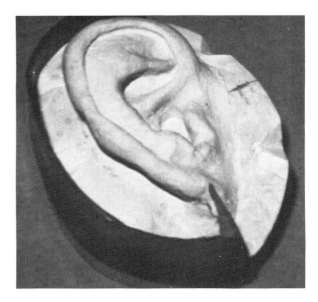

Fig. 17-64. Auricular pattern with boxed posterior segment and keyed master cast.

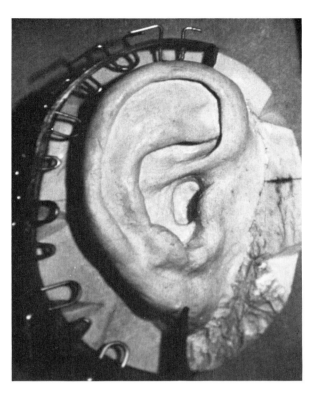

Fig. 17-65. Mechanical retention is provided with wire loops.

17. Melt linotype metal used in newspaper printing with a torch, at approximately 500° F (260° C).

18. Pour the metal into a vent, and use a torch to keep the metal molten. Hold the flame over the main sprue, and pass it down the sprue adjacent to the periphery of the mold.

19. Cool it for approximately 30 minutes, then immerse it in water, and brush it clean.

20. Cut the vents and sprues evenly to form a stand for the molds.

21. Fit the molds if necessary by spot grinding with articulating paper (Figs. 17-62 and 17-63).

Fabrication of three-piece auricular metal mold
PROCEDURE

1. For patterns with multiple undercuts, make the upper or external portion of the mold in two pieces.

2. Key the master cast.

3. Mark the crest of the helix around the periphery to beneath the lobe.

4. Box the area posterior to the helix and behind the ear (Figs. 17-64 and 17-65).

5. Make a separate boxing keyed to the posterior segment (Fig. 17-66).

6. Mix the alginate, pour it behind the helix, and key it (Fig. 17-67).

7. Place the remaining boxing, and pour the alginate (Fig. 17-68).

8. Back both boxings with stone (Fig. 17-69).

9. Remove the posterior crescent, box it, and pour it with gray investment (Fig. 17-70).

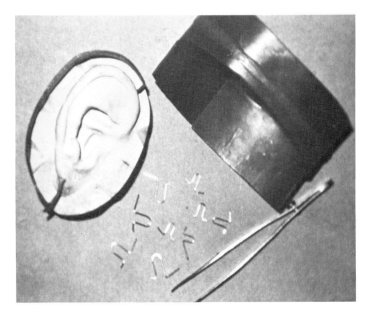

Fig. 17-66. Segmented boxing pattern is fabricated.

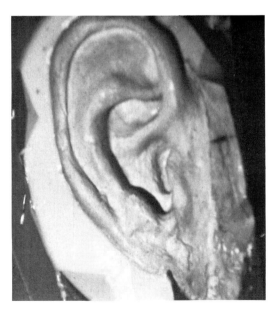

Fig. 17-67. Poured alginate with keys.

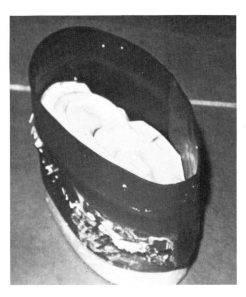

Fig. 17-68. Remaining boxing is placed for upper half of mold.

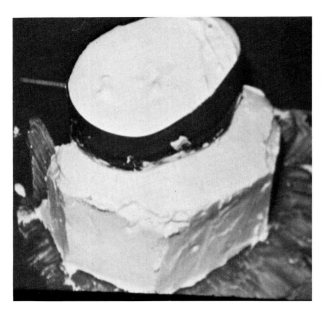

Fig. 17-69. Both segments are backed with stone to reinforce alginate.

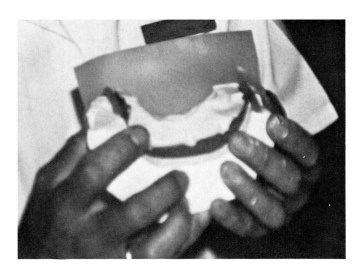

Fig. 17-70. Posterior crescent is removed and boxed.

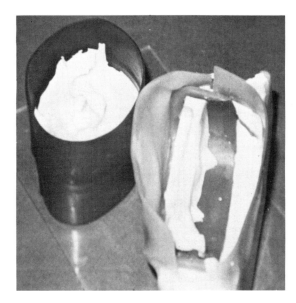

Fig. 17-71. Both segments of upper half of mold are ready for pouring with gray investment.

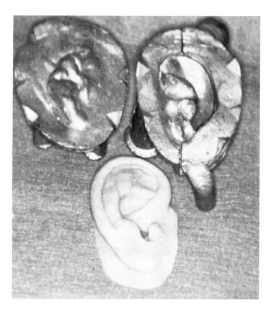

Fig. 17-72. Completed three-piece metal molds.

10. Box the remaining external segment, and pour it (Fig. 17-71).

11. Make the defect side in the same manner as the two-piece mold.

12. Make metal molds (Fig. 17-72).

Direct wax method of metal mold fabrication

An alternative to the metal mold procedure is a direct wax method of metal mold fabrication advocated by Vini et al. (1975).

PROCEDURE

1. Carefully paint molten baseplate wax directly onto the clay pattern and the master cast.

2. After proper cooling, remove the wax mold, and place the sculptured pattern into the wax form.

3. Fabricate the tissue side of the mold by painting wax to the wax mold with the pattern in place.

4. Then invest and cast both.

Stone mold fabrication
PROCEDURE

1. Position the clay pattern with the margins sealed and detail maintained.

2. Key the stone, and box it.

3. Apply a separator, such as soapy water or silicone, to the stone.

4. Vibrate additional stone into the mold.

5. Separate the molds.

6. If the mold is small enough, invest it in a denture flask, and then remove it from the flask for storage.

PROBLEM AREAS

Metal mold fabrication is technique critical, if maximum mold accuracy is desired. Refer to Table 17-7 for some common problems and solutions.

RADIATION APPLIANCE

Radiation therapy is a useful treatment modality for the control and management of cancer. Damage to normal tissues is a frequent side effect because many lesions are accessible only by radiating through normal structures. It is possible sometimes to minimize damage to the oral and paraoral structures by using various appliances that permit direct access to a lesion with a radiation source or a beam directed from a radiation source.

Requirements

The design must allow the therapist to achieve treatment plan goals for the particular tumor. It should be easy to place, relatively comfortable, able to be repositioned accurately with repeated application, light, easy to clean, rigid and stable, nonirritating, and durable with use. It is essential to consider the requirements of each patient prior to establishing a design (Delclos, 1965).

Materials

The material of choice depends on the requirements of the patient, but generally, chemically or thermally activated methyl methacrylate is preferable. Time is an important consideration when selecting the material. If there is need for a radiation source, a mockup of the source, such as rods or seeds, and a method of locating the source precisely within the appliance in relation to the lesion are essential. Regular laboratory processing and flasking equipment are important.

Fabrication of locator

A locator (cone locator and radiation source locator) is usually of acrylic resin and helps to position the cone or the tip of the machine with repeated accuracy in relation to the lesion.

PROCEDURE FOR CONE LOCATOR

1. Use maxillary and mandibular casts with a wax occlusal registration, preferably in the open position.

2. Mount the case on a simple hinge. The degree of opening depends on the vertical height of the cone.

3. Adapt baseplate wax over the ridge, but short of the peripheral roll. Overextension is undesirable.

4. If the lesion extends close to or over the ridge, keep the wax short of these areas.

5. Form a cylinder of wax slightly larger than the

Table 17-7. Metal mold

Problem	Probable cause	Solution
Discarding incorrect impression	Improper labeling of impression	Label impressions; review concept of mold fabrication
Lack of detail	Improper handling of soft investment	Modify investment to improve surface detail
Mold porosity	Improper sprue location	Place vents at highest pattern points and sprues at lowest
Investment fracture during pouring	Moisture retention	Use dry-heat oven for adequate time period
Improper fit of molds	Distortion of alginate	Fabricate proper stone core; pour gray investment as soon as possible to minimize alginate distortion

cone tip from the machine. Foil can be applied to the cone to prevent the wax from sticking. Place a wax stop in the tumor or tissue end of the cylinder so that the cone will not slip through.

6. Process the bases and cone positioner by investing them in a stone flask and compression-molding them. Trim the flash, and finish polishing it.

7. Return the case so that the clinician can position the cone support to the bases in relation to the position of the lesion.

8. Attach the three pieces with chemically activated resin, and polish them (Fig. 17-73). As an alternative, fabricate the cone locator from chemically activated resin.

Radiation source carrier

A radiation source carrier is an appliance that positions and holds a source of radiation in close proximity to a lesion for a specified period of time. An impression of the tumor and surrounding area must be obtained. Invest it in the appropriate manner. The design of the carrier depends on the anatomic location and size of the tumor.

Fabrication of nasopharyngeal carrier

It is impossible to reach the nasopharynx with externally applied radiation without producing side effects on normal tissues. If indicated, a nasopharyngeal carrier will minimize these effects.

PROCEDURE

1. Invest in stone an impression of the nasopharynx as advocated by Rudd et al. (1966) (Fig. 17-74).

2. Make an acrylic model that includes the area of the tumor (Fig. 17-75).

3. Determine the position of the source to find out whether to split the final appliance for ease and proper placement.

4. Reinvest the acrylic model, and split-pack it with clear resin if indicated, process it, recover it, and polish it.

5. Achieve final positioning of the source by using mockups (Fig. 17-76).

6. Fit the halves together easily, and secure them with a screw.

7. Place umbilical tape through the external nares for retention (Fig. 17-77).

Fabrication of palatal carrier

Some lesions of the palate may require radiation therapy. A removable appliance, such as a palatal carrier, may be used to place a source near these lesions.

PROCEDURE

1. Make casts of the lesion and corresponding arches.

2. Mount these casts on a hinge articulator in an open position to keep the normal tissues as far away from the radiation as possible.

3. Make a split resin base over the site of the lesion, and hold it together with screws or by some other method.

4. Place the source between the two bases, and hold it securely (Fig. 17-78).

5. Key or attach the base of the opposite arch to the other rim by acrylic bite blocks (Fig. 17-79).

6. Insert the case, and have the patient close against the rim for comfort.

PROBLEM AREAS

Proper radiation source positioning is very important for successful treatment. Table 17-8 reviews two problems.

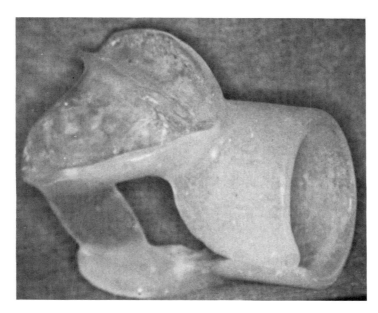

Fig. 17-73. Comfortable, completed one-piece intraoral cone locator that satisfies needs of particular treatment modality.

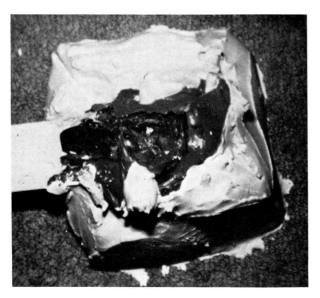

Fig. 17-74. Impression of nasopharynx made by using tongue blade with wire-reinforced compound and rubber base wash. This impression is invested in stone.

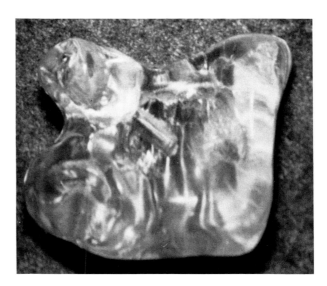

Fig. 17-75. Acrylic model formed from processed clear resin to determine position of radiation source.

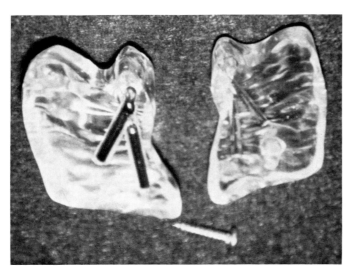

Fig. 17-76. Sources positioned appropriately in relation to tumor can be maintained securely by means of screw.

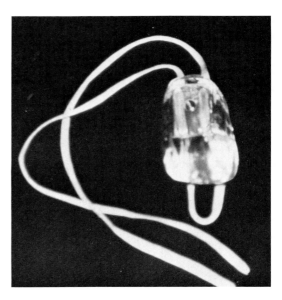

Fig. 17-77. Completed nasopharyngeal carrier with umbilical tape used for retention with nasopharynx.

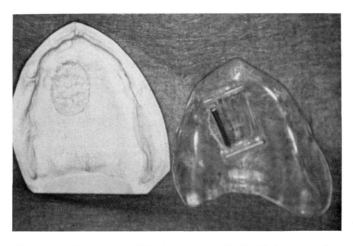

Fig. 17-78. Master cast with lesion circumscribed might be treated by placing radiation source in acrylic stent as shown.

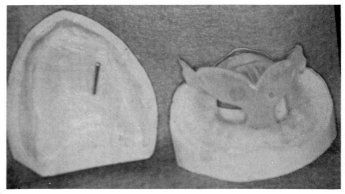

Fig. 17-79. Two-piece acrylic maxillary stents are secured together, and appliance is inserted with mandible of patient positioned by acrylic struts.

Table 17-8. Radiation appliance

Problem	Probable cause	Solution
Inaccurate cone position	Improper fit of cylinder	Use minimal relief and cone stop
	Inaccurate base-to-cone relationship	Reattach with chemically activated resin
Inaccurate source position	Improper split-packing or mold-sectioning	Refer to dosimetry chart to verify source placement

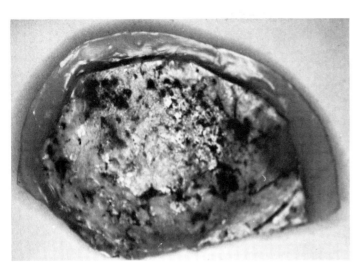

Fig. 17-80. Bone fragment with wax added to periphery ready to be duplicated in resin by investing it in stone, recovering the bone segment, and compression-molding an acrylic resin implant.

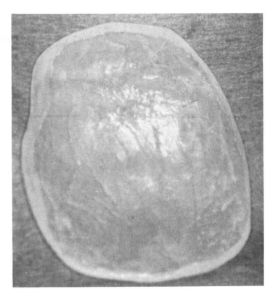

Fig. 17-81. Finished cranial implant prior to perforation and placement of retention holes. Note slight flange-like overextension around periphery to allow adjustments.

CRANIAL IMPLANTS

A cranial implant is positioned surgically and secured into a skull defect. The two principal indications for cranial implants are for defects secondary to trauma or infection. The implants are made of metal, such as stainless steel and acrylic resin.

Requirements

A cranial implant should restore contour and esthetics, as well as protect the brain from injury resulting from trauma. It should be stable, nontoxic, and nonirritating. Methyl methacrylate implants are the most common.

Materials

Clear, thermally activated acrylic resin is the material of choice. However, it is possible to use chemically activated acrylic resin for a rapid result.

PROCEDURE FOR IMMEDIATE CRANIAL IMPLANT

1. Duplicate a bone fragment in resin after adding wax to the periphery to compensate for loss of tissue, resulting from cutting the segment (Fig. 17-80).

2. This implant is reinserted on completion of a lengthy procedure.

PROCEDURE FOR DELAYED IMPLANT

1. Make an impression of the skull defect area, and pour it with stone. Have the hair short or shave that part of the head.

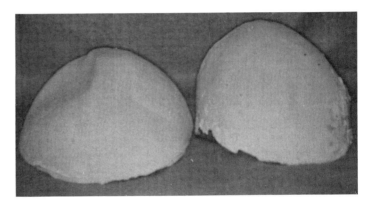

Fig. 17-82. Cast of patient's head before surgery, *left,* and after surgery, *right.*

2. Outline the defect with an indelible pencil and transfer this outline to the cast.

3. Relieve the cast to compensate for the approximate thickness of the soft tissues and skull plate. Generally, the skull is thicker toward the superior midline. The clinician who palpated the defect should perform the relief.

4. Make a wax or clay sculpting to restore the anatomic contour. Add a bevel or flange to the implant to compensate for any deficiencies in marginal extension.

5. Invest the implant, and process it. Frequently, a large flask may be essential.

6. After finishing the implant, perforate it only on request of the clinician (Fig. 17-81).

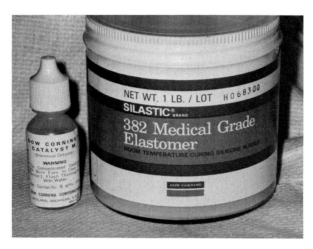

Fig. 17-83. Dow Corning Silastic 382 Medical Grade Elastomer.

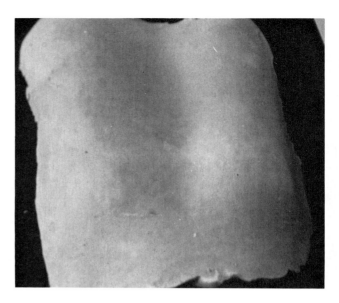

Fig. 17-84. Cast of chest made from reversible hydrocolloid impression to be used to fabricate Silastic implant to correct pectus excavatum defect.

7. Retentive holes are placed at the time of surgery, and the implant is fixed with stainless steel or tantalum wire, braided wire, or silk suture (Fig. 17-82) (Sabin, 1975).

SILASTIC IMPLANT

A Silastic implant is a surgically implanted prosthesis that restores or modifies body contour.

Requirements

Silastic implants should be nontoxic, tissue compatible, stable, durable, easy to fabricate, and able to be adapted accurately.

Materials

The material used for a Silastic implant is Dow Corning Silastic 382 medical-grade silicone (Fig. 17-83). It is room-temperature vulcanizing and easy to use.

PROCEDURE

1. Make an impression of the patient, and fabricate a cast (Fig. 17-84).
2. Make a clay pattern directly on the cast.
3. Return the pattern for trial positioning. Make any changes required directly on the patient.
4. Return the pattern, and make a stone mold by pouring stone over the pattern and on the periphery of the cast.
5. Mix the Silastic, and press it into place using the mold.

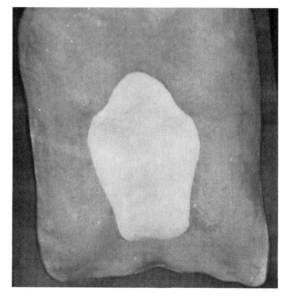

Fig. 17-85. Finished silicone implant prior to placement of retention holes and surgical implantation.

6. Perforate the inferior border with holes approximately the size of a No. 8 round bur for retention after trimming and smoothing (Fig. 17-85).

PROBLEM AREAS

This type of silicone is relatively simple to use when the proper technique is followed. (See Table 17-9.)

Table 17-9. Silastic implants

Problem	Probable cause	Solution
Silicone with embedded stone particles	Sticking during curing	Lubricate stone properly with soapy water
Porosity	Delayed packing	Pack and mold prosthesis before initiation of final set
Thick prosthesis	Improper compression	Do not place too much material in mold; use adequate compression force; do not delay too much during processing, thus allowing initial set

SUMMARY

This chapter presents some approaches useful to the technician who is involved in maxillofacial prosthetics. It is not all-inclusive; its purpose is primarily to stimulate imaginative and innovative ideas. Additional references listed contain information about other techniques.

REFERENCES

Ackerman, A. J.: The prosthetic management of oral and facial defects following cancer surgery, J. Prosthet. Dent. 5:413-432, 1955.

Ampil, J., Ellinger, C., and Rahn, A.: A temporary prosthesis for an edentulous patient following maxillary resection, J. Prosthet. Dent. 17:88-91, 1967.

Appleman, R. M.: The prosthetic repair of defects of the maxilla resulting from surgery, J. Prosthet. Dent. 1:424-437, 1951.

Aramany, M., Drane, J., and Anderson, K.: Radiation protection prostheses for edentulous patients, J. Prosthet. Dent. 22:292-296, 1972.

Boucher, L. J.: Prosthetic restoration of a maxilla and associated structures, J. Prosthet. Dent. 16:154-168, 1966.

Brown, K. E.: Fabrication of orbital prosthesis, J. Prosthet. Dent. 22:592-597, 1968.

Brown, K. E.: Fabrication of ear prosthesis, J. Prosthet. Dent. 21:670-676, 1969.

Brown, K. E.: Fabrication of an alloplastic cranioimplant, J. Prosthet. Dent. 24:213-224, 1970.

Canario, C.: A two-section metal mold for an ear prosthesis, J. Prosthet. Dent. 31:343-348, 1974.

Carl, W.: Preoperative and immediate postoperative obturators, J. Prosthet. Dent. 36:298-305, 1976.

Chalian, J., and Barnet, M.: A new technique for constructing a one-piece hollow obturator after partial maxillectomy, J. Prosthet. Dent. 28:448-453, 1972.

Chalian, J., Drane, J., and Standish, M.: Maxillofacial prosthetics, multidiscipline practice, Baltimore, 1972, The Williams & Wilkins Co.

Delclos, L.: Radiotherapy for head and neck cancer, J. Prosthet. Dent. 15:157-167, 1965.

Fine, L., Robinson, J. E., Sharett, T., et al.: Fabrication of a prosthesis for guiding and fixing radioactive sources in treatment of cancer of the floor of the mouth, J. Prosthet. Dent. 30:349-353, 1973.

Firtell, D. N.: Maxillofacial prosthesis: reproducible fabrication, J. Prosthet. Dent. 22:247-252, 1969.

Fonseca, E.: The importance of form, characterization and retention in facial prosthesis, J. Prosthet. Dent. 16:338-343, 1966.

Hahn, G. W.: A comfortable silicone bulb obturator with or without dentures, J. Prosthet. Dent. 28:313-317, 1972.

Hawkinson, R. T.: Development of skin surface texture in maxillofacial prosthetics, J. Prosthet. Dent. 15:929-937, 1965.

Malson, T. S.: Complete denture for the congenital cleft palate patient, J. Prosthet. Dent. 5:567-578, 1955.

Matalon, V.: A simplified method for making a hollow obturator, J. Prosthet. Dent. 36:580-582, 1976.

Moore, D., and Mitchell, D.: Rehabilitating dentulous hemimandibulectomy patients, J. Prosthet. Dent. 35:202-206, 1976.

Ohyama, T., Gold, H., and Pruzansky, S.: Maxillary obturator with silicone lined hollow extension, J. Prosthet. Dent. 34:336-341, 1975.

Ouellette, J. R.: Spray coloring of silicone elastomer maxillofacial prostheses, J. Prosthet. Dent. 22:271-275, 1969.

Parel, S., and Drane, J.: Reproducing the vertical lateral defect space in obturator construction, J. Prosthet. Dent. 35:314-318, 1976.

Rahn, A., and Boucher, L.: Maxillofacial prosthetics, principles and concepts, Philadelphia, 1970, The W. B. Saunders Co.

Robinson, J. E., and Rubright, W. C.: Use of a guide plane for maintaining the residual fragment in partial or hemimandibulectomy, J. Prosthet. Dent. 14:992-999, 1964.

Rudd, K. D., Green, A. E., Jr., Morrow, R. M., et al.: Radium source appliance for treatment of nasopharyngeal cancer, J. Am. Dent. Assoc. 72:862-866, 1966.

Sabin, H.: Cranial implant problems, J. Prosthet. Dent. 34:659-665, 1975.

Santiago, A.: Fabrication of an intraoral radiotherapy prosthesis, J. Prosthet. Dent. 33:212-215, 1975.

Schaaf, N.: Oral reconstruction for edentulous patients after partial mandibulectomies, J. Prosthet. Dent. 36:292-297, 1976.

Schuppe, N.: Cranioplasty prostheses for replacement of cranial bone, J. Prosthet. Dent. 19:594-597, 1965.

Swoope, C.: Prosthetic management of resected edentulous mandibles, J. Prosthet. Dent. 21:197-202, 1969.

Tanaka, Y., Gold, H., and Pruzansky, S.: A simplified technique for fabricating a lightweight obturator, J. Prosthet. Dent. 38:638-642, 1977.

Vini, R., Krill, R., and Aramany, M.: Direct wax method for fabrication of metallic facial mold, J. Prosthet. Dent. 33:85-88, 1975.

Wood, R., and Carl, W.: Hollow silicone obturators for patients after total maxillectomy, J. Prosthet. Dent. 38:643-651, 1977.

CHAPTER 18

LABORATORY PROCEDURES FOR IMMEDIATE OVERDENTURES

ROBERT M. MORROW

overdenture A complete denture constructed for placement over some remaining natural teeth and the residual ridges.
immediate overdenture An overdenture constructed for placement immediately after removal of the last hopeless teeth.

Interest in overdenture treatment procedures has continued to gain momentum and has resulted in more practitioners providing overdentures for their patients than ever before. As a result, it is appropriate that the laboratory procedures for immediate overdentures be described in detail. Construction of impression trays, baseplates, occlusion rims, and the procedures for setting the teeth and constructing the immediate overdenture will be presented in this chapter. Most overdenture procedures are similar to those for conventional immediate dentures; however, certain procedures are unique to overdentures and will be described in detail.

CONSTRUCTING IMPRESSION TRAYS

Making impressions for immediate overdentures is similar to that for conventional immediate dentures. One method found to be effective involves first making an impression of the posterior edentulous arch in a suitable impression material, using an autopolymerizing resin tray. The posterior impression is examined and replaced in the mouth, and an overall alginate impression made over the posterior edentulous impression and the anterior teeth (Fig. 18-1).

498

PROCEDURE

1. Stone casts of the involved arches are required. Examine the casts for undercuts, which should be blocked out with baseplate wax prior to constructing the impression tray. This will permit the completed impression tray to be removed from the cast without breaking either the cast or the tray.

2. Draw the impression tray outline on the cast. The tray extension should be approximately 2 mm short of the vestibular reflection on the cast (Fig. 18-2). The tray should extend posteriorly to the vibrating line.

3. Soften a sheet of baseplate wax, and adapt it to the cast (Fig. 18-3). Take care to avoid entrapment of air beneath the baseplate wax, and then trim the baseplate wax to the tray outline (Fig. 18-4).

4. Flow baseplate wax onto the lingual surfaces of the anterior teeth and into any spaces that exist between the teeth (Fig. 18-5). This provides relief and prevents the tray resin from extending into the spaces. If resin extends into the spaces, the teeth may be broken when the impression tray is removed from the cast.

5. Paint tinfoil substitute on the stone cast and over the baseplate wax (Fig. 18-6). Painting tinfoil substitute on the baseplate wax facilitates removal of the baseplate wax later when the dentist makes the final impression.

6. Proportion the autopolymerizing tray resin according to the manufacturer's recommendations, and mix it, and roll it to form a thin resin wafer (Fig. 18-7).

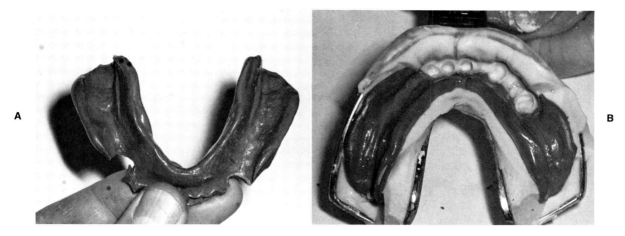

Fig. 18-1. A, Impression is made of posterior edentulous arch. **B,** Alginate impression is made over first impression and remaining natural teeth.

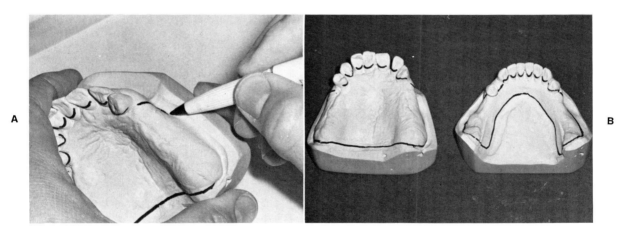

Fig. 18-2. A, Draw outline of impression tray on cast. Tray extensions should be approximately 2 mm short of borders of overdenture. **B,** Tray outlines have been drawn on maxillary and mandibular casts.

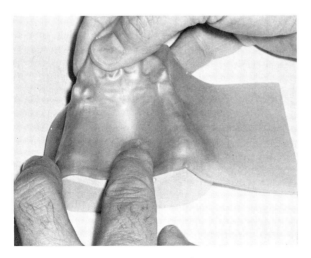

Fig. 18-3. Adapt sheet of baseplate wax to casts.

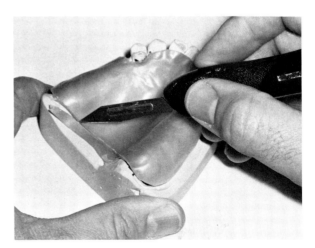

Fig. 18-4. Trim to tray outline.

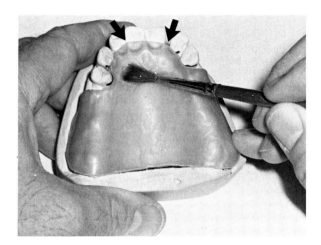

Fig. 18-5. Wax can extend onto and between anterior teeth (arrows) to provide relief.

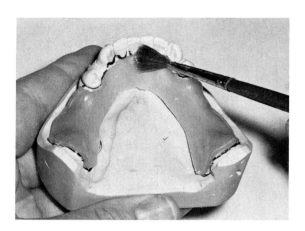

Fig. 18-6. Paint baseplate wax and cast with tinfoil substitute.

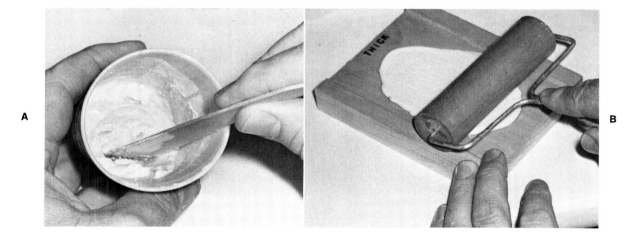

Fig. 18-7. A, Mix autopolymerizing tray resin. **B,** Roll resin into wafer before adapting it to cast.

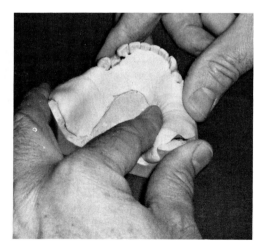

Fig. 18-8. Adapt resin to cast.

7. Place the resin wafer on the cast, and adapt it with finger pressure (Fig. 18-8). Take care when finger adapting to not overthin the tray material over the convex portions of the cast (Fig. 18-9). Continue to adapt the tray resin to the cast until the resin sets.

8. After the tray resin has set, remove the tray from the cast, and trim and smooth the impression tray with arbor bands and burs (Fig. 18-10). The tray borders should be finished even with the baseplate wax relief (Fig. 18-11). Be sure that no sharp or rough edges exist on the tray borders. The completed impression tray is stored on the cast until needed (Fig. 18-12).

PROBLEM AREAS

Principal problems associated with making an impression tray are failure to maintain uniform thickness of

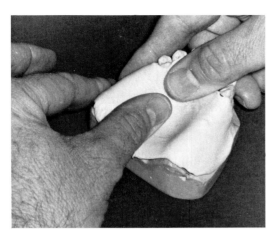

Fig. 18-9. Do not overthin at convex portions of ridges.

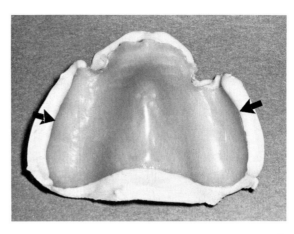

Fig. 18-10. Trim tray borders to level of relief wax (arrows). Space for compound will be made later by removing strip of wax from borders.

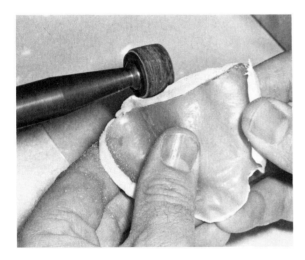

Fig. 18-11. Trim impression trays with lathe-mounted arbor band.

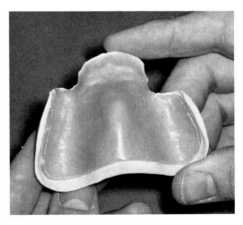

Fig. 18-12. Store trays on casts until needed at next appointment. Strip of wax 3 mm wide has been removed to create space for border molding compound.

Table 18-1. Impression trays

Problem	Probable cause	Solution
Impression tray too thick	Tray resin not rolled into thin wafer before adapting to cast	Roll resin into thin wafer before adapting to cast
Impression tray too thin over residual ridges	Tray resin thinned over convex portion of cast during adaptation	Use care when adapting resin to prevent overthinning
Teeth broken off cast during removal of impression tray	Tray resin contacted teeth on cast or projected into spaces between teeth	Block out spaces between teeth to provide relief

the impression tray during finger adaptation; making the impression tray too thick or too thin; allowing the tray resin to extend into spaces between the teeth, resulting in a broken cast; and failure to finish and smooth the borders of the completed tray (Table 18-1). Rolling the tray resin into a wafer with a roller will help achieve an impression tray of uniform thickness. Careful finger adaptation will minimize the tendency to overthin the tray over convex portions of the cast. Spaces between the teeth should be blocked out with wax prior to adapting the resin to prevent extrusion of the tray resin between the teeth. The tray border should be smoothed and finished with arbor bands and acrylic burs to remove sharp ridges or fins that might prove uncomfortable for the patient.

CONSTRUCTING BASEPLATES

Baseplates for immediate overdentures can be constructed of shellac baseplate material or autopolymerizing resin. Shellac baseplates can be constructed more quickly than resin baseplates; however, the dimensional stability of shellac baseplates is not as good as resin baseplates. The procedure for adapting shellac baseplates for immediate overdentures is similar to that for constructing baseplates for conventional immediate dentures (Chapter 4).

Shellac baseplates
PROCEDURE

1. Soak the cast in clear slurry water for a few minutes prior to adapting the shellac baseplate (Fig. 18-13).

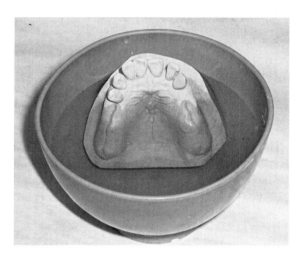

Fig. 18-13. Cast is soaked in slurry water for few minutes before adapting shellac baseplate.

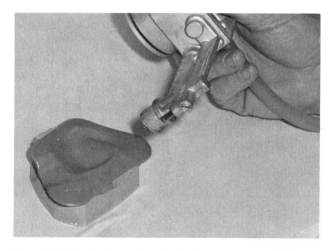

Fig. 18-14. Shellac baseplate is wilted onto wet cast with flame.

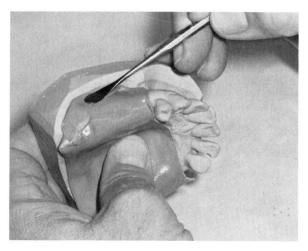

Fig. 18-15. Edges are folded over and blended into shellac material.

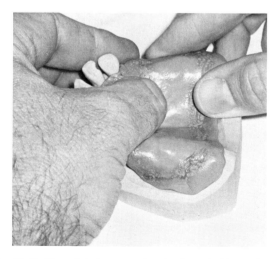

Fig. 18-16. Baseplate is warmed and adapted with wet fingers.

2. Wilt the shellac baseplate onto the wet cast with a flame (Fig. 18-14).

3. Fold the edges of the shellac material over, and blend them into the shellac baseplate material (Fig. 18-15).

4. Warm the baseplate, and continue to adapt it to the cast with wet fingers (Fig. 18-16). Remove the baseplate, and soften areas of the baseplate that extend into undercuts so that the baseplate can be removed and replaced on the cast without damaging the cast.

5. Add a wax occlusion rim, and seal it to the baseplate (Fig. 18-17). The maxillary and mandibular baseplates are complete (Fig. 18-18).

6. The mandibular shellac baseplate can be strengthened by embedding a heavy paper-clip wire into the lingual material from premolar to premolar area. The wire improves the rigidity of the baseplate.

PROBLEM AREAS

The principal problem associated with making shellac baseplates is related to maintaining dimensional stability of the baseplate once it is constructed. Shellac baseplate materials also tend to stick to dry casts during dry-heat adaptation (Table 18-2). It is important to wet the cast prior to adapting the baseplate material onto the cast with heat. Careful adaptation of the shellac baseplate to the wet cast will result in an excellent fit of the completed baseplate and minimize the tendency of the material to stick to the cast.

Resin baseplates

Autopolymerizing resin baseplates are preferred for immediate overdentures. Resin baseplates can be made thin over residual ridges, yet are reasonably rigid and dimensionally stable. This is an important consideration, since the baseplates will be used for setting teeth. In the procedure described, two types of autopolymerizing resins are used in constructing baseplates. A soft-setting autopolymerizing resin* is first placed in undercut areas, and conventional hard-setting autopolymerizing resin† is sprinkled over the soft resin to provide rigidity (Fig. 18-19). Soft resin in the undercuts becomes an integral part of the baseplate and will permit the baseplate to be

---

*Coe-soft, Coe Laboratories, Inc., Chicago, Ill.
†Caulk repair resin, The L. D. Caulk Co., Milford, Del.

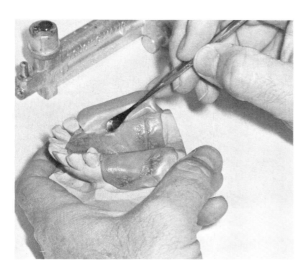

Fig. 18-17. Wax occlusion rims are added and sealed to baseplate.

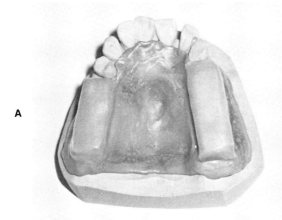

A

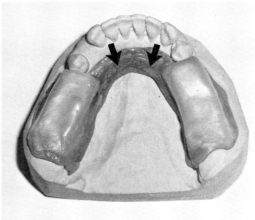

B

Fig. 18-18. A, Completed maxillary shellac baseplate. **B,** Completed mandibular shellac baseplate. This baseplate can be strengthened by embedding heavy paper-clip wire in lingual area from premolar area to premolar area (arrows).

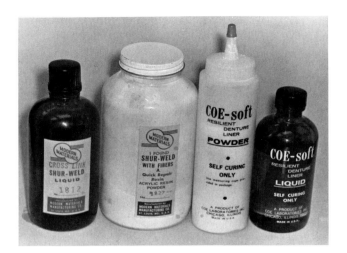

Fig. 18-19. Two types of autopolymerizing resin are used for baseplate construction. Soft-setting resin (Coe-soft) is placed in undercuts, and conventional hard-setting resin (Caulk Repair Resin) forms baseplate.

Table 18-2. Shellac baseplates

Problem	Probable cause	Solution
Shellac baseplate sticks to cast	Cast not wet before baseplate adapted	Soak cast in clear slurry water before adapting shellac baseplate
Shellac baseplate does not fit cast	Baseplate distorted during removal from cast	Replace baseplate on cast; readapt it
	Baseplate not properly adapted to cast	Adapt baseplate to cast with finger pressure

removed from moderate cast undercuts without damage to the cast or baseplate. However, severe undercuts require block-out with baseplate wax prior to the addition of soft resin.

PROCEDURE

1. Check the master cast carefully for undercuts. Undercuts are usually found on the buccal slope of residual ridges just posterior to canine abutments, in the tuberosity region of the maxillary cast, and in the posterior lingual region of mandibular casts (Fig. 18-20).

2. Undercuts should be blocked out with baseplate wax if they are severe. Soft-setting autopolymerizing resin is placed in minor to moderate undercuts; however, the soft resin will not compensate for severe undercuts.

3. Block out spaces existing between the teeth on the cast to prevent autopolymerizing resin from flowing between these teeth during baseplate construction (Fig. 18-21). As in the case of the impression tray, if resin extends into these spaces, the teeth may be fractured from the cast during baseplate separation.

4. Soak the master cast for a few minutes in clear slurry water (Fig. 18-22).

5. Paint tinfoil substitute onto the cast and over the previously placed blockout (Fig. 18-23).

6. Mix soft-setting resin monomer and polymer in a dappen dish, and apply the mixed resin to the previously identified undercuts (Fig. 18-24).

7. Completely fill the undercuts with the soft resin.

8. Warm the tip of a chip blower in a flame, and blow a gentle stream of warm air onto the soft-resin surface (Fig. 18-25). The warm airstream will produce a surface hardening effect, which will prevent the soft resin from flowing out of the undercut and into the cast border area where it is of no benefit (Fig. 18-26). In this manner, fill all undercuts with soft resin.

9. Using the sift-on technique, apply conventional hard-setting autopolymerizing resin polymer to the cast, and wet it with monomer (Fig. 18-27).

10. Add liquid and powder alternately to build up the desired baseplate thickness.

11. Tilt the cast to one side when sprinklng on the polymer to minimize pooling of the resin in the palate

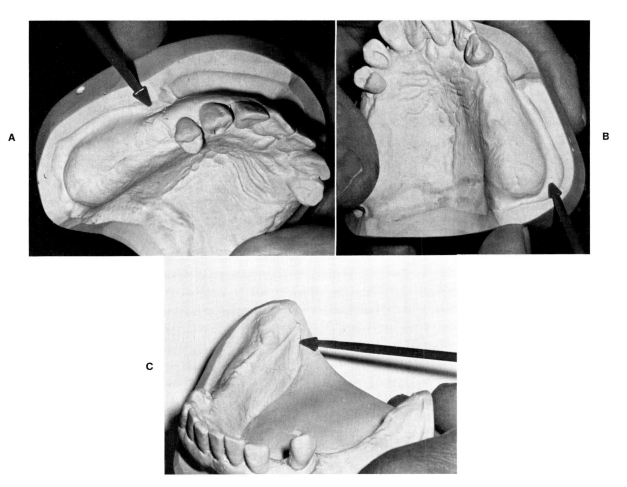

Fig. 18-20. A, Cast undercuts are commonly encountered distal to canine abutment teeth. **B,** Undercuts are often found lateral to tuberosity region. **C,** Undercuts commonly exist in posterior lingual region of mandibular casts. Failure to compensate for these undercuts can result in broken cast, fractured baseplate, or both.

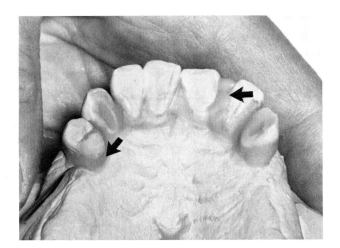

Fig. 18-21. Flow baseplate wax around and between teeth on cast (arrows). This will prevent resin from flowing into these areas, minimizing cast tooth breakage when baseplate is removed.

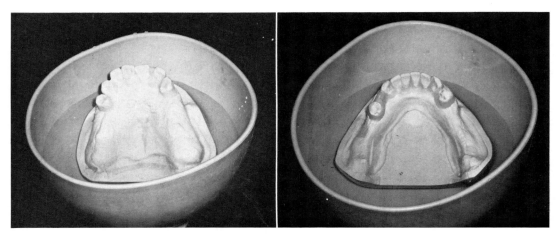

Fig. 18-22. Soak casts in clear slurry water for few minutes before coating with tinfoil substitute.

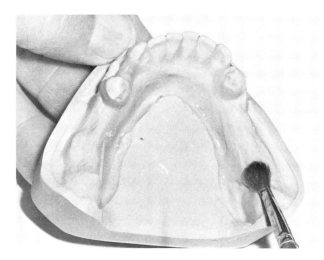

Fig. 18-23. Paint tinfoil substitute over cast and blockout wax. Be sure to cover teeth.

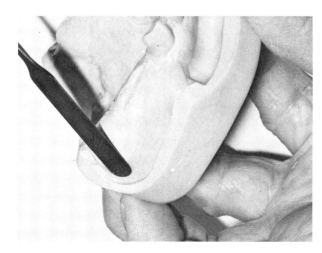

Fig. 18-24. Fill in cast undercuts with soft-setting autopolymerizing resin.

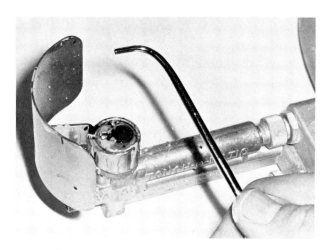

Fig. 18-25. Warm tip of chip blower over flame.

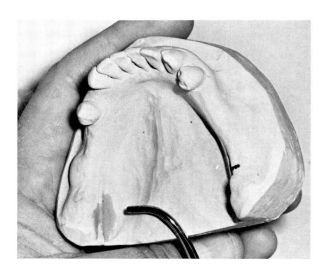

Fig. 18-26. Gently blow warmed air onto soft resin. This will produce surface "set" that retains soft resin in position in undercut. If not treated in this manner, soft resin tends to flow out of undercut into border area where it is of no benefit.

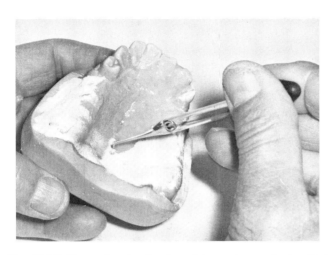

Fig. 18-27. Conventional autopolymerizing resin powder is sifted onto cast and over soft resin in undercuts. Polymer is wetted with monomer, and desired thickness of baseplate is built up in this manner.

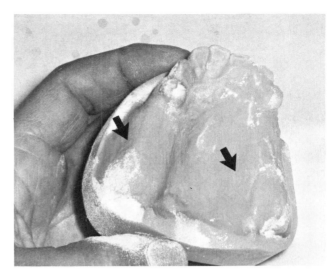

Fig. 18-28. Tilt cast to side when adding resin. Add powder and liquid to two upward-facing surfaces (arrows), then tilt cast in opposite direction and add to remaining surfaces.

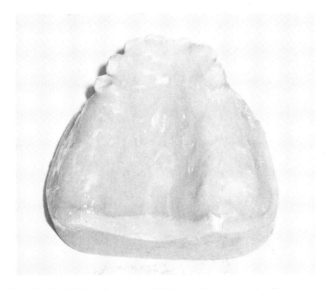

Fig. 18-29. Build up baseplate thickness in increments. Do not permit resin to pool in palate of maxillary casts, which will result in overly thick palate that will need to be thinned later.

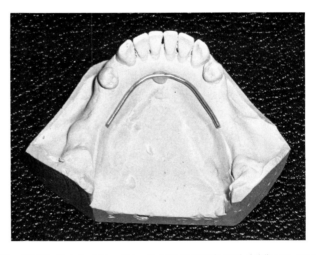

Fig. 18-30. Reinforcing wire will add strength and rigidity to completed baseplate.

of maxillary casts, resulting in an overthick baseplate (Fig. 18-28).

12. Allow the resin to extend onto the lingual surfaces of anterior teeth. This resin can be removed later if it interferes with the occlusion (Fig. 18-29).

13. Completely fill the border area of the cast to duplicate the thickness of the impression border. Be certain that the baseplate is adequately thick over the residual ridges to be sufficiently rigid. The mandibular baseplate can be strengthened, as with the shellac baseplate, by incorporating an adapted wire in the resin (Fig. 18-30).

14. Cure the baseplate under an inverted plaster bowl to reduce porosity (Fig. 18-31).

15. After hardening, remove the baseplate carefully from the cast, and examine it (Fig. 18-32).

16. After examining the baseplate, reduce overly thick areas with a bur or arbor band (Fig. 18-33).

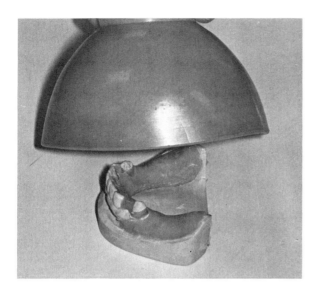

Fig. 18-31. Cure baseplate under inverted plaster bowl or in pressure pot to control porosity.

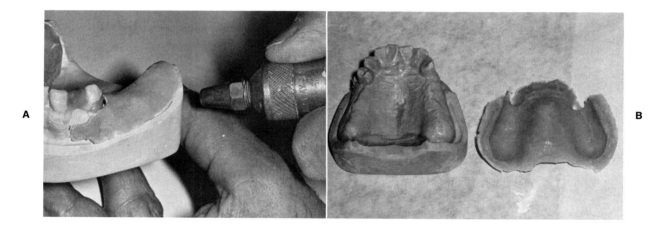

A

B

Fig. 18-32. A, Cured baseplate can sometimes be lifted off cast by directing stream of air under it. Be careful when prying baseplate from cast to prevent cast and baseplate breakage. **B,** Maxillary baseplate is separated and ready for trimming.

Fig. 18-33. Thick areas should be thinned with lathe-mounted arbor band. Note how band is positioned on chuck (arrow). Band extension will flex during trimming, reducing tendency to groove baseplate.

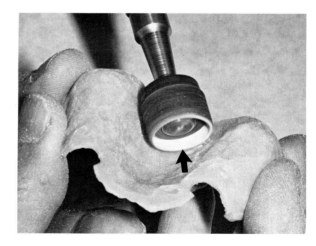

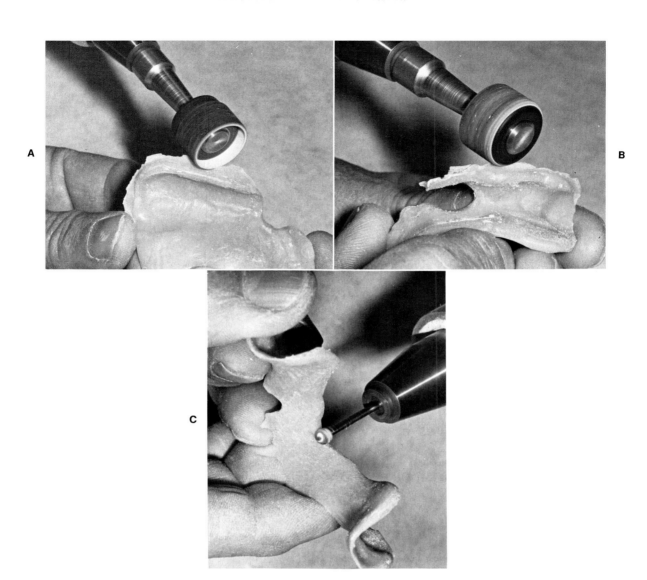

Fig. 18-34. Baseplate borders should be finished to contours dictated by impressions. Arbor bands **(A** and **B)** and burs **(C)** can be used to contour and smooth baseplate.

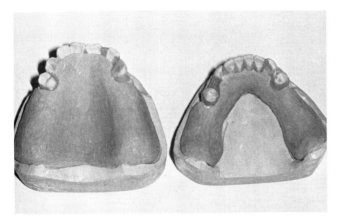

Fig. 18-35. Test baseplates for ease of placement and removal from cast. Adjust baseplate if necessary to facilitate placement on cast without undue flexing.

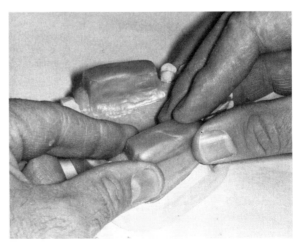

Fig. 18-36. Adapt baseplate wax to form occlusion rim.

17. The borders should be trimmed to form smooth rounded contours to prevent sharp edges that would abuse the patient's tissue (Fig. 18-34).

18. Pumice the border if required. However, a high polish is not desired. The finished baseplate should be approximately 2 to 3 mm thick, except over the ridges where it should not be thicker than 1 mm. The baseplate should be smooth, relatively rigid, and capable of being easily placed on or removed from the cast (Fig. 18-35).

Occlusion rims
PROCEDURE

1. Soften a sheet of baseplate wax, form it into a roll, and adapt it onto the baseplate to make an occlusion rim (Fig. 18-36). Seal the wax rim to the baseplate with a hot spatula (Fig. 18-37). The rim should be adapted over the residual ridges, be somewhat higher than the pro-posed occlusal plane, and be approximately 8 mm wide. It should extend posteriorly to the region of the second molar.

2. Smooth the wax of the occlusion rim, and replace the completed baseplate on the cast (Fig. 18-38).

PROBLEM AREAS

Principal problems associated with constructing baseplates of autopolymerizing resin are related to the difficulty in achieving a baseplate that is not too thick in some areas and too thin in others (Table 18-3). Porosity can also be a problem, and failure to block out the undercuts adequately can result in a broken cast and baseplate. Tilting the cast when sifting the resin powder minimizes pooling of the resin in the palate of maxillary casts. Examining the cast carefully prior to constructing the baseplate will identify severe undercuts that should be blocked out with baseplate wax. Baseplate resin

Table 18-3. Resin baseplates

Problem	Probable cause	Solution
Baseplate difficult to remove or fractures on removal from cast	Undercuts not identified and blocked out	Identify and block out undercuts before sifting resin on cast
	Tinfoil substitute not painted on cast	Paint tinfoil substitute on cast
	Soft resin used to block out severe undercuts	Block out severe undercuts with baseplate wax
	Soft resin flowed out of undercut	Warm surface of soft resin to produce surface set
Maxillary baseplate too thick in palate and too thin over ridges	Cast not tilted when sifting resin, permitting resin to pool in palate	Tilt cast to one side; sift resin on upward facing surfaces, then tilt to other side in similar manner
Cured baseplate porous	Baseplate not cured in pressure pot or under inverted plaster bowl	Cure baseplate in pressure pot or under inverted plaster bowl

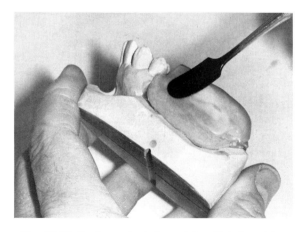

Fig. 18-37. Seal wax rim to baseplate with hot spatula.

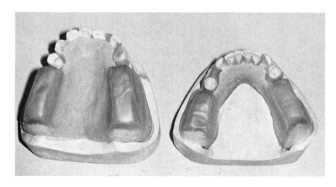

Fig. 18-38. Completed baseplates and occlusion rims are stored on casts until needed.

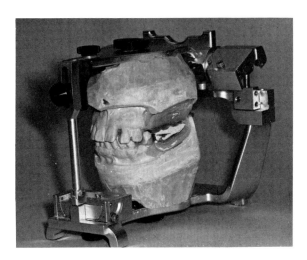

Fig. 18-39. Master casts mounted in articulator.

porosity can be controlled by curing the baseplate in a pressure pot or beneath an inverted plaster bowl.

SETTING THE TEETH

After the raw relation recording procedures are completed, the master casts are mounted in an articulator (Fig. 18-39). Anterior and posterior teeth are selected for the proposed overdenture, using the teeth on the cast as a guide for size and mold selection.

PROCEDURE

1. Measure the width and length of the central incisor and any other anterior teeth present on the cast (Fig. 18-40).

2. Check the shape of the natural teeth on the cast to determine the tooth form; square, tapering, ovoid, or combination. Based on these measurements and observations select *resin* anterior teeth that will closely approximate the size and shape of the patient's natural

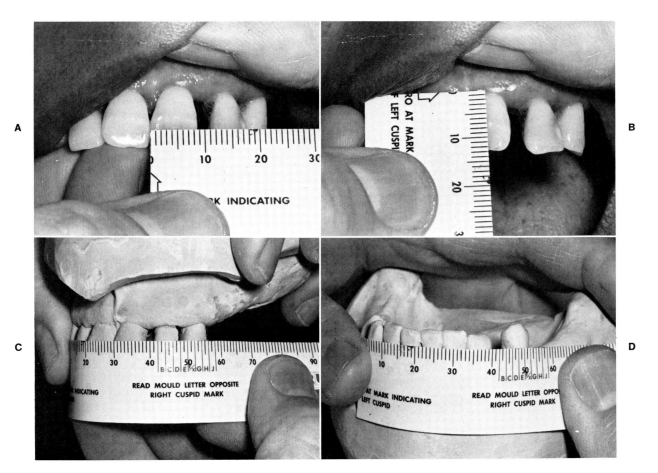

Fig. 18-40. A, Measure width of central incisor on cast and on patient. **B,** Measure length of central incisor. **C,** Measure combined width of maxillary anterior teeth using flexible plastic rule. Remember to allow for spaces between teeth. **D,** Measure mandibular anterior teeth.

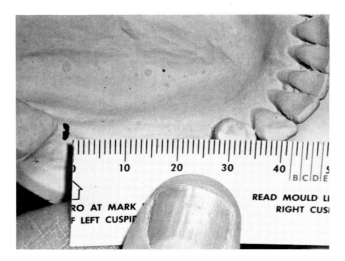

Fig. 18-41. Measure posterior arch length to determine size of posterior denture teeth.

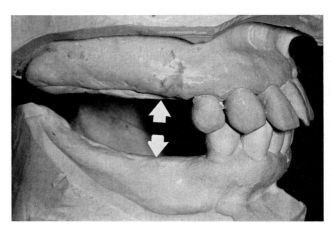

Fig. 18-42. Height of posterior tooth is determined by space available for teeth (arrows). Tooth length should be as long as possible.

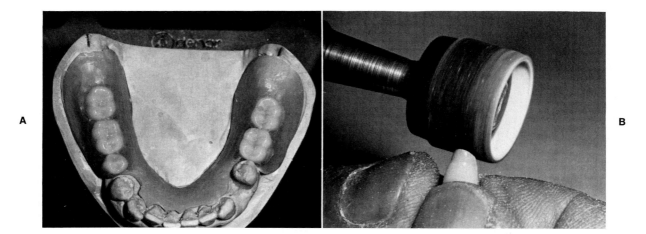

Fig. 18-43. A, Set posterior teeth on baseplate. **B,** Grind ridge laps if necessary when setting teeth.

teeth. It is important to use resin teeth in an immediate overdenture, since they contribute to a stronger overdenture.

3. Select the posterior teeth using a millimeter rule to measure from the distal surface of the canine on the cast to a point where the posterior occlusion would normally terminate (Fig. 18-41). In this manner the appropriate combined mesiodistal widths of the four posterior teeth can be selected.

4. Take the posterior shade from the anterior teeth so that the shade will be compatible.

5. Select the posterior tooth length by closing the articulator and observing the available denture space (Fig. 18-42). Select resin posterior teeth to provide a strong unitized overdenture that will resist breakage in service. The occlusal pattern of posterior teeth will depend on the preference of the dentist; however, anatomic or nonanatomic forms can be used. Anterior and posterior molds, shade, and type of tooth and material should be recorded in the laboratory records for future reference in the event of a fracture.

Setting the posterior teeth

If a try-in of the posterior teeth is desired, the posterior teeth are set on the baseplate before the anterior teeth are positioned.

PROCEDURE

1. Set the posterior teeth on the baseplate (Fig. 18-43, *A*). Often the space is minimal, and it is necessary to modify the teeth by grinding the ridge laps (Fig. 18-43, *B*).

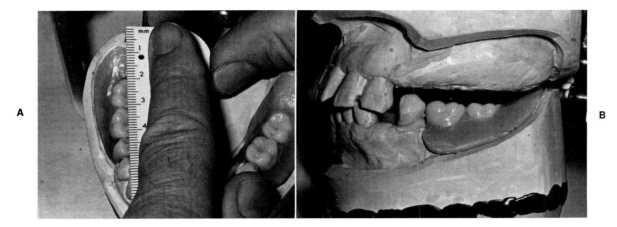

Fig. 18-44. A, Center posterior teeth over ridge. **B,** Posterior height of occlusal plane should be one half to two thirds height of pear-shaped pad.

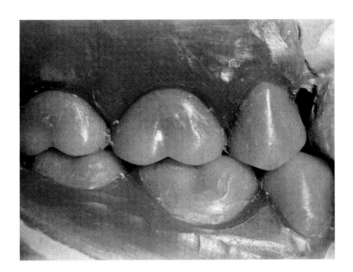

Fig. 18-45. Incorporate horizontal overlap in setup to minimize cheek biting.

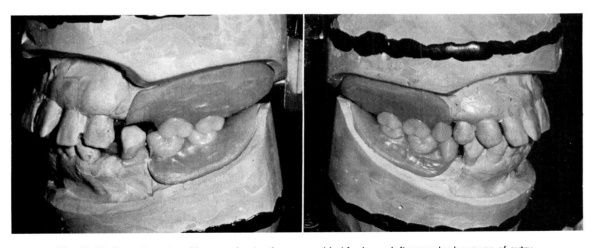

Fig. 18-46. Posterior setup. No opposing tooth was provided for lower left premolar because of extrusion. It will be removed when overdenture is inserted.

2. Center the mandibular posterior teeth over the residual ridge buccolingually and establish the posterior occlusal plane so that it is no higher than one half to two thirds the distance up the pear-shaped pad (Fig. 18-44).

3. Adjust each individual tooth position to develop the desired occlusion. Incorporate sufficient horizontal overlap to minimize the tendency for cheek biting (Fig. 18-45). After the posterior setup is complete, wax the posterior teeth securely to the baseplate, and wax the teeth for try-in (Fig. 18-46).

4. Check the occlusion with thin tissue or plastic tape after waxing, and adjust it if necessary before tri-in. Store the baseplate and wax-up on the cast in the articulator until needed.

Setting anterior teeth
PROCEDURE

1. Resin anterior teeth should be selected because, as previously stated, they bond to the overdenture base and result in a stronger overdenture. Selected teeth should approximate the size and shape of the natural teeth they are to replace.

2. With casts in the occluded position, use the incisal edges of the maxillary teeth as a guide and draw a line on the labial surface of the lower anterior teeth (Fig. 18-47). This line indicates the vertical overlap and is a guide for setting the maxillary teeth (Fig. 18-48).

3. Remove one anterior tooth, the central incisor if present, from the cast with a bur or saw (Fig. 18-49). Remove only one tooth at a time so that the adjacent tooth on the cast serves as a guide for positioning the denture tooth.

4. Contour the ridge of the cast so that it has a smooth rounded contour (Fig. 18-50). Do not, however, inlet the cast.

5. Position the denture tooth on the space formed by the removal of the tooth on the cast (Fig. 18-51). Usually the ridge lap of the denture tooth will require grinding to assure proper placement (Fig. 18-52). The ridge lap can be adjusted with an arbor band or a bur until the tooth can be placed in the same position as the natural tooth.

6. Duplicate the positions of the natural teeth if appropriate. However, overdenture patients may have malpositioned, extruded teeth, in which case duplication of these abnormal tooth positions may not be desirable. In these situations, modify the tooth position to improve esthetics and meet functional requirements (Fig. 18-53).

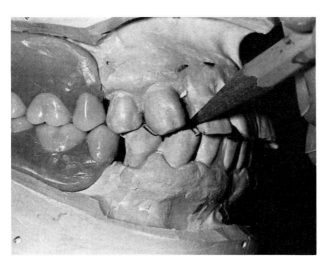

Fig. 18-47. Use incisal edges of maxillary teeth as guide; draw line on lower anterior teeth to indicate vertical overlap.

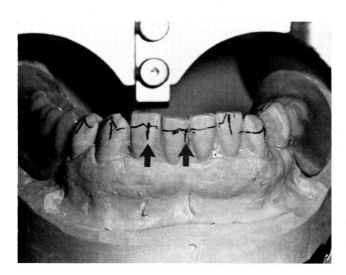

Fig. 18-48. Mark midline and contacts between maxillary teeth on lower teeth (arrows).

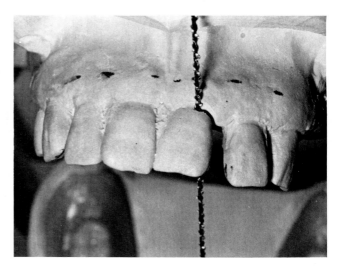

Fig. 18-49. One anterior tooth is removed from cast. Saw, bur, or knife can be used for this procedure.

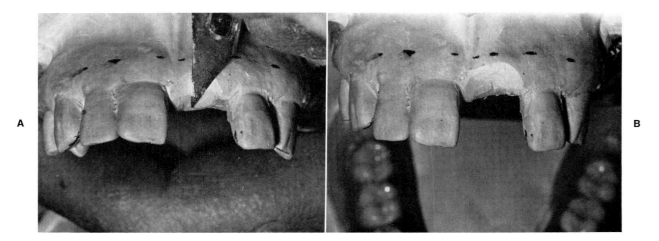

Fig. 18-50. A, Smooth ridge where tooth was removed but do not inlet cast. **B,** If tooth was severely periodontally involved with deep periodontal pockets, cast may be reduced slightly to compensate. This should be done by dentist.

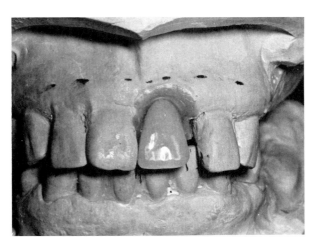

Fig. 18-51. Set denture tooth in position and grind if necessary.

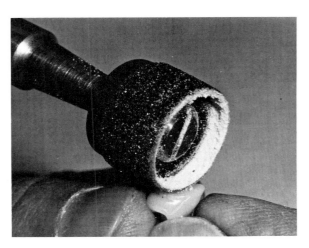

Fig. 18-52. Lathe-mounted arbor band can be used to grind tooth ridge lap. Use care and do not overshorten, which will compromise esthetics. Note position of band on chuck, which increases its flexibility.

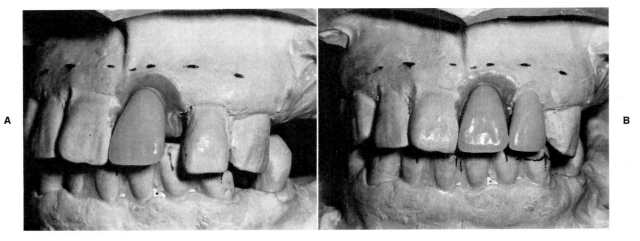

Fig. 18-53. A, Malpositioned teeth may be corrected in setup if desired. In this situation lateral incisor is extruded. **B,** Lateral incisor position has been corrected in setup.

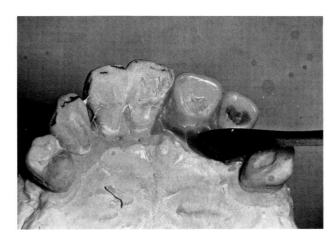

Fig. 18-54. Wax tooth to cast. Be sure to check occlusion and adjust tooth position as required.

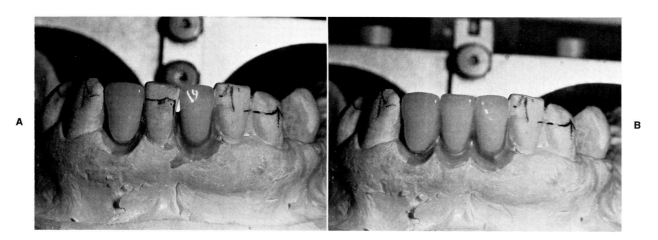

Fig. 18-55. A, Sequentially remove tooth from cast. **B,** Replace with corresponding denture tooth, using cast tooth as guide.

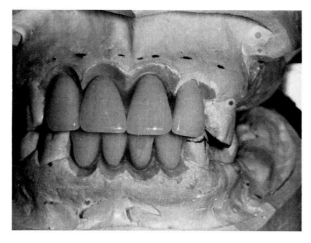

Fig. 18-56. All anterior teeth are set except abutment teeth.

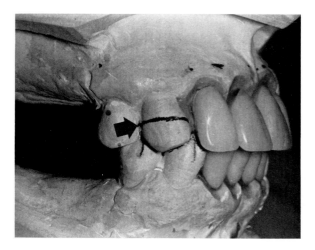

Fig. 18-57. Mark abutment tooth (arrow) to indicate amount of occlusogingival reduction.

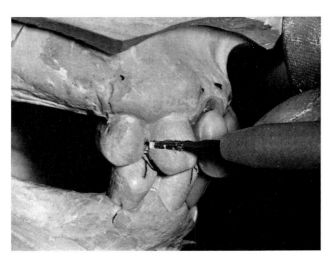

Fig. 18-58. Cut cast tooth with saw or No. 558 bur.

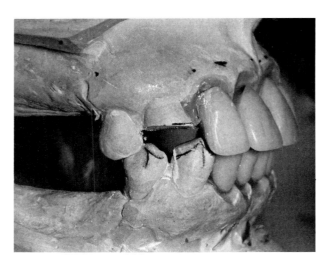

Fig. 18-59. Check occlusion to determine that 2- to 3-mm space exists between abutment and opposing teeth.

7. After the denture tooth has been modified so that it can be positioned properly, wax it to the cast (Fig. 18-54).

8. Remove another tooth from the cast, and replace it with a denture tooth as previously described. The sequence of removal and replacement should allow an adjacent tooth on the cast to serve as a guide for positioning the denture tooth (Fig. 18-55).

9. In this manner all anterior teeth, except the abutments, are set on the cast (Fig. 18-56). If maxillary and mandibular overdentures are being constructed, maxillary and mandibular anterior teeth are set.

Preparing cast abutments
PROCEDURE

1. The dentist should mark the cast abutment indicating the amount the tooth is to be reduced (Fig. 18-57). Shorten the cast abutment with a bur or saw (Fig. 18-58). The abutment should be shortened so that a minimum space of 2 to 3 mm exists between the abutment preparation and an opposing tooth (Fig. 18-59). A space of less than 2 to 3 mm will result in a resin thickness that will not be adequate to prevent breakage. Strength requirements for an overdenture exceed those for most conventional complete dentures. The presence of supporting natural teeth permits increased functional forces to be placed on the overdenture, and the indentations in the overdenture base to accommodate the abutment teeth can have a weakening effect on the overall structure. As a result, an overdenture needs to be stronger than a conventional complete denture to prevent breakage.

2. Prepare the abutment on the cast, removing stone from the facial, proximal, and lingual surfaces (Fig. 18-60). If faciolingual reduction of the cast abutment

is represented as a percentage, approximately 60% of the reduction should come from the facial surface, and about 40% from the lingual surface (Fig. 18-61). This reduction facilitates positioning of the denture tooth over the cast abutment. The basic purpose of the prepared cast abutment is to form an indentation in the overdenture that will be occupied by the natural abutment tooth. Thus it is very important when removing teeth from the cast and setting the denture teeth that *the abutment teeth are not inadvertently removed from the cast.* To prevent removal of the abutments, the teeth can be identified on the cast by writing "save" on the abutment tooth.

3. Hollow a resin denture tooth with a bur so that it can be positioned over the cast abutment. Use a large acrylic bur for gross reduction, and make refinements with a No. 8 round bur (Fig. 18-62). Usually the denture tooth should be modified so that it can be placed in the position of the natural tooth (Fig. 18-63).

4. Occasionally, because of drifting, abutment teeth may not be in a position compatible with an esthetic result (Fig. 18-64). In this instance the denture tooth can be modified so that it can be positioned either mesial or distal to the cast abutment and not directly over it (Fig. 18-65). The cast abutment is then positioned between two teeth on the overdenture. This is acceptable; however, sufficient wax must be placed over the interproximal area to provide at least a 2 mm thickness of denture base resin to prevent breakage.

WAXING THE IMMEDIATE OVERDENTURE

Waxing the immediate overdenture is similar to waxing a conventional immediate complete denture. Anatomic contours should be stimulated as discussed

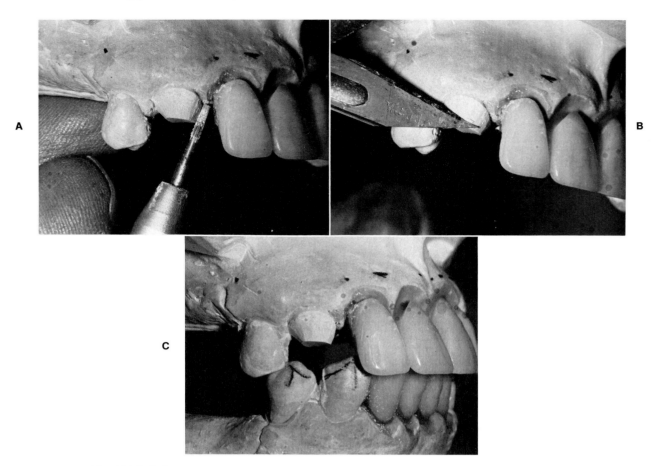

Fig. 18-60. A, Prepare cast abutment using bur for proximal reduction. **B,** Sharp knife can be used to shape abutment preparation on cast. **C,** Completed cast preparation.

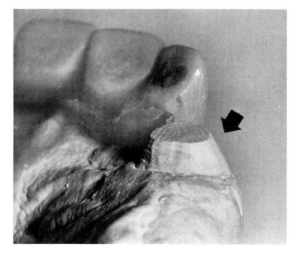

Fig. 18-61. When preparing cast abutment, remove more stone from facial surface than from lingual surface. This reduction (arrow) will facilitate placing denture tooth in correct position faciolingually.

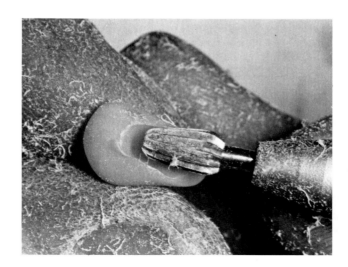

Fig. 18-62. Large acrylic bur is used for gross reduction.

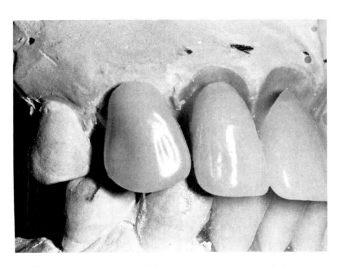

Fig. 18-63. Denture tooth is positioned over cast abutment.

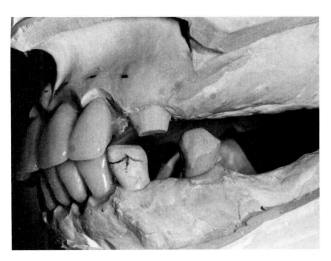

Fig. 18-64. If abutment tooth has drifted out of position, it may not be desirable to place denture tooth directly over it. In this situation, denture teeth may be positioned anterior and posterior to cast abutment. There is too much space mesial to cast abutment in this illustration.

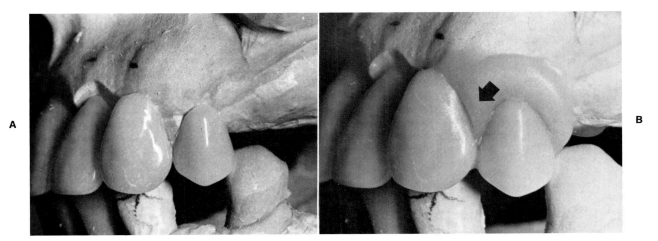

Fig. 18-65. A, Canine and premolar denture teeth have been positioned over canine cast abutment. **B,** Wax in interproximal area (arrow) in this situation should not be less than 2 mm thick.

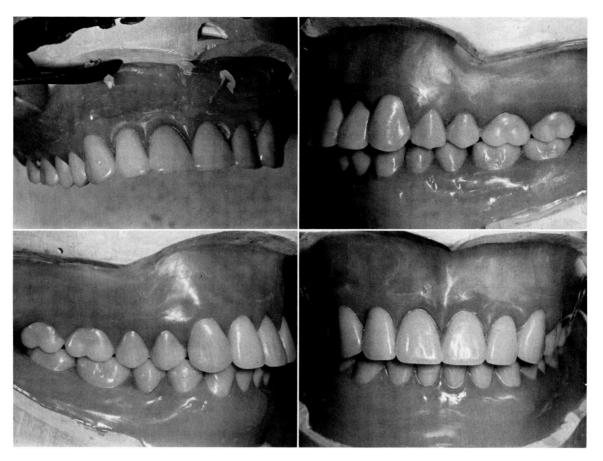

Fig. 18-66. Carve wax to simulate anatomic contours.

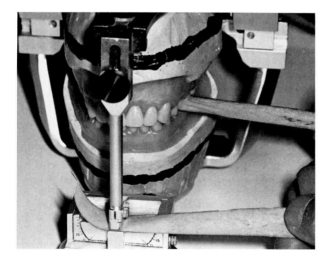

Fig. 18-67. Occlusion of wax denture should be checked with thin tissue before removing wax-up for processing. Be certain to check contact of incisal guide pin and incisal table at this time.

in Chapter 8, although overcharacterization is to be avoided. After the posterior teeth have been tried in and returned to the laboratory, the overdenture can be waxed for flasking, or the denture teeth may be removed from the baseplates, and the baseplates discarded. This is usually done when an anatomic palate form is to be used. In this situation the baseplates are no longer needed, and their presence on the cast can interfere with waxing. This is an optional procedure. Waxing of the overdenture is done in a conventional manner, and prior to flasking, the occlusion is checked with tape (Figs. 18-66 and 18-67). Waxing of the overdenture can cause teeth to move, resulting in occlusion error that should be corrected prior to flasking the overdenture.

FLASKING THE IMMEDIATE OVERDENTURE

Select denture flasks that do not rock when assembled, and flask the overdenture as described in Chapter 10 (Fig. 18-68). After the dentures have been flasked, eliminate the wax by placing the denture in boiling water for 5 minutes. After the wax has been eliminated,

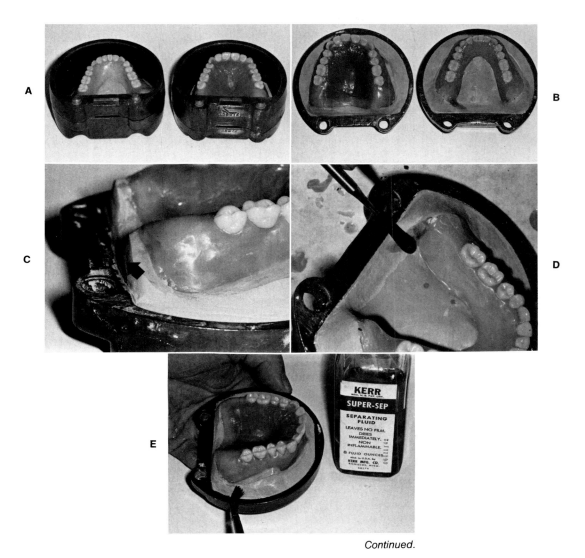

Continued.

Fig. 18-68. A, Place casts and wax-ups in lower half of flasks and place upper halves of flask in position. Be sure that there is enough space above incisal edges of teeth for stone cap. **B,** Invest casts and wax denture in lower part of flask using artificial stone. **C,** Check half-flasked overdentures for undercuts. Flasked maxillary overdenture is undercut (arrow). Note particularly heel region of mandibular cast, since undercuts are commonly encountered in this area. **D,** Undercuts can be obturated by flowing baseplate wax into undercut. Failure to do this may result in broken cast when separating flask halves after boilout procedures. **E,** Coat artificial stone in lower half of flask with separating medium. **F,** Brush artificial stone onto wax denture, using stiff brush to help prevent voids. **G,** When painting separating medium on stone surface in preparation for pouring stone cap, do not coat occlusal surfaces of teeth with separating medium. Certain separating media may stain resin teeth if they come in contact with teeth. **H,** Flasked overdentures are ready for caps. **I,** Lid is placed on flask and tapped into place. Stone is then allowed to set before being placed in boiling water to eliminate wax.

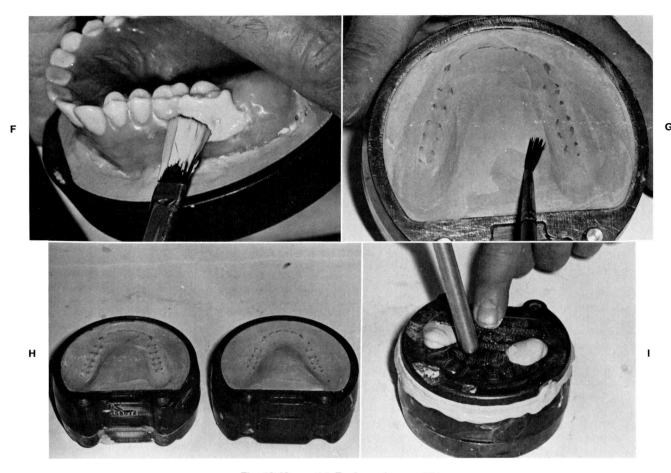

Fig. 18-68, cont'd. For legend see p. 521.

the molds are thoroughly flushed, and a final flush is completed with clean boiling water. The flasks are then placed upright to drain and cool.

Making an impression of the overdenture cast

It is a definite advantage for the dentist to have a cast of the abutment preparations to serve as a guide when the abutments are prepared in the mouth. This cast is easily obtained at this time.

PROCEDURE

1. Dip the lower half of the flask containing the overdenture cast in water to wet the cast.

2. Select an oversize rim lock tray (Fig. 18-69). Mix fast-setting alginate, and make an impression of the flasked cast (Fig. 18-70).

3. After the alginate has set, separate the impression, and pour it in artificial stone (Fig. 18-71). The resultant cast can then be used to fabricate a surgical template and can also serve as a guide for the dentist to ensure

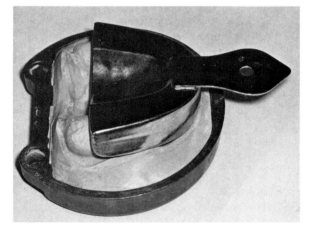

Fig. 18-69. Select oversize rim-lock tray.

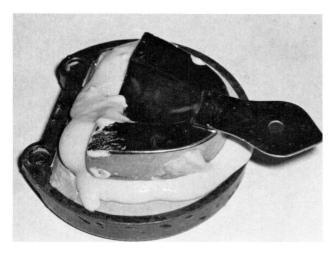

Fig. 18-70. Make impression of flasked cast using fast-setting alginate.

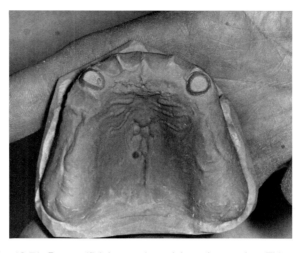

Fig. 18-71. Pour artificial stone into alginate impression. This cast will be used as guide for tooth preparation later.

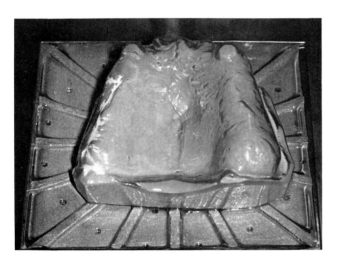

Fig. 18-72. Adapt sheet of clear resin over cast, using vacuum-adapting device to form surgical template.

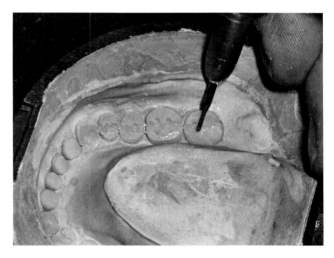

Fig. 18-73. Using No. 558 bur or No. 37 inverted cone bur, place grooves approximately 2 mm wide and 2 mm deep across mesiodistal width of resin posterior denture teeth.

that the abutment preparation in the mouth of the patient will be slightly smaller than the abutment preparation on the cast.

Making a surgical template

A clear resin template is often requested by the dentist and can be made using the above cast. The template is made by adapting a sheet of clear resin over the flask with a vacuum-adapter device as discussed in Chapter 4 (Fig. 18-72).

Preparing ridge laps

A stronger break-resistant overdenture can be obtained if the ridge laps of the resin posterior teeth are grooved mesiodistally with an inverted cone or cross-cut fissure bur to produce diatorics in these teeth.

PROCEDURE

1. Grooves, approximately 2 mm wide and where possible 2 mm deep, are cut in the ridge lap of the resin posterior teeth (Fig. 18-73). They should extend across the full width of the denture teeth. If minimal denture space necessitated shortening of the teeth for the setup, the teeth may be too thin to permit placement of the grooves. However, where space is available, grooves are placed to increase the bonding area, and the ridge of high-impact resin extending into the grooves imparts additional strength and rigidity to the overdenture.

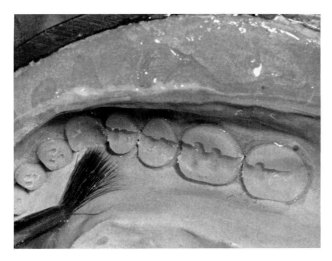

Fig. 18-74. Carefully paint tinfoil substitute over stone mold and cast. Take care to not get tinfoil substitute onto ridge laps of teeth. If tinfoil is inadvertently placed on ridge laps of teeth, it must be removed before denture base resin is added, or bond strength between denture base resin and denture tooth will be severely compromised.

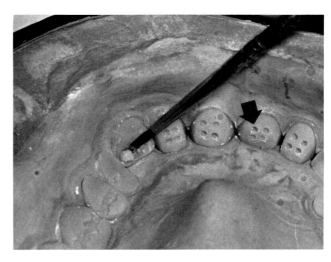

Fig. 18-75. Paint heat-curing tooth-shade resin into all abutment teeth. Dip brush first in monomer and then polymer, and transfer to abutment tooth. Do not overfill. Note indentations in anterior teeth (arrow).

2. Prepare the ridge laps after the wax has been eliminated from the mold, but before the tinfoil substitute has been applied. Be sure that the posterior palatal seal has been placed on the maxillary cast before the overdenture is packed.

3. Do not place grooves in the anterior teeth ridge laps, since grooves in these teeth can modify the shade. Pink denture base resin ridges may be visible through the relatively thin anterior tooth. Three to four shallow indentations made in the ridge laps of these teeth with a No. 6 round bur will improve attachment to the denture base resin.

4. Remove the glazed surface on the ridge laps of anterior teeth to facilitate bonding between the tooth and denture base resin. Ridge-lap modification, careful boilout procedures to assure complete wax removal, and the use of high-impact denture base resin will significantly reduce overdenture breakage.

Applying tinfoil substitute

Painting the mold with tinfoil substitute is an important step in achieving a successful overdenture.

PROCEDURE

1. Pour fresh tinfoil substitute in a paper cup, and carefully paint the stone mold.

2. Do not coat the ridge laps of the teeth with tinfoil substitute. If this is done inadvertently, remove it with a cotton swab (Fig. 18-74). If tinfoil substitute is allowed

to remain on the ridge laps of the resin teeth, a significant reduction of bond strength will occur. This reduced sterngth compromises overall overdenture strength and should be avoided. Be certain that all stone surfaces are coated with tinfoil substitute, and place the flask aside to dry.

3. Paint tooth-shade heat-curing resin into the hollowed-out denture teeth over the abutments, and wet it with monomer (Fig. 18-75).

PACKING THE OVERDENTURE
PROCEDURE

1. Pack the overdenture with a high-impact denture base resin.* Proportion the powder and liquid, and mix it according to the manufacturer's recommendations (Fig. 18-76).

2. After the resin has reached the dough stage, remove it from the mixing jar, and adapt it to the mold. Use plastic golves, or plastic sheets, to avoid contacting the resin with the hands (Fig. 18-77). Place a plastic sheet over the resin, assemble the flask, and close it slowly in a bench compress as in the case of the conventional complete denture. Be sure to allow adequate time for the resin to flow throughout the mold. Do not attempt to obtain metal-to-metal flask contact on the initial closing.

---

*Lucitone 199, The L. D. Caulk Co., Milford, Del.; Hircoe, Coe Laboratories, Inc., Chicago, Ill.; or equivalent.

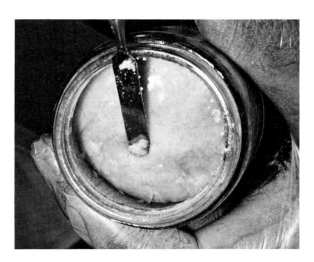

Fig. 18-76. Use high-impact denture base resin and proportion powder and liquid according to manufacturer's recommendations.

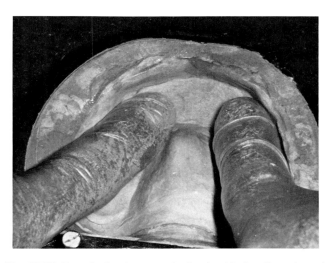

Fig. 18-77. Use plastic gloves or plastic sheet to handle resin and place resin into mold. Use of gloves prevents contamination of resin with skin oils and, more important, may prevent contact dermatitis as result of repeated contacts with resin.

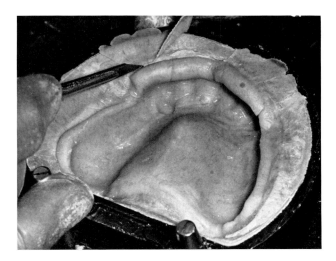

Fig. 18-78. Remove flask from bench press, open it, and trim excess resin flash with sharp No. 25 blade. Take care to not incorporate any stone particles from trimming into resin.

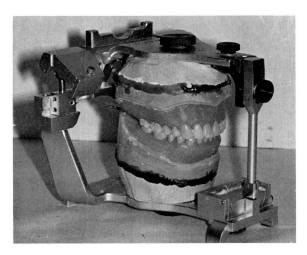

Fig. 18-79. Remount overdentures on casts in articulator, and determine amount of processing error.

3. Remove the flask from the bench press, open it, and trim the excess resin flash with a No. 25 blade in a Bard-Parker handle (Fig. 18-78). Take care to not incorporate stone particles in the resin as a result of trimming. Replace the plastic sheet, and make another trial closure. Remove the flask, separate the halves, and trim the excess as before. In this manner, make additional trial packs until resin flash within the mold no longer occurs, and metal-to-metal closure of the flask is obtained.

4. Place the packed dentures in a hand compress, and cure them according to the manufacturer's recommendations.

CORRECTING PROCESSING ERROR

After the overdentures have been retrieved from the flask, they are remounted in the articulator, and the amount of pin opening is determined (Fig. 18-79). Use articulating paper to indicate the deflective contacts on the occlusal surfaces of the teeth, and adjust the deflective contacts (Fig. 18-80). Some dentists may prefer

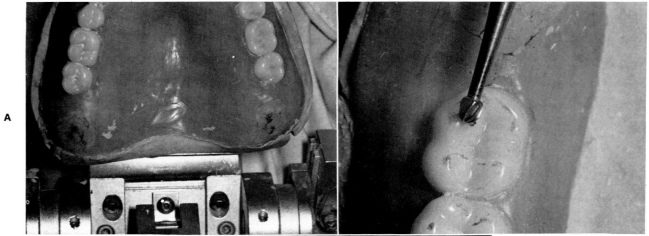

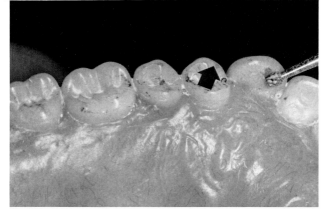

Fig. 18-80. A, Be certain that indicated processing error is not caused by contact of posterior extensions of overdenture. These areas are frequently waxed more heavily immediately before flasking and, as result, produce interferences once overdentures are remounted in articulator. B, In centric relation position, grind fossa of tooth unless opposing cusp is high not only in centric relation position but also in eccentric positions. C, Adjust inclines of buccal cusps of maxillary teeth (arrow) and lingual cusps of mandibular teeth to eliminate working side interferences.

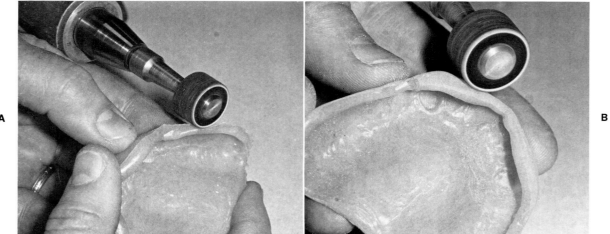

Fig. 18-81. A, Trim overdenture borders with arbor band mounted on lathe. B, Anterior flange of overdenture usually requires thinning, since portion of impression is not border molded. Do not overthin before dentist adjusts for undercuts.

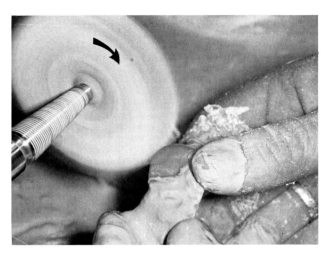

Fig. 18-82. Polish accessible areas of overdenture with lathe-mounted rag wheel in slurry of flour of pumice. (Arrow denotes direction of rotation.)

to make corrections after the remounting procedure. After the occlusion has been adjusted, an occlusal index of the maxillary overdenture can be made to preserve the face-bow record if a face-bow record was used to mount the maxillary cast.

POLISHING THE OVERDENTURE
PROCEDURE

1. Remove the overdentures carefully from the cast as previously discussed. A laboratory shell blaster can be used to remove stone from the interior of the overdenture. Otherwise, remove the stone in small sections, and do not attempt to pry the overdenture from the cast.

2. Trim overdenture borders with a lathe-mounted arbor band (Fig. 18-81).

3. Smooth accessible exterior surfaces of the overdenture with a lathe-mounted rag wheel and a slurry of flour of pumice (Fig. 18-82).

4. Smooth the palate and the region adjacent to the teeth with a handpiece-mounted brush and rubber prophy cup and flour of pumice (Fig. 18-83). The smaller

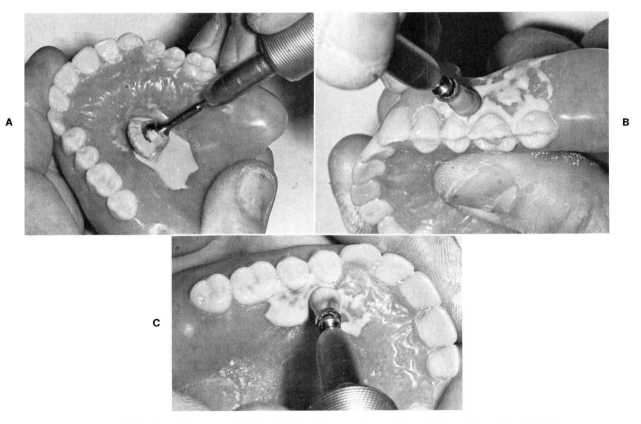

Fig. 18-83. Use handpiece-mounted brush **(A)**, rubber prophy cup **(B and C)**, and flour of pumice to polish areas of overdenture where access is limited. Use of larger wheel in these areas will obliterate anatomic contour.

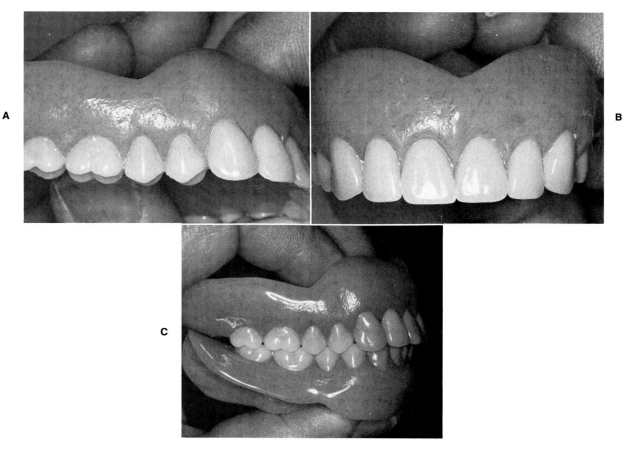

Fig. 18-84. A, Eggshell finish placed on overdenture is frequently esthetic because it breaks up light reflections. This finish is accomplished by first outlining finish area on overdenture with eyebrow pencil. In this overdenture canine is over abutment (arrow). **B,** No. 200 finishing bur is rotated against resin to create desired surface. Bur should be randomly moved over surface within outlined area with light pressure.

Fig. 18-85. Buff overdenture to produce high-luster surface. Note effect of finishing bur on surface.

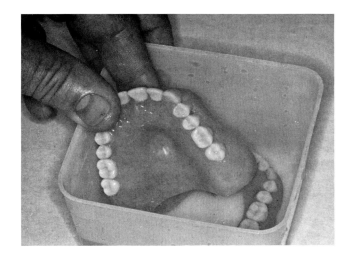

Fig. 18-86. Scrub polished all-resin overdenture with soap and water and store in water.

Table 18-4. Immediate overdentures

Problem	Probable cause	Solution
Immediate overdenture breaks repeatedly in service	High-impact resin not used	Use high-impact resin to pack the immediate overdenture
	Resin teeth not used	Use resin teeth on overdenture
Resin teeth did not bond to denture base resin	Wax not completely removed during boilout	Use boiling water, to which detergent has been added, to flush mold; follow with clean boiling-water flush
	Tinfoil substitute inadvertently painted on ridge laps of teeth	Take care to not paint tinfoil substitute on ridge laps of resin teeth; remove any placed inadvertently
	Ridge laps not grooved before packing resin	Place grooves in ridge laps of resin posterior teeth; place indentations in ridge laps of anterior teeth

rubber cup allows smoothing areas of the overdenture base without obliterating contours.

5. Stipple, or place an eggshell surface on the polished anterior and buccal surface of the overdenture with a finishing bur if desired (Fig. 18-84).

6. Buff the polished surface to a high luster with a lathe-mounted rag wheel and polishing medium* (Fig. 18-85).

7. Examine the interior of the overdenture, and remove any nodules or sharp fins that might prove uncomfortable for the patient.

8. Scrub the polished overdenture with soap and water to remove all traces of polishing compound. Rinse and store the overdenture in water, or seal it in a plastic bag containing water (Fig. 18-86).

---

*Ti-gleam No. 341, Ticonium Company, Albany, N.Y., or prepared chalk or equivalent polishing agent.

PROBLEM AREAS

Principal problems associated with constructing an immediate overdenture are related to failure to use a high-impact resin for construction of the overdenture; failure to use resin denture teeth; and failure to place retention grooves in the ridge laps of resin denture teeth, which will contribute to a weaker overdenture (Table 18-4). Using a high-impact resin, such as Lucitone 199 or Hircoe, using resin teeth in the overdenture, and the placement of retentive grooves in the ridge laps of the posterior teeth and retentive indentations in the anterior teeth, will contribute significantly to a stronger overdenture.

SUMMARY

Laboratory procedures incident to constructing immediate overdentures were discussed in this chapter. The procedures are similar to those for conventional immediate overdentures. Significant differences exist, however, and these relate to the method in which the teeth are set on the cast, the use of resin teeth for the denture, the method in which the resin teeth are grooved to provide additional bonding area, and the use of a high-impact resin to construct the denture. When constructing an immediate overdenture, it is important to remember to not remove all the teeth from the cast. Abutment teeth are prepared on the cast, and preparation can be accomplished by the dentist. Imme-

diate overdentures are finding widespread acceptance throughout the dental profession, and it is axiomatic that those involved in constructing immediate overdentures be knowledgeable in the procedures involved.

BIBLIOGRAPHY

Brewer, A. A., and Morrow, R. M.: Overdentures, St. Louis, 1975, The C. V. Mosby Co.

Morrow, R. M.: Handbook of immediate overdentures, St. Louis, 1978, The C. V. Mosby Co.

CHAPTER 19

DENTURE BASE TINTING

KENNETH D. RUDD and ROBERT M. MORROW

tinted denture base A denture base that simulates the coloring and shading of natural oral tissues.

TINTING THE DENTURE BASE

Several methods have been used to tint denture base resins to achieve a more natural appearance. Usually heat-curing or autopolymerizing resins of various shades or colors are painted on the denture base or are sifted onto the mold during denture construction to obtain a tinted denture. Skillful tinting procedures can produce excellent results, but it is equally true that poorly executed tinting can produce garish results, much worse than no tinting at all. Recently more denture base resins are available in different shades to meet individual patient needs. Denture base resins can be obtained in a range of colors and shades from deep pink brown to light pink (Fig. 19-1).* Denture base resins are also fibered or nonfibered and range in translucency from relatively translucent to moderately opaque. A major indication for special denture base shades and individualized tinting is for those patients with pigmented oral tissues. Methods for tinting the denture bases for these patients are described by Choudhary et al. (1975).

A method for tinting the denture base using heat-curing tinting resins† will be described in this chapter. This method is based on the sift-in technique of Pound (1951). A simple method for gaining experience and developing skill in tinting will also be described.

---

*Natural Coe-Lor Denture Resin, Coe Laboratories, Inc., Chicago, Ill.

†Kayon Denture Stains, Kay-See Dental Manufacturing Co., Kansas City, Mo.

PROCEDURE

Usually, five stains or tinting resins are adequate to characterize most dentures (Fig. 19-2):

H, basic color (light pink as in attached gingiva)

F, light red

A, medium red, use cautiously

E, purple, use sparingly in most dentures

B, brown, used for patients with heavy gingival pigmentation.

1. When waxing the denture, use care in carving appropriate contours on the denture base. Skillful contouring is probably more important for esthetics than tinting. Application of stains is related to carved contours (Fig. 19-3).

2. Flask and boil out the denture, paint it with tinfoil substitute, and allow to dry.

3. Modify a glass dropper by heating and drawing to create a smaller orifice and better monomer control (Fig. 19-4). Use heat-curing monomer to wet the resin.

4. Sift H resin over the facial aspect of the flasking stone in the region occupied by the attached gingiva, and saturate it with monomer (Figs. 19-3 and 19-5). Tint half the denture, then tint the other half.

5. Sift a light coat of F over the H, and extend the F higher on the flange (Fig. 19-6).

6. Sift E sparingly on the area of the attached gingiva/mucosa junction, and saturate it with monomer. Do not overwet the resin, or it may pool in the lower gingival areas.

7. Sift A higher on the flanges to the borders of the denture. Use care, since A is red (Fig. 19-7).

8. After tinting one side of the denture, complete the other side in the same manner. Continually refer to the

531

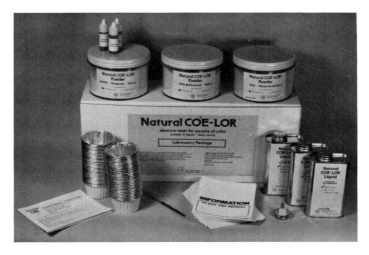

Fig. 19-1. Natural Coe-Lor denture resin. (Courtesy Coe Laboratories, Inc., Chicago, Ill.).

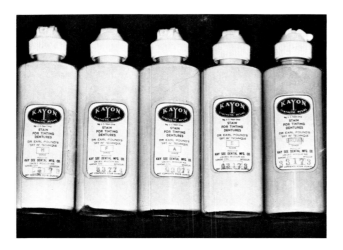

Fig. 19-2. Kayon stains: H, F, A, E, and Brown.

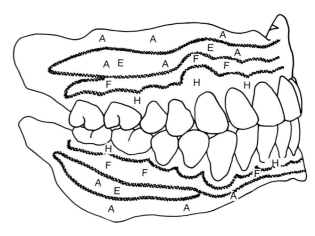

Fig. 19-3. Drawing indicates appropriate areas for each stain.

tinted side for comparison to avoid a pronounced difference in color and distribution of the tinting resin.

9. Place a plastic sheet over the tinted flask, and allow it to set for 15 to 20 minutes before packing the denture base. If the denture is packed too soon, the tinting resin can be squeezed out of the mold, or the distribution modified.

10. Cure the denture, and finish and polish it in the usual manner (Fig. 19-8).

PROBLEM AREAS

The principal problem with this technique is related to poor results because of improper application of the tinting resin (Table 19-1). The procedure must not be done hastily or in a slipshod manner. It is important to overlay each addition of tinting resin to produce a gradual color change, rather than a striped appearance. Experience is very important in achieving an acceptable result.

USE OF PRACTICE MOLD

In Chapters 8, 9, and 11, methods for using a flexible silicone mold material were discussed (Fig. 19-9). After the dentures are processed in the mold, the mold can be used for practice to improve tinting skills. The flexible silicone permits the tinting veneer to be removed from the mold and evaluated (Fig. 19-10). Thus the technician can see immediate results of the tinting proce-

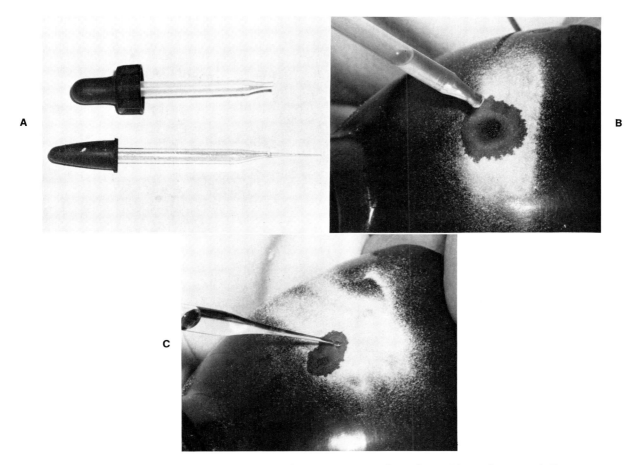

Fig. 19-4. A, Lower dropper has been modified to produce smaller orifice and better flow control. **B,** Large dropper orifice releases too much monomer. **C,** Smaller orifice permits excellent monomer flow control.

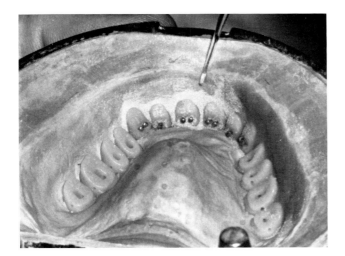

Fig. 19-5. Stain H has been applied and is wetted with monomer from small dropper.

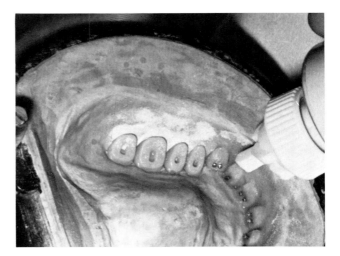

Fig. 19-6. Stain F is sifted over stain H and extended higher on flange.

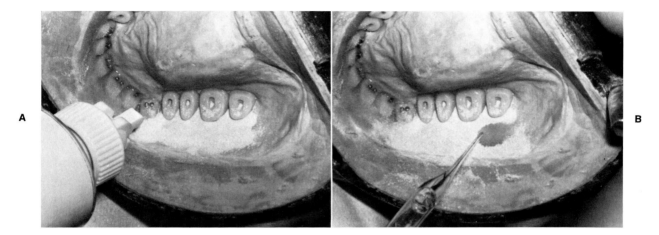

Fig. 19-7. A, Stain A is sifted over stain F and extends to denture border. **B,** Resin is wetted with monomer.

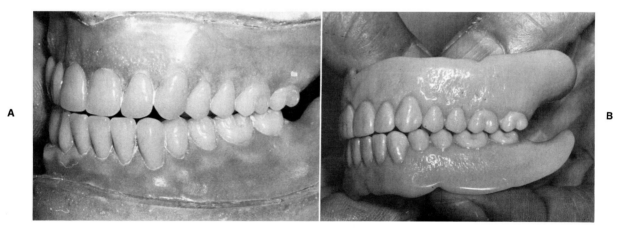

Fig. 19-8. A, Tinted dentures before removing from casts. **B,** Contour and texture of denture surfaces are important factors.

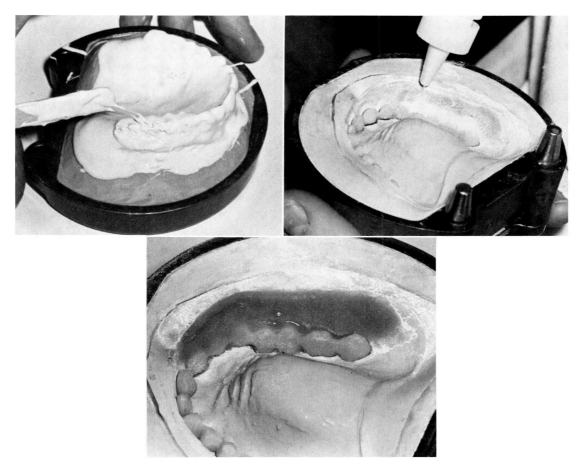

Fig. 19-9. Flexible silicone mold makes excellent practice mold. Autopolymerizing tooth-colored resin can be sifted into the mold first to simulate denture teeth.

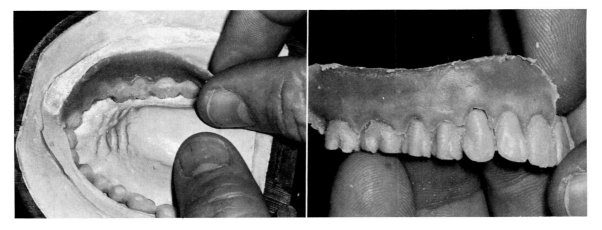

Fig. 19-10. Resin veneer can be easily removed for evaluation and study.

Table 19-1. Denture base tinting

Problem	Probable cause	Solution
Denture tinting too red and gaudy	Too much A applied	Apply less A
Denture has horizontal streaks of color	Tinting resins not blended or over-lapped	Overlap resins with each application to produce gradual color change
Stone adhered to tinted resin when deflasked	No coating of tinfoil substitute applied	Paint cast; flask stone with tinfoil substitute
	No coating of tinfoil substitute in spots or small areas because of retained wax on mold	Clean mold thoroughly with detergent during boilout to permit tinfoil substitute to react with gypsum mold
	Too much monomer added, permitting resin to penetrate investing stone	Control flow of monomer
Tinted surface is porous on de-flasking	Tinting resin monomer evaporated before denture was packed	Keep previously tinted surface slightly wet; cover tinting resin with sheet of plastic after application to reduce evaporation of monomer
Tinting resin squeezed out during trial packing	Resin not allowed to set for 15 to 20 minutes before packing	Permit tinting resin to set for 15 to 20 minutes before packing

dures. Different combinations of resins and the application sequence can be studied and practiced to improve skills.

SUMMARY

A method for characterizing the denture base by tinting was described in this chapter. It is important to remember that proper contouring of the denture base is even more critical to achieving an esthetic denture. Poorly executed tinting is usually worse than no tinting. Practice will usually result in vastly improved skills.

REFERENCES

Choudhary, S. C., Craig, J. F., and Suls, F. J.: Characterizing the denture base for non-Caucasian patients, J. Prosthet. Dent. **33**:73-79, 1975.

Johnson, H. B.: Techniques for packing and staining complete or partial denture bases, J. Prosthet. Dent. **6**:154-159, 1956.

Kemnitzer, D. F.: Esthetics and the denture base, J. Prosthet. Dent. **6**:603-615, 1956.

Pound, E.: Esthetic dentures and their phonetic values, J. Prosthet. Dent. **1**:98-111, 1951.

Powers, J. L.: Brush-on technique in natural coloring of cured cross-linked plastic artificial denture materials, J. Prosthet. Dent. **3**:350-353, 1953.

Proctor, H. H.: Characterization of dentures, J. Prosthet. Dent. **3**:339-349, 1953.

INDEX